W9-DIE-849

Metabolic Syndrome and Cardiovascular Disease

Metabolic Syndrome and Cardiovascular Disease

T. Barry Levine, MD

Professor of Medicine
Department of Cardiology
Drexel University College of Medicine

Vice Chairman
Department of Medicine
Allegheny General Hospital
Pittsburgh, Pennsylvania

Arlene Bradley Levine, MD

Consulting Staff
Division of Cardiology
Allegheny General Hospital
Pittsburgh, Pennsylvania

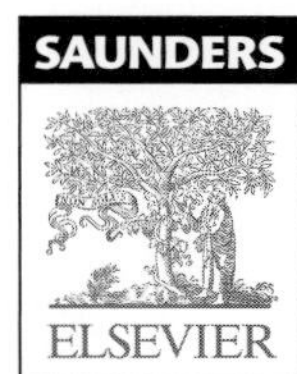

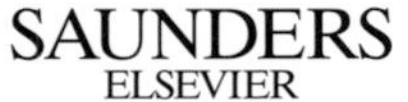

SAUNDERS
ELSEVIER

1600 John F. Kennedy Blvd.
Ste 1800
Philadelphia, PA 19103-2899

METABOLIC SYNDROME AND CARDIOVASCULAR DISEASE

ISBN-13: 978-1-4160-2545-0
ISBN-10: 1-4160-2545-6

Notice

Knowledge and best practice in this field are constantly changing. As new research and experience broaden our knowledge, changes in practice, treatment, and drug therapy may become necessary or appropriate. Readers are advised to check the most current information provided (i) on procedures featured or (ii) by the manufacturer of each product to be administered to verify the recommended dose or formula, the method and duration of administration, and contraindications. It is the responsibility of practitioners, relying on their own experience and knowledge of patients, to make diagnoses, to determine dosages and the best treatment for each individual patient, and to take all appropriate safety precautions. To the fullest extent of the law, neither the Publisher nor the Authors assume any liability for any injury and/or damage to persons or property arising out of or related to any use of the material contained in this book.

The Publisher

Library of Congress Cataloging-in-Publication Data
Levine, T. Barry.
Metabolic syndrome and cardiovascular disease / T. Barry Levine, Arlene B. Levine.–1st ed.
p. cm.
Includes bibliographical references.
ISBN 1-4160-2545-6
1. Metabolism–Disorders. 2. Cardiovascular system–Diseases. I. Levine, Arlene B. II. Title.

RC669.L44 2006
616.3'9–dc22
2005049981

Acquisitions Editor: Susan Pioli
Publishing Services Manager: Frank Polizzano
Project Manager: Lee Ann Draud
Design Direction: Gene Harris

Printed in the United States of America

Last digit is the print number: 9 8 7 6 5 4 3 2 1

We dedicate this book to our mothers

Brigitte L. Bradley, Ph.D.
Lillian Levine

Two women of valor

We would also like to acknowledge our children

Lionel Marc
Edlyn Victoria

for their contributions and support of this project.

Preface

The increasing global incidence of obesity and the metabolic syndrome threatens to become a worldwide public health disaster, extending beyond the epidemic of type 2 diabetes mellitus to include coronary, peripheral, and cerebrovascular disease; hypertension; heart failure; and an array of noncardiac "diseases of aging." The cardiovascular and metabolic complications arising from the metabolic syndrome need to be understood by the health care profession to formulate and enact effective preventive and therapeutic measures.

The definition of the metabolic syndrome encompasses overweight, hypertension, and disturbances in lipid and carbohydrate metabolism. To an outside observer, these manifestations of the metabolic syndrome are not intuitively related. Although the serious manifestations of the metabolic syndrome are cardiovascular in etiology, the subcellular mechanisms linking the metabolic to the vascular disturbances are not automatically apparent.

This multidisciplinary work seeks to present to the cardiovascular research and treatment community the molecular underpinnings of the known risk factors for the metabolic syndrome, spanning diverse factors such as genetics, diet, inactivity, overweight, stress, infection, inflammation, and oxidative stress. The book elucidates the mechanisms of end-organ involvement in the metabolic syndrome and the relationship to clinical disease. Lastly, mechanisms whereby exercise, weight loss, nutrition, and pharmacologic therapy beneficially affect the metabolic syndrome are explored.

The book has five sections. In its first section, the book provides a background of the mechanisms of insulin's metabolic, vascular, and mitogenic signaling.

The second section discusses the molecular links of oxidative stress and proinflammatory pathways to insulin resistance. Although genetics and the environment feed into the genesis of insulin resistance and the metabolic syndrome, insulin resistance arises primarily in a milieu of oxidative stress and inflammation. Pro-oxidant and proinflammatory stress signals engender a multiplicity of redundant and mutually reinforcing molecular pathways leading to insulin resistance. Insulin resistance is effectively the metabolic expression of inflammation. It is an essential host response that protects the energy requirements for an immune response: a beneficial acute reaction that turns detrimental when it becomes a chronic state. A variety of sources of inflammation are explored. Stress pathways aroused by omnipresent stresses of everyday life are investigated, determining their impact on inflammatory mediators, vascular function, and metabolism. In this respect, the effect of adipose tissue, in particular of visceral adipose tissue, is discussed, as it functions akin to an immune tissue tumor, inducing local and systemic insulin resistance.

The third and fourth sections address target end-organ effects deriving from inflammation and insulin resistance. Stress pathways link insulin resistance and vascular dysfunction. As endothelial dysfunction and insulin resistance reciprocally aggravate each other and deteriorate, they progress toward the full-blown manifestations of vascular and metabolic disease. However, inflammation and insulin resistance affect not only adipose tissue and the vasculature. They also have a profound impact on the metabolism of the liver and skeletal and cardiac muscle, engendering atherogenic dyslipidemia, exercise intolerance, and the metabolic underpinning to diabetic cardiomyopathy and other diseases.

The fifth section provides a detailed discussion of the mechanisms whereby established preventive and therapeutic lifestyle changes and pharmacologic interventions affect oxidative stress, inflammation, vascular function, and insulin resistance. Pharmacologic approaches are usually needed for the management of manifestations of the metabolic syndrome. However, lifestyle changes, including exercise and dietary modifications with some weight loss, are the most effective interventions for the prevention of cardiovascular and metabolic disease progression and can be anticipated to reduce the future risk of both microvascular and macrovascular complications.

This book is written by cardiologists for professionals engaged in cardiovascular medicine, be they physicians, nurses, exercise physiologists, nutritionists, or students. Its far-reaching multidisciplinary approach and detailed intervention section should be of interest to the research scientist and the clinical practitioner and to the interventionist and the internist with an interest in preventive cardiology.

The book is structured so that the information in each chapter is self-contained and can be read by itself. To that end, each chapter has its own table of contents and glossary. The text is broken up into small, easily readable sections. Sections and paragraphs are presented so that they lead with the important information. Take home points are high-lighted, allowing for quick skimming where desired.

It is our aim to provide cardiology professionals with an appreciation of the interaction of inflammation with insulin resistance and vascular and metabolic disease. It is our hope that such insights may lead to a more concerted effort at preventive and therapeutic interventions for individuals and populations at risk. We also hope that insights gained from this book may provide novel entry points for the development of new strategies to enhance the vascular and metabolic health of the general population and ultimately to benefit societal health status trends.

T. Barry Levine, MD, FACC
Arlene Bradley Levine, MD, FACC

Contents

Section I

Background

Insulin and Glucagon

1

Resistance to insulin signaling is a cardiovascular risk factor that underlies the pathophysiology of the metabolic syndrome. Although insulin in compensatory hyperinsulinemia has adverse mitogenic and proinflammatory effects, at normal physiologic concentrations, preserved sensitivity to insulin signaling has a protective effect on the vasculature.

ANABOLISM AND CATABOLISM

Metabolism comprises the highly coordinated and purposeful sum total of cellular enzymatic reactions concerning the synthesis, transformation, and degradation of molecules such as carbohydrates, proteins, nucleic acids, lipids, and other cell components. The two basic components of metabolism take place concurrently but are independently regulated:

1. Anabolism comprises the energy-requiring biosynthesis of macromolecular cell components from simple precursors. It is essential for cell growth and maintenance, as well as for the synthesis of storage fuels.
2. Catabolism encompasses the degradation of macromolecules derived from the cellular environment or from cellular nutrient storage depots into smaller, simpler molecules such as lactic acid, acetic acid, carbon dioxide, ammonia, or urea. Catabolism entails the hydrolysis and subsequent oxidation of macromolecules by which the chemical energy contained in the macromolecular bond structure is released and stored through generation of the physiologic high-energy currency adenosine triphosphate (ATP).[1]

During childhood and growth, anabolic pathways exceed catabolic pathways. In normal healthy adults, the two processes are balanced.[2-4]

CONTROL OF PLASMA GLUCOSE

Glucose provides the major source of metabolic energy for mammalian cells. Plasma glucose levels are maintained within a relatively narrow range, 72 to 126 mg/dL.

This range is a physiologic requisite. In normal, well-fed mammals, nervous tissue such as the brain uses plasma glucose exclusively as its energy source because it contains essentially no fuel reserves of glycogen or triacylglycerols. Neurons are intolerant of severe, acute hypoglycemia and are unable to use alternative energy sources such as free fatty acids to any significant extent. If blood glucose should fall to half its normal level, symptoms of brain dysfunction may supervene. Coma ensues as blood glucose concentration falls to 20 mg/dL. Conversely, the osmotic load of excessive plasma glucose levels is physiologically not tolerated.[1]

Blood glucose has the potential for varying widely. During the course of the day, intermittent, significant potential perturbations in blood sugar arise from a variety of venues for glucose entry and glucose clearance:

- Glucose entry into the circulation occurs postprandially from the gastrointestinal tract and postabsorptively from the liver and kidney.
- Glucose clearance from the circulation transpires via the energy demands of neuronal tissue, skeletal muscle, and the immune system and as a result of uptake by the splanchnic bed and adipose tissue.

Nevertheless, glucose levels are tightly regulated through exquisitely coordinated interactions between the liver, pancreatic beta cells, and peripheral insulin-sensitive tissues. The major site of glucose utilization during physiologic conditions such as exercise is skeletal muscle, where glucose is metabolized via aerobic oxidation or anaerobic glycolysis to generate ATP. Diet-derived glucose is primarily stored in adipose tissue as triacylglycerols and in the liver and skeletal muscle as glycogen.[2-4]

Pancreatic hormones, principally insulin and glucagon, are the dominant hormonal regulators of glucose metabolism.

INSULIN

Insulin is an essential hormone involved in the control of intermediary metabolism. It is an anabolic hormone, quintessential for normal glucose homeostasis. Insulin profoundly affects carbohydrate and lipid metabolism and has a significant influence on protein and mineral metabolism. Insulin also affects vascular function. In addition, it has anti-inflammatory and mitogenic effects.

Structure. Insulin is a relatively small protein with a molecular weight of approximately 6 kDa.

It is composed of two amino acid chains, A and B, connected via two disulfide bonds. The amino acid sequence is highly conserved among vertebrates. As a result, insulin from one mammal is physiologically active in another.[5]

Synthesis. Insulin is synthesized in the beta cells of the pancreatic islets of Langerhans.

A single amino acid chain, "preproinsulin," is translated from mRNA. "Proinsulin" is generated when the signal peptide is removed upon insertion of the insulin precursor into the cisternae of the endoplasmic reticulum. Within the endoplasmic reticulum, the single-chain proinsulin is exposed to endopeptidases. These enzymes excise the central portion of the peptide chain, called C peptide. The residual carboxy-terminal A chain and the amino-terminal B chain of the original peptide constitute the final insulin product, with both A and B peptide chains connected by two disulfide bonds.[5,6]

Secretion. On stimulation, insulin is secreted from the pancreatic beta cell via exocytosis.

Stimuli for Insulin Secretion. Secretion of insulin is initiated by numerous stimuli.

The stimulus for insulin secretion is primarily an elevation in blood glucose above the fasting level, which is between 80 and 90 mg/dL for most humans and mammals. Insulin secretion is also promoted by increased blood concentrations of other nutrient molecules such as amino acids and fatty acids, by certain gastrointestinal hormones such as incretins, and by neural stimuli such as the site and taste of food (Table 1-1).[5,6]

Insulin secretion can also be up-regulated by other hormones such as human growth hormone, placental lactogen, estrogens, and progestins, all of which increase preproinsulin mRNA, as well as the enzymes involved in processing the insulin precursor.[5]

Mechanism of Insulin Secretion. The trigger for insulin secretion appears to be a rise in cytoplasmic glucose.

Table 1-1. Stimuli for Insulin Secretion

Glucose
Amino acids
Free fatty acids
Gastrointestinal hormones
Neural stimuli

With increased plasma glucose levels, the intracellular glucose concentration increases as a result of facilitated glucose transmembrane transport via a low-affinity, high-K_M glucose transporter (GLUT), GLUT2. In combination with hexokinase, GLUT2 serves as part of the cellular glucose sensor.[7]

Mitochondrial glucose metabolism is crucial to linking the glucose stimulus to insulin secretion. Metabolism of the elevated intracellular glucose, specifically via glycolysis, elevates the ATP–adenosine 5′-diphosphate (ADP) ratio, which inhibits an ATP-sensitive K^+ channel. This effect ultimately leads to an alteration in membrane conductance, membrane depolarization, and the influx of extracellular Ca^{2+}.[5,6]

The resulting increase in cytoplasmic Ca^{2+} is thought to be the final trigger for exocytosis of insulin-containing secretory granules. However, there also appear to be Ca^{2+}-independent pathways for insulin secretion.

The stimuli for insulin secretion also induce transcription of the insulin gene and translation of its mRNA.[5,6]

Insulin Release. Insulin release into the portal circulation is biphasic. Upon glucose stimulation, an initial spike of plasma insulin reflecting the release of insulin stores is seen within minutes. Insulin stores are rapidly depleted. A secondary rise in plasma insulin occurs within 15 to 20 minutes of a glucose challenge and primarily represents newly synthesized insulin that is immediately released.[5,6]

Insulin diffuses from pancreatic islet capillary blood into the portal vein to be presented to the liver and the systemic circulation. The liver clears about 50% of insulin in the first pass.[5,6]

The Insulin Receptor. The insulin receptor, a heterotetrameric glycoprotein, is identical in all cells.

The receptor is composed of two domains, an extracellular, hormone-binding region, as well as an intracellular region that triggers the physiologic response. The extracellular, hormone-binding domain consists of two α-subunit chains. The intracellular domain is composed of two β-subunit chains that penetrate through the plasmalemma into the intracellular domain. Disulfide bonds link these chains.[8]

INSULIN RECEPTOR LOCATION—CAVEOLAE

Insulin transduces its physiologic effects via the insulin receptor, which is a plasmalemmal glycoprotein. The signaling molecules that convey the insulin signal intracellularly are indiscriminate; that is, they are common to signaling pathways of other receptors. Despite the promiscuity of these signaling molecules, insulin exerts specific metabolic effects on cells that are not shared by other receptor signaling pathways.[9]

Microdomains and Rafts. Rafts and microdomains are regions of spatial organization in the plasma membrane that may provide signaling specificity for receptors despite the indiscriminate nature of signaling pathways.

The plasma membrane, with relatively disordered, loosely packed phospholipids, is disrupted by highly ordered, hydrophobic microdomains. The plasmalemmal liquid-ordered phase of such regions packs together lipids to form dynamic rafts within the plane of the plasma membrane.[10]

Composition. Lipid rafts are relatively depleted of phospholipids. They are enriched in cholesterol and sphingolipids such as sphingomyelin and glycolipids, and their polar lipids contain predominantly saturated fatty acyl residues. Such lipids spontaneously aggregate to form the liquid-ordered membrane regions.[10]

Exoplasmic and Endoplasmic Raft Composition. Sphingolipids and glycosylphosphatidylinositol (GPI)-anchored proteins are typical constituents of rafts, but they are attached exclusively in the outer, exoplasmic leaflet of the plasma membrane bilayer. The lipid composition of the inner, cytoplasmic leaflet of rafts also appears to be enriched in saturated fatty acyl chains without stabilizing sphingolipids.[10]

Compartmentalization. Lipid rafts may provide specialized scaffolds, anchors, and adapter proteins to segregate signaling molecules into specific compartments. Rafts may either recruit or exclude specific signaling proteins.[9,11]

Rafts may often be enriched in GPI-anchored plasma membrane proteins, non-receptor tyrosine kinases, and caveolin. The physical segregation of raft proteins into such "microdomains" may have an impact on the accessibility of such proteins to regulatory or effector molecules. Examples of the structural bases for protein association with rafts include

- GPI anchors—for the folate receptor,
- dual fatty acylation by myristoylation and palmitoylation—for the Src family tyrosine kinases,
- transmembrane domain structure—for influenza hemagglutinin polypeptide,
- caveolins—for cholesterol binding, and
- caveolin-interacting proteins—for protein-protein interactions.

On the basis of their ability to sort proteins, rafts have been implicated in a number of cell functions, including

- membrane targeting in polarized cells,
- receptor signal transduction,
- endocytosis, and
- uptake of small molecules via potocytosis.[9]

Potocytosis is the ability to concentrate and internalize molecules such as ligand-bound folate receptors.

Caveolae. Caveolae ("little caves") are morphologic correlates of lipid rafts. They are omega-shaped invaginations, 50 to 100 nm in diameter, found in the plasma membrane. Caveolae are spatially restricted plasma membrane lipid domains that typically represent about 1% to 4% of the total myocyte sarcolemmal surface area, but they may occupy up to 30% of the cell surface in capillary endothelial cells.[12]

Caveolar Formation. Caveolae may form from the cholesterol- and sphingolipid-rich rafts in the plasma membrane. Caveolae are, in fact, a subset of lipid raft microdomains.

The structure and function of caveolae depend on the amount of cholesterol associated with the caveolae. High caveolar concentrations of cholesterol induce the caveolae to invaginate, whereas low cholesterol concentrations generate a flattened morphology.[13] The process that fashions caveolae requires the caveola-specific structural protein caveolin. Caveolin is found in plasma membranes, confined to caveolae, as well as intracellularly.

Caveolins. The caveolins (caveolins 1, 2, and 3 and flotillins) are a family of 21- to 25-kDa membrane proteins.

Caveolin-1 is abundantly expressed in endothelial cells, whereas caveolin-3 is expressed only in muscle cells. The tissue distribution of caveolin-2 appears to be similar to that of caveolin-1.

Structure. Caveolin-1 is composed of 178 amino acids.[14] An unusual hairpin structure of caveolin's membrane domain causes its amino- as well as its carboxy-terminal domains to face the cytoplasm, thereby allowing both domains to freely interact with cytosolic molecules.[9,15]

The short amino-terminal cytoplasmic region of caveolin-1 (residues 82 to 101) is termed the "scaffolding domain," and it can interact directly with receptors and signaling molecules.[16,17]

Caveolin Oligomerization. Caveolae consist largely of oligomerized caveolin proteins, which establish the coat structure of caveolae.

Caveolin actually undergoes two stages of oligomerization. Caveolin monomers first assemble into discrete, multivalent oligomers. Subsequently, via interactions between amino-terminal residues, these caveolin homo-oligomers react with each other and polymerize to form caveola-like structures.[9,15] Caveolae are assembled, or begin to assemble, in the Golgi.[18]

Scaffolding Function. Caveolin may function as a scaffolding protein for lipids as well as for signaling molecules within caveolar membranes.

Caveolins avidly bind cholesterol. This property may underlie their association with the liquid-ordered phase of the plasma membrane. Caveolin family members appear to organize and concentrate cholesterol, glycosphingolipids, and lipid-modified signaling proteins within the caveolae.[9,15]

Caveolar Distribution. Caveolae are present in most eukaryotic cell types and collect at actin-rich margins of the cell and along stress fibers. They are especially abundant in fully differentiated cells, such as

- adipocytes,
- fibroblasts,
- smooth muscle cells,
- skeletal myocytes,
- cardiac myocytes,
- endothelial cells, and
- type I pneumocytes.

Although other cell types also display caveolae, they are present at lower density.[9,15]

In adipocytes, caveolae increase in number in accordance with the degree of maturation. Multiple individual caveolae and clusters of caveolae organize into large, ring-shaped structures in the adipocyte plasma membrane. These structures can be visualized at both the electron microscopic and light microscopic levels.[19]

Caveolar Function. Caveolae may function as subcellular compartments. They were originally associated with cellular transport.[20] Caveolae have been implicated in functions analogous to those discharged by lipid rafts, such as

- transport functions:
  - vesicular internalization of small molecules, ions, and folate by the process of potocytosis,
  - endocytic and transcytotic movement of macromolecules, and
  - cholesterol transport,
- cellular Ca^{2+} regulation, and
- receptor signal transduction.[21]

Caveolae also mediate the desensitization of receptor signaling, the latter occurring via endocytic caveolar fission as caveolae are pinched off from the sarcolemma in a guanosine 5′-triphosphate (GTP)-dependent fashion, a process that leads to receptor sequestration.[20]

Caveolar Signal Transduction. Specific membrane domains, such as

- caveolae,
- focal adhesion sites, and
- sites of cell-cell contact,

are locations for the multiple molecular interactions that ensue as cells process information received from the environment.

Compartmentalization of Signal Transduction. Caveolae, in particular, have emerged as important regulators of signal transduction. They coordinate the interaction of receptors with downstream signal-transducing molecules as the latter translocate to the plasma membrane after cell stimulation. Caveolae also facilitate direct crosstalk between distinct signaling cascades.

Although many receptor agonists share common intracellular signaling pathways, distinct receptor-specific biologic responses are produced. Caveolae may act as switchboards that spatially compartmentalize signal transduction cascades at the plasma membrane to preserve the specificity and fidelity of receptor-specific signaling. The selective inclusion or exclusion of key signaling molecules within lipid rafts or caveolae, while storing inactive signaling molecules for subsequent regulated activation, may be one way of organizing a multitude of signals into distinct signaling cascades.[22]

Specific Caveola-Based Components of Signaling Pathways. A wide variety of components of intracellular signal transduction pathways have a caveolar location. Alternatively, redistribution to caveolin-containing subcellular fractions occurs for a variety of receptors and signaling molecules upon agonist stimulation. With most of the involved receptors located in or redistributed to caveolae, signal transduction is thus effectively spatially organized at the cell surface.

Organized signal transduction within caveolae occurs for

- growth factor receptors (e.g., epidermal growth factor, platelet-derived growth factor),
- the insulin receptor,
- G protein–coupled receptors (e.g., for acetylcholine, angiotensin II type 1 [AT_1] receptor, bradykinin, catecholamines, cholecystokinin, endothelin),
- nitric oxide synthase (NOS),
- tumor necrosis factor (TNF) receptor type 1,
- non-receptor tyrosine kinases (e.g., Fyn),

- Src family kinases,
- G proteins,
- components of the Ras, Raf, and Rho family GTPases,
- extracellular signal–regulated kinase (ERK)/ mitogen-activated protein kinase (MAPK) pathways,
- adenylate cyclase,
- several protein kinase C (PKC) isoforms, and
- other downstream elements (e.g., Son of Sevenless [SOS], Grb2, the regulatory subunit of phosphatidylinositol 3-kinase [PI3K], phosphatidylinositol 4,5-diphosphate).[16,21,23-26,]

Targeting of Signaling Molecules to Caveolae. Signaling molecules are targeted to caveolae by their lipid composition and molecular scaffolding:

- The lipid environment of the caveolar membrane plays an essential role in attracting and organizing receptors and signaling molecules.

  Many primary and secondary signaling proteins that operate from caveolae are covalently modified with lipids such as myristate, palmitate, and isoprenyl groups, and their acylation sites appear to be essential for protein translocation to the lipophilic microenvironment.[27]
- The caveolin scaffolding domain interacts directly with signaling molecules associated with caveolae.

  Caveolins generally appear to operate as kinase inhibitors. Caveolin interactions apparently sequester the proteins within caveolae, where they modulate or suppress their catalytic activities and hold them in an inactive state. The inactive signaling molecules may, in fact, form signal transduction units within caveola-like structures that are ready to be activated in the correct configuration during receptor stimulation by specific stimuli.[16,17]

  The cytoplasmic, amino-terminal scaffolding domain of caveolin-1 can interact directly with certain receptors and signaling molecules, for example,

  - receptor tyrosine kinases such as the insulin receptor,
  - endothelial NOS (eNOS),
  - signaling molecules present in caveolae such as Ras and Src.

  Many of these molecules contain caveolin-binding sites with a common motif through which they bind to the scaffolding domain of caveolin-1.[22]

Caveolar Cholesterol Content. Caveolae are highly enriched in cholesterol. Not only are the morphology and function of caveolae contingent on a sufficient level of cholesterol in the caveolae, the integrity of receptor signal transduction is also critically dependent on membrane cholesterol.[9] Because cholesterol directly binds to caveolin-1, cholesterol may influence the function of caveolin-1 as it interacts with and regulates many signaling molecules, including eNOS, the insulin receptor, G proteins, Src, and Ras.[28]

Cell Membrane Cholesterol. Cell membrane cholesterol content is important. Approximately 85% of free cholesterol is found within the plasma membrane of mammalian cells, and the majority of free cholesterol molecules are primarily situated on the cytoplasmic surface of the plasmalemma.[29]

The biophysical and biochemical microenvironment of caveolae, such as membrane fluidity and composition, significantly influences the function of signaling proteins. Cholesterol may regulate biophysical membrane properties such as fluidity and rigidity.[29]

However, the function of cholesterol is not limited to being a structural component of plasma membranes; it also actively participates in the regulation of cell physiology by modulating signal transduction through membrane lipid-ordered microdomains and gene expression through cholesterol-activated transcription factors.[29]

Plasmalemmal cholesterol is essential for the proper functioning of receptors and other membrane signaling proteins such as G proteins. Receptors for

- β-adrenergic agonists,
- insulin,
- 5-methyltetrahydrofolate,
- rhodopsin,
- oxytocin,
- cholecystokinin,

- transferrin, and
- acetylcholine

all require normal levels of plasmalemmal cholesterol for optimal functioning.

Depletion of cholesterol from caveolae correlates with disruption of caveolar structure. Caveolar cholesterol depletion also inhibits signaling functions, such as

- epidermal growth factor receptor transactivation,
- eNOS activation via shear stress in endothelial cells, and
- insulin signaling.[26,28]

The Insulin Receptor Location in Caveolae. **Upon stimulation, the insulin receptor appears to be situated in caveolae.** The receptor and important elements of the insulin signaling pathway are embedded in the plasma membrane of cells, where they phosphorylate and colocalize with the major structural component of caveolae, caveolin.

Caveolin-1 acts as a molecular chaperone that is essential for the proper stabilization and function of the insulin receptor in adipocytes in vivo.[9,14,30] The scaffolding domain of caveolin-1 binds to a specific motif within the kinase domain of the insulin receptor (residues 1193 to 1200). The caveolin scaffolding domain is required to stabilize the insulin receptor and to stimulate its signaling.[19,30,31] Interestingly, mutations within the caveolin-binding motif of the human insulin receptor (W1193L and W1200S) result in a syndrome of severe insulin resistance.[31]

Caveolae are critical for targeted, specific insulin receptor signaling. Other ligands may use components of the insulin signaling cascade without subsuming insulin's physiologic actions. For example,

- integrins, interferon, interleukins, and gastrin signal through the insulin receptor substrate-1 (IRS-1);
- numerous other ligands stimulate PI3K. Activation of PI3K with production of phosphatidylinositol 3,4,5-triphosphate (PIP3) is a ubiquitous signaling step to link cell surface receptors to their intracellular targets.

The selectivity in signaling within the microdomains is derived via receptor-encoded time courses and amplitudes of the resultant PIP3 signal.[32] Direct interactions between microdomain proteins (caveolin and flotillin-1) and insulin signaling molecules appear to organize these molecules in space and time to ensure faithful transduction of the specific metabolic insulin signal.[14]

Integrity of Caveolae and Insulin Signaling. In contrast to certain other caveolar receptors, **the insulin receptor appears to be critically dependent on caveolar cholesterol and caveolar integrity for its ability to signal.**[14] Depletion of cholesterol from the caveolar plasma membrane with attendant caveolar destruction leaves the insulin receptor itself intact but causes selective insulin resistance. The immediate downstream metabolic and vascular control by insulin is inhibited, whereas insulin signaling via the MAPK pathway remains unaffected.[9,33]

Caveolar Cholesterol Depletion and the Insulin Receptor. Depletion of plasma membrane cholesterol disrupts caveolar structure and function. Experimentally, extraction of plasma membrane cholesterol via cyclodextrin flattens the caveolar invaginations.[9]

Loss of caveolar structure has no impact on several aspects of insulin signaling, such as

- the number of insulin receptors in the membrane,
- their affinity for insulin,
- levels of plasma membrane caveolin,
- interaction of the insulin receptor with caveolin,
- insulin-stimulated tyrosine autophosphorylation of the insulin receptor,
- IRS-1 serine/threonine phosphorylation, and
- activation of the MAPK pathway by insulin.

However, **caveolar disruption via cholesterol depletion does inhibit the downstream activation of protein kinase B (PKB)/Akt kinase, thereby interfering with insulin-stimulated glucose uptake and eNOS activation.**[9,33] A parallel glucose uptake pathway, via Cbl-activating protein (CAP)/c-Cbl leading to activation of the small GTP-binding protein TC10, is also located in membrane microdomains and lipid rafts and is sensitive to their structural integrity.[34]

GLUCOSE UPTAKE

Glucose transport is the rate-limiting step in glucose metabolism. It is a highly regulated process.

Facilitated Diffusion. Glucose is transported into cells via facilitated diffusion.

Because the plasmalemmal phospholipid bilayer of cells is impermeable to carbohydrates, glucose entry into cells cannot occur through simple diffusion. Plasma membrane glucose transport is effected by a family of specific membrane-spanning hexose or glucose transporters, GLUTs. **GLUTs are proteins that form hydrophilic passages for glucose through the lipid bilayer of the cell membrane.**[3]

GLUT Proteins. The GLUT protein family is characterized by a single polypeptide of approximately 500 amino acids. As the protein traverses the cell membrane, both the amino-terminus and the carboxy-terminus are exposed to the cytosol. A gradient for unidirectional glucose transport is achieved as free cytosolic glucose is rapidly removed and phosphorylated by hexokinase into glucose 6-phosphate.[4]

Types of GLUT. GLUTs may either be constitutively expressed on the plasma membrane or be actively translocated to the plasma membrane in response to specific stimuli.[3] GLUTs differ in their subcellular localization and tissue expression. GLUTs specific for diverse tissues have differing kinetics of glucose transport.[4]

Numerous glucose transporters have been identified: GLUT1 to GLUT12, as well as GLUTX1 in the central nervous system and the myoinositol transporter HMIT1. GLUT1 handles basic glucose uptake and is ubiquitously expressed. GLUT2, with low glucose affinity, is located in the liver and pancreatic beta cells. GLUT2 transports glucose out of hepatocytes during glycogenolysis and gluconeogenesis. GLUT3, which has the highest glucose affinity, is expressed in fetal development and adult neurons. **GLUT4 is predominantly present in mature fat cells, as well as in striated skeletal and cardiac muscle.** It is also found in the brain and kidneys.[7,35]

GLUT4. GLUT4 is not constitutively expressed on the membrane but requires activation and membrane translocation. Insulin is one of its principal activators, and GLUT4 is the only glucose transporter controlled by insulin.

Because GLUT4 is the major glucose transporter for skeletal and cardiac muscle and adipose tissue, glucose uptake can be achieved only through stimulation of facilitated diffusion. Insulin-stimulated glucose uptake in these tissues is thus mediated by the isoform GLUT4.[3] In contrast, the liver, inflammatory cells, and the brain do not require insulin or other stimuli for intracellular glucose uptake.[7,35]

GLUT4 Basal State. The insulin-responsive GLUT4 in adipocytes and in skeletal and cardiac myocytes resides in a cytoplasmic, tubulovesicular system and is inactive in that location.

In the basal state, GLUT4 cycles slowly between one or more of these tubulovesicular compartments and the plasma membrane. Unstimulated, the vast majority of the transporters, 95% to 97%, reside within the cell interior.[34,35]

GLUT4 Stimulation. Binding of insulin to its receptor rapidly shifts the steady-state distribution of GLUT4 from the basal, intracellular location to the activated, cell surface location.

Insulin triggers a rise in the rate of GLUT4 vesicle exocytosis. As a result, GLUT4 vesicles accumulate at the cell surface, fuse with the plasma membrane, and then cause membrane insertion of the GLUT4 transporter.[4,19] This process is followed by a slower transition of GLUT4 to the caveola-rich regions of the plasma membrane, where glucose transport appears to take place. Insulin not only recruits transporters to the cell surface from the intracellular pool but also raises the intrinsic activity of the transporters, thereby engendering a net increase in glucose uptake.[14,36]

Stimuli other than insulin that instigate GLUT4 translocation to the plasma membrane are

- muscle contraction,
- hypoxia.

INSULIN SIGNALING

The same insulin receptor controls several different signaling pathways:

- **metabolic signaling for glucose, lipid, and amino acid transport and metabolism,**

- **vascular signaling for eNOS activation,**
- **the MAPK pathway for mitogenic control.**

Phosphatidylinositol 3-Kinase Metabolic Insulin Signaling. The intracellular part of the insulin receptor is itself an enzyme that initiates its physiologic response. The receptor functions as a tyrosine kinase. As such, it transfers a phosphate group from ATP to tyrosine residues of intracellular target proteins.

Insulin Receptor Autophosphorylation. On insulin binding, the insulin receptor autophosphorylates.

Specifically, as insulin binds to the extracellular α-subunits of the receptor, the receptor changes conformationally and initiates autophosphorylation of multiple tyrosine residues on its intracellular β-subunits.[8]

Tyrosine Kinase Activity of the Insulin Receptor. Insulin receptor autophosphorylation initiates the catalytic tyrosine kinase activity of the β-subunits.[8]

In the process, the β-subunits phosphorylate a number of intracellular targets to increase their physiologic activity. Some of the intracellular targets for tyrosine phosphorylation are docking proteins such as

- the insulin receptor substrates IRS-1, -2, -3, and -4,
- Shc,
- Gab-1,
- associated protein substrate (APS),
- p53/58,
- SIRP, and
- c-Cbl.

These docking proteins are themselves enzymes, which when activated by phosphorylation stimulate other enzymes to ultimately mediate the physiologic effects of insulin.[37]

Insulin Receptor Substrate. The IRS molecules contain multiple tyrosine phosphorylation sites. Phosphorylation of IRS proteins by the insulin receptor activates PI3K.[35]

There are different IRS isoforms. Although IRS family members share many similarities, the various isoforms have distinct distributions and maintain specificity with respect to insulin's biologic action[38]:

- IRS-1 is the main signaling molecule in skeletal muscle;
- IRS-2 is located in the liver and pancreatic beta cells.

Both IRS-1 and IRS-2 participate in modulating the metabolic and mitogenic responses to insulin in skeletal muscle, adipose tissue, and the liver.[35]

The subcellular distribution of IRS-1 and IRS-2 is regulated by insulin. Insulin releases the association of IRS-1 and IRS-2 with a cytoskeletal "scaffold" contiguous to the plasma membrane, which causes these molecules to move from the particulate to the cytosolic fraction and behave as soluble proteins.[39]

Phosphatidylinositol 3-Kinase. Phosphorylated IRS activates PI3K by docking with its p85 regulatory subunit, thus activating the p110 catalytic subunit of PI3K. PI3K catalyzes the production of

- PIP3 and
- phosphoinositide moieties

in the plasma membrane. These compounds activate 3-phosphoinositide–dependent kinases (PDKs), including PDK-1.[35]

Akt/Protein Kinase B. The downstream targets for PDK-1 are two classes of serine/threonine kinases,

- Akt, also known as PKB isoforms α/β, and
- the atypical PKC isoforms.

The is conflicting evidence regarding whether Akt is involved in the glucose transport signaling process, but one or the other of these kinases is implicated in stimulating GLUT4 translocation to the plasma membrane (Fig. 1-1).[35]

Protein Kinase C. Atypical PKCs serve as required terminal molecular switches for insulin-dependent and insulin-independent pathways stimulating

- glucose transport via GLUT4 translocation,
- glycogen synthesis, and
- protein synthesis.[3,40,41]

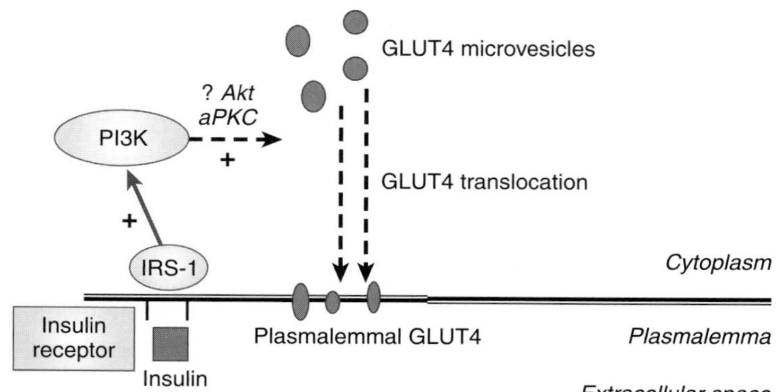

Figure 1–1. Phosphatidylinositol 3-kinase (PI3K)–Akt/atypical protein kinase C (aPKC) cellular glucose uptake pathway mediated by insulin. GLUT, glucose transporter; IRS, insulin receptor substrate. *(Adapted from Winder WW, Hardie DG. AMP-activated protein kinase, a metabolic master switch: possible roles in type 2 diabetes. Am J Physiol 1999;277:E1-E10.)*

Protein Kinase C Subgroups. PKCs are serine/threonine kinases. There are three structurally related PKC subgroups based on their respective cofactor requirements:

1. conventional PKCs (α, β_1, β_2, γ), which are dependent on Ca^{2+} and diacylglycerol (DAG) or phorbol ester for activity;
2. novel PKCs (δ, ε, θ), which are not dependent on Ca^{2+} but are activated by DAG and phorbol esters; and
3. atypical PKCs (ζ, ι), which are neither dependent on Ca^{2+} nor stimulated by DAG and phorbol esters.[42]

PROTEIN KINASE C	Ca^{2+} DEPENDENCE	DAG DEPENDENCE
Conventional	Yes	Yes
Novel	No	Yes
Atypical	No	No[42]

The DAG- and Ca^{2+}-independent, atypical PKCs are, instead, activated by

- acidic phospholipids,
- PIP3, and
- phosphatidic acid.

The atypical PKC isoforms can function interchangeably within the insulin signaling pathway.[3,40,41]

In contrast to atypical PKCs, conventional PKCs are not required for facilitated glucose transport. Rather, they serve as negative feedback inhibitors of insulin signaling.[3]

Proto-oncogene c-Cbl Metabolic Insulin Signaling. Additional insulin signaling events independent of PI3K may be essential for glucose transport. **Insulin stimulation of GLUT4 translocation requires at least two parallel, but distinct, insulin receptor–mediated signals:**

- **one leading to activation of PI3K, discussed earlier, and**
- **one causing activation of the small GTP-binding protein TC10.**

The latter is a proto-oncogene pathway, the components of which are localized to the caveolin-enriched lipid microdomains of the plasma membrane. It functions independently of the PI3K pathway and is implicated in GLUT4 translocation (Table 1-2).[22,37]

The c-Cbl Pathway. In parallel with PI3K-dependent signaling, insulin activates the small GTP-binding protein TC10.

Specifically, insulin-dependent phosphorylation of the Cbl-activating protein CAP recruits the proto-oncogene product c-Cbl to the microdomains. There, coupled to the insulin

Table 1-2. Parallel Signaling Events Mediating Insulin-Stimulated Glucose Transport

Insulin receptor autophosphorylation
Activation of IRS molecules
PI3K recruitment to sarcolemma
Phosphoinositide-dependent protein kinase activation
Akt/PKB and PKC-δ/λ activation
↓
GLUT4 translocation to sarcolemma
↑
Insulin receptor phosphorylation of CAP
Activation of proto-oncogene c-Cbl

CAP, Cbl-activating protein; GLUT, glucose transporter; IRS, insulin receptor substrate; PI3K, phosphatidylinositol 3-kinase; PKC, protein kinase C.

receptor via APS, c-Cbl is tyrosine-phosphorylated by the insulin receptor. This CAP-Cbl interaction results in dissociation of Cbl from the insulin receptor, thereby allowing CAP to bind to flotillin in the microdomains. Through a small adapter protein, CrkII, the tyrosine-phosphorylated Cbl protein recruits the guanyl nucleotide exchange factor C3G for the small GTP-binding protein TC10, a member of the Rho family. Ultimately, insulin stimulation converts TC10 from the inactive, guanosine 5′-diphosphate (GDP)-bound to the active, GTP-bound state.[22,37]

Activation of TC10 leads to cellular glucose uptake. In the process, TC10 at the lipid raft subdomains of the plasma membrane modulates the cytoplasmic actin structure. Via downstream effector proteins, insulin activation of TC10 leads to the formation of phosphatidylinositol 3-phosphate, which promotes the plasma membrane translocation of GLUT4.[19,43,44]

TC10. TC10 is a member of the Rho family that is constitutively localized to plasmalemmal microdomains. Although TC10 has a high degree of sequence homology with Rac, Rho, and Cdc42, it differs from the Rho protein family in other respects.

Most Rho family members contain a single carboxy-cysteine residue appropriate for geranylgeranylation that may prevent their interaction with the intracellular Golgi apparatus and direct their association to the plasma membrane.[22]

In contrast, the carboxy-terminal region of TC10 resembles that of H-Ras in that it encodes for both farnesylation and palmitoylation. Farnesylation and the subsequent palmitoylation of H-Ras and TC10 allow for their insertion and trafficking throughout the secretory membrane system. TC10 thus cycles through the perinuclear recycling endosome compartment while en route to the caveolin-enriched plasmalemmal microdomains.[22]

Glucose Uptake. Upon insulin stimulation, both the PI3K and c-Cbl pathways function in concert to control the actin dynamics regulating GLUT4 translocation. Connection of actin to the microtubular cytoskeleton is implicated in the regulation of GLUT4 trafficking.[7,37]

Insulin stimulation of GLUT4 translocation requires intact lipid raft microdomains or caveolae. Spatial separation and distinct compartmentalization of the PI3K and c-Cbl signaling pathways are essential. **With disruption of the lipid raft microdomains, TC10 lipid raft localization is impaired, and insulin stimulation of GLUT4 translocation does not occur.**[22]

Insulin-Mediated Glucose Disposal. Insulin lowers plasma glucose levels not only by mediating glucose uptake but also by stimulating glucose utilization and storage.

Insulin

- stimulates glycogenesis,
- inhibits glycogenolysis, and
- inhibits hepatic gluconeogenesis.

The serine-threonine kinase Akt is a principal target of insulin signaling that inhibits hepatic glucose output when glucose is available from food.

Insulin Impact on Gluconeogenesis. Insulin suppresses hepatic gluconeogenesis.

Gluconeogenesis is the formation of glucose from nonhexose substrates such as amino acids and glycerol. Upon insulin receptor binding with resultant Akt kinase activation, Akt phosphorylates a transcription factor called the forkhead transcription factor 1 (Foxo1) in the cytoplasm. The resultant decrease in cytoplasmic, unphosphorylated Foxo1 triggers the dissociation of nuclear Foxo1 from a coactivator molecule, thereby blocking the transcription of gluconeogenic genes. As a result, gluconeogenesis is attenuated and hepatic glucose output is reduced.[45]

Lipogenesis. Insulin promotes lipogenesis with the intake of surplus calories.

Hepatic Lipogenesis. Insulin stimulates hepatic lipogenesis. **With food intake, after saturation of hepatic glycogen stores, any additional glucose taken up by hepatocytes is shunted into fatty acid synthesis.**

Lipogenesis incorporates glucose into fatty acids and triglycerides. In the process, a carbohydrate response element–binding protein initiates a chain reaction that expresses the necessary enzymes to catalyze the transformation of excess glucose into fatty acids. Specifically, insulin activates enzymes such as

- acetyl–coenzyme A (CoA) carboxylase and
- fatty acid synthase

by inducing phosphorylation.

Glucose is also metabolized to glycerol. Glycerol, along with the fatty acids in the cell, then serves as substrate for the formation of triacylglycerols. In the process, insulin stimulates the requisite esterification process whereby three fatty acid chains attach to glycerol.

Insulin regulates the metabolism of free fatty acids and the production of triglyceride-rich particles. It is an important factor in the intracellular degradation of freshly translated apolipoprotein B-100, thus acutely suppressing the total production and release of large very-low-density lipoprotein (VLDL) particles.[46]

Fatty Acid Uptake in Adipose Tissue. Fatty acids are exported from the liver as triacylglycerols, or triglycerides, in triglyceride-rich lipoproteins such as VLDL. In the sated state, lipoproteins provide fatty acids to other tissues such as adipocytes for storage.

Lipoprotein Lipase. Insulin facilitates fatty acid uptake by adipose tissue and skeletal muscle.

Insulin stimulates lipoprotein lipase (LPL) activity by increasing LPL mRNA.[46] LPL is the primary enzyme that hydrolyzes triglycerides in chylomicrons and VLDLs, thereby catalyzing the key step in removal of triglycerides from the circulation to generate fatty acids for adipose tissue storage or skeletal muscle oxidation.

Fatty Acid Uptake. Insulin-stimulated free fatty acid uptake into adipocytes is more than 90% transporter mediated.

Induction of fatty acid transport proteins (FATPs) 1 and 4 occurs during adipocyte differentiation. Within minutes of receptor stimulation, insulin induces the translocation of FATPs from the intracellular, perinuclear compartment to the plasma membrane to increase the uptake of long-chain fatty acids.[47]

Adipocyte Lipogenesis. Glucose taken up by adipocytes is used to synthesize glycerol. Adipocytes use glycerol together with the fatty acids delivered by lipoproteins to resynthesize triacylglycerols, or storage fat.

Within adipose tissue, insulin blocks the breakdown of triacylglycerols by inhibiting intracellular, hormone-sensitive lipase. Thus, insulin actions that favor fat deposition include

- an increase in glucose uptake for the synthesis of fatty acids and glycerol,
- stimulation of enzymes that synthesize fatty acids from glucose,
- an increase in fatty acid uptake into adipocytes,
- enhanced fatty acid esterification to form triacylglycerols, and
- inhibition of intracellular lipolysis.

Amino Acid Uptake. In addition to its effect on plasma glucose and lipids, insulin also stimulates the uptake of amino acids and thus contributes to an overall anabolic effect with the generation of structural protein. Insulin action on protein synthesis includes

- the promotion of amino acid transport into cells,
- an increase in the rate of protein synthesis, and
- inhibition of protein degradation.

Excess amino acids are, however, also diverted to gluconeogenesis and lipogenesis.

Insulin-eNOS Interaction. Insulin activates eNOS, which has a favorable impact on endothelial function and inflammatory activation.

Endothelial Function. Activation of the PI3K pathway by insulin is associated not only with metabolic regulatory effects. **Insulin at physiologic and pharmacologic concentrations induces NO release via the same PI3K and Akt signaling pathway that also mediates GLUT4 translocation. Insulin also enhances NOS expression in endothelial cells and exerts a vasodilatory effect via NO release from the endothelium.**[48]

The mechanism underlying insulin vasodilation appears to be as follows: insulin activation of NOS initiates the cyclic 3′,5′-guanosine monophosphate (cGMP) signaling cascade. cGMP-dependent protein kinase (cGK) I is a downstream effector of the cGMP signaling pathway. cGK I inactivates the small GTPase RhoA directly by increasing RhoA phosphorylation and impairing its isoprenylation. It thus inhibits RhoA membrane translocation and activation. As a result, Rho kinase activation by RhoA is undercut, and vascular smooth muscle cell myosin-bound phosphatase activity is enhanced. Increased phosphatase activity lowers myosin light chain phosphorylation, and vascular smooth muscle cell relaxation ensues (Fig. 1-2).[49]

Enhanced Insulin Sensitivity. It is not only insulin that increases NOS expression and activity. In reciprocal fashion, the NOS-cGMP pathway also enhances cellular sensitivity to insulin signaling. cGK I, as a downstream effector of the cGMP signaling pathway, enhances insulin signaling by

- limiting Rho kinase activation and
- inhibiting the association of Rho kinase with IRS-1.[49]

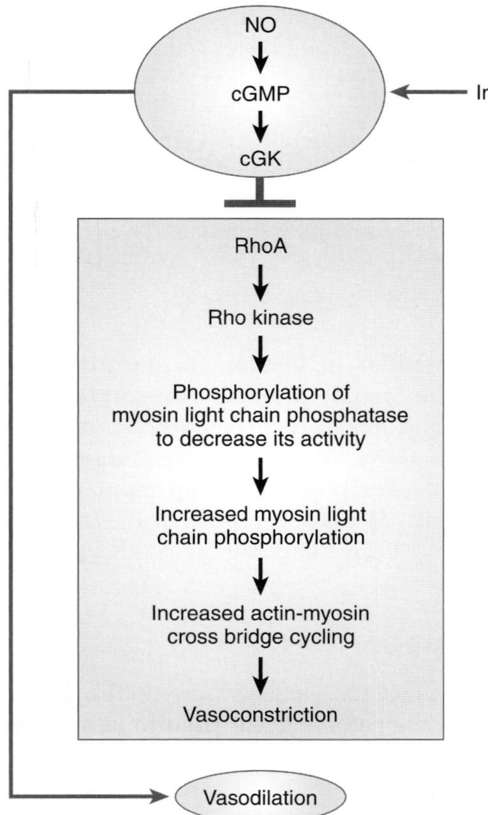

Figure 1–2.
Insulin causes vasodilation by modulating myosin light chain phosphorylation. Insulin activation of nitric oxide (NO) synthase initiates the guanosine 3′,5′-cyclic monophosphate (cGMP) signaling cascade. cGMP-dependent protein kinase (cGK) inactivates the small GTPase RhoA, thus inhibiting RhoA activation and Rho kinase stimulation. As a result, vascular smooth muscle cell myosin-bound phosphatase activity is enhanced, which lowers myosin light chain phosphorylation, and vascular smooth muscle cell relaxation ensues.

Anti-inflammatory Effects. Insulin has anti-inflammatory effects that are dependent on NO production.[50]

Insulin exerts a nuclear factor kappaB (NFκB) suppressive effect and constrains the intranuclear content of NFκB.[51] In human aortic endothelial cells, insulin inhibits the expression of NFκB, intracellular adhesion molecule-1 (ICAM-1), and monocyte chemoattractant protein-1 (MCP-1), three major proinflammatory mediators reduced in parallel with an increase in eNOS expression.[50] Similarly, insulin decreases the generation of reactive oxygen species by polymorphonuclear leukocytes and mononuclear cells and lowers C-reactive protein (CRP) levels.[52] Insulin suppresses TNF-α and interleukin-6.[53]

In ventilated, intensive care unit patients, the majority without diabetes, an insulin infusion to normalize blood glucose may reduce markers of inflammation and, ultimately, mortality.[54]

Insulin Mitogenic Effects. Insulin signal transduction occurs not only via the metabolic-vascular pathways but also via MAPK signaling cascades (Fig. 1-3).

Impact of Insulin-Activated MAPK. Insulin activation of MAPK is associated with mitogenic effects. In the vasculature, MAPK activation ultimately leads to vascular cell growth and proliferation, atherogenesis, and thrombogenesis.[55]

MAPK activation may also modulate the activity of glucose transport. Insulin stimulation of p38 MAPK may lead to GLUT4 activation (Fig. 1-4).[56]

MAPK activation by insulin modulates transcriptional activity by altering the cell content of numerous mRNAs and producing changes in protein expression.[56] It is associated with

- cell growth,
- DNA synthesis,
- cell proliferation,

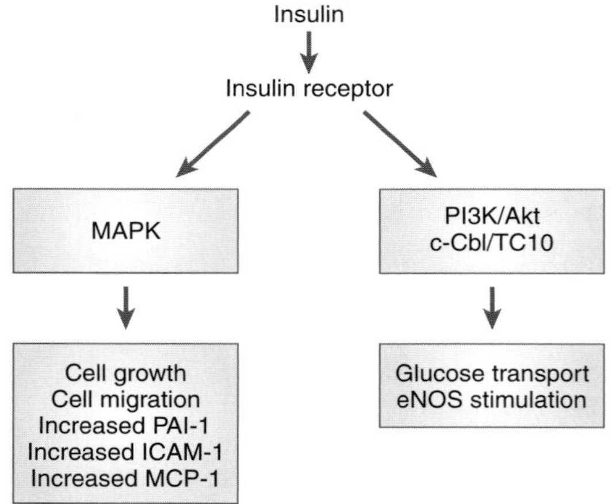

Figure 1–3.
Insulin-stimulated mitogen-activated protein kinase (MAPK) and phosphatidylinositol 3-kinase (PI3K) pathways mediating mitogenic and metabolic-vascular stimulation, respectively. eNOS, endothelial nitric oxide synthase; ICAM, intercellular adhesion molecule; MCP, monocyte chemoattractant protein; PAI, plasminogen activator inhibitor. *(Adapted from Hsueh WA, Quinones WA. Role of endothelial dysfunction in insulin resistance. Am J Cardiol 2003;92:10J-17J.)*

- vascular remodeling,
- endothelin-1 overexpression,
- plasminogen activator overexpression,[57,58]
- plasminogen activator inhibitor-1 (PAI-1) gene transcription,[46]
- prenylation of Ras and Rho proteins,
- vascular cell adhesion molecule-1 (VCAM-1) overexpression,
- endothelial-selectin (E-selectin) overexpression, and
- increased rolling interactions of monocytes with endothelial cells.[59]

Insulin Activation of MAPK. Insulin activates MAPK via two possible mechanisms, activation of Ras or PKC:

1. *Ras.* The ubiquitous IRS-1 protein plays a major role in the transduction of insulin's proliferative effects by activating Ras.

   IRS-1 has multiple tyrosine phosphorylation residues, which allows it to interact with other signaling molecules to convey mitogenic signals. These molecules include PI3K regulatory subunits and Grb2, an adapter protein that interacts with the exchange factor SOS and induces activation of the GTPase Ras. Ras, in turn, functions as an activator of the small GTPase Raf, which ultimately activates MAPK kinase (MAPKK) to enable phosphorylation and stimulation of MAPK.

   Most mitogenic signals initiated by tyrosine kinase receptors such as the insulin receptor converge on MAPK through Ras activation.[42] Insulin receptor substrates other than IRS-1/2, such as Shc and Gab, also appear to mediate insulin's mitogenic actions (Fig. 1-5).[38]
2. *PKC.* Insulin can stimulate MAPK by activating PKC, thereby bypassing Ras.

   PKC is activated after cell surface receptor stimulation. Binding of insulin to its receptor triggers phospholipase activity and the production of DAG. DAG binds to and activates PKC. PKC-mediated signaling systems control numerous cell functions and may stimulate Raf independently of Ras to achieve MAPKK/MAPK activation.[42]

Other Activities of Insulin. Insulin also promotes the renal tubular reabsorption of sodium and enhances sympathetic nervous system activity. Insulin causes significant increases in renin release. It up-regulates the angiotensin II AT_1 receptor with crosstalk between the insulin and angiotensin II signaling pathways.[60]

GLUCAGON

Many of glucagon's effects oppose the effects of insulin. Its net effect is a rise in plasma glucose concentration. As such, it complements insulin in the control of steady plasma glucose levels.

Cessation of Insulin Secretion. As the plasma glucose concentration falls, insulin secretion ceases.

In the absence of insulin, most body cells become unable to take up glucose and, in the short term, derive glucose from glycogen reserves. The absence of insulin during the fasting state pushes the metabolic balance to catabolism

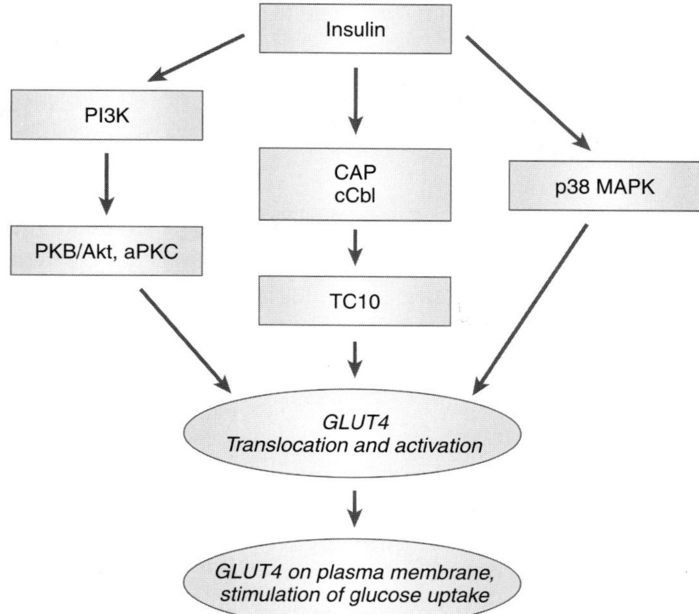

Figure 1–4.
Insulin stimulation of glucose uptake by the phosphatidylinositol 3-kinase (PI3K)/Akt, proto-oncogene c-Cbl/TC10, and p38 mitogen-activated protein kinase (MAPK) pathways. aPKC, atypical protein kinase C; CAP, Cbl-activating protein; GLUT, glucose transporter; PKB, protein kinase B. *(Adapted from Furtado LM, Somwar R, Sweeney G, et al. Activation of the glucose transporter GLUT4 by insulin. Biochem Cell Biol 2002;80:569-578.)*

with degradation of intracellular glycogen, fat, and protein. Glycogenolysis is complemented by hepatic gluconeogenesis, which is essential for survival during prolonged fasting or starvation because it supplies tissues such as the insulin-independent nervous system with a continuing, constant supply of glucose. Other tissues that are not dependent on glucose switch to alternative fuels such as fatty acids for energy generation.[61]

Secretion of Glucagon. Glycogenolysis and gluconeogenesis are stimulated not only by the absence of insulin but also by the action of glucagon, which is secreted as plasma glucose levels fall below normal.

Glucagon is a 29–amino acid, linear protein with conserved structure among vertebrates. It is synthesized in the alpha cells of the pancreatic islets as proglucagon and is then proteolytically processed.

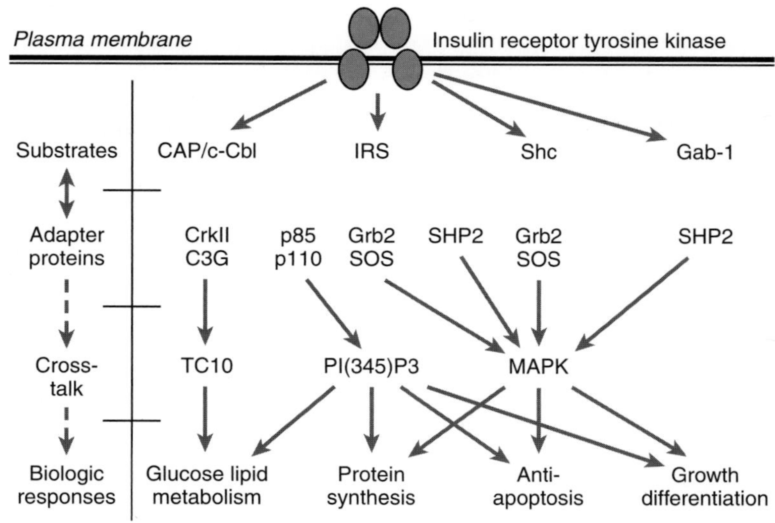

Figure 1–5.
Insulin signaling pathways leading to various metabolic and mitogenic biologic responses. *(Modified from Kanzaki M, Pessin JE. Signal integration and the specificity of insulin action. Cell Biochem Biophys 2001;35:191-209.)*

Glucagon is secreted in response to

- hypoglycemia,
- elevated blood levels of amino acids, as seen after the consumption of a protein-rich meal, and
- exercise.

With a fall in plasma glucose levels below the normal range, glucagon is secreted into the portal vein and thereafter into the systemic circulation.

Glucagon secretion is inhibited

- directly by hyperglycemia and
- indirectly by insulin's inhibitory effect on glucagon secretion.[61]

Hepatic and Adipose Tissue Effects of Glucagon. Glucagon has several effects on the liver and adipose tissue.

It has strong gluconeogenic actions on the liver. In the liver, glucagon

- blocks glycogen synthesis,
- stimulates glycogenolysis, and
- activates gluconeogenesis.

Additionally, glucagon

- decreases hepatic protein synthesis and
- promotes hepatic protein degradation.

In adipose tissue, glucagon

- decreases triglyceride synthesis and
- enhances triglyceride lipolysis

in order to preserve glucose by providing fatty acids as fuel to cells.[61]

CONCLUSION

Insulin receptor signaling appears to be initiated from specialized plasmalemmal caveolar microdomains. Caveolae are present in adipocytes, smooth muscle cells, skeletal and cardiac myocytes, and endothelial cells, all tissues that are very sensitive to the intact functioning of metabolic and vascular insulin signaling. Caveolae function as switchboards for large arrays of receptor signaling pathways. Given the proximity of molecular pathways for eNOS, insulin, TNF-α, angiotensin II, or endothelin-1, to name a few, crosstalk or interactions between insulin signaling and other pathways appear to be quite feasible. One such positive interaction pertains to the reciprocal, positive interaction between eNOS and the insulin receptor, which has a favorable impact on endothelial function and insulin sensitivity. There are corresponding, potentially negative interactions between cytokine/vasoconstrictor pathways and insulin signaling that may play a role in mediating insulin resistance.

Not only do caveolae expose insulin signaling to potentially adverse receptor crosstalk, but the caveolar microenvironment is also potentially vulnerable and may jeopardize the integrity of insulin signaling. Derangements in caveolar cholesterol content or caveolin scaffolding, as may occur with dyslipidemia, jeopardize some, but not all of the insulin signaling cascades. Specifically, with perturbation of caveolar integrity, metabolic and vascular insulin signaling is disrupted; however, the mitogenic insulin pathway remains undisturbed. The resulting imbalance in insulin signaling would be expected to lead to selective insulin resistance and the metabolic syndrome.

Conceivably, caveolae may play a multifaceted, but central role in the pathogenesis of clinical insulin resistance. A more detailed understanding of the role of caveolar integrity and receptor crosstalk in insulin signaling may have beneficial implications for a targeted, therapeutic approach to insulin resistance.

GLOSSARY

ADP	adenosine 5′-diphosphate
APS	associated protein substrate
AT_1	angiotensin II type 1
ATP	adenosine triphosphate
CAP	Cbl-activating protein
cGK	cGMP-dependent protein kinase
cGMP	cyclic 3′,5′-guanosine monophosphate
CoA	coenzyme A
CRP	C-reactive protein
DAG	diacylglycerol
eNOS	endothelial nitric oxide synthase

ERK	extracellular signal–regulated kinase
E-selectin	endothelial-leukocyte adhesion molecule-1, or endothelial-selectin
FATP	fatty acid transport protein
Foxo1	forkhead transcription factor 1
GDP	guanosine 5′-diphosphate
GLUT	glucose transporter
GPI	glycosylphosphatidylinositol
GTP	guanosine 5′-triphosphate
ICAM-1	intracellular adhesion molecule-1
IRS	insulin receptor substrate
LPL	lipoprotein lipase
MAPK	mitogen-activated protein kinase
MAPKK	MAPK kinase
MCP-1	monocyte chemoattractant protein-1
NFκB	nuclear factor kappaB
NOS	nitric oxide synthase
PAI-1	plasminogen activator inhibitor-1
PDK	3-phosphoinositide–dependent kinase
PI3K	phosphatidylinositol 3-kinase
PIP3	phosphatidylinositol 3,4,5-triphosphate
PKB	protein kinase B
PKC	protein kinase C
SOS	Son of Sevenless
TNF	tumor necrosis factor
VCAM-1	vascular cell adhesion molecule-1
VLDL	very-low-density lipoprotein

REFERENCES

1. Lehninger AL. Biochemistry, 2nd ed. New York, Worth Publishers, 1975
2. Guerre-Millo M, Rouault C, Poulain P, et al. PPAR-alpha-null mice are protected from high-fat diet–induced insulin resistance. Diabetes 2001;50:2809-2814
3. Farese RV. Function and dysfunction of aPKC isoforms for glucose transport in insulin-sensitive and insulin-resistant states. Am J Physiol Endocrinol Metab 2002; 283:E1-E11
4. Khayat ZA, Patel N, Klip A. Exercise- and insulin-stimulated muscle glucose transport: distinct mechanisms of regulation. Can J Appl Physiol 2002;27:129-151
5. Meglasson MD, Matschinsky FM. Pancreatic islet glucose metabolism and regulation of insulin secretion. Diabetes Metab Rev 1986;2:163-214
6. Malaisse WJ. Physiology, pathology and pharmacology of insulin secretion: recent acquisitions. Diabetes Metab 1997;23(suppl 3):6-15
7. Khan AH, Pessin JE. Insulin regulation of glucose uptake: a complex interplay of intracellular signaling pathways. Diabetologia 2002;45:1475-1483
8. Youngren JF, Keen S, Kulp JL, et al. Enhanced muscle insulin receptor autophosphorylation with short-term aerobic exercise training. Am J Physiol Endocrinol Metab 2001;280:E528-E533
9. Bickel PE. Lipid rafts and insulin signaling. Am J Physiol Endocrinol Metab 2002;282:E1-E10
10. Stulnig TM, Huber J, Leitinger N, et al. Polyunsaturated eicosapentaenoic acid displaces proteins from membrane rafts by altering raft lipid composition. J Biol Chem 2001;276:37335-37340
11. Muller G. Dynamics of plasma membrane microdomains and cross-talk to the insulin signaling cascade. FEBS Lett 2002;531:81-87
12. Goligorsky MS, Li H, Brodsky S, Chen J. Relationships between caveolae and eNOS: everything in proximity and the proximity of everything. Am J Physiol Renal Physiol 2002;283:F1-F10
13. Uittenbogaard A, Shaul PW, Yuhanna IS, et al. High density lipoprotein prevents oxidized low density lipoprotein–induced inhibition of endothelial nitric-oxide synthase localization and activation in caveolae. J Biol Chem 2000;275:11278-11283
14. Gustavsson J, Parpal S, Karlsson M, et al. Localization of the insulin receptor in caveolae of adipocyte plasma membrane. FASEB J 1999;13:1961-1971
15. Couet J, Sargiacomo M, Lisanti MP. Interaction of a receptor tyrosine kinase, EGF-R, with caveolins. Caveolin binding negatively regulates tyrosine and serine/threonine kinase activities. J Biol Chem 1997;272:30429-30438
16. Muller G, Jung C, Wied S, et al. Redistribution of glycolipid raft domain components induces insulin-mimetic signaling in rat adipocytes. Mol Cell Biol 2001;21:4553-4567
17. Park H, Go YM, Darji R, et al. Caveolin-1 regulates shear stress–dependent activation of extracellular signal–regulated kinase. Am J Physiol Heart Circ Physiol 2000;278:H1285-H1293
18. Kincer JF, Uittenbogaard A, Dressman J, et al. Hypercholesterolemia promotes a CD36-dependent and endothelial nitric-oxide synthase–mediated vascular dysfunction. J Biol Chem 2002;277:23525-23533
19. Watson RT, Shigematsu S, Chiang S-H, et al. Lipid raft microdomain compartmentalization of TC10 is required for insulin signaling and GLUT4 translocation. J Cell Biol 2001;154:829-840
20. Dessy C, Kelly RA, Balligand JL, Feron O. Dynamin mediates caveolar sequestration of muscarinic cholinergic receptors and alteration in NO signaling. EMBO J 2000;19:4272-4280
21. Veldman RJ, Maestre N, Aduib OM, et al. A neutral sphingomyelinase resides in sphingolipid-enriched microdomains and is inhibited by the caveolin-scaffolding domain: potential implications in tumour necrosis factor signalling. Biochem J 2001;355(Pt 3):859-868
22. Saltiel AR, Pessin JE. Lipid raft microdomain compartmentalization of TC10 is required for insulin signaling and GLUT4 translocation. J Cell Biol 2001;154:829-840
23. Shaul PW. Regulation of endothelial nitric oxide synthase: location, location, location. Annu Rev Physiol 2002;64:749-774
24. Bernier SG, Haldar S, Michel T. Bradykinin-regulated interactions of the mitogen-activated protein kinase pathway with the endothelial nitric-oxide synthase. J Biol Chem 2000;275:30707-30715
25. Michaely PA, Mineo C, Ying YS, Anderson RG. Polarized distribution of endogenous Rac1 and

RhoA at the cell surface. J Biol Chem 1999;274: 21430-21436
26. Ushio-Fukai M, Hilenski L, Santanam N, et al. Cholesterol depletion inhibits epidermal growth factor receptor transactivation by angiotensin II in vascular smooth muscle cells: role of cholesterol-rich microdomains and focal adhesions in angiotensin II signaling. J Biol Chem 2001;276:48269-48275
27. Liu P, Wang P, Michaely P, et al. Presence of oxidized cholesterol in caveolae uncouples active platelet-derived growth factor receptors from tyrosine kinase substrates. J Biol Chem 2000;275:31648-31654
28. Park H, Go YM, St John PL, et al. Plasma membrane cholesterol is a key molecule in shear stress–dependent activation of extracellular signal–regulated kinase. J Biol Chem 1998;273:32304-32311
29. Le Lay S, Krief S, Farnier C, et al. Cholesterol, a cell size–dependent signal that regulates glucose metabolism and gene expression in adipocytes. J Biol Chem 2001;276:16904-16910
30. Cohen AW, Combs TP, Scherer PE, Lisanti MP. Role of caveolin and caveolae in insulin signaling and diabetes. Am J Physiol Endocrinol Metab 2003;285:E1151-E1160
31. Cohen AW, Razani B, Wang XB, et al. Caveolin-1–deficient mice show insulin resistance and defective insulin receptor protein expression in adipose tissue. Am J Physiol Cell Physiol 2003;285:C222-C235
32. Kim F, Gallis B, Corson MA. TNF-alpha inhibits flow and insulin signaling leading to NO production in aortic endothelial cells. Am J Physiol Cell Physiol 2001;280:C1057-C1065
33. Parpal S, Karlsson M, Thorn H, Stralfors P. Cholesterol depletion disrupts caveolae and insulin receptor signaling for metabolic control via insulin receptor substrate-1, but not for mitogen-activated protein kinase control. J Biol Chem 2001;276:9670-9678
34. Kanzaki M, Pessin JE. Signal integration and the specificity of insulin action. Cell Biochem Biophys 2001;35:191-209
35. Ryder JW, Chibalin AV, Zierath JR. Intracellular mechanisms underlying increases in glucose uptake in response to insulin or exercise in skeletal muscle. Acta Physiol Scand 2001;171:249-257
36. Gustavsson J, Parpal S, Stralfors P. Insulin-stimulated glucose uptake involves the transition of glucose transporters to a caveolae-rich fraction within the plasma membrane: implications for type II diabetes. Mol Med 1996;2:367-372
37. Mora S, Pessin JE. An adipocentric view of signaling and intracellular trafficking. Diabetes Metab Res Rev 2002;18:345-356
38. Montagnani M, Ravichandran LV, Chen H, et al. Insulin receptor substrate-1 and phosphoinositide-dependent kinase-1 are required for insulin-stimulated production of nitric oxide in endothelial cells. Mol Endocrinol 2002;16:1931-1942
39. James DJ, Cairns F, Salt IP, et al. Skeletal muscle of stroke-prone spontaneously hypertensive rats exhibits reduced insulin-stimulated glucose transport and elevated levels of caveolin and flotillin. Diabetes 2001;50: 2148-2156
40. Zierath JR. Exercise effects of muscle insulin signaling and action. Invited review: Exercise training–induced changes in insulin signaling in skeletal muscle. J Appl Physiol 2002;93:773-781
41. Henriksen EJ. Exercise effects of muscle insulin signaling and action. Invited review: Effects of acute exercise and exercise training on insulin resistance. J Appl Physiol 2002;93:788-796
42. Formisano P, Oriente F, Fiory F, et al. Insulin-activated protein kinase C beta bypasses Ras and stimulates mitogen-activated protein kinase activity and cell proliferation in muscle cells. Mol Cell Biol 2000;20: 6323-6333
43. Litherland GJ, Hajduch E, Hundai HS. Intracellular signaling mechanisms regulating glucose transport in insulin-sensitive tissues (review). Mol Membr Biol 2001;18:195-204
44. Maffucci T, Brancaccio A, Piccolo E, et al. Insulin induces phosphatidylinositol-3-phosphate formation through TC10 activation. EMBO J 2003;22:4178-4189
45. Puigserver P, Rhee J, Donovan J, et al. Insulin-regulated hepatic gluconeogenesis through FOXO1–PGC-1alpha interaction. Nature 2003;423:550-555
46. Ruotolo G, Howard BV. Dyslipidemia of the metabolic syndrome. Curr Cardiol Rep 2002;4:494-500
47. Stahl A, Evans JG, Pattel S, et al. Insulin causes fatty acid transport protein translocation and enhanced fatty acid uptake in adipocytes. Dev Cell 2002;2:477-488
48. Aljada A, Dandona P. Effect of insulin on human aortic endothelial nitric oxide synthase. Metabolism 2000;49: 147-150
49. Begum N, Sandu OA, Ito M, et al. Active Rho kinase (ROK-alpha) associates with insulin receptor substrate-1 and inhibits insulin signaling in vascular smooth muscle cells. J Biol Chem 2002;277:6214-6222
50. Aljada A, Saadeh R, Assian E, et al. Insulin inhibits the expression of intercellular adhesion molecule-1 by human aortic endothelial cells through stimulation of nitric oxide. J Clin Endocrinol Metab 2000;85:2572-2575
51. Dandona P, Aljada A, Mohanty P, et al. Insulin inhibits intranuclear nuclear factor kappa B and stimulates IkappaB in mononuclear cells in obese subjects: evidence for an antiinflammatory effect? J Clin Endocrinol Metab 2001;86:3257-3265
52. Aljada A, Ghanim H, Saadeh R, Dandona P. Insulin inhibits NFκB and MCP-1 expression in human aortic endothelial cells. J Clin Endocrinol Metab 2001;86:450-453
53. Dandona P, Aljada A, Mohanty P. The anti-inflammatory and potential anti-atherogenic effect of insulin: a new paradigm. Diabetologia 2002;45:924-930
54. van den Berghe G, Wouters P, Weekers F, et al. Intensive insulin therapy in the critically ill patients. N Engl J Med 2001;345:1359-1367
55. Carel K, Kummer JL, Schubert C, et al. Insulin stimulates mitogen activated protein kinase by a Ras independent pathway in 3T3-L1 adipocytes. J Biol Chem 1996;271:30625-30630
56. Furtado LM, Somwar R, Sweeney G, et al. Activation of the glucose transporter GLUT4 by insulin. Biochem Cell Biol 2002;80:569-578
57. Federici M, Menghini R, Mauriello A, et al. Insulin-dependent activation of endothelial nitric oxide synthase is impaired by O-linked glycosylation modification of signaling proteins in human coronary endothelial cells. Circulation 2002;106:466-472
58. Cusi K, Maezono K, Osman A, et al. Insulin resistance differentially affects the PI 3-kinase– and MAP kinase–mediated signaling in human muscle. J Clin Invest 2000;105:311-320
59. Montagnani M, Golovchenko I, Kim I, et al. Inhibition of phosphatidylinositol 3-kinase enhances mitogenic actions of insulin in endothelial cells. J Biol Chem 2002;277: 1794-1799
60. Zeng G, Quon MJ. Insulin-stimulated production of nitric oxide is inhibited by wortmannin. J Clin Invest 1996;98:894-898
61. Jiang G, Zhang BB. Glucagon and regulation of glucose metabolism. Am J Physiol Endocrinol Metab 2003;284: E671-E678

Section II

Causes of Insulin Resistance

Oxidative Stress 2

BACKGROUND

Oxidative stress reflects an imbalance between the production and degradation of reactive, pro-oxidant substances. Several types of reactive species, in the form of free radicals or nonradicals, are generated in the body as a result of metabolic reactions. These pro-oxidant species may be either oxygen derived, termed reactive oxygen species (ROS), such as

- superoxide anion radical ($O_2^{\bullet -}$),
- hydroxyl radical ($OH^{\bullet}$),
- hydrogen peroxide (H_2O_2), and
- lipid peroxides,

or nitrogen derived, termed reactive nitrogen oxide species (RNOS), such as

- peroxynitrite ($ONOO^-$) (Table 2-1).

Oxidative stress may derive from excessive production of ROS and RNOS or from reduced antioxidant activity. In health, pro-oxidants are balanced by antioxidants. In the absence of an appropriate, compensatory endogenous antioxidant response, a shift in this balance toward pro-oxidants gives rise to oxidative stress. Depending on the extent of the shift, oxidative stress may be either mild, moderate, or severe.[1,2]

Acute and Chronic Oxidative Damage. Acutely, immunologic host defense and microbial killing are major physiologic roles for potent ROS and RNOS.

In the absence of a compensatory endogenous antioxidant response, however, **high levels of ROS and RNOS may not only serve as host defense but may also cause collateral injury both directly and indirectly:**

- Directly, pro-oxidant molecules damage cellular macromolecules by oxidizing and damaging proteins, lipids, and the nucleic acids DNA and RNA, thereby impairing cellular function.
- Indirectly, ROS and RNOS damage tissues by activating cellular stress-sensitive signaling pathways.

Table 2-1. Biologically Important Reactive Species

TYPE	FREE RADICALS	NONRADICALS
Reactive oxygen species	Superoxide, $O_2^{\cdot-}$ Hydroxyl, $OH^{\cdot}$ Peroxyl, $RO_2^{\cdot}$ Hydroperoxyl, $HO_2^{\cdot-}$	Hydrogen peroxide, H_2O_2 Hydrochlorous acid, HOCl
Reactive nitrogen species	Nitric oxide, $NO^{\cdot}$ Nitrogen dioxide, $NO_2^{\cdot-}$	Peroxynitrite, $OONO^-$ Nitrous oxide, HNO_2

Modified from Evans JL, Goldfine ID, Maddux BA, Grodsky GM. Oxidative stress and stress-activated signaling pathways: a unifying hypothesis of type 2 diabetes. Endocr Rev 2002;23:599-622.

Clinical Sequelae of Chronic Stress Pathway Activation. Chronically sustained oxidative stress pathways are implicated in the pathogenesis and progression of a multiplicity of disorders, such as

- cardiovascular disease,
- insulin resistance,
- impaired insulin secretion,
- type 2 diabetes mellitus (DM),
- late diabetic end-organ complications,
- skin ailments,
- neurologic diseases,
- renal diseases,
- liver diseases,
- respiratory diseases,
- aging,
- malignancies,

and other protracted inflammatory conditions.[1,2]

All common risk factors for vascular disease are attended by the increased production of free oxygen radicals. In the vasculature, persistently activated stress pathways are implicated in endothelial dysfunction, adhesion molecule expression, intimal proliferation, apoptosis, and lipid peroxidation, all of which eventuate in clinical vascular disease.[3] Correspondingly, **chronic oxidant stress leads to insulin resistance and thereby engenders clinical metabolic disease** (Fig. 2-1).[1,2]

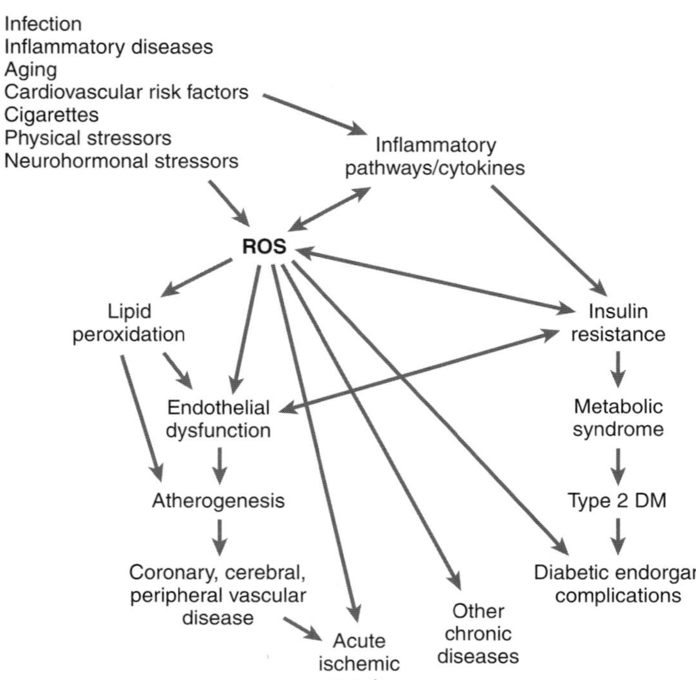

›› **Figure 2-1.** All risk factors for cardiovascular disease are associated with increased production of reactive oxygen species (ROS), which leads to endothelial dysfunction, insulin resistance, and vascular and metabolic disease. DM, diabetes mellitus.

ENDOGENOUS ANTIOXIDANTS

The first line of defense against ROS occurs through enzymatic inactivation. Inactivation of ROS is achieved mainly by endogenous antioxidants. Cellular exposure to oxidants may initiate adaptive intracellular antioxidant responses via the induction of antioxidant gene expression to protect against oxidative stress.[4]

The major antioxidant enzymes are

1. glutathione peroxidase and reductase, which reduce peroxynitrites and hydrogen and lipid peroxides;
2. superoxide dismutase, which targets superoxide; and
3. catalase, which inactivates hydrogen peroxide, thereby preventing the generation of hydroxyl radicals by the Fenton reaction.[2]

Other endogenous antioxidants are minerals such as Se, Mn, Cu, and Zn and vitamins such as vitamins A, C, and E. Additional compounds with antioxidant activity include flavonoids, bilirubin, and uric acid.[2]

Glutathione Peroxidases. Glutathione peroxidases with glutathione constitute the principal antioxidant defense system regulating the intracellular redox state and protecting cells from injury caused by oxygen free radicals.

There are at least four different glutathione peroxidases, all of which contain selenocysteine at their active sites. Of these, glutathione peroxidase 1 is the ubiquitous intracellular form and is the key antioxidant enzyme within most cells, including the endothelium. It thus preserves endothelial function in arteries exposed to oxidative stress. Correspondingly, glutathione depletion impairs nitric oxide (NO) bioavailability from endothelial cells.[5]

Glutathione peroxidase 1 uses glutathione to

- reduce hydrogen peroxide to water,
- reduce lipid peroxides to their respective alcohols, and
- reduce peroxynitrite to NO, thereby acting as a peroxynitrite reductase.[5]

Superoxide Dismutase. Superoxide dismutase is ubiquitously expressed. There are three different enzymatic forms that convert superoxide anion to hydrogen peroxide:

1. cytosolic copper- and zinc-containing superoxide dismutase,
2. mitochondrial manganese-containing superoxide dismutase, and
3. extracellular superoxide dismutase.

Extracellular superoxide dismutase is most active in the vessel wall. It enhances the availability of NO by scavenging superoxide anion.[5]

SOURCES OF OXIDATIVE STRESS

Oxidative stress is generated via normal oxidative metabolism and during an inflammatory response. Oxidative stress also arises from neurohormonal activation, cardiovascular risk factors, and physical stimuli.

Oxidative Phosphorylation as a Source of Oxidants. Normal oxidative metabolism produces low levels of ROS and RNOS as byproducts.

Molecular oxygen is essential during mitochondrial respiration for the complete metabolism of glucose, fatty acids, and other substances, during the course of which adenosine triphosphate (ATP) is generated. In normal oxidative phosphorylation, 0.4% to 4% of all oxygen consumed is converted to the free radical superoxide. Superoxide can either be eliminated by antioxidant defenses or be converted to other forms of ROS or RNOS.[1]

Oxidases Stimulated during Inflammation. Inflammatory reactions constitute a significant source of oxidative stress and are implicated in both its initiation and progression.

Sources of increased vascular oxidative stress are manifold and derive from plasmalemmal and intracellular oxidases within

- **leukocytes,**
- **endothelial cells,**
- **vascular smooth muscle cells, and**
- **adventitial cells.**[6]

Plasmalemmal Oxidases. The membrane-bound oxidative enzymes responsible for superoxide generation and increased oxidative stress in the vessel wall include

- nicotinamide adenine dinucleotide phosphate (NADH/NADPH) oxidase,
- xanthine oxidase,
- inducible nitric oxide synthase (iNOS), and
- uncoupled, constitutive endothelial NOS (eNOS) itself.[7]

Intracellular Oxidases. Intracellular oxidative enzymes implicated in the production of oxidants are

- myeloperoxidase,
- lipoxygenases,
- cyclooxygenases (COXs),
- cytochrome P-450 enzymes, and
- ceramide-activated protein kinases.[8]

Plasmalemmal NADH/NADPH Oxidase. NADH/NADPH is located in all layers of the vascular wall. In the vasculature, leukocyte and vascular cell NADH/NADPH oxidase is the enzyme primarily responsible for the generation of superoxide anion.

NADH/NADPH Constituents and Activation. The neutrophil/macrophage NADH/NADPH enzyme is a membrane-associated enzyme complex with cytosolic constituents. Translocation of the cytosolic, regulatory subunits to the plasma membrane is a prerequisite for oxidase activation and ROS production. The oxidase generates superoxide during the respiratory burst by catalyzing the transfer of electrons from NADPH to molecular oxygen.[9,10]

The active, multicomponent enzyme complex consists of

- the membrane-bound flavocytochrome b_{558}, which is the redox center of the enzyme. Flavocytochrome *b* is a heterodimer composed of gp91 phagocyte oxidase (phox) and p22*phox*.
- the three cytosolic subunits p47*phox*, p67*phox*, and p40*phox*. Membrane-bound flavocytochrome *b* appears to be activated upon binding of the regulatory cytosolic p47*phox* and p67*phox* subunits. p47*phox* serves as a carrier for p67*phox* to the membrane. Interaction of p67*phox* with flavocytochrome *b* is essential for electron flow from NADPH to O_2 to form superoxide.
- two small guanosine 5′-triphosphate (GTP)ases, Rap1A and Rac. These enzymes are involved in regulating the NADH/NADPH oxidase complex. Rac1 also serves as a carrier for p67*phox* to the membrane flavocytochrome.[9-11]

Up-regulation of Oxidant Output. The low-molecular-weight plasmalemmal guanine nucleotide–binding proteins Rac1, Rac2, and Rap1A up-regulate NADH/NADPH activity. Rac is essential for high-level superoxide production.

A critical process in activation of NADH/NADPH oxidase is prenylation of Rac at its carboxy-terminal domain, which determines its translocation to the membrane and the exchange of guanosine diphosphate for GTP at its regulatory site.[9,10] The GTP-bound form of Rac binds to p67*phox* and probably also to flavocytochrome *b* in the assembled oxidase complex.[9,10]

Superoxide and Other Reactive Oxygen Species. Superoxide formation by NADH/NADPH oxidase is a critical, proximal step in the generation of other ROS and RNOS.

After the generation of superoxide, H_2O_2 can be generated via a two-electron oxidation of oxygen or via dismutation of superoxide either spontaneously or by superoxide dismutase. H_2O_2 generation is followed by the generation of other toxic molecules (Fig. 2-2). Peroxynitrite is the reaction product of NO and superoxide.

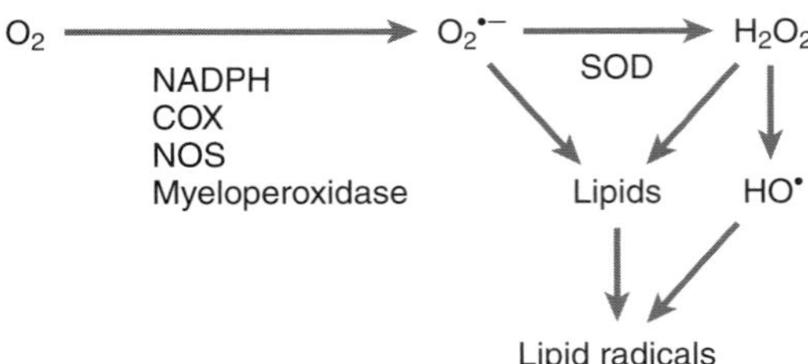

▸▸ **Figure 2–2.**
Oxidases generate superoxide from molecular oxygen. Superoxide dismutates into hydrogen peroxide via superoxide dismutase (SOD), which devolves into the hydroxyl radical. All these reactive oxygen species can oxidize lipid moieties. COX, cyclooxygenase; NADPH, nicotinamide adenine dinucleotide phosphate; NOS, nitric oxide synthase. *(Modified from Harrison D, Griendling KK, Landmesser U, et al. Role of oxidative stress in atherosclerosis. Am J Cardiol 2003;91[suppl]:7A-11A.)*

Further actions of peroxidases and superoxide dismutases generate other ROS such as lipid- and carbon-centered, thiyl, and hydroxyl radicals. Via these oxidants, physical forces and inflammatory cytokines can further increase tissue ROS levels by acting on numerous substrates.[3]

Plasmalemmal Uncoupled eNOS. eNOS itself may contribute to oxidative stress. With reduced availability of L-arginine as eNOS substrate or tetrahydrobiopterin (BH_4) as NOS cofactor, eNOS produces superoxide anion.

In the absence of BH_4, electron transfer within eNOS is shunted to molecular oxygen, the preferred substrate for NOS, whereupon the eNOS reaction produces superoxide through the uncoupled NADH/NADPH oxidase reaction (Fig. 2-3).[12] Superoxide instead of NO is also generated upon oxidation of the Zn-thiolate complex of eNOS by ROS such as peroxynitrite.[8]

Plasmalemmal iNOS. iNOS increases oxidative stress. It can be induced in a multiplicity of tissues, including macrophages, skeletal and cardiac muscle, fat, and liver.

iNOS induction is calcium independent and results in high-output production of NO. NO, reacting with superoxide, generates the potent oxidant peroxynitrite. Peroxynitrite modulates cellular functions through oxidative protein modifications such as the nitration of amino acid residues.[13]

Convergent signals from cytokine-activated pathways such as Janus kinase (JAK), mitogen-activated protein kinase (MAPK), and IκB kinase (IKK) induce iNOS expression through the binding of transcription factors to the iNOS gene promoter.[13]

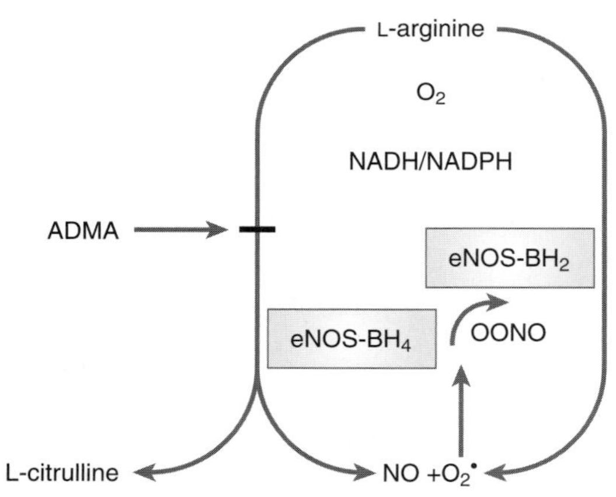

Figure 2-3.
Endothelial nitric oxide synthase (eNOS) coupled with tetrahydrobiopterin (BH_4) generates nitric oxide (NO) and L-citrulline. Asymmetric dimethylarginine (ADMA) is an endogenous, competitive inhibitor of NOS. Oxidative consumption of NO, as through the interaction with superoxide, produces the potent nitrating oxidant peroxynitrite, OONO. BH_4 is very susceptible to oxidation by peroxynitrite, whereupon dihydrobiopterin (BH_2) is produced. In the absence of BH_4, electron transfer is shunted to molecular oxygen, and the eNOS reaction produces superoxide through the uncoupled nicotinamide adenine dinucleotide phosphate (NADH/NADPH) oxidase reaction.

Intracellular Myeloperoxidase. The intracellular leukocyte-derived hemoprotein myeloperoxidase is a considerable source of oxidant stress. Normally playing a role in innate host defenses as a microbicidal enzyme, myeloperoxidase is implicated in proatherogenic and other pathogenic mechanisms.

Myeloperoxidase is released by activated neutrophils or monocytes and catalyzes the halogenation reaction of H_2O_2 with Cl^-, which results in the formation of hypochlorous acid (HOCl) and Cl_2. These substances have oxidant activity and generate further oxidative products such as other chlorinating agents, RNOS, and tyrosyl radicals and their cytotoxic reactions.

The myeloperoxidase-H_2O_2-chloride system of phagocytes

- catalytically consumes endothelium-derived NO, thereby reducing NO bioavailability and its vasodilatory and anti-inflammatory functions;
- stimulates neutrophil adherence to endothelial cells, thereby inducing the production of further ROS by neutrophils, interleukin-8 formation by monocytes, and an increase in platelet aggregation;
- activates matrix metalloproteinases and other protease cascades, which leads to destabilization and rupture of the atherosclerotic plaque surface; and
- promotes the formation of advanced glycosylated end products (AGEs), which participate in vascular disease.[14]

Clinical Correlates. The myeloperoxidase-H_2O_2-chloride system is an important in vivo oxidant that is intimately implicated in the atherosclerotic process.

Enzymatically active myeloperoxidase and hypochlorite-modified lipoproteins are present in human atherosclerotic lesions, where they colocalize with macrophages and endothelial cells.[15] Myeloperoxidase is elevated in persons with angiographically documented cardiovascular disease and has also recently been shown to serve as an independent predictor of atherosclerotic risk in subjects undergoing coronary angiography.[16] In emergency department patients with chest pain, the initial measurement of plasma myeloperoxidase independently predicts the early risk for myocardial infarction, as well as the risk for major adverse cardiac events in the ensuing 30-day and 6-month periods in the absence of myocardial necrosis.[17] In patients with acute coronary syndromes, myeloperoxidase serum levels predict an increased risk for subsequent cardiovascular events, thus complementing traditional biochemical markers.[18] Autopsy studies of subjects after sudden death reveal intense immunostaining for myeloperoxidase within fissured or ruptured culprit lesions.[17]

Stimulants for Oxidative Stress. Aside from the generation of ROS with oxidative phosphorylation and inflammation, **oxidant stress is also induced by neurohormonal activation, cardiovascular risk factors, and physical stimuli.**

Angiotensin II. Angiotensin II is one of the most potent endogenous stimuli for the generation of superoxide. Activation of the angiotensin II type 1 receptor (AT_1) serves as an oxidant stimulus via induction of NADH/NADPH oxidase.[19]

In the vascular endothelium as well as in vascular smooth muscle cells, activation of the AT_1 receptor stimulates intermediates such as protein kinase C (PKC), phospholipase D, and Src. As a result, p47*phox* is phosphorylated and, with the other NADH/NADPH subunits, translocates to the plasmalemma where it associates with flavocytochrome b_{558} and forms the active NADH/NADPH oxidase. Activated NADH/NADPH oxidase causes the increased production of oxygen radicals.[3,11]

Angiotensin II also activates transcription factors such as nuclear factor kappaB (NFκB), which in turn mediate the induction of proinflammatory genes. Angiotensin II stimulates stress-activated signaling pathways through p38 MAPK, c-Jun NH_2-terminal kinase (JNK), stress-activated protein kinase (SAPK), and AGEs.[3,11]

Aldosterone. Aldosterone, another product of the renin-angiotensin-aldosterone system (RAAS), likewise induces oxidative stress at vascular and nonvascular sites.

Chronic exposure of rats to aldosterone causes sustained activity of NADH/NADPH oxidase, with 3-nitrotyrosine generation by endothelial cells and inflammatory cells leading to a proinflammatory and fibrogenic vascular injury response.[20]

Hyperlipidemia. Hyperlipidemia increases oxidant stress. It is associated with higher AT_1 receptor density and increased angiotensin II–derived superoxide production via NADH/NADPH oxidase.

Lipoproteins undergo oxidant modifications. The myeloperoxidase-H_2O_2-chloride system of activated phagocytes initiates lipid peroxidation in vivo. The system is implicated in the conversion and oxidation of low-density lipoprotein (LDL) to an oxidized, high-uptake form that is cytotoxic and thrombogenic. Oxidized LDL is avidly taken up by macrophages. It participates in foam cell formation and the development of lipid-laden, soft atheromata.[15]

Free Fatty Acids. Elevated levels of free fatty acids cause oxidative stress as a result of increased metabolic ROS production induced by increased mitochondrial uncoupling and beta oxidation.[1]

Hyperglycemia. Elevated glucose causes oxidative stress as a result of increased production of mitochondrial superoxide, nonenzymatic glycation of proteins, and glucose auto-oxidation.[1]

Vascular Stretch. Vascular stretch is a potent, physical stimulus for the production of ROS by the endothelium and vascular smooth muscle cells.[21,22]

CELLULAR STRESS-SENSITIVE PATHWAYS

In addition to directly oxidizing macromolecules and interfering with their function, oxidants such as superoxide, hydrogen peroxide, and other ROS activate intracellular, proinflammatory pathways that culminate in cellular hypertrophy, proliferation, and apoptosis.[14]

Stress-sensitive systems include

- NFκB,
- JNK/SAPK,
- p38 MAPK,
- JAK/signal transducer and activator of transcription (STAT),
- hexosamine, and
- signaling cascades.[14]

Nuclear Factor KappaB. The inflammatory response to oxidants is effectively launched with the release of NFκB.

A major target activated by oxidative stress is the transcription factor NFκB. NFκB translocates from the cytosol into the nucleus to initiate the transcription of genes essential for the generation of proinflammatory mediators, such as

- cytokines,
- chemokines,
- adhesion molecules,
- interferons,
- growth factors,
- iNOS,
- cyclooxygenase-2, and
- acute phase proteins

that will initiate, augment, and sustain the inflammatory process.[23]

Stress-Activated Protein Kinases. Cellular stressors such as ROS and inflammatory cytokines trigger signal transduction cascades that induce changes in cellular function.

Cells respond to diverse forms of cellular stress by activating SAPKs, which are key elements for signal transduction from the cell surface to the nucleus. SAPKs have central roles in cellular proliferation, differentiation, growth arrest, and apoptosis.[1]

SAPK pathways can be initiated by

- activation of the small GTP-binding protein Ras. Activated Ras recruits the kinase Raf-1 to the plasma membrane, which leads to Raf-1 phosphorylation and ultimately to phosphorylation and activation of SAPKs;
- stimulation of G protein–coupled receptors, independent of Ras. The resulting PKC-dependent phosphorylation of Raf-1 stimulates the SAPKs.[1,24]

SAPK pathways within cells are

- JNK/SAPK,
- p38 MAPK, and
- JAK/STAT.[25]

NH_2-Terminal Jun Kinase/Stress-Activated Protein Kinase. Activated JNK/SAPKs phosphorylate the transcription factor c-Jun, which together with other members of the c-Fos and c-Jun families is one component of the activator protein-1 (AP-1) transcription factor complex. As a result, with oxidant stress there is enhanced expression of genes with AP-1 recognition sites, including the gene for c-Jun, thus creating a positive feedback loop. A major role of the JNK/SAPK pathway is the mediation of apoptosis.[1]

p38 Mitogen-Activated Protein Kinase. p38 MAPK is a serine/threonine protein kinase. When activated, p38 MAPK phosphorylates downstream elements, which leads to the modulation of gene transcription. It influences inflammation, immunity, cell growth, and apoptosis.

p38 MAPK also has an effect on cytoskeletal arrangements. Activation of the p38 MAPK pathway leads to tyrosine 14 phosphorylation of caveolin-1. Caveolin-1, a 21- to 24-kDa integral membrane protein, functions as one of the scaffolding proteins to concentrate and organize cholesterol, sphingolipids, and signaling molecules within the plasma membrane of cell surface caveolae.[25]

Janus Kinases and Signal Transducers and Activators of Transcription. JAKs are associated with cytokine receptors. Many cytokines elicit biologic effects through the stimulation of JAK. JAKs, in turn, tyrosine-phosphorylate and thus activate a specific family of transcription factors known as signal transducers and activators of transcription, the STATs. STATs reside latently in the cytoplasm. In response to tyrosine phosphorylation and activation, STATs form dimers and translocate to the nucleus where they bind to specific DNA targets and induce the transcription of responsive genes. Some members of the STAT family play a role in cellular proliferation. Abnormal STAT regulation may be involved in oncogenic transformation.[26]

ENDOTHELIAL DYSFUNCTION WITH OXIDATIVE STRESS

Oxidative stress is a central cause of endothelial dysfunction in atherosclerosis.[27] **Exposure of the endothelium to oxidative stress impairs endothelial NO bioavailability and causes endothelial dysfunction** (see Fig. 2-1). **Mechanisms are multifactorial and may differ for diverse situations.**[28]

eNOS Expression and Activity. ROS may affect eNOS expression, oxidant-sensitive eNOS cofactors, and its catalytic action.

eNOS Expression. eNOS mRNA stability and eNOS expression may be decreased by oxidized/modified LDL, which plays a key role in the development of atherosclerosis.[8]

eNOS Activity. Oxidative consumption of essential eNOS cofactors, such as BH_4, impairs NO production at the expense of further ROS generation.[12] Oxidized LDL also leads to the reduced formation of NO as a result of the limited availability of L-arginine.[8]

Asymmetric Dimethylarginine. ROS increase plasma levels of asymmetric dimethylarginine (ADMA). ADMA is an endogenous, competitive inhibitor of NOS. Increased levels of ADMA are thus associated with endothelial dysfunction (see Fig. 2-3).

The activity of dimethylarginine dimethylaminohydrolase (DDAH), an enzyme involved in ADMA catabolism, appears to be critical for control of ADMA levels. DDAH is sensitive to oxidative stress. Oxidation or nitrosylation of a sulfhydryl moiety in the DDAH catalytic site, which is required for enzymatic activity, impairs enzyme functionality. By lowering DDAH activity, oxidative stress increases ADMA accumulation, thereby contributing to endothelial cell dysfunction.[12,29]

Caveolae. ROS are potent disrupters of caveolae, the 50- to 100-nm invaginations of the plasma membrane that modulate signal transduction processes. Preservation of the structural integrity of caveolae is essential for normal eNOS function, as is proper interaction of eNOS with caveolin, a caveolar scaffolding protein.

eNOS-caveolin interactions may be perturbed via several oxidative mechanisms:

- Oxidation of plasmalemmal cholesterol may alter caveolar structure and cause caveolin to shuttle back to the Golgi membranes.
- eNOS-caveolin protein-protein interactions may be disturbed by the oxidation of critical amino acids.
- ROS activation of signal transduction events may alter eNOS phosphorylation and subcellular localization.[14,30]
- Endothelial cells exposed to oxidized LDL lose caveola-associated cholesterol with subsequent translocation of both eNOS and caveolin-1 from the plasma membrane to internal membranes.[15]

Thus, inhibition of endothelial NO formation by hypochlorite-oxidized LDL is associated with a reduction of eNOS in the plasma membrane, a striking intracellular redistribution of eNOS, and disintegration of the perinuclear Golgi localization.[15]

Nitric Oxide Bioavailability and Signaling. Oxidative stress suppresses NO bioavailability by reducing the half-life of NO.

Oxidative consumption of NO, as through the interaction with superoxide, produces the potent nitrating oxidant peroxynitrite (see Fig. 2-3). Peroxynitrite anion induces lipid peroxidation and nitrosation of tyrosine moieties, thereby disrupting caveolae, cell membranes, cell signaling, and cell survival.[31]

Both superoxide and peroxynitrite also potently inhibit soluble guanylate cyclase and as a result interfere with the eNOS–NO–guanosine 3′,5′-cyclic monophosphate (cGMP) signaling pathway.[8]

OXIDATIVE STRESS AND VASCULAR DISEASE

Oxidative stress is implicated in early vascular disease. It underlies all phases of the atherosclerotic process (see Fig. 2-1). **Enhanced oxidative stress occurs within the arterial wall of atherosclerotic vessels, and multiple distinct oxidation products are enriched within human atherosclerotic plaque.**[16] **Animal models of atherosclerosis have documented that all the constituents of atheromatous plaque produce and use ROS.**[32]

A deficiency in endogenous antioxidants may be associated with the increased oxidative stress of vascular disease. In a prospective cohort of patients with angiographically documented coronary heart disease (CHD), erythrocyte intracellular glutathione peroxidase 1 activity was inversely associated with future fatal and nonfatal cardiovascular events. The relationship between glutathione peroxidase 1 and future cardiovascular events was independent of other risk factors and clinical features.[5]

Atheromatous lesion formation is associated with

- inactivation of NO with resultant endothelial dysfunction,
- induction of inflammatory genes,
- accumulation of lipid peroxidation products, and
- increased growth of smooth muscle cells.[32]

Oxidants enhance platelet-derived growth factor (PDGF)-induced smooth muscle proliferation and increase the expression of several gene products associated with atherogenesis, including

- vascular cell adhesion molecule-1 (VCAM-1),
- monocyte chemotactic protein-1 (MCP-1),
- monocyte colony-stimulating factor (M-CSF), and
- matrix metalloproteinase-9 (MMP-9).[32,33]

OXIDATIVE STRESS, INSULIN RESISTANCE, AND TYPE 2 DIABETES MELLITUS

Obesity and insulin resistance are linked to a rise in oxidative stress. In populations at risk for the development of type 2 DM, elevated oxidative stress precedes the subsequent development of insulin resistance (Fig. 2-4).[34] **Ultimately, oxidative stress, worsened by the effects of hyperglycemia and elevations in free fatty acid levels, leads not only to insulin resistance but also to impaired insulin secretion and the development of type 2 DM.**[1]

Mechanism of Oxidant Impairment of Insulin Signaling. **Oxidative stress interferes with metabolic insulin signaling.**

Oxidative stress causes insulin resistance in a multiplicity of tissues, such as

- the vasculature,
- skeletal and cardiac muscle,
- fibroblasts, and
- adipose tissue.

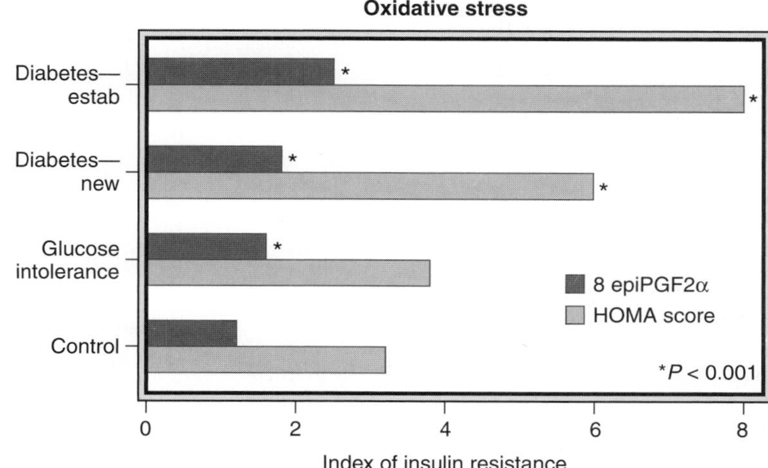

Figure 2–4. In Mauritian Indians, a population at risk for the development of type 2 diabetes mellitus, elevated oxidative stress, as measured by plasma F2 isoprostane 8-epiPGF2α, precedes the subsequent development of insulin resistance, as measured by the Homeostasis Model Assessment (HOMA) score. *(Modified from Gopaul NK, Manraj MD, Hebe A, et al. Oxidative stress could precede endothelial dysfunction and insulin resistance in Indian Mauritians with impaired glucose metabolism. Diabetologia 2001;44:706-712.)*

Serine/Threonine Phosphorylation. Oxidant stress interferes with insulin signaling and the stimulation of glucose transport by inhibiting the enzymatic function of the insulin receptor and its insulin receptor substrate (IRS).[1,35]

Stress-sensitive kinase activity induced by oxidative stress, such as via NFκB activating kinases, p38 MAPK, JNK/SAPK, and PκC isoforms, activates multiple serine/threonine kinase cascades. These cascades phosphorylate discrete serine or threonine sites of enzymes pertaining to the insulin signaling pathway. Serine/threonine phosphorylation of the insulin receptor and IRS proteins inhibits the tyrosine phosphorylation of these proteins induced by insulin receptor binding. In the absence of the requisite tyrosine phosphorylation, insulin signaling fails to occur (Fig. 2-5).

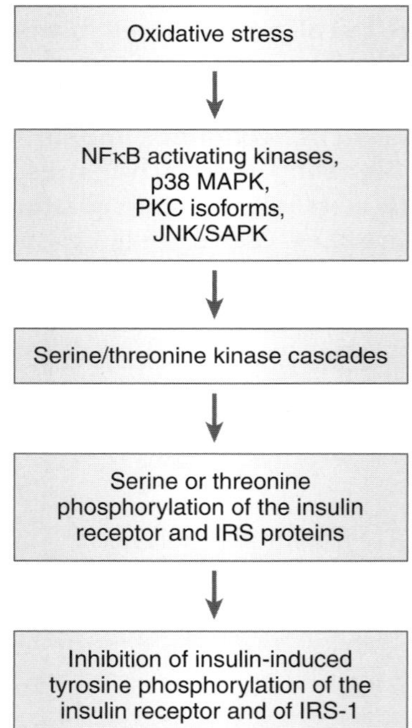

▸▸ **Figure 2–5.**
Oxidative stress and stress-sensitive kinase activity activate serine/threonine kinase cascades. Serine/threonine phosphorylation of the insulin receptor and the insulin receptor substrate (IRS) protein inhibits their insulin-induced tyrosine phosphorylation, which is a requisite for insulin signaling to occur. JNK, NH_2-terminal Jun kinase; MAPK, mitogen-activated protein kinase; NF, nuclear factor; PKC, protein kinase C; SAPK, stress-activated protein kinase.

Increased Oxidative Stress Pathways with Insulin Resistance. Oxidative stress not only interferes with insulin signaling and causes insulin resistance. **In a vicious circle, insulin resistance increases levels of free radicals and ROS, which will in turn cause further impairment of metabolic and vascular insulin signaling** (see Fig. 2-1).

Insulin resistance and the metabolic syndrome engender dyslipidemia, elevated circulating levels of free fatty acids, and prediabetic hyperglycemia, all of which further increase ambient oxidative stress by stimulating the production of ROS and RNOS.[36]

The higher concentration of pro-oxidants in insulin resistance is caused by increased oxidase activity, endothelial dysfunction, and decreased antioxidant capacity. Specifically, there is

- increased NADH/NADPH oxidase activity,
- a deficiency in antioxidant defense with decreased tissue levels of glutathione,
- an uncoupling of eNOS with deficient vascular NO production and increased vascular superoxide elaboration,
- increased lipid peroxidation, protein carbonylation, and orthotyrosine and metatyrosine formation.[36]

Hexosamine Pathway. In the setting of insulin resistance, the hexosamine biosynthetic pathway, stimulated by increased levels of ROS and excessive flux of glucose or free fatty acids into cells, further impairs sensitivity to insulin signaling.

Activation of the hexosamine pathway shifts glucose metabolism toward increased glucosamine production, which contributes to endothelial dysfunction. The hexosamine pathway also effects *O*-linked glycosylation modification of serine/threonine residues of insulin signaling proteins, which has a negative impact on the insulin receptor response.[1,37]

Advanced Glycosylated End Products. Oxidative stress increases the formation of AGEs. In turn, AGEs, which are associated with prediabetic hyperglycemia, may also augment oxidative stress.[1]

Oxidant stress is increased

- during the formation of AGEs by the generation of hydrogen peroxide and
- as a result of the interaction of AGEs with receptors for advanced glycosylation end products (RAGEs).

AGEs are a heterogeneous group of proteins, lipids, and nucleic acids that are nonenzymatically glycosylated.[1] AGEs are initially formed via glucose addition reactions with proteins, followed by further reactions, rearrangements, dehydrations, and cleavages that eventually generate brown, insoluble cross-linked complexes termed AGEs. AGE formation releases hydrogen peroxide through

- the 1,2-enolization pathway, whereby 3-deoxyglucosone forms hydrogen peroxide and glucosone; and
- the 2,3-enolization pathway, whereby 1-deoxyglucosone and 1,4-deoxyglucosone ultimately release hydrogen peroxide and carboxymethyllysine.[33]

As AGEs interact with their specific cell surface receptors, the RAGEs, postreceptor signaling generates intracellular oxygen free radicals and thus induces oxidative stress. NFκB signal transduction is initiated, thereby creating a chronically active, inflammatory state. The presence of AGEs further up-regulates RAGEs.[33]

Some AGE pathway intermediates are highly reactive. They are potent cross-linkers and polymerize proteins to AGEs. **Highly cross-linked proteins, such as collagen, increase vascular rigidity and decrease compliance of the arterial vessel wall. This process ultimately leads to systolic hypertension, left ventricular hypertrophy, and diastolic dysfunction.**[33]

There are also advanced fructosylation end products (AFEs). They follow a similar pattern in the production of ROS and bind with even greater affinity to proteins than AGEs do.[33]

Pancreatic Islet Beta Cell Insufficiency. Redox-sensitive cellular signaling also plays a role in injury to pancreatic islet beta cells. Oxidant stress is implicated in the remodeling and development of islet amyloid, a process that engenders space-occupying lesions and defective beta cell insulin secretion. It is an early event in the evolution of type 2 DM.[1]

TESTS FOR OXIDATIVE STRESS

Assays for oxidative stress have not been standardized. A number of indirect indicators of oxidative stress, such as oxidative modification of macromolecules or the antioxidant response, have been used in research and clinical studies.

Oxidatively Damaged DNA. The plasma or urine concentration of 8-hydroxy-2′-deoxyguanosine, an adduct of oxidatively damaged DNA, is one of the most commonly used markers for evaluating oxidative DNA damage and is used as an index of oxidative stress.[38]

Oxidatively Damaged Proteins. Plasma levels of protein-bound chlorotyrosine, nitrotyrosine, dityrosine, and orthotyrosine are systemic markers specific for protein oxidative modification caused by oxidant pathways that are up-regulated in atheromatous disease. These markers can be determined by mass spectrometry.[16]

Oxidized Lipoproteins. In vivo oxidation of LDL can be assessed by autoantibodies to model epitopes of oxidized LDL, including malondialdehyde-modified LDL and copper-oxidized LDL. Malondialdehyde-modified LDL is a stable, terminal metabolite of oxidized lipids, an index of oxidative stress. Elevated plasma levels of LDL particles containing oxidation-specific epitopes and immunoglobulin G (IgG) autoantibody titers to epitopes of oxidized LDL have been directly correlated with the severity of CHD, but the predictive value of these indices is unclear.[39]

Antioxidant Response. Plasma thioredoxin is also a marker of oxidative stress. Thioredoxin is induced by oxidative stress and is secreted by cells. It is a small protein with a redox-active dithiol/disulfide at its active site, critical for the redox regulation of protein function. Cytosolic thioredoxin has numerous functions, including protection against oxidative stress, control of cell growth, and modulation of apoptosis. Plasma/serum levels of thioredoxin are elevated in oxidative stress–associated disorders.[40]

Isoprostanes. Promising biomarkers for oxidative stress are plasma F2 isoprostanes such as total plasma 8-epiPGF2α.[39]

CONCLUSION

Oxidative mechanisms play an essential role not only in oxidative metabolism but also in defeating injury or infection. During host defense, a pro-oxidant milieu is readily generated given the simplicity of its derivation, and the damage to pathogens effected by oxidative stress can be considerable. In fact, with ineffective generation of oxidative stress, an organism is prone to chronic infections.

As with most mechanisms in physiology, an excessive and protracted measure of oxidative stress will cease to be beneficial and turn harmful. This situation is further aggravated as oxidative stress begets more oxidative stress in a vicious circle. Chronic oxidative stress can in fact be devastating when that damage is wrought as "friendly fire" against the host's own tissues.

The vasculature is one of the lines of engagement for host defense. It stands to reason that increased oxidative stress in the vasculature would adversely affect blood vessels as innocent bystanders.

Oxidative stress has a negative effect on endothelial function with loss of the vasodilatory and anti-inflammatory endothelium-dependent NO-cGMP signaling pathway. All common risk factors for vascular disease are attended by the increased production of free oxygen radicals. Oxidants are implicated in the pathogenesis, development, progression, and final destabilization of vascular lesions in atherosclerosis.

ROS play a pivotal role in the genesis of insulin resistance as well. Oxidative stress pathways directly interfere with molecular aspects of the metabolic and vascular insulin signaling pathways. The compromise in insulin's vasoactive effects in the vasculature is expected to aggravate the metabolic impairment by impairing microvascular glucose and insulin delivery to the skeletal musculature. Oxidative stress is implicated not only in insulin resistance mechanisms but also in the evolving metabolic syndrome, the development of type 2 DM, and the late vascular and neurologic complications of DM.

Oxidative stress underlies not only vascular and metabolic disease but a whole host of other inflammatory conditions, malignancies, and the aging process as well. Antioxidant venues to redress a pro-oxidant milieu have been keenly pursued. However, the majority of antioxidant trials have been disappointing. A number of difficulties are apparent from such studies. For any particular pathophysiology, the major pro-oxidant pathway needs to be identified. The antioxidant intervention must suit the chemical kinetics of the oxidant stress. Appropriate measures of oxidant stress need to be assessed at baseline and in follow-up to ascertain efficacy of the intervention. Only with evidence of effective antioxidant impact can inferences be drawn on the efficacy of a particular antioxidant approach on cardiovascular and metabolic end points.

At present, a number of promising antioxidant lifestyle and pharmacologic approaches are apparent that may enhance endogenous antioxidants or lessen the impact of exogenous stressors:

- Cessation of cigarette smoking, mild to moderate exercise, and the consumption of dietary flavonoid antioxidants are of benefit.
- Antagonism of the RAAS counteracts angiotensin II– and aldosterone-mediated oxidative stress.
- Statins interfere with the mechanism for isoprenylation of the small GTPases needed for up-regulating NADH/NADPH superoxide output.
- In general, metabolic control of the lipid profile, with a reduction in free fatty acid levels and avoidance of hyperglycemia, will further mitigate the pro-oxidant milieu.

GLOSSARY

ADMA	asymmetric dimethylarginine
AFE	advanced fructosylation end product
AGE	advanced glycosylation end product
AP-1	activator protein-1
AT_1	angiotensin II type 1
ATP	adenosine triphosphate
BH_4	tetrahydrobiopterin
cGMP	guanosine 3′,5′-cyclic monophosphate
CHD	coronary heart disease

COX	cyclooxygenase
DDAH	dimethylarginine dimethylaminohydrolase
DM	diabetes mellitus
eNOS	endothelial nitric oxide synthase
GTP	guanosine 5′-triphosphate
H_2O_2	hydrogen peroxide
Ig	immunoglobulin
IKK	IκB kinase
iNOS	inducible nitric oxide synthase
IRS	insulin receptor substrate
JAK	Janus kinase
JNK	c-Jun NH2-terminal kinase
LDL	low-density lipoprotein
MAPK	mitogen-activated protein kinase
MCP-1	monocyte chemotactic protein-1
M-CSF	monocyte colony-stimulating factor
MMP-9	matrix metalloproteinase-9
NADH/NADPH	nicotinamide adenine dinucleotide phosphate oxidase
NFκB	nuclear factor kappaB
NO	nitric oxide
NOS	nitric oxide synthase
$O_2^{\cdot -}$	superoxide
$OH^{\cdot}$	hydroxyl radical
$ONOO^-$	peroxynitrite
PDGF	platelet-derived growth factor
phox	phagocyte oxidase
PKC	protein kinase C
RAAS	renin-angiotensin-aldosterone system
RAGE	receptor for advanced glycosylation end products
RNOS	reactive nitrogen oxide species
ROS	reactive oxygen species
SAPK	stress-activated protein kinase
STAT	signal transducer and activator of transcription
VCAM-1	vascular cell adhesion molecule-1

REFERENCES

1. Evans JL, Goldfine ID, Maddux BA, Grodsky GM. Oxidative stress and stress-activated signaling pathways: a unifying hypothesis of type 2 diabetes. Endocr Rev 2002;23: 599-622
2. Irshad M, Chaudhuri PS. Oxidant-antioxidant system: role and significance in human body. Indian J Exp Biol 2002;40:1233-1239
3. Harrison D, Griendling KK, Landmesser U, et al. Role of oxidative stress in atherosclerosis. Am J Cardiol 2003;91(suppl):7A-11A
4. Nakamura S-I, Sugiyama S, Fujioka D, et al. Polymorphism in glutamate-cysteine ligase modifier subunit gene is associated with impairment of nitric oxide–mediated coronary vasomotor function. Circulation 2003;108: 1425-1427
5. Blankenberg S, Rupprecht HJ, Bickel C, et al. Glutathione peroxidase 1 activity and cardiovascular events in patients with coronary artery disease. N Engl J Med 2003;349: 1605-1613
6. Cai H, Harrison DG. Endothelial dysfunction in cardiovascular disease: the role of oxidant stress. Circ Res 2000;87:840-844
7. McCord JM. Oxygen-derived radicals: a link between reperfusion injury and inflammation. Fed Proc 1987; 46:2402-2406
8. Munzel T, Feil R, Mulsch A, et al. Physiology and pathophysiology of vascular signaling controlled by cyclic guanosine 3′,5′-cyclic monophosphate–dependent protein kinase. Circulation 2003;108:2172-2183
9. Kim C, Dinauer MC. Rac2 is an essential regulator of neutrophil nicotinamide adenine dinucleotide phosphate oxidase activation in response to specific signaling pathways. J Immunol 2001;166:1223-1232
10. Maack C, Kartes T, Kilter H, et al. Oxygen free radical release in human failing myocardium is associated with increased activity of Rac1-GTPase and represents a target for statin treatment. Circulation 2003;108:1567-1574
11. Schiffrin EL, Touyz RM. Multiple actions of angiotensin II in hypertension: benefit of AT1 receptor blockade. J Am Coll Cardiol 2003;42:911-913
12. Cooke JP. Does ADMA cause endothelial dysfunction? Arterioscler Thromb Vasc Biol 2000;20:2032-2037
13. Marette A. Mediators of cytokine-induced insulin resistance in obesity and other inflammatory settings. Curr Opin Clin Nutr Metab Care 2000;5:377-383
14. Jaimes EA, Sweeney C, Raij L. Effects of the reactive oxygen species hydrogen peroxide and hypochlorite on endothelial nitric oxide production. Hypertension 2001;38:877-883
15. Nuszkowski A, Grabner R, Marsche G, et al. Hypochlorite-modified low density lipoprotein inhibits nitric oxide synthesis in endothelial cells via an intracellular dislocalization of endothelial nitric-oxide synthase. J Biol Chem 2001;276:14212-14221
16. Shishehbor MH, Brennan M-L, Aviles RJ, et al. Statins promote potent systemic antioxidant effects through specific inflammatory pathways. Circulation 2003;108:426-431
17. Brennan M-L, Penn MS, Van Lente F, et al. Prognostic value of myeloperoxidase in patients with chest pain. N Engl J Med 2003;349:1595-1604
18. Baldus S, Heeschen C, Meinertz T, et al. Myeloperoxidase serum levels predict risk in patients with acute coronary syndromes. Circulation 2003;108:1440-1445
19. Diep QN, Amiri F, Touyz RM, et al. PPARalpha activator effects on Ang II–induced vascular oxidative stress and inflammation. Hypertension 2002;40:866-871

20. Sun Y, Zhang J, Lu L, et al. Aldosterone-induced inflammation in the rat heart: role of oxidative stress. Am J Pathol 2002;161:1773-1781
21. Hishikawa K, Luscher TF. Pulsatile stretch stimulates superoxide production in human aortic endothelial cells. Circulation 1997;96:3610-3616
22. Hishikawa K, Oemar BS, Yang Z, et al. Pulsatile stretch stimulates superoxide production and activates nuclear factor-kappa B in human coronary smooth muscle. Circ Res 1997;81:797-803
23. Tham DM, Martin-McNulty B, Wang Y-X, et al. Angiotensin II is associated with activation of NF kappaB–mediated genes and downregulation of PPARs. Physiol Genomics 2002;11:21-30
24. Bernier SG, Haldar S, Michel T. Bradykinin-regulated interactions of the mitogen-activated protein kinase pathway with the endothelial nitric-oxide synthase. J Biol Chem 2000;275:30707-30715
25. Volonte D, Galbiati F, Pestell RG, Lisanti MP. Cellular stress induces the tyrosine phosphorylation of caveolin-1 (Tyr(14)) via activation of p38 mitogen-activated protein kinase and c-Src kinase. Evidence for caveolae, the actin cytoskeleton, and focal adhesions as mechanical sensors of osmotic stress. J Biol Chem 2001;276:8094-8100
26. Faruqi TR, Gomez D, Bustelo XR, et al. Rac1 mediates STAT3 activation by autocrine IL-6. Proc Natl Acad Sci U S A 2001;98:9014-9019
27. Keany JF Jr. Atherosclerosis, oxidative stress, and endothelial function. In Keany JF Jr (ed): Oxidative Stress and Vascular Disease. Boston, Kluwer Academic, 2000, pp 155-181
28. Schindler TH, Nitzsche EU, Munzel T, et al. Coronary vasoregulation in patients with various risk factors in response to cold pressor testing. J Am Coll Cardiol 2003;42:814-822
29. Stühlinger MC, Oka RK, Graf EE, et al. Endothelial dysfunction induced by hyperhomocyst(e)inemia. Role of asymmetric dimethylarginine. Circulation 2003;108: 933-938
30. Peterson TE, Poppa V, Ueba H, et al. Opposing effects of reactive oxygen species and cholesterol on endothelial nitric oxide synthase and endothelial cell caveolae. Circ Res 1999;85:29-37
31. Drexler H. Endothelial dysfunction: clinical implications. Prog Cardiovasc Dis 1997;4:287-324
32. Griendling KK, FitzGerald GA. Oxidative stress and cardiovascular injury. Part II: Animal and human studies. Circulation 2003;108:2034-2040
33. Uemura S, Matsushita H, Li W, et al. Diabetes mellitus enhances vascular matrix metalloproteinase activity: role of oxidative stress. Circ Res 2001;88: 1291-1298
34. Gopaul NK, Manraj MD, Hebe A, et al. Oxidative stress could precede endothelial dysfunction and insulin resistance in Indian Mauritians with impaired glucose metabolism. Diabetologia 2001;44:706-712
35. Rakugi H, Kamide K, Ogihara T. Vascular signaling pathways in the metabolic syndrome. Curr Hypertens Rep 2002;4;105-111
36. Kesavulu MM, Rao BK, Giri R, et al. Lipid peroxidation and antioxidant enzyme status in type 2 diabetics with coronary heart disease. Diabetes Res Clin Pract 2001;53:33-39
37. Federici M, Menghini R, Mauriello A, et al. Insulin-dependent activation of endothelial nitric oxide synthase is impaired by O-linked glycosylation modification of signaling proteins in human coronary endothelial cells. Circulation 2002;106:466-472
38. Goto C, Higashi Y, Kimura M, et al. Effect of different intensities of exercise on endothelium-dependent vasodilation in humans: role of endothelium-dependent nitric oxide and oxidative stress. Circulation 2003;108: 530-535
39. Engler MM, Engler MB, Malloy MJ, et al. Antioxidant vitamins C and E improve endothelial function in children with hyperlipidemia. Endothelial Assessment of Risk from Lipids in Youth (EARLY) Trial. Circulation 2003;108:1059-1063
40. Hirai N, Kawano H, Yasue H, et al. Attenuation of nitrate tolerance and oxidative stress by an angiotensin II receptor blocker in patients with coronary spastic angina. Circulation 2003;108:1446-1450

Inflammation 3

Inflammation is essential in an organism's response to pathogens, irritants, or trauma. Inflammation creates a hostile environment to isolate or kill a pathogen. Innate, nonseletive immunity with the production of oxidant molecules, phagocytic leukocytes, activated complement, and proinflammatory cytokines is rapidly mobilized in response to pathogens or irritants. This action is followed by an adaptive immune response modulated by immunoregulatory cytokines with the activation of T lymphocytes and antibody formation.[1]

In addition to its pivotal role in host defense, inflammation plays a role in the pathogenesis, progression, and complications of atherosclerosis and diabetes mellitus (DM), as borne out by observations in biochemistry and vascular biology and in clinical and epidemiologic studies. **Cytokines appear to provide the underlying link between inflammation, endothelial dysfunction, and insulin resistance that ultimately leads to the generation of a dysregulated metabolism and atherosclerotic vascular disease.**[2]

SELECTED PARTICIPANTS IN THE INFLAMMATORY RESPONSE

The inflammatory process is initiated by nuclear factor kappaB (NFκB). NFκB is instrumental in the generation of a multiplicity of inflammatory cytokines, or humoral mediators that direct the inflammatory response of tissues. Small guanosine 5′-triphosphatases (GTPases) such as Rho and Rac transduce the initial intracellular steps of biochemical pathways activated by inflammatory mediators.

Nuclear Factor KappaB. NFκB is the collective name for inducible dimeric transcription factors of the Rel family of DNA-binding proteins. NFκB is widely expressed and found in essentially all cell types.

The inflammatory response is initiated with activation of NFκB transcription factors. These transcription factors exert a positive regulatory effect on the expression of genes for several cytokines and cell adhesion molecules. **NFκB activates a large number of genes in response to infection and inflammation. It mediates inflammatory and immune responses, as well as apoptosis.**[3]

Activators of Nuclear Factor KappaB. NFκB can be activated by a multiplicity of stimuli (Fig. 3-1) **encompassing oxidative stressors and proinflammatory mediators,** such as

- reactive oxygen species (ROS),
- reactive nitrogen oxide species (RNOS),
- tumor necrosis factor-alpha (TNF-α),
- interleukin-1beta (IL-1β),
- angiotensin II,
- advanced glycosylated end products (AGEs) binding to cell surface receptors for AGEs (RAGEs), and
- p38 mitogen-activated protein kinase (MAPK).[3]

NF kappaB activators

NF kappaB can be activated by a multiplicity of stimuli:

ROS, RNOS, TNF-α, IL-1β, Angiotensin II, AGEs binding to RAGEs, p38 MAPK

›› **Figure 3–1.**
Nuclear factor (NF) kappaB activators. AGEs, advanced glycosylation end products; IL, interleukin; MAPK, mitogen-activated protein kinase; RAGEs, receptors for AGEs; RNOS, reactive nitrogen oxide species; ROS, reactive oxygen species; TNF, tumor necrosis factor. *(Modified from Evans JL, Goldfine ID, Maddux BA, Grodsky GM. Oxidative stress and stress-activated signaling pathways: a unifying hypothesis of type 2 diabetes. Endocr Rev 2002;23:599-622.)*

Nuclear Factor KappaB Composition. NFκB is a dimeric transcription factor composed of

1. transactivator subunits: Rel A (p65) and c-rel, as well as
2. DNA-binding subunits: NFκB1 (p50) and NFκB2 (p52).

These subunits form various intracellular homodimers and heterodimers.[3]

Nuclear Factor KappaB Stimulation. In the resting cell, NFκB subunits are retained in the cytoplasm, complexed with an inhibitory protein IκB, which masks the nuclear localization signal of NFκB.[3]

Stimulation of NFκB entails the activation of a serine kinase cascade of upstream activating kinases such as protein kinase (PKC) isoforms and MAPK kinase kinases (MAPKKK). These kinases phosphorylate IκB via IκB kinase-beta (IKK-β). Phosphorylation of IκB induces ubiquitination of it by the proteolytic ubiquitin-proteasome pathway, which leads to proteolytic proteasome–mediated degradation of IκB. IκB degradation disinhibits and thus activates

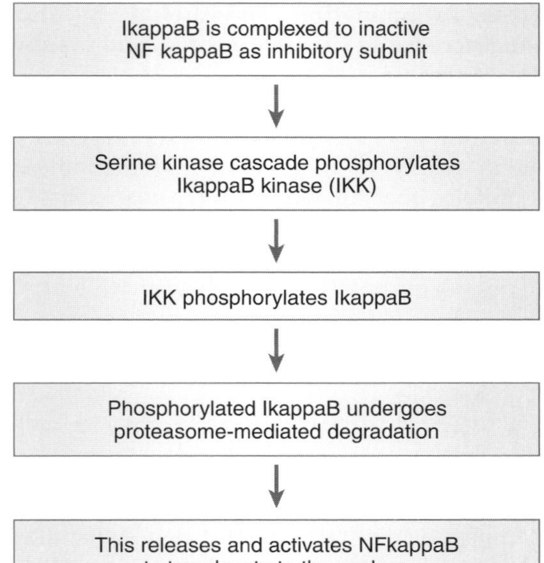

Figure 3–2.
Nuclear factor (NF) kappaB activation. *(Modified from Evans JL, Goldfine ID, Maddux BA, Grodsky GM. Oxidative stress and stress-activated signaling pathways: a unifying hypothesis of type 2 diabetes. Endocr Rev 2002;23: 599-622.)*

cytosolic NFκB, thereby allowing it to translocate to the nucleus (Fig. 3-2).[4] A Rho protein–dependent signal is also necessary to induce the nuclear transport of NFκB.[5]

In the nucleus, NFκB activates the transcription of target genes. The promoters of such genes contain binding sites for NFκB. On binding to such recognition elements in the promoter region of proinflammatory genes, **NFκB acts as their dominant regulator to induce or increase gene transcription of proinflammatory cytokines, chemokines, interferons, growth factors, and other inflammatory**[3,6] **mediators** such as

- cyclooxygenase-2 (COX-2),
- endothelial selectin (E-selectin),
- inducible nitric oxide synthase (iNOS),
- intercellular adhesion molecule-1 (ICAM-1),
- macrophage colony-stimulating factor (M-CSF),
- monocyte chemotactic protein-1 (MCP-1),
- proinflammatory cytokines (TNF-α, IL-1β, IL-6),
- RAGEs,
- vascular cell adhesion molecule-1 (VCAM-1), and
- vascular endothelial growth factor (VEGF) (Table 3-1).[7]

Table 3–1. Nuclear Factor KappaB–Mediated Gene Transcription of Proinflammatory Mediators

Cyclooxygenase-2 (COX-2)
Endothelial-selectin (E-selectin)
Inducible nitric oxide synthase (iNOS)
Intercellular adhesion molecule-1 (ICAM-1)
Macrophage colony-stimulating factor (M-CSF)
Monocyte chemotactic protein-1 (MCP-1)
Proinflammatory cytokines (tumor necrosis factor-α, interleukin-1β, interleukin-6)
Receptor for advanced glycosylation end products (RAGE)
Vascular cell adhesion molecule-1 (VCAM-1)
Vascular endothelial growth factor (VEGF)

The transcription factor NFκB mediates immune and inflammatory responses and apoptosis by translocating to the nucleus and regulating the expression of genes for the mediators presented. Modified from Evans JL, Goldfine ID, Maddux BA, Grodsky GM. Oxidative stress and stress-activated signaling pathways: a unifying hypothesis of type 2 diabetes. Endocr Rev 2002;23: 599-622.

Many of these gene products in turn activate NFκB in a positive feedback loop.[7]

Cytokines. Cytokines are relatively low-molecular-weight, soluble polypeptides. Inflammatory cytokines are elaborated by immune system cells and by adipocytes. There are more than 200 cytokines. Cytokines have a hierarchy, with certain cytokines modulating the elaboration and activity of others. Different families of cytokines and their receptors share a characteristic structure.[8]

Cytokines serve as humoral mediators to alter a cell's own function (autocrine) or the function of adjacent cells (paracrine). Individual cytokines have a multiplicity of biologic effects, and different cytokines may share the same activity, thus causing significant redundancy. **Cytokines modulate**

- **the inflammatory cascade,**
- **carbohydrate and fat metabolism,**
- **hematopoiesis, and**
- **immunoregulation.**[9,10]

They recruit and activate inflammatory cells to initiate the process of inflammation.[7]

Key cytokine mediators of inflammation are

- **TNF-α,**
- **IL-1,**
- **IL-6, and**
- **interferon.**

TNF-α and IL-1 are the cytokines principally responding to bacterial infection, IL-1 is the primary mediator of noninfectious inflammation, and interferon is primarily activated by viral infection.[11] IL-6 mediates B-cell maturation, complement activation, and further cytokine release.[1]

Acute Phase Response. During infection and inflammation, a wide range of alterations in metabolism occur, termed the acute phase response. It is the role of cytokines such as TNF-α, IL-1, and IL-6 to initiate these metabolic changes.

TNF-α may induce the release of IL-1. **These "messenger" cytokines, specifically IL-6, stimulate hepatocytes to produce large, systemic amounts of acute phase response proteins such as**

1. **C-reactive protein (CRP),**
2. **fibrinogen, and**
3. **serum amyloid A (SAA).**[1]

These acute phase reactants are termed "positive" because their levels dramatically increase with inflammation. The function of acute phase response proteins is to

1. protect against further injury,
2. minimize the extent of tissue damage,
3. facilitate repair by directly neutralizing foreign agents, and
4. participate in tissue regeneration.

Concurrent with the acute phase response, levels of "negative" acute phase proteins such as

1. albumin,
2. retinal binding protein, and
3. transferrin

decrease.[11]

Rho, Rac, and Other GTPase Molecules. The small GTPase proteins participate in the early steps of numerous intracellular inflammatory pathways. Rho and Rac GTPases are implicated in mediating oxidative stress, inflammation, endothelial dysfunction, increase in vasomotor tone, and insulin resistance.

Structure and Function. Small GTPases constitute a family of more than 100 monomeric G proteins that function as molecular switches in cellular signaling. Small GTPases are structurally classified into five subfamilies:

1. Ras,
2. Rho,
3. Rab,
4. Arf, and
5. Ran.

Ras and Rho family members play key roles in gene induction and cytoskeletal rearrangement. Members of the Rab, Arf, and Ran subfamilies function primarily in vesicular and nuclear/cytoplasmic trafficking and spindle microtubule assembly events.

Signaling pathways used by the small GTPases to elicit cellular transformation involve the activation of a variety of kinases, reactive oxygen intermediates, and transcription factors.[12]

Activation and Deactivation. Small GTPases cycle between an active, GTP-bound and an inactive, guanosine diphosphate (GDP)-bound state.

A number of molecular interactions modulate the nucleotide status of small GTPases, such as

1. specific guanine nucleotide exchange factors (GEFs), which stimulate the exchange of GTP for GDP, and
2. GTPase-activating proteins, which stimulate GTP hydrolysis.[12]

Rho GTPases. The Rho GTPases are members of the Ras superfamily of small GTP-binding proteins. There are three Rho GTPase subclasses based on homology to the three prototypic members:

1. RhoA,
2. Rac1, and
3. Cdc42Hs.

These prototypic members encompass seven distinct proteins, including

1. Rho (A, B, and C isoforms),
2. Rac (1, 2, and 3 isoforms),

3. Cdc42 (Cdc42Hs and G25K isoforms),
4. RhoD,
5. RhoG,
6. RhoE, and
7. TC10.[13,14]

Location and Activation of Rho GTPases. Caveolae are an obligatory site for RhoA to bind its targets and complete its signaling event.

Caveolar Location. The GDP-GTP exchange process for the Rho family members entails translocation of Rac1 and RhoA to the plasma membrane as a prerequisite for nucleotide exchange. Rac1 and RhoA have a polarized distribution at the cell surface. They are concentrated in caveolae, which are the plasma membrane domains associated with actin-rich regions of cells. Agonist stimulation induces the recruitment of additional Rac1, RhoA, or both to these caveolar fractions.[13,14]

Prenylation. Rho family proteins are targeted from the cytosol to caveolae through prenylation.

Prenylation is a mechanism for protein localization to caveolae. Thus proteins containing the carboxy-terminal consensus site for Rac1 and RhoA prenylation are constitutively targeted to caveolar fractions. Most Rho family members contain a single COOH-cysteine residue specifically appropriate for geranylgeranylation. For RhoA, geranylgeranylation by the isoprenoid geranylgeraniol is essential for its translocalization to the caveolar membranes and for its biologic functions. The association of RhoA with endothelial caveolar domains probably also occurs through physical interaction with caveolin-1.[13-15]

Role of Rho GTPases. Rho GTPases are intracellular signaling proteins that regulate cytoskeletal and inflammatory responses.

Cytoskeletal Organization. Rho GTPases were initially identified as regulators of cellular functions requiring cytoskeletal alterations via actin filament rearrangements, such as

- platelet aggregation,
- smooth muscle cell contraction, and
- cell migration.

Rac1 and RhoA regulate membrane ruffling and stress fiber formation.

Cell Response to Inflammatory Mediators. Rho family GTPase activity is essential for the inflammatory response to infection.

When cells are exposed to growth factors and cytokines, G proteins of the Rho family function as intermediary molecular switches. As such, **Rho GTPases transfer signals from stimulated receptors and their associated kinases to downstream effectors** in response to the exchange of GDP for GTP. Rho GTPases act as important intermediaries in the implementation of a diversity of proinflammatory responses through

- gene expression,
- gene transcription,
- cell growth,
- cell proliferation, and
- superoxide production

in response to cell surface stimulation.[16]

All these RhoA-regulated cellular functions are important in the pathogenesis of vascular disease because they eventuate in neointimal proliferation, vascular remodeling, and platelet aggregation.[13,14]

Rho GTPase Activators. Diverse inflammatory, vasoconstrictive, and growth factor stimuli activate Rho family GTPase recruitment.

Recruitment of Rac1 and RhoA to caveolae in response to stimulants occurs in concert with tyrosine phosphorylation of multiple substrates in caveolae and activation of a resident population of MAPKs—all critical molecular interactions required for cytoskeletal reorganization and signal transduction.[13,15]

Activators of Rho include

- α_1-adrenergic agonists,
- angiotensin II,
- endothelin-1,
- growth factors,
- iNOS
- leptin,
- thrombin,
- thromboxane A_2,
- TNF-α.[13,15,17-20]

α-Agonists and angiotensin II activate the Rho-Rho kinase pathway via the α_1-adrenoceptor-G_q and the angiotensin II type 1 (AT_1) receptors, respectively. RhoA activation by TNF-α occurs via the TNFR1 receptor subtype. The leptin signaling pathway, which depends on activation of trimeric G proteins and phosphoinositide 3-kinase, entails activation of Rho and Rac GTPases. Treatment with growth factors stimulates the recruitment of additional Rac1 and RhoA to caveolar fractions. iNOS interacts with Rac GTPases.[13,15,17,20-22]

RhoA GTPase Effect on Vascular Smooth Muscle. The RhoA-dependent signaling pathway controls vascular smooth muscle cell functions such as

- **contraction,**
- **migration, and**
- **proliferation.**

Many RhoA effects are mediated by its downstream effector RhoA kinase.

Normal Vascular Smooth Muscle Contraction. Classically, in vascular smooth muscle, the following events need to transpire for contraction to occur:

1. an increase in cytoplasmic calcium,
2. activation of the calcium-calmodulin–dependent enzyme myosin light chain kinase (MLCK),
3. MLCK phosphorylation of the 20-kDa myosin light chain,
4. myosin/actin filament interaction, and
5. initiation of smooth muscle contraction.

Vascular smooth muscle tone is dependent on the level of myosin light chain phosphorylation. The degree of myosin light chain phosphorylation is controlled by a balance between the competing activities of

1. calcium-calmodulin–dependent MLCK and
2. myosin phosphatase.

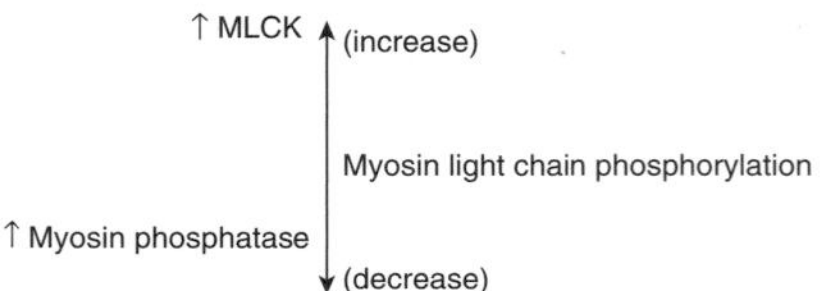

Vascular Smooth Muscle Calcium Sensitization and Desensitization. Although smooth muscle tone is expected to rise with incremental cytoplasmic calcium concentrations, the relationship between cytosolic calcium and myosin light chain phosphorylation can vary depending on

1. calcium sensitization—increased myosin light chain phosphorylation and higher tension occur at lower calcium levels; and
2. calcium desensitization—decreased myosin light chain phosphorylation and diminished tension occur despite higher calcium levels.

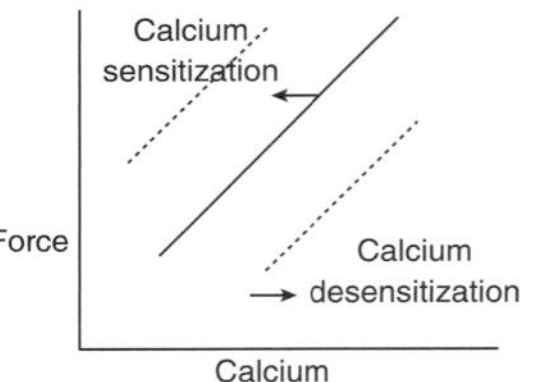

Vascular Smooth Muscle Contractile Agonists and Receptors. Vasoconstriction characterized by calcium sensitization occurs with many contractile agonists.

In vascular smooth muscle, the receptors for various contractile agonists are coupled to G_q/G_{11} or G_{12}/G_{13} proteins.

Many agonists, such as norepinephrine and thromboxane A_2, act via G_q protein–coupled receptors. They stimulate phospholipase C, which mobilizes an initial rise in cytoplasmic free calcium concentration with activation of MLCK and the initial development of tension. Calcium sensitization characterizes the subsequent, sustained contraction.

$G_{12/13}$ protein–coupled receptor agonists, such as endothelin-1 and thrombin, may stimulate smooth muscle contraction primarily and exclusively through calcium sensitization independent of an initial rise in cytoplasmic calcium.[23]

RhoA as a Smooth Muscle Calcium Sensitizer. Numerous contractile agonists induce activation of RhoA in vascular cells, and calcium sensitization mediated by RhoA and its target Rho kinase constitutes the major component of the sustained vasomotor tone induced by vasoconstrictors.[23,24]

RhoA serves as a molecular switch to enhance the calcium sensitivity of vascular smooth muscle contractile proteins in response to stimulation by vasoconstrictive, heterotrimeric G protein receptor agonists. Inhibition of myosin phosphatase by RhoA is a major contributor to myofibrillar calcium sensitization.[23]

In smooth muscles, the calcium-dependent and calcium-independent contractile effects of RhoA are mediated by activation of Rho-dependent kinase, or Rho kinase. Rho kinase phosphorylates the 110-kDa myosin-targeting subunit of smooth muscle myosin phosphatase at threonine (Thr) 695 (Thr696 in human isoform), thereby inhibiting the activity of the catalytic subunit of myosin phosphatase.

In addition, Rho kinase phosphorylates and activates a smooth muscle–specific inhibitor of myosin phosphatase, the phosphoprotein CPI-17, at Thr38, which may also participate in RhoA/Rho kinase–mediated myofibrillar calcium sensitization.[17,18]

Inhibition of myosin phosphatase increases the degree of myosin light chain phosphorylation and enhances smooth muscle contraction for any given level of cytoplasmic calcium consistent with calcium sensitization of the myofilaments.[17,18]

Rho GTPase Effect on Endothelial Function. Rho-induced Rho kinase impairs endothelial function by inactivating endothelial nitric oxide synthase (eNOS).

Specifically, Rho/Rho kinase suppresses eNOS activity as well as eNOS gene expression, thereby engendering both a rapid and a sustained decline in nitric oxide (NO) production.[25]

RhoA GTPase Effect on Insulin Resistance. Activation of RhoA with stimulation of Rho kinase, via growth factors, cytokines, and vasoconstrictors, inhibits insulin signaling.

Rho kinase is a serine/threonine protein kinase. Increased activation of Rho kinase causes serine phosphorylation of the insulin receptor substrate-1 (IRS-1). As a consequence, insulin-mediated IRS-1 tyrosine phosphorylation is impaired, as is association of the p85 subunit of phosphatidylinositol 3-kinase (PI3K) with IRS-1 and insulin signaling via the PI3K enzymatic pathway.[17]

Stimulation of RhoA by protracted neurohormonal and inflammatory stress activation induces sustained up-regulation of Rho kinase activity. As a result, an increased Rho kinase/IRS-1 association would be expected to chronically inhibit insulin signaling via the IRS-1/PI3K cascade, thus ultimately thwarting insulin metabolic and vascular NO/guanosine 3′,5′-cyclic monophosphate (cGMP) signaling.[17]

Other Rho Kinase Cellular Functions. Several other Rho-regulated cellular functions are mediated by Rho kinase, such as

- cytoskeletal rearrangement,
- cytokinesis,
- dephosphorylation of protein kinase B (PKB), and
- c-fos expression.[25]

Clinically, Rho kinase is implicated in

- **vascular inflammation,**
- **vascular remodeling,**
- **endothelial permeability,**
- **coronary artery spasm,**
- **hypertension,**
- **effort angina, and**
- **myocardial cell hypertrophy.**[23]

Other Downstream Rho Effectors. Other downstream effectors of Rho's critical role in gene expression, cell growth, migration, and contraction are

- PKC-related protein kinases,
- citron kinase,
- phosphatidylinositol pentaphosphate (PIP5) kinase, and
- protein kinase N (PKN).[23,26]

Rac1 GTPase Roles. The small Rho family GTPase Rac1 plays a role in various cellular processes, including

- **the production of ROS,**
- **cytoskeletal rearrangement,**
- **gene transcription, and**
- **malignant transformation.**

Rac1 and Rac3 are expressed in a wide variety of tissues. Rac2 is a hematopoietic-specific Rho family GTPase that shares 92% amino acid homology with Rac1.[14]

Rac and ROS Production. Rac is a component of the nicotinamide adenine dinucleotide phosphate (NADH/NADPH) oxidase complex of both leukocytes and vascular endothelial cells. NADH/NADPH oxidase is a major source of ROS production in endothelial cells under hemodynamic stress. **Rac, along with other components, is required for NADH/NAPDH oxidase activity and is essential for enhanced superoxide elaboration.**

Rac-dependent NADH/NADPH oxidase acts as an upstream activator for cyclic strain-induced MCP-1 expression in endothelial cells.[27]

Rac1, IL-6, and Malignancy. Persistent Rac1 activity may induce malignant transformation.

Activation of NFκB by Rac1 GTPases leads to transcriptional induction of the IL-6 gene. IL-6, in turn, stimulates the Janus kinase (JAK)/signal transducer and activator of transcription-3 (STAT-3) signal pathway, which has been identified as a potential oncogene. This stimulation occurs in an autocrine fashion via the IL-6 receptor.[12]

THE RENIN-ANGIOTENSIN-ALDOSTERONE SYSTEM AND INFLAMMATION

Inflammation is an independent risk factor for the development and progression of cardiovascular disease and type 2 DM by contributing to an oxidant-rich, inflammatory milieu that induces phenotypic changes in cells. Although inflammation is clearly multifactorial in etiology, the renin-angiotensin-aldosterone system (RAAS) plays an important, contributory role.

In fact, inflammation can become a self-sustaining process through a biologic positive feedback loop involving the RAAS. Angiotensin II promotes the secretion of IL-6, a cytokine that induces the synthesis of angiotensinogen in the liver. Increased angiotensinogen production, in turn, supplies more substrate for further angiotensin II elaboration. This positive feedback mechanism is also supported as active inflammatory cells express angiotensin-converting enzyme (ACE).[28]

The Systemic and Local Renin-Angiotensin-Aldosterone System. RAAS has traditionally been regarded as a systemic hormonal system.

Prorenin is produced by renal juxtaglomerular cells in response to stimuli such as reduced renal perfusion pressure, reduced tubular sodium delivery at the macula densa, or sympathetic activation. Active renin is released from its prohormone and acts on the acute phase reactant angiotensinogen of predominantly hepatic origin to produce the relatively inactive decapeptide angiotensin I. The latter is converted to angiotensin II by ACE in the pulmonary circulation.

Local tissue RAASs are widely distributed. Tissue-bound ACE may account for up to 90% of ACE activity found in the body.[29] RAASs are present in numerous tissues, including

- adipose tissue,
- adrenal glands,
- brain,
- kidneys, and
- the vasculature.[1]

The local vascular RAAS appears to play a major role in vascular pathophysiology. ACE is expressed at the shoulder region of atherosclerotic plaque, and ACE activity is enhanced in unstable plaque.

Angiotensin II. Angiotensin II is produced locally by the activated vascular RAAS of inflamed vessels.

Angiotensin II is a highly pluripotential hormone in vascular smooth muscle cells. It stimulates multiple signaling pathways, including the Src family kinases, MAPKs, and Akt/PKB. Angiotensin and its congeners, such as angiotensin II, IV, and (1-7), mediate the principal physiologic effects. Although most of these actions are transacted via the angiotensin II type 1 (AT_1) receptors, type 2, 4, and (1-7) receptors may also play a role. The receptors belong to the superfamily of G protein–coupled receptors with seven transmembrane regions. They all have distinct signal transduction pathways. The AT_1 receptor is present in many tissues and organs, including the myocardium, vasculature, kidney, and adipose tissue.[1]

Acting via the AT_1 receptor on endothelial and vascular smooth muscle cells, angiotensin II

- stimulates NADH/NADPH,
- activates Rho/Rho kinase,
- activates PKC, and
- activates MAPKs.

Through these pathways, **angiotensin engenders clinical hypertension, vascular hypertrophy, remodeling, inflammation, and**

Table 3-2. Angiotensin II Effects on the Vasculature

Inflammation
Increased expression of MCP-1, TNF-α, IL-6, VCAM, ICAM
Activation of NADH/NADPH oxidase
Production of superoxide anions
Activation of monocyte and macrophage cytokine production
Vasoconstriction
Stimulation of AT_1 receptors
Increased destruction of NO
Enhanced release of norepinephrine and endothelin
Decreased baroreceptor sensitivity
Reduced vasodilatory prostaglandins
Compliance
Increased destruction of NO
Increased fibrosis
Increased inflammation
Decreased vasodilatory prostaglandins
Remodeling
Stimulation of matrix glycoproteins and metalloproteinase production
Stimulation of vascular smooth muscle cell hypertrophy, migration, and proliferation
Increased expression of growth factors
Increased fibrosis
Thrombosis
Increased platelet activation, aggregation, and adhesion
Stimulation of PAI-1 synthesis
Reduced tPA production
Alteration of the tPA/PAI-1 ratio
Increased inflammation

AT_1, angiotensin II type 1 receptor; ICAM, intercellular adhesion molecule; IL-6, interleukin-6; MCP-1, monocyte chemotactic protein-1; NADH/NADPH, nicotinamide adenine dinucleotide phosphate; NO, nitric oxide; PAI-1, plasminogen activator inhibitor-1; TNF, tumor necrosis factor; tPA, tissue plasminogen activator; VCAM, vascular cell adhesion molecule. Modified from McFarlane SI, Kumar A, Sowers JR. Mechanisms by which angiotensin-converting enzyme inhibitors prevent diabetes and cardiovascular disease. Am J Cardiol 2003;91(suppl): 30H-37H.

thrombosis, as well as myocardial hypertrophy and remodeling (Table 3-2).

Specifically, angiotensin II mediates a multiplicity of effects:

- oxidative stress,
- activation of several phospholipases,
- stimulation of calcium influx,
- stimulation of calcium release from intracellular stores,
- vasoconstriction,
- vascular smooth muscle migration,
- vascular smooth muscle proliferation,
- vascular smooth muscle hypertrophy,
- extracellular matrix formation,
- opposition to the local actions of NO,
- elaboration of matrix metalloproteinases (MMPs),
- production of plasminogen activator inhibitor-1 (PAI-1),
- production of cellular adhesion molecules, and
- release of thromboxane A_2.[1,30]

The AT_1 receptor dynamically accesses the caveolar specialized signaling domain in vascular smooth muscle cells. Because of the multitude of signaling and coupling proteins localized in caveolae, caveola–AT_1 receptor interaction is probably an important focus for dynamic receptor-receptor communication and signaling.[1,30]

Dyslipidemia. There is crosstalk between the vascular RAAS and dyslipidemia. **Expression of local RAAS components is enhanced by lipid accumulation in the vessel wall, and activation of the local RAAS stimulates the accumulation of oxidized low-density lipoprotein (LDL).**[31]

Proinflammatory Effects. Angiotensin II has multiple significant proinflammatory actions.

- **Angiotensin II activates NFκB** with increases in both the p52 and p65 NFκB subunits, which results in the induction of NFκB-dependent proinflammatory and pro-oxidant genes to promote the production of ROS, inflammatory cytokines, chemokines, and adhesion molecules.[3]
- Via NFκB, **angiotensin II promotes the synthesis and secretion of IL-6**, which induces the hepatic synthesis of angiotensinogen in the liver through a JAK/STAT-3 pathway to further enhance angiotensin II elaboration.[28]
- **Angiotensin II enhances apoptosis** via activation of the c-Jun NH_2-terminal kinase (JNK)/stress-activated protein kinase (SAPK) pathways.[7]
- **Angiotensin II is a major deleterious generator of oxidative stress by activating the**

potent membrane NADH/NADPH oxidase to produce the superoxide anion.[1]

- **Angiotensin II down-regulates both peroxisome proliferator–activated receptor (PPAR) alpha and gamma** mRNA and protein, which may attenuate the anti-inflammatory potential of the PPARs and further contribute to enhanced vascular inflammation.[3]

Hypercoagulability. Angiotensin II promotes hypercoagulability via prothrombotic effects and impaired fibrinolysis.

- Enhanced thromboxane A_2 production causes increased platelet aggregation.
- Formation of PAI-1 antagonizes fibrinolysis.
- ACE-mediated degradation of bradykinin lowers the production of tissue plasminogen activator (tPA) by endothelial cells.

Profibrogenic Effects. Angiotensin II has a profibrogenic effect. It stimulates cell growth with extracellular matrix deposition of collagen and fibronectin, thus increasing vascular rigidity and myocardial stiffness.

Increased PAI-1 elaboration with angiotensin II increases fibrosis.[32] In an angiotensin II–infused rat model, connective tissue growth factor staining is increased with overexpression of the extracellular matrix. Angiotensin II increases the endogenous production of connective tissue growth factor by inducing its mRNA expression and protein production via PKC activation, ROS, and transforming growth factor-β.[33]

The Mineralocorticoid Aldosterone. Another RAAS product, aldosterone, is primarily known to mediate water and electrolyte balance by acting on mineralocorticoid receptors in the kidneys. However, **aldosterone is also generated locally in the vasculature and the myocardium. The enzymes required for aldosterone biosynthesis are expressed in these locations, and mineralocorticoid receptors are present in these locations as well.**[34]

Aldosterone exerts adverse cardiovascular effects mediated by local mineralocorticoid receptors, including

- oxidative stress,
- inflammation,
- endothelial dysfunction,
- hypertension,
- reduced fibrinolysis,
- cardiac and vascular fibrosis,
- left ventricular hypertrophy,
- congestive heart failure, and
- cardiac arrhythmias.[34]

Chronic exposure of rats to aldosterone causes sustained activation of

- NADH/NADPH oxidase with 3-nitrotyrosine generation,
- NFκB activation,
- COX-2 mRNA expression,
- MCP-1 mRNA expression, and
- osteopontin mRNA expression

in endothelial and inflammatory cells, thereby leading to severe vascular inflammatory lesions. The proinflammatory/fibrogenic vascular injury response is characterized by monocyte/macrophage infiltration and focal ischemic and necrotic changes. Aldosterone mineralocorticoid receptor antagonism attenuates these responses, as well as the ensuing vascular and myocardial damage.[35-37]

CARBOHYDRATE METABOLISM AND DYSLIPIDEMIA IN ACUTE INFLAMMATION

Inflammatory pathways affect carbohydrate and lipid metabolism. The inflammatory response initiates **metabolic adaptations initiates to service the increased energy needs of the perceived "injured organ" and the reactive inflammatory cells. The result is insulin resistance, glucose intolerance, and an atherogenic dyslipidemia characterized by hypertriglyceridemia, low levels of high-density lipoprotein (HDL), and the formation of small, dense LDL, which is prone to oxidation.**

Carbohydrate and Protein Metabolism with Inflammation. Inflammation, as occurs with sepsis, trauma, and extensive muscle injury, alters carbohydrate metabolism acutely in order to benefit the host response.

Glucose and glutamine are the major energy sources for the cells of the immune system.

During infection and sepsis, the need for glucose as fuel for the immune system rises significantly. Glucose uptake and utilization increase in inflammatory cells, and endogenous glucose production is up-regulated.[10]

Insulin Resistance. To accommodate the energy requirements of the immune response, proinflammatory cytokines stimulate gluconeogenesis and impair systemic insulin sensitivity, thereby engendering insulin resistance. As a result, glucose uptake by insulin-dependent tissues is compromised, but glucose availability for the non–insulin-dependent immune cells is enhanced.[10]

Protein Catabolism. Proinflammatory cytokines mediate the catabolic breakdown of muscle in acute inflammation. Catabolism of muscle protein releases glutamine, which serves as a fuel for immune cells. Glutamine also opposes insulin action, thus favoring gluconeogenesis upon amino acid release.[38] Hypoglycemia or hyperglycemia may supervene with inflammation, depending on the severity of the inflammatory response and the fuel supply (Table 3-3).[10]

Changes in Lipid Metabolism. Infection and inflammation perturb lipid metabolism. Catabolic, cytokine-induced changes in lipid metabolism are part of the acute immune response and may benefit the host's reaction to the traumatic insult.

Proliferating immune cells derive fatty acids as fuel mainly from the triacylglycerols in adipose tissue. Immune stimulation with catabolic hormone production and decreased insulin sensitivity prompts lipolysis and the release of fatty acids for provisioning the immune response. Fatty acids are then redistributed to the cells involved in immune defense or tissue repair.[11,38,39]

Lipoproteins and apolipoproteins themselves may contribute to host defense:

- Lipoproteins bind and target parasites for destruction.
- Lipoproteins compete with viruses for cellular receptors.
- Lipoproteins bind toxic agents to neutralize their harmful effects.
- Apolipoproteins may lyse parasites and neutralize viruses.[40]

Hypertriglyceridemia. A consistent feature of inflammation is hypertriglyceridemia. This effect is mediated via cytokines such as TNF-α, IL-1, IL-6, and interferon and occurs as a result of

- an increase in very-low-density lipoprotein (VLDL) synthesis and secretion and/or
- a decrease in VLDL clearance.

Cytokines rapidly stimulate hepatic fatty acid synthesis, which results in increased VLDL production, hepatic triglyceride secretion, and hypertriglyceridemia.[41]

Hypertriglyceridemia is accentuated because **IL-6 additionally inhibits lipoprotein lipase activity and fatty acid uptake into adipocytes.** Although the cytokine activation pathways differ for diverse causes of inflammation, the effects on triglyceride metabolism are similar.[11]

Small, Dense Low-Density Lipoproteins. During acute inflammation, LDL levels are typically not elevated and may actually be reduced. Reductions in LDL levels during inflammation may occur as a result of decreased hepatic production, increased catabolism of these lipoproteins, or both mechanisms.

LDL is converted to small, dense LDL particles because of the prevalence of triglyceride-rich lipoproteins. The latter exchange their triglyceride for LDL cholesteryl ester via cholesterol ester transfer protein (CETP). Subsequent lipolysis of LDL triglyceride

Table 3-3. Cytokine- and Stress-Induced Modifications of Glucose Metabolism

Stress-induced increase in cytokines
Noninflammatory tissue insulin resistance
Increased inflammatory tissue glucose transport
Increased inflammatory tissue glucose utilization
Stress hormone release with metabolic effects
Increased gluconeogenesis
Skeletal muscle catabolism and amino acid release
Increased azotemia
Anorexia

Modified from Avignon A, Monnier L. Insulinosensibilite et situations de stress. Diabetes Metab (Paris) 2001;27:233-238.

renders the lipoprotein small and dense.[42] **Small, dense LDL is particularly susceptible to oxidation induced by the host response.** In addition, small dense LDL has poor binding affinity to LDL receptors, which leads to decreased clearance of it.[11]

Sphingolipid-Laden Lipoproteins. During acute inflammation, VLDL and LDL are enriched in sphingolipids such as sphingomyelin and ceramide.

The increase in the sphingolipid content of lipoproteins derives from cytokine-induced up-regulation of serine palmitoyltransferase, the rate-limiting enzyme in sphingolipid synthesis in the liver. As a result, hepatic sphingomyelin and ceramide production is increased. Sphingomyelin is a substrate for cytokine-induced ceramide formation by activated arterial wall macrophages and endothelial cell sphingomyelinases.[11]

An increase in the sphingolipid content of lipoproteins has also been proposed to increase the atherogenicity of VLDL and LDL. For example, an increase in LDL ceramide levels

- facilitates LDL aggregation,
- stimulates LDL uptake by macrophages,
- favors foam cell formation,
- retards the clearance of triglyceride-rich lipoproteins, and
- enhances arterial wall accumulation of proatherogenic remnant particles.[11]

High-Density Lipoprotein Changes. Inflammatory cytokines reduce HDL cholesterol levels, in part via

- reduced lecithin-cholesterol acyltransferase (LCAT) activity,
- increased plasma phospholipid transfer protein (PLTP) activity, and
- increased CETP activity.[43]

In the circulation, CETP is associated with HDL. The increased plasma levels of triglyceride-rich VLDL, in the presence of CETP, can interact with HDL and, via CETP, cause exchange of HDL cholesteryl esters for triglycerides. This process lowers the cholesterol concentration of HDL while rendering HDL rich in triglycerides. Furthermore, a cytokine-induced decrease in lipoprotein lipase and hepatic lipase activity may lower clearance of triglyceride-rich lipoprotein particles.[11,44] Thus, HDL during infection and inflammation is

- depleted in cholesteryl ester,
- enriched in triglyceride, and
- enriched in sphingolipids.

In addition to the lipid changes in HDL, attendant alterations take place in the HDL apolipoprotein, enzyme, and transfer protein composition. Inflammation causes a decrease in HDL-associated

- apolipoprotein A-I and
- paraoxonase levels.

In contrast, there is an increase in HDL-associated

- ceruloplasmin,
- apolipoprotein J, and
- SAA levels.

SAA is an acute phase reactant that binds to HDL during an inflammatory response. SAA may

- displace apolipoprotein A-I, which increases the catabolism of HDL,
- inhibit LCAT, which leads to lower levels of esterified cholesterol in HDL, and
- directly impair endothelial function.[45]

These inflammation-induced changes lower HDL levels and have an adverse impact on HDL functions such as reverse cholesterol transport, prevention of LDL oxidation, and protection of endothelial function.[11,46]

INFLAMMATION AND CHRONIC DISEASES

An acute inflammatory response is critical for a successful host defense against a pathogen. **Despite the initial benefits of acute inflammation, the metabolic changes attending inflammation, if protracted, can have detrimental consequences for the host.**

Potential triggers for a chronic vascular and systemic inflammatory response may include ongoing

- mental and emotional stress,
- chronic pain,
- mechanical strain,
- smoke exposure,

- hypercholesterolemia,
- hyperhomocysteinemia, and
- chronic infection.[47]

Chronic inflammation underlies ailments as diverse as

- **abnormal lipid and carbohydrate metabolism,**
- **the metabolic syndrome,**
- **type 2 DM,**
- arthritis,
- collagen vascular diseases,
- inflammatory bowel diseases,
- fibrotic lung disease,
- Alzheimer's disease,
- selected cancers, and
- asthma.

An increase in inflammatory mediators and oxidative stress, triggered by proinflammatory transcription factors, is associated with incident macrovascular disease such as stable

- **coronary heart disease (CHD),**
- **peripheral arterial disease, and**
- **cerebrovascular disease.**

An inflammatory process with pro-oxidant stress is also implicated in the pathogenesis of atherothrombotic, acute ischemic syndromes through plaque rupture and thrombosis of the inflamed, diseased arterial vessel as occurs in

- myocardial infarction (MI) and
- stroke.

INFLAMMATION AND ENDOTHELIAL DYSFUNCTION

Inflammation of the arterial wall causes endothelial dysfunction, and endothelial dysfunction sets the stage for the atherosclerotic process.

Intact functional endothelium releases NO, a potent vasodilator that mitigates and inhibits key processes in atherogenesis such as monocyte adhesion, platelet aggregation, and vascular smooth muscle proliferation. The reduced endothelium-derived NO activity of dysfunctional endothelium may contribute to the initiation and progression of vascular disease and atherosclerosis.[48,49]

The mechanisms of endothelial dysfunction in inflammation are probably multifactorial. Neurohormonal and cytokine mediators of inflammation, such as TNF-α, IL-6, CRP, and angiotensin II, interfere directly and indirectly with endothelial function.

Tumor Necrosis Factor-α Impact on Endothelial Function. TNF-α, one of the principal proinflammatory cytokines, impairs endothelial function in a multiplicity of ways.

eNOS Expression and Activity. TNF-α reduces the expression and activity of e-NOS in a dose-dependent fashion.[50]

- TNF-α down-regulates the expression of eNOS in endothelial cells by destabilizing eNOS mRNA, thus reducing its half-life.[50,51]
- TNF-α inhibits both insulin- and fluid shear stress–mediated eNOS activation via IRS-1 serine phosphorylation.[52]
- TNF-α appears to selectively inhibit receptor-mediated endothelial NO release.[53]

Asymmetric Dimethylarginine. Asymmetric dimethylarginine (ADMA) is an endogenous competitive inhibitor of eNOS. TNF-α–induced endothelial dysfunction may in part derive from reduced degradation of ADMA.

A number of cells, including human endothelial cells, elaborate ADMA. ADMA is metabolized by the enzyme dimethylarginine dimethylaminohydrolase (DDAH). Although TNF-α does not change DDAH expression, it reduces DDAH activity, thus lowering ADMA degradation.[54]

Free Fatty Acids. TNF-α indirectly contributes to endothelial dysfunction by increasing plasma levels of free fatty acids.

TNF-α stimulates lipolysis, thereby resulting in an increase in plasma free fatty acid levels. Free fatty acids impair endothelial function.[55]

Other Effects. TNF-α stimulates vascular smooth muscle endothelin-1 and angiotensin II production with adverse sequelae for the endothelium.[56,57]

Angiotensin II. Angiotensin II contributes to endothelial dysfunction.

It decreases the activity of the NO/cGMP/cGMP-dependent protein kinase (cGK) pathway. By stimulating the activity and expression of phosphodiesterase, angiotensin II increases cGMP hydrolysis, thus decreasing cGMP levels and cGK action.

Additionally, angiotensin II increases vasomotor tone by enhancing vascular smooth muscle sensitivity to calcium.[58]

C-Reactive Protein. There is a negative association between CRP levels and endothelial function.

CRP decreases eNOS mRNA, protein abundance, and enzyme activity, in essence causing a direct reduction in NO bioavailability with endothelial dysfunction.[59] Elevated CRP levels are associated with impaired endothelially mediated vasoreactivity in healthy children, in adults with atherosclerosis, and after percutaneous coronary intervention.[60-62]

Other Agents. IL-6 and other cytokines adversely affect endothelial function. Like TNF-α, they increase adipocyte lipolysis, which raises free fatty acid levels with attendant endothelial dysfunction.[55]

ADMA levels are also increased with oxidized LDL and homocysteine, and endothelial function is consequently impaired.[54]

Rho-Rho Kinase. From a molecular perspective, activation of Rho/Rho kinase may constitute a final common pathway whereby inflammatory and neurohormonal activities impair endothelial function. Rho/Rho kinase causes endothelial dysfunction by suppressing eNOS activity and gene expression and thus achieving both a rapid and a sustained decrease in NO production.

After receptor stimulation by inflammatory mediators, geranylgeranylation of the small GTPase Rho activates Rho/Rho kinase.[63] As a result,

- inactivation of PKB/Akt by Rho kinase prevents eNOS phosphorylation and activation;
- in a convergence of downstream cellular actions, Rho/Rho kinase and PKC downregulate eNOS expression by disrupting eNOS mRNA stability.[25]

Activated Rho/Rho kinase is also essential for the basal production of endothelin-1, a potent vasoconstrictor and mitogen that regulates vascular tone and remodeling.[25]

Anti-inflammatory Cytokines and Endothelial Function. Proinflammatory pathways that impair endothelial function have counterbalancing, anti-inflammatory factors.

Whereas IL-1, IL-6, IL-12, and IL-18 are all proinflammatory cytokines, IL-10 is an anti-inflammatory cytokine. **Anti-inflammatory cytokines are protective of endothelial function. It may ultimately be the balance between proinflammatory and anti-inflammatory cytokines that determines endothelial function.** Serum levels of the anti-inflammatory cytokine IL-10 are independent predictors of the endothelium-mediated forearm vasodilator response in patients with CHD. Interestingly, elevated IL-10 levels counteract the impairment in systemic endothelial function associated with increased CRP levels (Fig. 3-3).[64,65]

IL-10, which is predominantly secreted by activated monocytes, macrophages, and lymphocytes, has multifaceted anti-inflammatory properties, including

- inhibition of the inflammatory transcription factor NFκB, which leads to suppressed cytokine production,
- inhibition of TNF-α expression,
- inhibition of IL-8,
- inhibition of matrix-degrading metalloproteinases,
- reduction of tissue factor expression,
- inhibition of apoptosis of macrophages and monocytes after infection, and
- reduction of vascular wall oxidative stress.[64,65]

INFLAMMATION AND ATHEROSCLEROSIS

Half of all MIs and strokes occur in individuals without elevated cholesterol levels, thus suggesting other underlying pathophysiologic processes.[66]

Virchow proposed the inflammatory theory of atherosclerosis, referring to it as "endarteritis deformans."[67] Atherosclerotic plaques have histologically been likened to healing inflammatory

Figure 3–3.
The balance of prominent proinflammatory and anti-inflammatory mediators may determine vascular and metabolic health or disease. CRP, C-reactive protein; HDL, high-density lipoprotein; IL, interleukin; MCP, monocyte chemoattractant protein; MMP, matrix metalloproteinase; NF, nuclear factor; NSAIDs, nonsteroidal anti-inflammatory drugs; PPAR, peroxisome proliferator–activated receptor; RAAS, renin-angiotensin-aldosterone system; TNF, tumor necrosis factor. *(Adapted from Mills R, Bhatt DL. The yin and yang of arterial inflammation. J Am Coll Cardiol 2004;44:50-52.)*

Proinflammatory mediators		Anti-inflammatory mediators
CRP IL-1 IL-6 TNF-α CD40 Myeloperoxidase MCP-1 IL-18 MMP-9 NF kappaB Interferon-γ Phospholipase A2 Estrogen replacement Smoking Vascular disease Metabolic syndrome Periodontal disease	vs	IL-10 Adiponectin PPAR-γ agonists PPAR-α agonists HDL Moderate exercise Weight loss Moderate alcohol consumption Mediterranean diet Smoking cessation Aspirin NSAIDs RAAS antagonists Statins

lesions by Russell Ross, who proposed a "response to injury" hypothesis. Although atherosclerosis has been considered a disorder of lipid metabolism and lipid deposition, atherosclerosis is a chronic inflammatory disease, and **the pathophysiology of linking dyslipidemia to atherogenesis involves an inflammatory process.**[68] **Inflammation underlies the beginning, the progression, and the thrombotic complications of the atheromatous process. Furthermore, exacerbations of inflammation are associated with clinical events.**[69]

Increased vascular risk is heralded by a diverse range of inflammatory markers encompassing nonspecific inflammatory indicators, such as increased

- plasma viscosity,
- erythrocyte sedimentation rate, and
- leukocyte count;

acute phase reactants, such as elevated levels of

- CRP,
- SAA,
- fibrinogen, and
- reduced serum albumin;

and cytokines and soluble adhesion molecules, such as

- IL-6,
- ICAM-1, and
- VCAM-1.[47]

Systemic signs of inflammation are detectable in the majority of patients with acute coronary syndromes or the metabolic syndrome. **The presence of detectable markers of systemic inflammation adversely affects the long-term prognosis for**

- **disease-free individuals,**
- **individuals with CHD, and**
- **individuals with the metabolic syndrome.**[70]

Inflammation in the Vessel Wall. In the permissive environment of endothelial dysfunction, inflammatory processes initiate incipient atherogenesis.

Cytokines. Circulating inflammatory cytokines are implicated in mediating endothelial dysfunction, and inflammatory markers such as CRP, IL-6, and TNF-α are independent risk factors for CHD. **The vascular wall is, however, not merely a passive responder to circulating inflammatory stimuli. There is, in fact, overexpression of several cytokines and cell adhesion molecules by the dysfunctional vascular endothelial and smooth muscle cells in response to proinflammatory cytokines** such as

- TNF-α,
- IL-1β,

- IL-6, and
- IL-18.

These inflammatory mediators are, in turn, systemically amplified by the acute phase response of the liver whereby SAA and CRP are generated.[69,71]

Endothelial-Leukocyte Adhesion Molecule-1 (E-Selectin). Both acute and chronic forms of inflammation involve endothelial-leukocyte interactions.

Proinflammatory cytokines induce the endothelial expression of adhesion molecules to attract the cellular component of the inflammatory response. Endothelial and other cells at an inflammatory site elaborate chemoattractant cytokines, or chemokines. Chemokines, members of a large family of small proteins, attract inflammatory cells with the appropriate chemokine receptor to the site of inflammation.[2]

Endothelial-leukocyte adhesion molecule-1, or E-selectin, is one such chemokine elaborated by endothelial cells during inflammation. Interaction of E-selectin with carbohydrate ligands on leukocytes causes them to adhere to endothelial cells with the subsequent extravasation of leukocytes into the subjacent tissue. **E-selectin and neutrophils are associated with acute inflammation, a short-term response to infection or injury.**[72]

Adhesion Molecules. As a protracted response to infections or injury, **chronic inflammation entails the endothelial expression of an immunoglobulin superfamily of proteins, such as**

- **VCAM-1 and**
- **ICAM-1,**

which interact with the $\alpha4\beta1$ integrin receptors and the $\beta2$ integrin receptors on leukocytes, respectively. VCAM-1 and monocytes are generally associated with chronic inflammation.[72] **These adhesion molecules bind to monocytes and lymphocytes, first allowing the rolling and then the adhesion of such phagocytes and T cells to the vascular endothelium to form an inflammatory nidus and a nascent atheromatous plaque.**[2,69,71]

Monocytes and macrophages elaborate surface receptors for platelet-activating factor (PAF), a proinflammatory substance mediating effects via a PAF receptor. PAF contributes to further cytokine production, leukocyte recruitment, and LDL oxidation.[73]

T Lymphocytes. The cellular, vascular immune process also entails the recruitment, activation, and proliferation of immune system cells such as T lymphocytes and dendritic cells, which colocalize in atheromatous lesions.

Major chemoattractants for T-lymphocyte recruitment are the interferon-γ–induced cysteine–X amino acid–cysteine (CXC) chemokines released by endothelial cells, such as

- interferon-inducible protein of 10 kDa (IP-10),
- monokine induced by interferon-γ (MIGγ), and
- interferon-inducible T cell–alpha chemoattractant (I-TAC).[2]

Dendritic cells are potent antigen-presenting cells. These cells have costimulatory surface molecules such as CD80 and CD86 and secrete the proinflammatory IL-12, which plays a key role in polarizing acquired immune responses.

T lymphocytes, as well as monocytes/macrophages, are the predominant cells present at sites of plaque rupture. They are active in further promoting the inflammatory response and enhancing plaque thrombogenicity by inducing the release of tissue factor.[2]

Although type 1 T cells predominate in vascular atheromata, type 2 T cells may mitigate lesion development via production of IL-10, which down-regulates the type 1 response.[73]

Atherogenesis. Atherogenesis entails the progression of inflammation within the vessel wall and its remodeling.

Fatty Streak. Transmigration of endothelially bound leukocytes into the intima occurs when other chemokine signals are produced by endothelial and smooth muscle cells after stimulation by cytokines. Such signals are

- MCP-1, which provides the signal to allow bound leukocytes to extravasate and enter the intima; and

- M-CSF, which acts as a comitogen for inflammatory cells and induces intimal monocytes to express scavenger receptors.

Once extravasated, **inflammatory cells promote the inflammatory response within the vessel wall.** Macrophages within plaques establish contact with activated T cells and actively advance inflammation. Scavenger receptors cause monocytes to engulf oxidized lipoprotein particles and thus to mature into the macrophage foam cells of the fatty streak, the early lesion of atherosclerosis.[69,71]

Activated mast cells also accumulate in plaques, where they are most abundant in the shoulder regions of a lesion.[74]

Low-Density Lipoprotein. LDL excess is a known risk factor for atherosclerosis. In particular, **the small, dense LDL associated with inflammation is more proatherogenic than regular LDL is** because it

- can penetrate the endothelium and bind to intima proteoglycans more effectively than large buoyant LDL can, thereby resulting in arterial wall retention of lipid[11];
- is preferentially taken up by the macrophage scavenger receptor pathway, thereby contributing to atherogenesis; and
- is particularly susceptible to oxidative modification and glycation.

Oxidized LDL and lipid accumulation in the vessel wall can further foment the inflammatory response by inducing the endothelial expression of VCAM-1 and by enhancing the expression of vascular RAAS.[31,69,71]

Fibrous Metaplasia. Other signals from the ongoing vascular inflammatory process cause fibrous metaplasia of the fatty streak.

The usually quiescent vascular smooth muscle cells start to divide and also to generate an extracellular matrix. Additionally, medial smooth muscle cells migrate into the intima. As a result, the fibrofatty streak with fibrous plaque cap, the intermediate lesion of atherosclerosis, is generated. Concomitantly, there is outward growth of the lesion with vascular remodeling and preservation of the vascular lumen.[69,71]

Table 3-4. Histopathologic Characteristics of Atheromatous Plaque That Is Vulnerable to Rupture

Thin fibrous cap with
- Reduced collagen content
- Reduced smooth muscle cell density
- Increased macrophage density and activity
- Increased activated T-cell infiltration

Large, soft, acellular lipid-laden core occupying close to half the plaque volume

Adventitial changes with
- Increased vasa vasorum
- Cellular inflammatory infiltrate
- Remodeling and outward expansion of large plaque

Modified from Shah PK. Pathophysiology of plaque rupture and the concept of plaque stabilization. Cardiol Clin 2003;21:303-314.

Atherothrombosis. Continued inflammation structurally destabilizes the atheromatous lesion by eroding the extracellular matrix. **Breach of the fibrous cap leads to thrombotic complications and acute ischemic syndromes** (Table 3-4).

T lymphocytes resident in lesions express cytokines such as interferon-γ, TNF-α, IL-1, and the CD40 ligand.[2] These cytokines

- interfere with further smooth muscle collagen synthesis;
- activate macrophages to secrete proteolytic enzymes such as MMPs to degrade the collagen, fibrin, and elastin constituents of the extracellular matrix[3,69]; and
- induce tissue factor expression.[2]

This continued intralesional inflammation appears to play a role in

- thinning of the fibrous cap,
- plaque rupture, and
- thrombosis.[3,69]

Matrix Metalloproteinases. Derangement of MMP regulation is a critical factor in the development of vascular lesions and plaque instability.

Metalloproteinase expression is regulated by the proinflammatory transcription factor activator protein-1 (AP-1), which in turn is regulated by the transcription factor Egr-1 and other proinflammatory factors. MMPs are Zn^{2+}- and Ca^{2+}-dependent endopeptidases that are secreted largely by macrophages as proenzymes and activated by proteolytic cleavage.[75]

The major MMPs are

- MMP-1, an interstitial collagenase,
- MMP-2, a gelatinase,
- MMP-3, a stromelysin, and
- MMP-9, a gelatinase.[76]

MMPs are essential for cellular migration and tissue remodeling in both physiologic and pathologic conditions. They are involved in monocyte invasion and vascular smooth muscle cell migration within the vessel wall. MMPs degrade and digest the extracellular matrix components and the fibrous cap of the atheromatous plaque, generating the advanced lesion of atherosclerosis, which is rendered biomechanically unstable and susceptible to plaque rupture.[77]

Tissue Factor. Tissue factor appears to play an important role in the thrombotic complications of plaque rupture. Disruption of the physical integrity of the vascular atheroma exposes tissue factor to blood with supervening thrombosis.

Tissue factor is present in lipid-rich plaque and is expressed on the surface of monocytes, macrophages, and foam cells in lesions after activation of the cell surface receptor CD40.[2] It is regulated by Egr-1 in addition to other proinflammatory transcription factors.[78] Tissue factor is involved in cellular migration and angiogenesis processes.[69]

Within the lipid core of atheromata, **tissue factor is the major procoagulant protein that initiates thrombus formation.** Tissue factor activates factor VII, which leads to the formation of thrombin. Thrombin initiates further signaling cascades by which platelet aggregation is activated and fibrinogen is converted to fibrin. These clotting cascades set the stage for local thrombogenesis overlying the atheromatous plaque, thereby **resulting in vessel occlusion with the clinical manifestations of acute ischemic syndromes.**[69]

Plasminogen Activator Inhibitor-1 and Fibrinogen. The balance between plaque thrombosis and thrombolysis is also mediated in part by factors such as tPA and PAI-1. **Elevated levels of PAI-1 are associated with accelerated atherosclerosis and plaque rupture.**[32] **They contribute to the thrombotic process in unstable atheromata by inhibiting plasmin and diminishing fibrinolytic activity.**[78]

PAI-1 interferes with the clot dissolution mediated by tPA. It is the primary physiologic inhibitor of clot lysis and is produced predominantly by endothelial cells and regulated by the proinflammatory transcription factors NFκB and Egr-1. PAI-1 is thus a byproduct of activated proinflammatory pathways.[70,79]

Circulating PAI-1 levels are elevated in patients with CHD. PAI-1 levels in the highest quintile are predictive of future coronary ischemic events and mortality.[80,81]

PAI-1 is also increased in insulin resistance and type 2 DM. Insulin resistance and hyperinsulinemia increase levels of both tPA and PAI-1, but the impact on PAI-1 is more pronounced. PAI-1 levels increase in stepwise fashion with increasing insulin resistance.[82]

Insulin resistance is also associated with elevated levels of fibrinogen. The metabolic syndrome thus causes a net increase in markers of hypercoagulability, which increases the risk for atherothrombotic events.[83]

CHRONIC INFLAMMATION AND THE METABOLIC SYNDROME

Atherosclerosis and the metabolic syndrome share similar pathophysiologic mechanisms, mainly caused by the action of two major proinflammatory cytokines, TNF-α and IL-6. Increased transcription rates of TNF-α and IL-6 are associated with

- deranged lipid metabolism with hypertriglyceridemia and low HDL;
- deranged carbohydrate metabolism with insulin resistance and the metabolic syndrome, with eventual development of type 2 DM; and
- endothelial dysfunction, vascular inflammation, and atherosclerosis.[84]

Inflammation is associated with insulin resistance and hyperinsulinemia,[70,84] **and the metabolic syndrome is a low-level, chronic inflammatory state.**[84]

Markers of Inflammation and the Metabolic Syndrome. Acute inflammation with elevation of TNF-α and other proinflammatory cytokines induces insulin resistance in a variety of catabolic states such as cancer, sepsis, and trauma.[52] **Chronic dysregulation of the inflammatory axis as a result of a prolonged infectious or inflammatory process similarly predicts the development of insulin resistance and the metabolic syndrome.** Chronic inflammation may be a trigger for the development of insulin resistance in genetically or metabolically predisposed individuals,[85] and TNF-α and other proinflammatory cytokines may constitute some of the links between inflammation and the genesis of metabolic syndrome.[86]

Obesity and the metabolic syndrome are linked to increased production and increased plasma concentrations of proinflammatory cytokines such as

- IL-1
- IL-6,
- TNF-α,
- TNF receptor, and
- interferon-γ.[4]

The key proinflammatory transcription factor NFκB is chronically activated in peripheral monocytes with insulin resistance.[84] Acute phase reactants and adhesion molecules are highly correlated with elevated insulin levels.[87] PAI-1 release from adipose tissue is enhanced in metabolic syndrome.[81]

The appearance of chronic inflammation is an early process in the pathogenesis of metabolic disease. Insulin-resistant individuals in whom DM develops in follow-up have higher levels of inflammatory proteins than do subjects who remain nondiabetic in follow-up.[88] Type 2 DM in elderly men is related to an ongoing COX-related low-grade inflammatory process reflected by enhanced prostaglandin formation.[89] Data from 121,700 women enrolled in the Nurses' Health Study indicated that baseline median levels of inflammatory biomarkers such as E-selectin, ICAM-1, and VCAM-1 were significantly higher in subjects in whom type 2 DM subsequently developed.[90] In the Atherosclerosis Risk in Communities Study, chronic activation of the innate immune system was associated with the metabolic syndrome, and markers of inflammation and endothelial dysfunction predicted the development of DM.[91]

Correspondingly, low levels of the anti-inflammatory cytokine IL-10 are associated with the metabolic syndrome in obese women.[65]

The Metabolic Syndrome and Atherogenesis. Inflammation appears to be the "common ground" underlying both CHD and type 2 DM.[92] Increased activation of inflammatory markers engenders both worsening of insulin resistance and progression of cardiovascular disease with CHD mortality.

Inflammation is an integral part of atherogenesis in patients with type 2 DM.[92] Because of the enhanced oxidative stress, inflammation, and thrombogenesis in metabolic syndrome, atheromatous plaques in affected patients tend to be particularly unstable and prone to rupture.[93]

C-REACTIVE PROTEIN IN VASCULAR DISEASE AND THE METABOLIC SYNDROME

Cytokine and Cytokine Receptor Assays. Histopathologic assessment of inflammation within tissues is clinically impractical. Plasma levels of circulating markers of inflammation, such as proinflammatory cytokines, are low but detectable and may reflect the activity of an underlying inflammatory process.

Circulating cytokine receptors have a longer half-life than do cytokines themselves. Cytokine receptor levels are more constant over time, and measurement of them may provide additional information on the activity of a chronic inflammatory process. Clinically, the soluble TNF receptors are excellent indicators of inflammatory processes. Elevated levels of TNF receptors are associated with obesity, insulin resistance, CHD, and angina severity.[94]

Elevated levels of IL-6, TNF-α, and TNF soluble receptor 1 may be seen with clinical cardiovascular disease, with cytokine levels in the highest tertile reflecting odd ratios of 2.35, 2.05, and 1.99 for MI, congestive heart failure, and stroke, respectively.[95] In a nested case-control study of post-MI men, the multivariable-adjusted relative risk for recurrent coronary events was 2.5 for patients whose TNF-α levels exceeded the 95th percentile.[96] Several other studies have examined the relationship between elevated levels of cytokines and the risk for CHD.[97,98]

Cytokine versus C-Reactive Protein Assay. When compared with assays of circulating cytokines, high-sensitivity CRP (hsCRP) is a more convenient measure of inflammation. It is inexpensively measured and has significant specificity for the prediction of cardiovascular disease.[99]

C-Reactive Protein. CRP, a complex, pentameric β-globulin, is a prototypic, nonspecific, but highly sensitive marker for systemic inflammation and tissue damage.[61,65,100]

CRP was initially described as an acute phase reactant that binds pneumococcal capsular polysaccharide. CRP is mainly synthesized and secreted by hepatocytes 6 hours after acute stimulation by elevated levels of, for example, IL-6.[70] Its levels can exceed 500 mg/L in a variety of acute and chronic, systemic inflammatory conditions.[101] In contrast, **CRP levels that reflect the presence of a low-grade inflammatory response range from 1 to 10 mg/L.**[102]

Relationship of C-Reactive Protein to IL-6 and TNF-α. Because CRP reflects the amplification of inflammatory cytokine activation,[70] **clinically, proinflammatory cytokines, including IL-6 and TNF-α, circulate at much lower concentrations than hsCRP does.**

The level of CRP, released as an acute phase reactant by the liver, is largely regulated by the concentration of circulating IL-6 released by macrophages or other inflammatory cells. **Levels of CRP, albeit amplified, are thus significantly related to those of IL-6 and TNF-α.**[70]

TNF-α levels can be very low and unstable. IL-6 has greater diurnal variability and a shorter half-life (2 to 4 hours) than hsCRP does (19 to 20 hours),[103] which has no diurnal variation and is stable over prolonged periods.[99]

C-Reactive Protein as a Predictive Marker for Coronary Heart Disease. In contrast to the other indicators of inflammation, hsCRP may be a more specific marker of cardiovascular risk.

hsCRP is of prognostic value in predicting the risk for CHD, MI, and stroke.[104] It is an independent predictor for the development of MI and other cardiovascular events in cardiac patients, as well as in healthy men and women, with a multivariable-adjusted relative risk of 1.68 for CHD.[105-107]

In fact, **hsCRP may be a stronger predictor of cardiovascular events than the plasma level of LDL is** (Fig. 3-4). hsCRP adds prognostic information to Framingham cardiovascular risk scoring (Fig. 3-5).[99,108] The relationship between hsCRP and cardiovascular risk is largely independent of cholesterol levels,[66] which is not surprising in view of the response of LDL levels to inflammation.

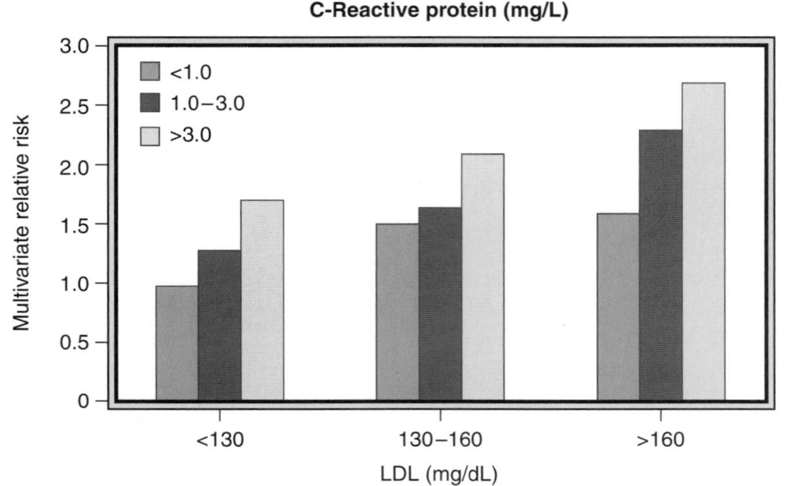

▸▸ **Figure 3–4.** Multivariable-adjusted relative risk for cardiovascular disease according to high-sensitivity C-reactive protein levels within categories of low-density lipoprotein (LDL). (Modified from Ridker PM, Rifai N, Rose L, et al. Comparison of C-reactive protein and low-density lipoprotein cholesterol levels in the prediction of first cardiovascular events. N Engl J Med 2003;347: 1557-1565.)

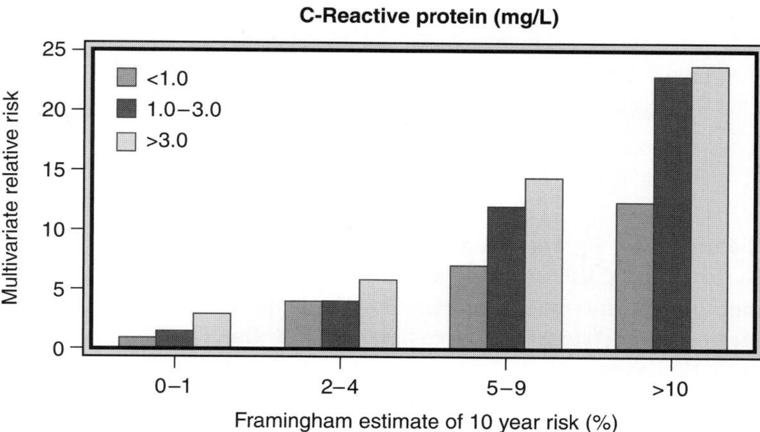

Figure 3–5.
Multivariable-adjusted relative risk for cardiovascular disease according to high-sensitivity C-reactive protein level and Framingham risk score. *(Modified from Ridker PM, Rifai N, Rose L, et al. Comparison of C-reactive protein and low-density lipoprotein cholesterol levels in the prediction of first cardiovascular events. N Engl J Med 2003;347:1557-1565.)*

	hsCRP RISK LEVEL FOR CORONARY HEART DISEASE
<1 mg/L	Low risk
1-3 mg/L	Intermediate risk
3-10 mg/L	High risk
>10 mg/L	Repeat test in 1 month, exclude other processes

Modified from Yeh ET, Willerson JT. Coming of age of C-reactive protein: using inflammation markers in cardiology. Circulation 2003;107:370-371.

C-Reactive Protein as a Vascular Inflammatory Mediator. Although CRP has been considered an inactive, systemic, downstream marker of inflammation, it may actually directly participate in aspects of atherogenesis.

Location. CRP is localized in atheromatous lesions.

Immunohistochemical staining of atherosclerotic plaque colocalizes CRP with complement proteins and macrophages. Serum levels of CRP correlate with the amount of CRP in atheromata and with anatomic features of plaque destabilization.[103] Furthermore, smooth muscle cells of atherosclerotic lesions with active disease may produce CRP independent of the traditional hepatic pathways.[109,110]

Endothelial Effects. CRP compromises NO bioavailibility.

CRP impairs vascular eNOS expression and attenuates the production of NO. CRP may increase the susceptibility of endothelial cells to destruction by cell lysis.[66]

CRP also reduces eNOS expression in endothelial progenitor cells. Endothelial progenitor cell–induced angiogenesis in response to ischemia is dependent on the presence of NO. In cultured human endothelial progenitor cells, CRP treatment, at concentrations associated with adverse vascular outcomes, causes a decrease in eNOS mRNA expression, thus directly inhibiting progenitor cell differentiation, survival, and function.[111]

Inflammatory Effects. CRP has diverse proinflammatory effects. It activates a number of inflammatory pathways that promote vascular inflammation, platelet aggregability, and thrombogenesis.

Specifically, CRP

- is a complement activator and complexes with complement;
- interacts with LDL[2];
- may induce NFκB and thereby lead to induction of MCP-1, IL-6, and iNOS gene expression;
- may activate MAPK[112];
- increases iNOS activity;
- increases nitration of prostacyclin (PGI_2) synthase via peroxynitrite, which impairs the release of PGI_2, a potent vasodilator and inhibitor of platelet aggregation[113];
- increases coronary endothelial expression of ICAM-1;
- is chemotactic for monocytes;
- activates tissue factor by mononuclear cells[114,115];

- potentiates the effects of angiotensin II by up-regulating the expression of angiotensin receptors on vascular smooth muscles;
- increases endothelin-1 production; and
- sensitizes endothelial cells to destruction by cytotoxic CD4-bearing T cells.[65]

C-Reactive Protein and the Metabolic Syndrome. CRP may be a hallmark of the metabolic syndrome, a marker for the inflammation underlying insulin resistance and diabetic diseases.

C-Reactive Protein and Obesity. CRP is elevated with total and central obesity.[116,117]

Visceral adiposity may act as a promoter of low-grade chronic inflammation.[118] Akin to the process of atheroma formation, in the presence of endothelial dysfunction, macrophages infiltrate adipose tissue in obese persons, where they induce a low-grade inflammatory state, release cytokines, and cause insulin resistance in adipocytes, especially those in visceral adipose tissue.[102,119] Consequently, the higher amounts of cytokines released by inflamed adipose tissue in obese persons augment the production of CRP by the liver, although CRP mRNA is also expressed by adipose tissue.[117]

As a result, CRP levels are significantly correlated with

- body mass index,
- total adiposity,
- waist size, and
- abdominal fat.[84,88,117]

C-Reactive Protein and Insulin Resistance. There appears to be an independent relationship between adiposity, CRP concentration, and insulin resistance.

CRP is elevated with central obesity and an elevated insulin resistance score.[116] Increased amounts of cytokines are released by visceral adipose tissue in obese persons, with the metabolic syndrome engendering greater hepatic production of CRP.[120] **In the general, nondiabetic population, elevations in markers of inflammation, such as CRP, the white blood cell count, and fibrinogen, are all significantly associated with increased fasting insulin levels and insulin resistance.**[84] In 3037 subjects with a mean age of 54 years monitored for 7 years, mean age-adjusted CRP levels for those with 0, 1, 2, 3, 4, or 5 criteria of the metabolic syndrome were 2.2, 3.5, 4.2, 6.0, or 6.6 mg/L, respectively (P trend < .0001).[121] CRP levels are significantly correlated with

- fasting glucose,
- fasting insulin,
- insulin sensitivity,
- higher triglyceride,
- lower HDL and apolipoprotein A-I, and
- systolic blood pressure.[84,88,117]

Insulin resistance may itself contribute to the hepatic release of acute phase reactants. With impaired insulin signaling, insulin's impact on hepatic protein synthesis is lost, thereby resulting in enhanced expression of acute phase proteins with lower albumin but higher fibrinogen and CRP synthesis and release.[122,123]

C-Reactive Protein and the Risk for Development of Type 2 Diabetes Mellitus. The metabolic syndrome is associated with increased levels of CRP, particularly in individuals at risk for the development of type 2 DM.[124]

In nondiabetic women, the elderly, and the general population, elevations in CRP, PAI-1, and IL-6 correlate with the development of type 2 DM (Fig. 3-6).[88,125-128] In the Women's Health Study, elevated CRP and IL-6 levels predicted the development of type 2 DM independent of body mass index, family history of DM, smoking, exercise, alcohol use, and hormone replacement therapy.[128] In the Monitoring of Trends and Determinants in Cardiovascular Disease study, men who had CRP levels in the highest quartile (≥2.91 mg/L) had a 2.7-fold higher risk for the development of DM.[129]

C-Reactive Protein and Risk for Coronary Heart Disease in Metabolic Syndrome. In the presence of the metabolic syndrome, an elevated hsCRP level has predictive power not only for new-onset DM but also for CHD events.[130] hsCRP and CHD risk factors are increased with an elevated insulin resistance score.[116] CRP adds prognostic information to the severity of the metabolic syndrome. The association of hsCRP with the metabolic

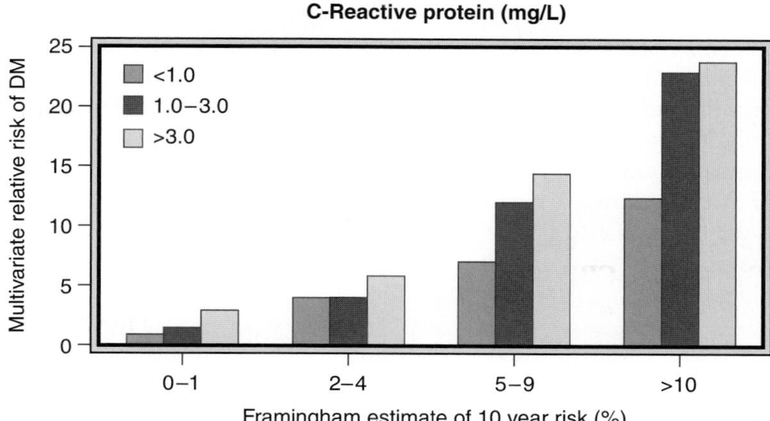

Figure 3–6.
Incidence of type 2 diabetes mellitus (DM) when stratified by quartiles of fibrinogen, high-sensitivity C-reactive protein level, and plasminogen activator inhibitor-1 level. *(Modified from Ridker PM, Rifai N, Rose L, et al. Comparison of C-reactive protein and low-density lipoprotein cholesterol levels in the prediction of first cardiovascular events. N Engl J Med 2003;347:1557-1565.)*

syndrome may account for some of its predictive value.[99]

Urinary albumin excretion, a marker for endothelial dysfunction and risk factor for vascular disease, is increased with insulin resistance and the metabolic syndrome. High levels of hsCRP, reflective of underlying inflammation, significantly raise the incidence of albuminuria and cardiovascular risk in the metabolic syndrome (Fig. 3-7).[131]

Both CRP and the metabolic syndrome are independent predictors of new CHD events. In 3037 subjects monitored for 7 years, the presence versus absence of the metabolic syndrome and baseline highest versus lowest CRP quartile were both related to an increased incidence of CHD events, with hazard ratios of 2.1 and 2.2, respectively.[121] In a study of the interrelationships between CRP, the metabolic syndrome, and incident cardiovascular events, 14,719 apparently healthy women were monitored for an 8-year period. Twenty-four percent of the cohort had the metabolic syndrome at study entry. Of these 3597 individuals with the metabolic syndrome, age-adjusted cardiovascular event rates per 1000 person-years were 3.4 for a CRP level lower than 3 mg/L and 5.9 for a CRP level higher than 3 mg/L, $P < .001$. At all levels of severity of metabolic syndrome, CRP levels higher than 3 mg/L added prognostic information on subsequent cardiovascular risk.[132]

CAUSES OF SYSTEMIC INFLAMMATION

The cause of the systemic inflammation associated with metabolic syndrome is not known. Although oxidized LDL is a stimulus for chronic

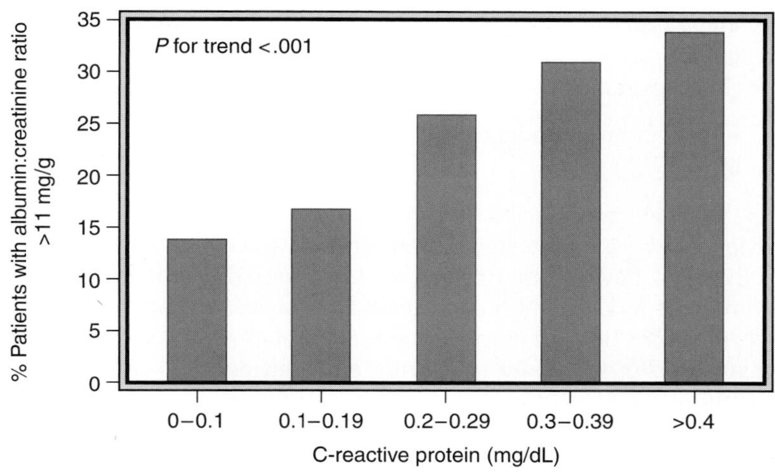

Figure 3–7.
Percentage of patients with a high urinary albumin-creatinine ratio greater than 11 mg/g across the range of high-sensitivity C-reactive protein levels. *(Modified from Messerli AW, Seshadri N, Pearce GL, et al. Relation of albumin/creatinine ratio to C-reactive protein and to the metabolic syndrome. Am J Cardiol 2003;92:610-612.)*

inflammation, the argument could be made that the lipid disturbance is a manifestation of an inflammatory process and the metabolic syndrome and, though contributing to ongoing inflammation, may not be its primary instigator. Similar arguments can be made about activation of stress pathways by free fatty acids because it would appear to be the lipolysis of an inflammatory state that released them in the first place.

Chronic Inflammatory Diseases. Chronic inflammation underlies a number of disabling chronic medical conditions such as cardiovascular disease, DM, Alzheimer's disease, selected cancers, and asthma.

Just as acute inflammation causes insulin resistance, lipid disturbances, and endothelial dysfunction, **chronic inflammatory diseases serve as potential triggers for the metabolic syndrome.** There is indeed a higher incidence of insulin resistance and the metabolic syndrome with

- dilated cardiomyopathy,
- rheumatoid arthritis,
- systemic lupus erythematosus, and
- psoriasis.[133-138]

Chronic Infectious Diseases. Various infectious etiologies have been examined as potential causes of a low-grade, systemic proinflammatory state. As with CHD and carotid vascular disease,[139-144] numerous infectious agents such as

- *Chlamydia pneumoniae,*
- *Helicobacter pylori,*
- *Mycoplasma pneumoniae,*
- cytomegalovirus,
- herpesviruses,
- human immunodeficiency virus, and
- influenza virus,

as well as nonspecific chronic periodontal, respiratory, gastrointestinal, and urinary tract infections, have been implicated as potential stimuli for inflammation and metabolic disease. Chronic infections may trigger systemic inflammatory processes. They have thus emerged as potential contributing factors to the systemic inflammatory disturbances that underlie vascular disease and the metabolic syndrome.[133,134]

Not surprisingly, it appears that the precipitating infection needs to be persistent and chronic rather than transient. In the Helsinki Heart Study of 4081 dyslipidemic, middle-aged men monitored for 8.5 years, persistently, but not transiently elevated *C. pneumoniae* immunocomplex–bound immunoglobulin A (IgA) or serum IgA and human heat shock protein p60 IgA antibodies, especially when present together with an elevated hsCRP level, predicted CHD events.[145]

However, the specific roles that these pathogens may play in the genesis of vascular and metabolic disorders remain contradictory.[70]

***Chlamydia pneumoniae. C. pneumoniae* is an example of an organism that may participate in an indolent, protracted inflammatory process.** The organism can be cultured from atheromata. Monocyte/macrophages harbor the organism in a persistent state that is inaccessible to antibiotic therapy.[146]

There appears to be immunomodulatory crosstalk between infected and uninfected cells, with reciprocal activation between macrophages and vascular smooth muscle cells. Membrane-bound RhoA and Rac1 expression and activity are increased in infected vascular smooth muscle cells. Rho GTPases and functional NADH/NADPH oxidase are required for *C. pneumoniae*–induced activation of NFκB.[16] Via NFκB activation, infected, activated cells produce cytokines, chemokines, and adhesion molecules, which in turn recruit and activate inflammatory cells and initiate the inflammatory process locally, with potential systemic ramifications.[147]

Periodontitis. Chronic periodontitis has emerged as a potential contributing factor to the systemic inflammation leading to vascular disease and the metabolic syndrome.

Periodontitis is another example of an indolent, chronic infectious process that is difficult to eradicate. The systemic inflammatory response derived from chronic periodontitis has the potential to elicit dyslipidemia and insulin resistance, thereby potentiating the metabolic disturbances inherent in metabolic syndrome.[148,149] Poor oral health, periodontitis, and incident tooth loss have been associated with peripheral artery disease in the 45,136-person Health Professionals Study.[150] Periodontal disease is a strong and independent predictor of elevated CRP levels and is common in patients with acute MI.[151] Periodontitis is twice as prevalent in diabetic individuals as in nondiabetics.[152]

Local Periodontal Infection. Periodontitis is caused by a small group of gram-negative bacteria that coat the surfaces of dental roots as biofilms. The biofilm configuration of periodontal pathogens is poorly amenable to antibiotic therapy. Lipopolysaccharide (LPS) and other microbial substances gain access to gingival tissues and initiate and perpetuate local immunoinflammation, which results in the production of high regional levels of proinflammatory cytokines.[152]

Systemic Manifestations. Periodontitis is more than a localized oral infection. It generates increased levels of circulating inflammatory mediators.

LPS, viable gram-negative bacteria from biofilms, and proinflammatory cytokines from inflamed periodontal tissues may enter the circulation in pathogenic quantities.[152] In particular, *Porphyromonas gingivalis,* one of the microorganisms responsible for periodontitis, is able to invade endothelial cells and is a potent signal for monocyte and macrophage activation.[153]

Periodontitis-induced bacteremia and endotoxemia cause systemic elevations of serum proinflammatory cytokines such as

- IL-1β,
- IL-6, and
- TNF-α.

These cytokines may produce alterations in lipid and carbohydrate metabolism that lead to dyslipidemia and insulin resistance.[153]

hsCRP levels are significantly elevated in middle-aged adults with periodontal disease who are otherwise healthy. hsCRP levels increase as a function of the extent and severity of periodontal pockets.[153]

Impact of Antibiotic Therapy on Inflammatory Markers. In selected instances, antibiotic therapy may reduce inflammatory markers.

Antibiotic treatment targeted at *C. pneumoniae* and *H. pylori* do reduce inflammatory markers, a prothrombotic disposition, and adverse cardiac events in patients with acute coronary syndromes over a 1-year period, independent of seropositivity.[154]

Similarly, effective antimicrobial therapy for periodontitis may significantly reduce the number of microorganisms in periodontal pockets and cause a significant reduction in

- circulating TNF-α levels and
- fasting insulin levels,

thus suggesting that successful eradication of an infectious nidus, if identified and amenable to treatment, may decrease inflammatory markers and improve the metabolic disturbances.[155,156]

However, pathogenic biofilms and other persistence modes for infectious agents may render host immune responses, as well as antibiotic therapy, ineffectual. The chronic presence of an infectious nidus stimulating severe, systemic inflammation would then continue to have an adverse impact on both vascular and metabolic homeostasis.

CHRONIC INFLAMMATION AND THE LEWIS ANTIGEN SYSTEM

Systemic signs of inflammation are manifest in the majority of patients with acute ischemic syndromes or metabolic syndrome. The presence of systemic inflammation adversely affects the long-term prognosis for individuals with and without cardiometabolic disease.[70] **A multitude of genetic factors may determine the activity of inflammation and modulate the attendant metabolic disturbance.** For example, single-nucleotide polymorphisms in the NFκB gene appear to alter the magnitude of the host defense response.[157] The Lewis antigenic system is a genetically determined blood group system that may also modify host responses to infections and to a number of systemic disorders.

The blood group ABO secretor phenotype or Lewis (Le) blood group status, or both, can drastically alter the carbohydrates present in body fluids and secretions and can thus profoundly affect microbial attachment and persistence. These ABO blood group antigens function as tumor markers and as receptors for parasites, bacteria, and viruses. They interact with immunologically active proteins. Individual differences in ABO secretor status and the Lewis blood groups may underlie

- aspects of the immune response,
- autoimmunity,

- insulin resistance and the metabolic syndrome,
- prothrombotic tendencies, and
- vascular disease.[158]

Secretor Status. The classic ABO blood group antigens, termed substances, are secreted in body fluids such as

- saliva,
- gastrointestinal secretions,
- mucus,
- sweat,
- tears,
- semen, and
- serum.

Antigens are secreted according to their specific blood group:

BLOOD GROUP	ANTIGEN SECRETED INTO BODY FLUIDS
Group O secretors	H antigen
Group A secretors	A and H antigens
Group B secretors	B and H antigens

Individuals are physiologically described as ABO secretors or nonsecretors, depending on qualitative and quantitative differences in the components of their secretions. The secretor genotype is controlled by two alleles, Se (secretor) and se (nonsecretor). Se is dominant and se is recessive, such that

1. Se/Se and Se/se are ABO secretors and
2. se/se represents ABO nonsecretors.

Approximately 80% of people are secretors (Se/Se or Se/se); the remainder are nonsecretors (se/se). In all instances, the ABO Se-secretor genotype causes the secretion of H substance.[158]

Generation of the H, A, B, and Lewis Antigens. The H antigen for blood group O is a fucose-containing glycan unit. It is encoded by a fucosyltransferase gene on chromosome 19 (*FUT1*). The H antigen serves as a precursor for synthesis of the A, B, and Lewis antigens. Specifically, this fucosylated glycan serves as a substrate for the glycosyltransferases encoded by secretor gene *FUT2* on chromosome 19q13.3 that generate the A, B, and Lewis blood group antigens in individuals who express the corresponding epitope. The antigenic specificity is expressed in the nonreducing end of the carbohydrate moiety and resides either on cell membrane glycolipids or on mucin glycoproteins in secretions.[158]

The Lewis Antigen. The allelic genes of the Lewis system are Le and le. The genotypes

1. Le/Le and Le/le (Lewis-positive type) produce Lewis antigen, termed Lewis a (Le^a), and
2. le/le (Lewis-negative type) produces no Lewis antigen

for secretion into body fluids.

The Lewis antigens are structurally related to the blood group determinants of the ABO system. Le^a resembles the H substance and differs only in the position of the fucose group.

The presence of the ABO Se-secretor genotype causes the addition of a second fucose group to Le^a, which converts Le^a to Lewis b (Le^b). Accordingly, ABO secretors, who are Lewis positive, are always Le (a–b+) because they convert all their Le^a antigen to Le^b. Correspondingly, Lewis-positive ABO nonsecretors are always Le (a+b–) because Le^a is not converted to Le^b.

Thus two broad phenotypes of Lewis blood type exist:

1. Lewis positive, either Le (a+b–) (nonsecretor) or Le (a–b+) (secretor),
2. Lewis negative, Le (a–b–) (irrespective of secretor status).

	LEWIS POSITIVE: a+ or b+	LEWIS NEGATIVE: a–/b–
Secretor		
Se/Se	Le (a–b+)	Le (a–b–)
Se/se	Le (a–b+)	Le (a–b–)
Nonsecretor		
se/se	Le (a+b–)	Le (a–b–)

Lewis-negative (le/le) individuals appear to have unique interactions with certain disease states.[158]

Host-Defense Implications of Antigen and Secretor Status. From an immunologic perspective, there may be an advantage to having large and diverse quantities of ABO and

Lewis antigen substances secreted into organic secretions.

The antigenic carbohydrate structures may aggregate infectious agents via adhesive mechanisms.[159] Secretor mucins have a significantly higher quantity and diversity of carbohydrate than do nonsecretor mucins. First-line host defense against pathogens may thus be more efficacious for secretors than for nonsecretors. An analogous argument appears to apply for Lewis positivity versus Lewis negativity.[158]

Implications of Lewis Blood Type. Lewis negativity may be associated with a higher incidence of cardiovascular and metabolic disease.

Coronary Heart Disease. The Lewis-negative phenotype may be associated with an increased risk for heart disease.

In the Copenhagen Male Study, 8% of men with the Lewis-negative Le (a–b–) phenotype had a history of nonfatal MI versus 4% of Lewis-positive men. Le (a–b–) men had an increased risk of death from heart disease when adjusted for age, with a relative risk of 4.4, $P < .001$, when compared with Lewis-positive men.[160]

The National Heart, Lung and Blood Institute Family Heart Study also showed a higher risk of CHD for Le (a–b–) than for other Lewis groups, with an odds ratio of 2.0.[161] In contrast, the Lewis-positive secretor phenotype Le (a–b+) was found to be a genetic marker of resistance to the development of CHD.[162,163]

Lewis positivity may, however, have adverse effects as well, possibly by enhancing the inflammatory response. In a 1-year follow-up of 54 patients with unstable angina, multivariate analysis showed the highest cardiac event rate in patients with seropositivity for *C. pneumoniae* who had the Lewis-positive secretor phenotype Le (a–b+) and those with hsCRP levels greater than 3 mg/L. hsCRP levels were higher in Le (a–b+) than in Le (a+b–) patients who were seropositive for *C. pneumoniae*.[164]

The Metabolic Syndrome. The Lewis-negative Le (a–b–) phenotype is associated with the metabolic syndrome. Le (a–b–) men exhibit features of the metabolic syndrome, such as higher

- body mass index,
- fasting levels of serum insulin,
- plasma glucose, and
- systolic blood pressure.[165]

Lewis-negative Le (a–b–) individuals also have significantly higher

- triglycerides,[166] and
- prothrombotic tendencies.[167]

Lewis Negativity and Genetic Linkages. Some of the determinants for the metabolic syndrome and Lewis negativity share a close genetic relationship.

Specifically, on chromosome 19, the Lewis genes are located in proximity to the genes for

- the LDL receptor,
- glycogen synthase, and
- the insulin receptor.[160]

Four mutations, T59G, T1067A, T202C, and C314T, of the human *FUT3* gene account for the vast majority of Lewis negative Le (a–b–) phenotypes in white individuals.[168] The Le (a–b–) phenotype might thus be a genetic marker for the metabolic syndrome.[169] These mutations are associated with higher hsCRP levels and may also be linked with an increased risk for CHD.[168]

Lewis Negativity and Alcohol. Alcohol may be of benefit with Lewis negativity.

In Lewis-negative Le (a–b–) men, a group genetically at high risk for metabolic syndrome and CHD, alcohol consumption appears to be especially protective and may ameliorate manifestations of the metabolic syndrome.[170]

CONVERGENCE AND DIVERGENCE OF VASCULAR DISEASE AND THE METABOLIC SYNDROME

Converging Effects. CHD and the metabolic syndrome have an inflammatory etiology and are characterized by vascular dysfunction.

A chronic inflammatory response is intimately linked to metabolic and vascular disease states. Atherosclerosis, the metabolic syndrome, and type 2 DM may share the same

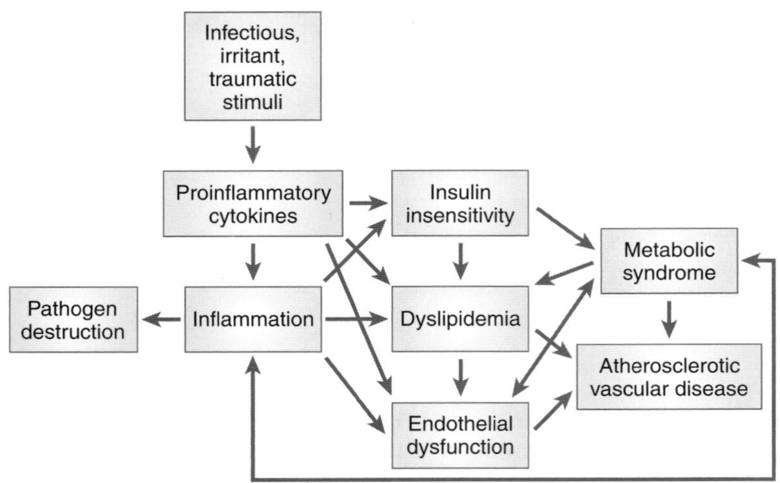

Figure 3–8. Inflammatory responses to pathogens, metabolic changes, and relationship to chronic cardiovascular and metabolic diseases. *(Modified from Grimble RF. Inflammatory status and insulin resistance. Curr Opin Clin Nutr Metab Care 2002;5:551-559.)*

inflammatory basis. Sustained, low-grade inflammation and vascular dysfunction may, in fact, underlie the convergence of insulin resistance, the metabolic syndrome, and cardiovascular disease (Fig. 3-8).[38]

Individuals with CHD and the metabolic syndrome have widespread vascular dysfunction. Diffuse endothelial dysfunction develops at an early stage in cardiovascular disease, as well as in metabolic syndrome.[171]

Diverging Manifestations. However, **there are clear-cut, divergent manifestations of vascular and metabolic disease:**

- patients with large vessel disease may show few signs of the full-blown metabolic syndrome;
- some individuals with the metabolic syndrome may be free of clinical conduit vessel disease.

Large and Small Vessel Heterogeneity. Whereas inflammation and dysfunctional endothelium play a central role in the atherogenesis of large and medium-sized arteries, an inflammatory response and vascular dysfunction at the arteriolar and capillary level may lead to insulin resistance and the associated features of metabolic syndrome. **Metabolic syndrome might thus be viewed as the consequence of an inflammatory process in the peripheral, microvascular bed.**[172]

As observed in studies of endothelial function, large vessel reactivity may diverge from small vessel reactivity. For example, brachial artery flow-mediated dilation may not correlate with resistance vessel microvascular function as measured by infusion studies. **This suggests differential regulation of vascular tone in conduit and resistance vessels.**[173]

Endothelial cells in diverse vascular loci may be dissimilar in morphology and function. The number of caveolae may differ at disparate vascular locations.[174] Whereas eNOS signaling may play a major role in larger vessels, endothelial hyperpolarizing factor and non–endothelium-dependent vasodilators may be of greater import in the microvasculature. There are clear, site-specific differences in the sensitivity of endothelial cells to injury mediated by activated neutrophils.[175,176] Such variations may contribute to the diverse reactivity of large and small vessels and the pathophysiologic distinctions between primary vascular and metabolic disease.[173]

In 2701 participants in the Framingham Offspring Study, the relationships of markers of inflammation to brachial flow-mediated dilation, a measure of conduit artery vasodilator function, and to reactive hyperemia, a measure of microvascular vasodilator function, were investigated. There were modest, unadjusted correlations between flow-mediated dilation and the inflammatory markers, which were rendered insignificant after adjustment for coronary risk factors. There were, however, statistically significant, risk factor–adjusted correlations between CRP, IL-6, and ICAM-1, as markers of inflammation, and reactive hyperemia.[177]

Site of Origin of Inflammation. Vascular disease and the metabolic syndrome may have divergent origins of inflammation.

Although vascular disease is a systemic process, the initial manifestations tend to be confined to conduit vessels and occur focally in sites of flow disturbance. As discussed in the Framingham Offspring Study, traditional cardiovascular risk factors induce a state of inflammation that impairs endothelial function in the conduit vessels. **Endothelial dysfunction induced by cardiovascular risk factors may be the primary driving force for conduit vessel dysfunction and the pathogenesis and clinical expression of large vessel atherosclerosis.** For flow-mediated dilation, there was no evidence that inflammation had additional effects beyond those attributable to traditional risk factors.[177]

In that same study, the incremental contribution of inflammatory markers to impaired reactive hyperemia above and beyond known risk factors suggested that systemic inflammation contributes to impaired vasomotor function in microvessels. Inflammation, in fact, had a predominant effect on the microvasculature rather than on conduit vessels. **Some source of inflammation, in addition to traditional risk factors, might contribute to microvascular dysfunction.**[177]

Metabolic syndrome is linked with infections such as periodontitis, with obesity-linked inflammation, and with systemic inflammatory disorders. The resultant systemic elevations in proinflammatory cytokines may cause a generalized, not focal vascular exposure to inflammation that appears to preferentially target the microvasculature. Microvascular dysfunction has an adverse impact on the metabolism of subjacent tissues such as skeletal muscle and adipose tissue. The ensuing insulin resistance of these tissues further aggravates systemic inflammation and eventually leads to systemic resistance to insulin signaling and the metabolic syndrome.

Reconvergence. Although insulin resistance may arise from a disordered microcirculation, ultimately an accelerating, systemic inflammatory process will involve coronary and systemic medium to large arteries with obstructive, atherosclerotic disease and atherothrombotic ischemic complications.

Just as the inflammatory milieu of end-stage heart failure begets systemic insulin resistance and ultimately type 2 DM, it is conceivable that worsening systemic inflammation associated with aggressive vascular disease may increasingly assume features of not only insulin resistance but also the full metabolic syndrome.

CONCLUSION

Inflammation and the immune response encompass a multitude of physiologic pathways, the majority of which have not been addressed in this chapter. They are essential survival mechanisms critical for an effective host response to infectious pathogens, injury, or trauma. Not surprisingly, inflammatory pathways incorporate many redundancies and numerous positive feedback loops.

Seropositivity toward infectious agents is abundant in the adult population, although the frequency thereof does not match the incidence of systemic markers of inflammation and the attendant metabolic and vascular disturbances. A multitude of genetic factors may determine the activity of inflammation. It is conceivable that the host response to underlying infections and infectious agents, for example, as modulated by the Lewis antigenic system and other genetic factors, may determine the degree and the duration of the inflammatory response.

The metabolic and vascular changes initiated by inflammation are geared to support the immune system. Inflammation engenders insulin resistance, with effects on lipid and carbohydrate metabolism, to provide fuel to the immune tissues. Neurohormonal mediators of inflammation cause endothelial dysfunction and vasoconstriction to preserve blood pressure in the setting of trauma or sepsis and to economize on nutritive perfusion to tissues not essential to the immune response. In effect, inflammation is the common foundation for insulin resistance and vascular disease. It underlies not only incipient disease, but also the progression and complications of atherosclerosis and the metabolic syndrome.

From a molecular perspective, neurohormonal and cytokine mediators of inflammation appear to effect endothelial dysfunction, as well as oxidative and inflammatory pathways, via Rac/Rho/Rho kinase. These small GTPases are simple, but potent molecular switches with a multiplicity of effects.

Interference with Rho and Rac prenylation, as well as with other inflammatory pathways, appears to underlie the potent, lipid-independent, beneficial impact of 3-hydroxy-3-methylglutaryl–coenzyme A (HMG-CoA) reductase inhibitors, or statins, on inflammation and endothelial function. Similarly, pharmacologic RAAS antagonists act not only as vasodilators and afterload reducers. Their pleiotropic effects also derive from antagonizing the proinflammatory and oxidant effects of angiotensin II and aldosterone.

Given the adverse health impact of a chronic inflammatory state, nonpharmacologic lifestyle measures with an anti-inflammatory focus may be of benefit. In that respect, smoking cessation would be appropriate, as would effort at reducing visceral obesity, increasing physical fitness, and consuming appropriate dietary choices. Additionally, it may be of benefit to aggressively avoid, minimize, or eliminate the impact of chronic foci of infection, such as periodontitis. In view of the significant cardiometabolic risk associated with chronic inflammatory disorders such as rheumatoid arthritis or systemic lupus erythematosus, a low threshold for using agents such as statins or RAAS antagonists bears consideration.

GLOSSARY

ACE	angiotensin-converting enzyme
ADMA	asymmetric dimethylarginine
AGE	advanced glycosylated end product
AP	activator protein
AT_1	angiotensin II type 1 receptor
CETP	cholesterol ester transfer protein
cGK	cyclic GMP–dependent protein kinase
cGMP	guanosine 3′,5′-cyclic monophosphate
CHD	coronary heart disease
CoA	coenzyme A
CRP	C-reactive protein
COX	cyclooxygenase
CXC	cysteine X–amino acid–cysteine
DDAH	dimethylarginine dimethylaminohydrolase
DM	diabetes mellitus
eNOS	endothelial nitric oxide synthase
E-selectin	endothelial-leukocyte adhesion molecule-1, or endothelial-selectin
FUT	fucosyltransferase
GDP	guanosine diphosphate
GEF	guanine nucleotide exchange factor
GTP	guanosine 5′-triphosphate
HDL	high-density lipoprotein
HMG	3-hydroxy-3-methylglutaryl
hsCRP	high-sensitivity C-reactive protein
ICAM-1	intercellular adhesion molecule-1
Ig	immunoglobulin
IκB	inhibitory protein kappaB
IKK	IκB kinase
IL	interleukin
iNOS	inducible nitric oxide synthase
IP10	interferon-inducible protein of 10κDa
IRS	insulin receptor substrate
I-TAC	interferon-inducible T cell–alpha chemoattractant protein
JAK	Janus kinase
JNK	c-Jun NH_2-terminal kinase
LCAT	lecithin-cholesterol acyltransferase
LDL	low-density lipoprotein
Le	Lewis
Le^a	Lewis a
Le^b	Lewis b
LPS	lipopolysaccharide
MAPK	mitogen-activated protein kinase
MAPKKK	MAPK kinase kinase
MCP-1	monocyte chemotactic protein-1
M-CSF	macrophage colony-stimulating factor
MI	myocardial infarction
MIG-γ	monokine induced by interferon-γ
MLCK	myosin light chain kinase
MMP	matrix metalloproteinase
NADH/NADPH	nicotinamide adenine dinucleotide phosphate oxidase

NFκB	nuclear factor kappaB	RAGE	receptor for advanced glycosylation end products
NO	nitric oxide	RNOS	reactive nitrogen oxide species
NOS	nitric oxide synthase	ROS	reactive oxygen species
PAF	platelet-activating factor	SAA	serum amyloid A
PAI-1	plasminogen activator inhibitor-1	SAPK	stress-activated protein kinase
PGI_2	Prostacyclin	STAT	signal transducer and activator of transcription
PI3K	phosphatidylinositol 3-kinase	Thr	threonine
PIP5	phosphatidylinositol pentaphosphate	TNF	tumor necrosis factor
PKB	protein kinase B	tPA	tissue plasminogen activator
PKC	protein kinase C	VCAM-1	vascular cell adhesion molecule-1
PKN	protein kinase N	VEGF	vascular endothelial growth factor
PLTP	phospholipid transfer protein	VLDL	very-low-density lipoprotein
PPAR	peroxisome proliferator–activated receptor		
RAAS	renin-angiotensin-aldosterone system		

REFERENCES

1. Schieffer B, Drexler H. Role of 3-hydroxy-3-methylglutaryl coenzyme A reductase inhibitors, angiotensin-converting enzyme inhibitors, cyclooxygenase-2 inhibitors, and aspirin in antiinflammatory and immunomodulatory treatment of cardiovascular disease. Am J Cardiol 2003; 91(suppl):12H-18H
2. Plutzky J. The potential role of peroxisome proliferator–activated receptors on inflammation in type 2 diabetes mellitus and atherosclerosis. Am J Cardiol 2003; 92(suppl):34J-41J
3. Tham DM, Martin-McNulty B, Wang Y-X, et al. Angiotensin II is associated with activation of NF kappaB–mediated genes and downregulation of PPARs. Physiol Genomics 2002;11:21-30
4. Marette A. Mediators of cytokine-induced insulin resistance in obesity and other inflammatory settings. Curr Opin Clin Nutr Metab Care 2000;5:377-383
5. Hippenstiel S, Schmeck B, Seybold J, et al. Reduction of TNF-alpha related nuclear factor-kappaB (NF-kappaB) translocation but not inhibitor kappa-B (Ikappa-B)-degradation by Rho protein inhibition in human endothelial cells. Biochem Pharmacol 2002;64:971-977
6. Xu X, Otsuki M, Saito H, et al. PPARalpha and GR differentially down-regulate the expression of nuclear factor-kappaB–responsive genes in vascular endothelial cells. Endocrinology 2001;142:3332-3339
7. Evans JL, Goldfine ID, Maddux BA, Grodsky GM. Oxidative stress and stress-activated signaling pathways: a unifying hypothesis of type 2 diabetes. Endocr Rev 2002;23:599-622
8. Coppack SW. Pro-inflammatory cytokines and inflammatory tissue. Proc Nutr Soc 2001;60:349-356
9. Van Stick J. Interleukin-6: an overview. Annu Rev Immunol 1990;8:253-278
10. Avignon A, Monnier L. Insulinosensibilite et situations de stress. Diabetes Metab (Paris) 2001;27:233-238
11. Khovidhunkit W, Memon RA, Feingold KR, Grunfeld C. Infection and inflammation-induced proatherogenic changes of lipoproteins. J Infect Dis 2000;181:S462-S472
12. Faruqi TR, Gomez D, Bustelo XR, et al. Rac1 mediates STAT3 activation by autocrine IL-6. Proc Natl Acad Sci U S A 2001;98:9014-9019
13. Michaely PA, Mineo C, Ying YS, Anderson RG. Polarized distribution of endogenous Rac1 and RhoA at the cell surface. J Biol Chem 1999;274:21430-21436
14. Kim C, Dinauer MC. Rac2 is an essential regulator of neutrophil nicotinamide adenine dinucleotide phosphate oxidase activation in response to specific signaling pathways. J Immunol 2001;166:1223-1232
15. Gingras D, Gauthier F, Lamy S, et al. Localization of RhoA GTPase to endothelial caveolae-enriched membrane domains. Biochem Biophys Res Commun 1998;247: 888-893
16. Dechend R, Maass M, Gieffers J, et al. *Chlamydia pneumoniae* infection of vascular smooth muscle and endothelial cells activates NFκB and induces tissue factor and PAI-1 expression. Circulation 1999;100:1369-1373
17. Begum N, Sandu OA, Ito M, et al. Active Rho kinase (ROK-α) associates with insulin receptor substrate-1 and inhibits insulin signaling in vascular smooth muscle cells. J Biol Chem 2002;277:6214-6222
18. Sakurada S, Takuwa N, Sugimoto N, et al. Ca^{2+}-dependent activation of Rho and Rho kinase in membrane depolarization-induced and receptor stimulation-induced vascular smooth muscle contraction. Circ Res 2003;93: 548-556
19. Suematsu N, Satoh S, Kinugawa S, et al. Alpha1-adrenoceptor-Gq-RhoA signaling is upregulated to increase myofibrillar Ca^{2+} sensitivity in failing hearts. Am J Physiol Heart Circ Physiol 2001;281: H637-H646
20. Hunter I, Cobban HJ, Vandenabeele P, et al. Tumor necrosis factor-alpha–induced activation of RhoA in airway smooth muscle cells: role in the Ca^{2+} sensitization of myosin light chain20 phosphorylation. Mol Pharmacol 2003;63:714-721
21. Attoub S, Noe V, Pirola L, et al. Leptin promotes invasiveness of kidney and colonic epithelial cells via phosphoinositide 3-kinase-, rho-, and rac-dependent signaling pathways. FASEB J 2000;14:2329-2338
22. Mareel M, Leroy A. Clinical, cellular, and molecular aspects of cancer invasion. Physiol Rev 2003;83:337-376
23. Seko T, Ito M, Kureishi Y, et al. Activation of RhoA and inhibition of myosin phosphatase as important

components in hypertension in vascular smooth muscle. Circ Res 2003;92:411-418
24. Sauzeau V, Rolli-Derkinderen M, Lehoux S, et al. Sildenafil prevents change in RhoA expression induced by chronic hypoxia in rat pulmonary artery. Circ Res 2003;93:630-637
25. Barandier C, Ming XF, Rusconi S, Yang Z. PKC is required for activation of ROCK by RhoA in human endothelial cells. Biochem Biophys Res Commun 2003;304:714-719
26. Ito M, Barandier C, Rathgeb L, et al. Thrombin suppresses endothelial nitric oxide synthase and upregulates endothelin-converting enzyme-1 expression by distinct pathways. Role of Rho/ROCK and mitogen-activated protein kinase. Circ Res 2001;89:583-590
27. Wung BS, Cheng JJ, Shyue SK, Wang DL. NO modulates monocyte chemotactic protein-1 expression in endothelial cells under cyclic strain. Arterioscler Thromb Vasc Biol 2001;21:1941-1947
28. Brasier AR, Recinos A 3rd, Eledrisi MS. Vascular inflammation and the renin-angiotensin system. Arterioscler Thromb Vasc Biol 2002;22:1257-1266
29. Dzau VJ. Tissue renin-angiotensin system in myocardial hypertrophy and failure. Arch Intern Med 1993;153: 937-942
30. Ishizaka N, Griendling KK, Lassegue B, Alexander W. Angiotensin II type 1 receptor: relationship with caveolae and caveolin after initial agonist stimulation. Hypertension 1998;32:459-466
31. Singh BM, Mehta JL. Interactions between the renin-angiotensin system and dyslipidemia: relevance in the therapy of hypertension and coronary heart disease. Arch Intern Med 2003;163:1296-1304
32. McFarlane SI, Kumar A, Sowers JR. Mechanisms by which angiotensin-converting enzyme inhibitors prevent diabetes and cardiovascular disease. Am J Cardiol 2003;91(suppl):30H-37H
33. Rupérez M, Lorenzo O, Blanco-Colio LM, et al. Connective tissue growth factor is a mediator of angiotensin II–induced fibrosis. Circulation 2003;108:1499-1505
34. Stier CT Jr, Koenig S, Lee DY, et al. Aldosterone and aldosterone antagonism in cardiovascular disease: focus on eplerenone (inspra). Heart Dis 2003;5:102-118
35. Sun Y, Zhang J, Lu L, et al. Aldosterone-induced inflammation in the rat heart: role of oxidative stress. Am J Pathol 2002;161:1773-1781
36. Rocha R, Funder JW. The pathophysiology of aldosterone in the cardiovascular system. Ann N Y Acad Sci 2002;970:89-100
37. Rocha R, Rudolph AE, Frierdich GE, et al. Aldosterone induces a vascular inflammatory phenotype in the rat heart. Am J Physiol Heart Circ Physiol 2002;283: H1802-H1810
38. Grimble RF. Inflammatory status and insulin resistance. Curr Opin Clin Nutr Metab Care 2002;5:551-559
39. Pond CM, Mattacks CA. The source of fatty acids incorporated into proliferating lymphoid cells in immune-stimulated lymph nodes. Br J Nutr 2003;89:375-383
40. Feingold KR, Hardardottir I, Grunfeld C. Beneficial effects of cytokine induced hyperlipidemia. Z Ernahrungswiss 1998;37(suppl 1):66-74
41. Rouzer CA, Cerami A. Hypertriglyceridemia associated with *Trypanosoma brucei brucei* infection in rabbits: role of defective triglyceride removal. Med Biochem Parasitol 1980;2:31-38
42. Memon RA, Staprans I, Noor M, et al. Infection and inflammation induce LDL oxidation in vivo. Arterioscler Thromb Vasc Biol 2000;20:1536-1542
43. Pussinen PJ, Metso J, Malle E, et al. The role of plasma phospholipid transfer protein (PLTP) in HDL remodeling in acute-phase patients. Biochim Biophys Acta 2001; 1533:153-163
44. Feingold KR, Memon RA, Moser AH, et al. Endotoxin and interleukin-1 decrease hepatic lipase mRNA levels. Atherosclerosis 1999;142:379-387
45. Salazar Soler A, Pinto Sala X, Mana Rey J, Pujol Farriols R. Inflammatory response, cholesterol metabolism, and arteriosclerosis. An Med Interna 2001;18:100-104
46. Khovidhunkit W, Shigenaga JK, Moser AH, et al. Cholesterol efflux by acute-phase high density lipoprotein: role of lecithin:cholesterol acyltransferase. J Lipid Res 2001;42:967-975
47. Mazzone A, De Servi S, Ricevuti G, et al. Increased expression of neutrophil and myocyte adhesion molecules in unstable coronary artery disease. Circulation 1993;88:358-363
48. Sinisalo J, Paronen J, Mattila KJ, et al. Relation of inflammation to vascular function in patients with coronary heart disease. Atherosclerosis 2000;149:403-411
49. Hingorani AD, Cross J, Kharbanda RK, et al. Acute systemic inflammation impairs endothelium-dependent dilatation in humans. Circulation 2002;102:994-999
50. Aljada A, Ghanim H, Assian E, Dandona P. Tumor necrosis factor-alpha inhibits insulin-induced increase in endothelial nitric oxide synthase and reduces insulin receptor content and phosphorylation in human aortic endothelial cells. Metabolism 2002;51:487-491
51. Paz Y, Frolkis I, Pevni D, et al. Effect of tumor necrosis factor-alpha on endothelial and inducible nitric oxide synthase messenger ribonucleic acid expression and nitric oxide synthesis in ischemic and nonischemic isolated rat hearts. J Am Coll Cardiol 2003;42:1299-1305
52. Kim F, Gallis B, Corson MA. TNF-alpha inhibits flow and insulin signaling leading to NO production in aortic endothelial cells. Am J Physiol Cell Physiol 2001; 280:C1057-C1065
53. Greenberg S, Xie J, Wang Y, et al. Tumor necrosis factor-alpha inhibits endothelium-dependent relaxation. J Appl Physiol 1993;74:2394-2403
54. Ito A, Tsao PS, Adimoolam S, et al. Novel mechanism for endothelial dysfunction: dysregulation of dimethylarginine dimethylaminohydrolase. Circulation 1999;99: 3092-3095
55. Steinberg HO, Tarshoby M, Monestel R, et al. Elevated circulating free fatty acid levels impair endothelium-dependent vasodilation. J Clin Invest 1997;100:1230-1239
56. Kahaleh MB, Fan PS. Effect of cytokines on production of endothelin by endothelial cells. Clin Exp Rheumatol 1997;15:163-167
57. Brasier AR, Li J, Wimbish KA. Tumor necrosis factor activates angiotensinogen gene expression by the Rel A transactivator. Hypertension 1996;27:1009-1017
58. Munzel T, Feil R, Mulsch A, et al. Physiology and pathophysiology of vascular signaling controlled by cyclic guanosine 3′,5′-cyclic monophosphate–dependent protein kinase. Circulation 2003;108:2172-2183
59. Venugopal SK, Devaraj S, Yuhanna I, et al. Demonstration that C-reactive protein decreases eNOS expression and bioactivity in human aortic endothelial cells. Circulation 2002;106:1439-1441
60. Jarvisalo MJ, Harmoinen A, Hakanen M, et al. Elevated serum C-reactive protein levels and early arterial changes in healthy children. Arterioscler Thromb Vasc Biol 2002;22:1323-1328
61. Fichtlscherer S, Rosenberger G, Walter DH, et al. Elevated C-reactive protein levels and impaired endothelial vasoreactivity in patients with coronary artery disease. Circulation 2000;102:1000-1006
62. Blum A, Schneider DJ, Sobel, BE, Dauerman HL. Endothelial dysfunction and inflammation after

percutaneous coronary intervention. Am J Cardiol 2004;94:1420-1423
63. Laufs U, Endres M, Liao JK. Regulation of endothelial NO production by Rho GTPase. Med Klin (Munich) 1999;94:211-218
64. Fichtlscherer S, Breuer S, Heeschen C, et al. Interleukin-10 serum levels and systemic endothelial vasoreactivity in patients with coronary artery disease. J Am Coll Cardiol 2004;44:44-49
65. Mills R, Bhatt DL. The yin and yang of arterial inflammation. J Am Coll Cardiol 2004;44:50-52
66. Ridker PM. High-sensitivity C-reactive protein and cardiovascular risk: rationale for screening and primary prevention. Am J Cardiol 2003;92(suppl):17K-22K
67. Ventura HO. Rudolph Virchow and cellular pathology. Clin Cardiol 2002;23:550-552
68. Ross R. Atherosclerosis: an inflammatory disease. N Engl J Med 1999;340:115-126
69. Libby P. Vascular biology of atherosclerosis: overview and state of the art. Am J Cardiol 2003;91(suppl):3A-6A
70. Yudkin JS, Stehouwer CD, Emeis JJ, Coppack SW. C-reactive protein in healthy subjects: associations with obesity, insulin resistance, and endothelial dysfunction: a potential role for cytokines originating from adipose tissue? Arterioscler Thromb Vasc Biol 1999;19:972-978
71. Libby P. Inflammation in atherosclerosis. Nature 2002; 420:868-874
72. Jackson SM, Parhami F, Xi XP, et al. Peroxisome proliferator–activated receptor activators target human endothelial cells to inhibit leukocyte-endothelial cell interaction. Arterioscler Thromb Vasc Biol 1999;19:2094-2104
73. Duval C, Chinetti G, Trottein F, et al. The role of PPARs in atherosclerosis. Trends Mol Med 2002;8:422-430
74. Kaartinen M, Pentilla A, Kovanen PT. Accumulation of activated mast cells in the shoulder region of coronary atheroma, the predilection site of atheromatous rupture. Circulation 1994;90:1669-1678
75. Benbow U, Brinckerhoff CE. The AP-1 site and MMP gene regulation: what is all the fuss about? Matrix Biol 1997:15:519-526
76. Ardehali H. The inflammatory progression of an atherosclerotic plaque. Cardiol News Issues New Millennium 2004;4:3-4
77. Uemura S, Matsushita H, Li W, et al. Diabetes mellitus enhances vascular matrix metalloproteinase activity: role of oxidative stress. Circ Res 2001;88:1291-1298
78. Dandona P, Aljada A. A rational approach to pathogenesis and treatment of type 2 diabetes mellitus, insulin resistance, inflammation, and atherosclerosis. Am J Cardiol 2002;90(suppl):27G-33G
79. Mackman N. Regulation of the tissue factor gene. FASEB J 1995;9:883-889
80. Folsom AR. Fibrinolytic factors and atherothrombotic events: epidemiological evidence. Ann Med 2000;32 (suppl 1):85-91
81. Carroll MF, Schade DS. Timing of antioxidant vitamin ingestion alters postprandial proatherogenic serum markers. Circulation 2003;108:24-31
82. Festa A, D'Agostino R, Mykkanen L, et al. Relative contribution of insulin and its precursors to fibrinogen and PAI-1 in a large population with different states of glucose tolerance: the Insulin Resistance Atherosclerosis Study (IRAS). Arterioscler Thromb Vasc Biol 1999;19:562-568
83. Meigs JB, Mittleman MA, Nathan DM, et al. Hyperinsulinemia, hyperglycemia, and impaired hemostasis: The Framingham Offspring Study. JAMA 2000;283:221-228
84. Festa A, D'Agostino RJ, Howard G, et al. Chronic subclinical inflammation as part of the insulin resistance syndrome: the Insulin Resistance Atherosclerosis Study (IRAS). Circulation 2000;102:42-47
85. Pickup JC, Crook MA. Is type II diabetes mellitus a disease of the innate immune system? Diabetologia 1998;41: 1241-1248
86. Marette A. Mediators of cytokine-induced insulin resistance in obesity and other inflammatory settings. Curr Opin Clin Nutr Metab Care 2000;5:377-383
87. Hak AE, Pols HA, Stehouwer CD, et al. Markers of inflammation and cellular adhesion molecules in relation to insulin resistance in nondiabetic elderly: the Rotterdam study. J Clin Endocrinol Metab 2001;86: 4398-4405
88. Festa A, Hanley AJG, Tracy RP, et al. Inflammation in the prediabetic state is related to increased insulin resistance rather than decreased insulin secretion. Circulation 2003;108:1822-1830
89. Helmersson J, Vessby B, Larsson A, Basu S. Association of type 2 diabetes with cyclooxygenase-mediated inflammation and oxidative stress in an elderly population. Circulation 2004;109:1729-1734
90. Meigs JB, Hu FB, Rifai N, Manson JE. Biomarkers of endothelial dysfunction and risk of type 2 diabetes mellitus. JAMA 2004;291:1978-1986
91. Duncan BB, Schmidt MI. Chronic activation of the innate immune system may underlie the metabolic syndrome. Sao Paulo Med J 2001;119:122-127
92. Stern MP. Diabetes and cardiovascular disease: the "common soil" hypothesis. Diabetes 1995;44:369-374
93. Hsueh WA, Law R. The central role of fat and effect of peroxisome proliferator–activated receptor-gamma on progression of insulin resistance and cardiovascular disease. Am J Cardiol 2003;92(suppl):3J-9J
94. Dibbs Z, Thornby J, White BG, Mann DL. Natural variability of circulating cytokines and cytokine receptors in patients with heart failure: implications for clinical trials. J Am Coll Cardiol 1999;33:1935-1942
95. Cesari M, Penninx BWJH, Newman AB, et al. Inflammatory markers and cardiovascular disease (the Health, Aging and Body Composition (Health ABC) Study). Am J Cardiol 2003;92:522-528
96. Ridker PM, Rifai N, Pfeffer M, et al. Elevation of tumor necrosis factor-alpha and increased risk of recurrent coronary events after myocardial infarction. Circulation 2000;101:2149-2153
97. Cesari M, Penninx BW, Newman AB, et al. Inflammatory markers and onset of cardiovascular events: results from the Health ABC study. Circulation 2003;108: 2317-2322
98. Pradhan AD, Manson JE, Rossouw JE, et al. Inflammatory biomarkers, hormone replacement therapy, and incident coronary heart disease: prospective analysis from the Women's Health Initiative observational study. JAMA 2002;288:980-987
99. Ridker PM, Rifai N, Rose L, et al. Comparison of C-reactive protein and low-density lipoprotein cholesterol levels in the prediction of first cardiovascular events. N Engl J Med 2003;347:1557-1565
100. Lundman P, Eriksson MJ, Silveira A, et al. Relation of hypertriglyceridemia to plasma concentrations of biochemical markers of inflammation and endothelial activation. Am J Cardiol 2003;91:1128-1131
101. Pepys MB, Hirschfield GM. C-reactive protein: a critical update. J Clin Invest 2003;111:1805-1812
102. Tall AR. C-reactive protein reassessed. N Engl J Med 2004;350:1450-1452
103. Kinlay S, Schwartz GG, Olsson AG, et al. High-dose atorvastatin enhances the decline in inflammatory markers in patients with acute coronary syndromes in the MIRACL Study. Circulation 2003;108:1560-1566
104. Pearson TA, Mensah GA, Alexander RW, et al. Markers of inflammation and cardiovascular disease: application

to clinical and public health practice: a statement for healthcare professionals from the Centers for Disease Control and Prevention and the American Heart Association. Circulation 2003;107:499-511
105. Yeh ET, Willerson JT. Coming of age of C-reactive protein: using inflammation markers in cardiology. Circulation 2003;107:370-371
106. Ridker PM, Haughie P. Prospective studies of C-reactive protein as risk factor for cardiovascular disease. J Invest Med 1988;46:391-395
107. Pai JK, Pischon T, Ma J, et al. Inflammatory markers and the risk of coronary heart disease in men and women. N Engl J Med 2004;351:2599-2610
108. Koenig W, Lowel H, Baumert J, Meisinger C. C-reactive protein modulates risk prediction based on the Framingham Score: implications for future risk assessment: results from a large cohort study in Southern Germany. Circulation 2004;109:1349-1353
109. Blake GJ, Ridker PM. Inflammatory bio-markers and cardiovascular risk prediction. J Intern Med 2002; 252:283-294
110. Jabs WJ, Theissing E, Nitschke M, et al. Local generation of C-reactive protein in diseased coronary artery venous bypass grafts and normal vascular tissue. Circulation 2003;108:1428-1431
111. Verma S, Kuliszewski MA, Li S-H, et al. C-reactive protein attenuates endothelial progenitor cell survival, differentiation, and function. Further evidence of a mechanistic link between C-reactive protein and cardiovascular disease. Circulation 2004;109:2058-2067
112. Hattori Y, Matsumura M, Kasai K. Vascular smooth muscle cell activation by C-reactive protein. Cardiovasc Res 2003;58:186-195
113. Venugopal SK, Devaraj S, Jialal I. C-reactive protein decreases prostacyclin release from human aortic endothelial cells. Circulation 2003;108:1676-1678
114. Danesh J, Whincup P, Walker M, et al. Low-grade inflammation and coronary heart disease: prospective study and updated meta-analysis. BMJ 2000;321:199-204
115. Pasceri V, Willerson JT, Yeh ET. Direct proinflammatory effect of C-reactive protein on human endothelial cells. Circulation 2000;102:2165-2168
116. Chambers JC, Eda S, Bassett P, et al. C-reactive protein, insulin resistance, central obesity, and coronary heart disease risk in Indian Asians from the United Kingdom compared with European whites. Circulation 2001; 104:145-150
117. Greenfield JR, Samaras K, Jenkins AB, et al. Obesity is an important determinant of baseline serum C-reactive protein concentration in monozygotic twins, independent of genetic influences. Circulation 2004; 109:3022-3028
118. Forouhi NG, Sattar N, McKeigue PM. Relation of C-reactive protein to body fat distribution and features of the metabolic syndrome in Europeans and South Asians. Int J Obes Relat Metab Disord 2001;25:1327-1331
119. Weisberg SP, McCann D, Desai M, et al. Obesity is associated with macrophage accumulation in adipose tissue. J Clin Invest 2003;112:1796-1808
120. Pannacciuli N, Cantatore FP, Minenna A, et al. C-reactive protein is independently associated with total body fat, central fat, and insulin resistance in adult women. Int J Obes Relat Metab Disord 2001;25:1416-1420
121. Rutter MK, Meigs JB, Sullivan LM, et al. C-reactive protein, the metabolic syndrome, and prediction of cardiovascular events in the Framingham Offspring Study. Circulation 2004;110:380-385
122. De Feo P, Volpi E, Lucidi P, et al. Physiological increments in plasma insulin concentrations have selective and different effects on synthesis of hepatic proteins in normal humans. Diabetes 1993;42:995-1002
123. Campos SP, Baumann H. Insulin is a prominent modulator of the cytokine-stimulated expression of acute-phase plasma protein genes. Mol Cell Biol 1992;12:1789-1797
124. Frohlich M, Imhof A, Berg G, et al. Association between C-reactive protein and features of the metabolic syndrome: a population based study. Diabetes Care 2000;23:1835-1839
125. Festa A, D'Agostino R, Tracy RP, Haffner SM. Elevated levels of acute-phase proteins and plasminogen activator inhibitor-1 predict the development of type 2 diabetes mellitus: the Insulin Resistance Atherosclerosis Study (IRAS). Diabetes 2002;51:1131-1137
126. Barzilay JI, Abraham L, Heckbert SR, et al. The relation of markers of inflammation to the development of glucose disorders in the elderly: the Cardiovascular Health Study. Diabetes 2001;50:2384-2389
127. Folsom AR, Wu KK, Rosamond WD, et al. Prospective study of hemostatic factors and incidence of coronary heart disease: the Atherosclerotic Risk in Communities (ARIC) Study. Circulation 1997;96:1102-1108
128. Pradhan AD, Manson JE, Rifai N, et al. C-reactive protein, interleukin-6, and risk of developing type 2 diabetes mellitus. JAMA 2001;286:327-334
129. Thorand B, Lowel H, Schneider A, et al. C-reactive protein as a predictor for incident diabetes mellitus among middle-aged men: results from the MONICA Augsburg cohort study, 1984-1998. Arch Intern Med 2003;163:93-99
130. Sattar N, Gaw A, Scherbakova O, et al. Metabolic syndrome with and without C-reactive protein as a predictor of coronary heart disease and diabetes in the West of Scotland Coronary Prevention Study. Circulation 2003;108:414-419
131. Messerli AW, Seshadri N, Pearce GL, et al. Relation of albumin/creatinine ratio to C-reactive protein and to the metabolic syndrome. Am J Cardiol 2003;92: 610-612
132. Ridker PM, Buring JE, Cook NR, Rifai N. C-reactive protein, the metabolic syndrome, and risk of incident cardiovascular events: an 8-year follow-up of 14 719 initially healthy American women. Circulation 2003; 107:391-397
133. Lowe GD. The relationship between infection, inflammation, and cardiovascular disease: an overview. Ann Periodontol 2001;6:1-8
134. Toplak H, Wascher TC, Weber K, et al. Increased prevalence of serum IgA *Chlamydia* antibodies in obesity. Acta Med Austriaca 1995;22:23-24
135. Swan JW, Walton C, Godsland IF, et al. Insulin resistance in chronic heart failure. Eur Heart J 1994;15:1528-1532
136. Taegtmeyer H, McNulty P, Young ME. Adaptation and maladaptation of the heart in diabetes, part I: general concepts. Circulation 2002;105:1727-1733
137. Dessein PH, Stanwix AE, Joffe BI. Cardiovascular risk in rheumatoid arthritis versus osteoarthritis: acute phase response related decreased insulin sensitivity and high-density lipoprotein cholesterol as well as clustering of metabolic syndrome features in rheumatoid arthritis. Arthritis Res 2002;4:R5
138. Witteles RM, Tang WHW, Jamali AH, et al. Insulin resistance in idiopathic dilated cardiomyopathy: a possible etiologic link. J Am Coll Cardiol 2004;44:78-81
139. Kiechl S, Egger G, Mayr M, et al. Chronic infections and the risk of carotid atherosclerosis: prospective results from a large population study. Circulation 2001;103: 1064-1070

140. Pasceri V, Cammarota G, Patti G, et al. Association of virulent *Helicobacter pylori* strains with ischemic heart disease. Circulation 1998;97:1675-1679
141. Folsom AR, Nieto FJ, Sorlie P, et al. *Helicobacter pylori* seropositivity and coronary heart disease incidence. Atherosclerosis Risk in Communities (ARIC) Study Investigators. Circulation 1998;98:845-850
142. Fryer RH, Schwobe EP, Woods ML, et al. Chlamydia species infect human vascular endothelial cells and induce procoagulant activity. J Invest Med 1997;45:168-174
143. Moazed TC, Kuo C, Grayston JT, et al. Murine models of *Chlamydia pneumoniae* infection and atherosclerosis. J Infect Dis 1997;175:883-890
144. Saikku P, Leinonen M, Mattila K, et al. Serological evidence of an association of a novel *Chlamydia*, TWAR, with chronic coronary heart disease and acute myocardial infarction. Lancet 1988;2:983-986
145. Huittinen T, Leinonen M, Tenkanen L, et al. Synergistic effect of persistent *Chlamydia pneumoniae* infection, autoimmunity, and inflammation on coronary risk. Circulation 2003;107:2566-2570
146. Ramirez JA, *Chlamydia pneumoniae*/Atherosclerosis Study Group. Isolation of *Chlamydia pneumoniae* from the coronary artery of a patient with coronary atherosclerosis. Ann Intern Med 1996;125:979-982
147. Dechend R, Gieffers J, Dietz R, et al. Hydroxymethylglutaryl coenzyme A reductase inhibition reduces *Chlamydia pneumoniae*–induced cell interaction and activation. Circulation 2003;108:261-265
148. Iacopino AM. Periodontitis and diabetes interrelationships: role of inflammation. Ann Periodontol 2001;6:125-137
149. Donahue RP, Wu T. Insulin resistance and periodontal disease: an epidemiologic overview of research needs and future directions. Ann Periodontol 2001;1:119-124
150. Hung H, Willett W, Merchant A, et al. Oral health and peripheral arterial disease. Circulation 2003;107: 1152-1157
151. Deliargyris E, Madianos P, Kadoma W, et al. Periodontal disease in patients with acute myocardial infarction: prevalence and contribution to elevated C-reactive protein levels. Am Heart J 2004;147:1005-1009
152. Page RC. The pathobiology of periodontal diseases may affect systemic diseases: inversion of a paradigm. Ann Periodontol 1998;3:108-120
153. Slade GD, Ghezzi EM, Heiss G, et al. Relationship between periodontal disease and C-reactive protein among adults in the Atherosclerosis Risk in Communities Study. Arch Intern Med 2003;163:1172-1179
154. Stone AFM, Mendall MA, Kaski JC, et al. Effect of treatment for *Chlamydia pneumoniae* and *Helicobacter pylori* on markers of inflammation and cardiac events in patients with acute coronary syndromes. South Thames Trial of Antibiotics in Myocardial Infarction and Unstable Angina Pectoris (STAMINA). Circulation 2002;106:1219-1223
155. Iwamoto Y, Nishimura F, Nakagawa M, et al. The effect of antimicrobial periodontal treatment on circulating tumor necrosis factor-alpha and glycated hemoglobin level in patients with type 2 diabetes. J Periodontol 2001;72:774-778
156. Grossi SG. Treatment of periodontal disease and control of diabetes: an assessment of the evidence and need for future research. Ann Periodontol 2001;6:138-145
157. Hegazy DM, O'Reilly DA, Yang BM, et al. NFkappaB polymorphisms and susceptibility to type 1 diabetes. Genes Immun 2001;2:304-308
158. D'Adamo PJ, Kelly GS. Metabolic and immunologic consequences of ABH secretor and Lewis subtype status. Altern Med Rev 2001;6:390-405
159. Rad R, Gerhard M, Lang R. The *Helicobacter pylori* blood group antigen–binding adhesion facilitates bacterial colonization and augments a nonspecific immune response. J Immunol 2002;168:3033-3041
160. Hein HO, Sorensen H, Suadicani P, Gyntelberg F. The Lewis blood group—a new genetic marker of ischaemic heart disease. J Intern Med 1992;232:481-487
161. Ellison RC, Zhang Y, Myers RH, et al. Lewis blood group phenotype as an independent risk factor for coronary heart disease (the NHLBI Family Heart Study). Am J Cardiol 1999;83:345-348
162. Zhiburt BB, Chepel' AI, Serebrianaia NB, et al. The Lewis antigen system as a marker of IHD risk. Ter Arkh 1997;69:29-31
163. Slavchev S, Tsoneva M, Zakhariev Z. The secretory type of persons who have survived a myocardial infarct. Vutr Boles 1989;28:31-34
164. Angiolillo DJ, Liuzzo G, Pelliccioni S, et al. Combined role of the Lewis antigenic system, *Chlamydia pneumoniae*, and C-reactive protein in unstable angina. J Am Coll Cardiol 2003;41:546-550
165. Clausen JO, Hein HO, Suadicani P, et al. Lewis phenotypes and the insulin resistance syndrome in young healthy white men and women. Am J Hypertens 1995;11:1060-1066
166. Petit JM, Morvan Y, Mansuy-Collignon S, et al. Hypertriglyceridaemia and Lewis (A–B–) phenotype in non–insulin-dependent diabetic patients. Diabetes Metab 1997;23:202-204
167. Green D, Jarrett O, Ruth KJ, et al. Relationship among Lewis phenotype, clotting factors, and other cardiovascular risk factors in young adults. J Lab Clin Med 1995;125:334-339
168. Salomaa V, Pankow J, Heiss G, et al. Genetic background of Lewis negative blood group phenotype and its association with atherosclerotic disease in the NHLBI family heart study. J Intern Med 2000;247: 689-698
169. Petit JM, Morvan Y, Viviani V, et al. Insulin resistance syndrome and Lewis phenotype in healthy men and women. Horm Metab Res 1997;29:193-195
170. Hein HO, Sorensen H, Suadicani P, Gyntelberg F. Alcohol consumption, Lewis phenotypes, and risk of ischaemic heart disease. Lancet 1993;341:392-396
171. Caballero AE, Arora S, Saouaf R, et al. Microvascular and macrovascular reactivity is reduced in subjects at risk for type 2 diabetes. Diabetes 1999;48:1856-1862
172. Pinkney JH, Stehouwer CD, Coppack SW, Yudkin JS. Endothelial dysfunction: cause of the insulin resistance syndrome. Diabetes 1997;46(suppl 2):S9-S13
173. Widlansky ME, Gokce N, Keaney JJ, Vita JA. The clinical implications of endothelial dysfunction. J Am Coll Cardiol 2003;42:1149-1160
174. Park H, Go YM, St John PL, et al. Plasma membrane cholesterol is a key molecule in shear stress–dependent activation of extracellular signal–regulated kinase. J Biol Chem 1998;273:32304-32311
175. Murphy HS, Bakopoulos N, Dame MK, et al. Heterogeneity of vascular endothelial cells: differences in susceptibility to neutrophil-mediated injury. Microvasc Res 1998;56:203-211
176. Otto M, Bittinger F, Kriegsmann J, Kirkpatrick CJ. Differential adhesion of polymorphous neutrophilic granulocytes to macro- and microvascular endothelial cells under flow conditions. Pathobiology 2001;69:159-171
177. Vita JA, Keaney JF, Larson MG, et al. Brachial artery vasodilator function and systemic inflammation in the Framingham Offspring Study. Circulation 2004;110: 3604-3609

Mental Stress and the Metabolic Syndrome

4

A stressor is an endogenous or exogenous stimulus that constitutes a perceived or a real threat to an individual's well-being. Stressors disturb the physiologic or psychological homeostasis of an individual and engender emotional and physiologic distress responses.[1]

Stressors are omnipresent in our world. The cover story of *Time Magazine* for June 6, 1983, termed stress "The Epidemic of the Eighties." Clearly, the impact of stress has continued to grow over the ensuing decades. Stress may pervade the home, personal and family relationships, the workplace, and financial and economic issues, as well as regional, national, and international sociopolitical situations. Job stress is the leading source of stress for adults, but stress levels have also escalated for the elderly, as well as for children, teenagers, and students, for whom academic and peer pressure plays a significant role. Media attention to national and international accidents, crime, violence, terror, conflicts, natural disasters, and other challenges to personal safety has drastically increased external stressors. Personal coping mechanisms have been undermined as a result of social isolation and loneliness arising from the erosion of family ties, the loss of stable neighborhoods, and pervasive moral and religious relativism exacerbating an individual's stress experience. **Contemporary stress, devolving primarily from a psychological reaction to threat, is more insidious, pervasive, and persistent than the temporary stress response to the physical menaces of the past.**[1]

Physiologic stress responses are, however, elicited not only in response to extraordinarily stressful events. There is a natural, underlying diurnal rhythm to stress responses, and banal factors such as interrupted sleep, exercise, alcohol consumption, or smoking elicit a hormonal stress response.[1]

ACUTE AND CHRONIC STRESS

The stress response temporarily empowers an individual to confront stressful challenges.

Physiologic Changes with Acute Stress. The distress response musters speedy and effective responses to acute environmental threats in order to reestablish physiologic and psychological balance and homeostasis. As a result of these physiologic changes, there is ready fuel available for the hyperdynamic cardiovascular response and for the immune tissues to implement an effective fight-or-flight response.[1] With acute stress, there is

- a catecholamine and angiotensin II surge,
- impaired arterial compliance,
- an attendant increase in pulse pressure,
- tachycardia,
- shallow respiration,
- an increase in insulin resistance,
- inducible nitric oxide (NO) release,
- alteration in immune function,
- interruption of nonessential functions such as growth, and
- enhancement of mental alertness, memory, and sensory perception.

Pathophysiologic Effects of Chronic Stress. Although the acute stress reaction to a sudden menace is of survival benefit, it turns maladaptive when chronically sustained in response to protracted, stressful stimuli and prolonged mental stress.[1]

Stress-Sensitive Conditions. Chronic stress responses do not cause specific diseases. However, **chronic stress pathways may variably contribute to the pathogenesis, exacerbation, and prolongation of stress-sensitive pathologies** underlying

- chronic anxiety,
- depression,
- memory impairment,
- chronic fatigue syndrome,
- sexual dysfunction,
- overweight,
- hypertension,
- osteoporosis,
- irritable colon,
- Graves' disease,
- multiple sclerosis,
- fibromyalgia,
- myofascial pain syndrome, and
- rheumatoid arthritis.

There are also psychosomatic underpinnings to conditions such as

- asthma,
- peptic ulcers, and
- allergies,

and stress-induced impairment of the immune system may render an individual more vulnerable to infections and malignancy.[1]

Cardiometabolic Diseases. Chronic stress plays a role in cardiovascular and metabolic diseases.

Coronary Heart Disease. The presence of psychosocial stressors is associated with an increased risk for coronary heart disease (CHD) and acute myocardial infarction.

In animal models, stress causes the development of atherosclerosis.[2] From an epidemiologic perspective, stress has an adverse impact on the development and progression of CHD and carotid artery disease.[3,4] The National Health and Nutrition Examination Survey (NHANES) I and the National Health Examination Survey (NHES) suggested an association between stress caused by a lack of control at work plus a low decision latitude and an increased prevalence of myocardial infarction.[1] In a case-control study of 11,119 patients with a first myocardial infarction and 13,648 age- and sex-matched controls from five continents, psychosocial stress related to work, home, financial issues, and major life events was assessed. Patients with myocardial infarction had a higher prevalence of all four stress factors ($P < .0001$). Permanent stress had a greater impact than periodic stress did. These differences applied to men and women and were consistent across all regions and ethnic groups. Odds ratios for acute myocardial infarction were 2.14, 2.12, 2.17, 1.33, 1.48, and 1.55 for permanent stress related to work, home, home and work, finances, life events, and depression, respectively.[5] The association of mental stress with ischemic events has been supported by a number of other studies.[6-8]

The Metabolic Syndrome. Environmental pressure may contribute to overweight and the metabolic syndrome.[9,10] Since the 1990s, rather than being a coincidental finding, the association between abdominal obesity and insulin resistance has been thought to have an underlying neuroendocrine basis. In genetically susceptible individuals, the cause of metabolic syndrome is psychosocial factors in 5% to 37% of cases and health-related behavior in only 5% to 15%.[11]

Individual Variability in Stress Sensitivity. There are clearly significant differences among individuals regarding their sensitivity to stress. Whereas one person may thrive under a particular set of circumstances, another may develop or suffer an exacerbation of a stress-related condition. Furthermore, purportedly stress-related conditions are rather diverse. **The physiologic stress response and the pathologic manifestations of stress may vary,** depending on an individual's

- genetic makeup,
- intrauterine and early childhood experiences,
- upbringing and education,
- age,
- sex,
- emotional status,
- diverse sensitivity to stressors,
- social acceptability,
- coping mechanisms, and
- comorbid conditions.[1,12,13]

STRESS RESPONSES

Neuroendocrine Stress Responses. Hypothalamic arousal by physical or mental stressors will result in the "fright-flight-fight" response. It may, however, make a difference what response is engendered by the "fright" arousal.

Active Response. An active, defensive "fight" response with regained control is mediated via

- vagal withdrawal,
- sympathetic pathways with catecholamine release,
- activation of the renin-angiotensin system, and
- cortisol secretion,

in order to increase circulatory hemodynamic readiness and mobilize the supporting energy substrate.[14] In animal models, testosterone secretion is increased in males[12] and has an effect on the animal's appearance: a successful, dominant male lion has the darkest mane.

Passive Response. In contrast to the active "fight" response, a passive, "fright"-engendered "flight" response gives rise to loss of control, submission, and a defeatist, depressive reaction characterized by

- hyperactivity of the hypothalamic-pituitary-adrenal (HPA) axis,
- hypercortisolism, and
- impairment of sex hormone function.[14]

A defeatist stress reaction occurs in a chronically stressed mouse model.[15] In a primate animal model, mild, yet continuous psychosocial stress caused by failed rank-order challenges in monkeys at the bottom of the social hierarchy engenders

- abdominal ponderosity,
- insulin resistance,
- hyperlipidemia,

- hypertension,
- early signs of diabetes mellitus (DM), and
- cardiovascular disease.[16]

Mental Stress Pathways. Stress engages the central nervous system by activation of physiologic and behavioral responses. There is involvement of the hippocampus and amygdala in the limbic system,[14] as well as the hypothalamus and brainstem.

The Hippocampus. The hippocampus participates in modulating contextual memory of strong emotional import. Hippocampal analysis serves a triage function. It analyzes the threat potential of a stimulus to determine whether the HPA axis requires activation or inhibition. Intact function of the hippocampus is critical for negative glucocorticoid feedback control to be effective.[17]

The Amygdala. The amygdala is the principal mediator of the stress response. It is involved in the perception and response to fear-provoking stimuli and is central to aggression. As the sensory and higher reasoning centers in the cerebral cortex perceive a threat, they communicate with the amygdala to coordinate stress and aversive behavior and modulate memory in a fear-producing context.[18]

The Hypothalamus and Brainstem. Centrally perceived stress is processed by two pathways:

1. the parvicellular corticotropin-releasing hormone (CRH)/arginine vasopressin (AVP) neurons of the paraventricular nuclei of the hypothalamus and
2. the noradrenergic neurons of the locus ceruleus/norepinephrine nuclei of the brainstem.

The hypothalamic CRH/AVP and the brainstem noradrenergic loci, in turn, stimulate

- the mesocorticolimbic dopaminergic system to mediate anticipatory and award phenomena and
- the amygdala.

As the name implies, **the CRH/AVP neuronal response to stress generates increased paraventricular nuclear–hypothalamic secretion of**

- **corticotropin-releasing hormone**: CRH activates the HPA axis and stimulates the pituitary production of corticotropin, also termed adrenocorticotropic hormone (ACTH). ACTH, in turn, stimulates the adrenal production of cortisol.[1]
- **arginine vasopressin**: AVP suppresses urine production, supports hemodynamic stability, and serves to potentiate CRH activity.

The noradrenergic neurons of the locus ceruleus/norepinephrine nuclei of the brainstem stimulate the sympathoadrenal system (Fig. 4-1).

These CRH-hypothalamic and noradrenergic brainstem pathways also innervate and stimulate each other to effect the peripheral physiologic responses mediated by the autonomic nervous system, the adrenals, or the gonads.[17,19] Thus, CRH activates not only the HPA axis but also the sympathoadrenal system: CRH increases norepinephrine synthesis by enhancing tyrosine hydrolase activity, and it increases both the firing rate and norepinephrine release from the locus ceruleus.[1] **Both the hypothalamic and brainstem loci effectively improve arousal, mood, memory, and attention during the acute response to stress.**

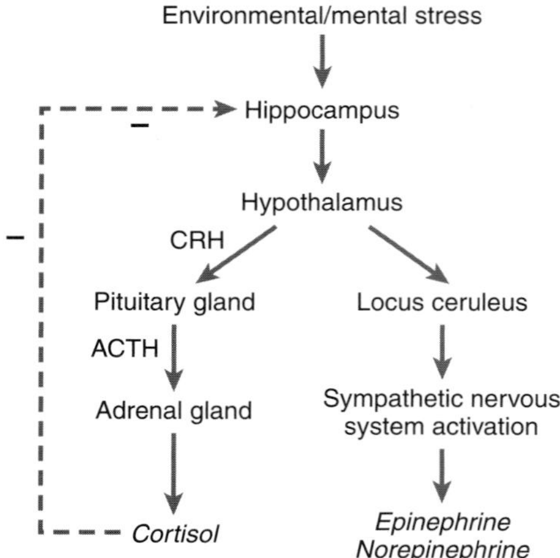

▸▸ **Figure 4–1.**
Activation of the hypothalamic-pituitary-adrenal axis and the sympathetic nervous system by mental stress in the hypothalamic and hippocampal regions of the brain. ACTH, adrenocorticotropic hormone; CRH, corticotropin-releasing hormone. *(Modified from Bjoerntorp P, Holm G, Rosmond R. Neuroendocrine disorders cause stress-related disease. "Civilization syndrome" is a growing health problem. Lakartidningen 1999;8:893-896.)*

STRESS AND THE HYPOTHALAMIC-PITUITARY-ADRENOCORTICAL AXIS

Normal Hypothalamic-Pituitary-Adrenocortical Function. Normal HPA function is characterized by a high variability of diurnal cortisol secretion. There are high morning, low evening plasma cortisol levels, with small, discrete elevations in response to feeding, and a sensitive dexamethasone suppression test.[20]

Stimulants of Hypothalamic-Pituitary-Adrenocortical Activation. In addition to the normal stimulants of diurnal HPA axis activation, **significant causes of HPA activation and sensitization are stress responses characterized by a sense of helplessness, defeat, depression, or anxiety. Physical stressors such as pain, cold, starvation, physical exertion, chronic infection, and toxins such as excessive alcohol and cigarette consumption are also implicated.**[20]

Interestingly, interleukin-6 (IL-6) as an inflammatory mediator stimulates the HPA axis.[21]

Chronic Hypothalamic-Pituitary-Adrenocortical Activation: Sensitization and Deterioration of the Axis. With sustained stress activation of the HPA axis, increased stress-related cortisol secretion engenders ponderosity with anthropometric and metabolic perturbations suggestive of the early metabolic syndrome. The HPA axis itself becomes hypersensitive as the ACTH and secondary cortisol responses to CRH and AVP become exaggerated.[20]

Over time, the HPA axis deteriorates. Observations in chronically stressed animals demonstrate a progressive change in HPA function. As a result of a protracted reaction to stress, HPA function is eventually characterized by low variability. Morning cortisol levels are low; in contrast, the evening nadir becomes elevated, and there is a rigid cortisol secretion pattern throughout the day with only small feeding responses and a blunted dexamethasone suppression test.[20] However, **time-integrated diurnal cortisol secretion is increased.**[19]

Sequelae of Hypothalamic-Pituitary-Adrenocortical Dysfunction over Time. The metabolic milieu of a dysfunctional HPA axis with effective hypercortisolism is conducive to the development of ponderosity, insulin resistance, and the metabolic syndrome.[1,19] There are associated metabolic alterations with elevations in

- plasma insulin,
- glucose,
- triglycerides,
- low-density lipoprotein (LDL) cholesterol,
- blood pressure, and
- heart rate,

whereas high-density lipoprotein (HDL) levels are low.[20] Furthermore, there is inhibition of the growth, thyroid, and reproductive axes and a rise in the plasma leptin concentration.[11,22]

The hormonal impact of a dysfunctional HPA axis may change over time. **Whereas hypercortisolism plays a role early on, with long-standing stress the HPA axis may eventually "burn out" and engender a decline in cortisol secretion. At that point, diminished sex and human growth hormone levels may adversely affect insulin resistance.**[20]

Hypothalamic-Pituitary-Adrenocortical Axis Feedback with Stress. Normally, excessive systemic cortisol secretion is prevented by negative feedback regulation of the HPA stress axis. Glucocorticoids and mineralocorticoids, acting via hippocampal receptors, modulate and regulate trough CRH and ACTH secretion.[1]

Excessive acute stress with relative glucocorticoid excess can impair hippocampal integrity. In the process, memory-mediating pathways, as well as feedback control mechanisms, are compromised.[1]

Although this acute injury to hippocampal structures and function is reversible, **chronic stress can precipitate irreversible hippocampal atrophy. As a result of chronic stress, the HPA regulatory mechanisms undergo progressive degradation, and the normal, receptor-mediated corticosteroid feedback regulation is overridden.** Thus, with chronic stress, dexamethasone suppression of CRH and ACTH release fails.[1]

Impairment of negative glucocorticoid feedback may occur as a result of

- early life stress,
- chronic emotional or physical stress, and
- old age

and engender dysfunction of the HPA axis. **The compromise in HPA feedback gives rise to relative hypercortisolism.**[19]

METABOLIC EFFECTS OF HYPOTHALAMIC-PITUITARY-ADRENOCORTICAL ACTIVATION AND THE METABOLIC SYNDROME

With chronic stress activation, contradictory aspects of the process are apparent:

- Inflammatory markers increase with stress; however, the immune response is blunted.
- Glucocorticoids are anti-inflammatory and increase some insulin responses. However, overall insulin sensitivity is compromised by glucocorticoids.

The characteristic features of glucocorticoid action underlie these apparent contradictory observations.

Glucocorticoid Tissue Effect. Tissue glucocorticoid effects are augmented with chronic HPA activation. The dysfunctional axis, together with impaired feedback control, can cause relative systemic hypercortisolism. Salivary cortisol or urinary cortisol metabolite excretion may thus be increased.[14]

Even in the absence of elevated glucocorticoid levels, persistent stressors enhance steroid tissue effects. With mean daily steroid concentrations unchanged, the dysfunctional HPA axis, characterized by reduced peak steroid levels, effectively leads to an elevation in circadian trough glucocorticoid levels. As a result, the prolonged daily occupancy of the glucocorticoid receptor engenders a change in metabolism analogous to a mild version of Cushing's syndrome.[11,22]

The resulting glucocorticoid tissue effects inhibit the growth hormone, thyroid, and reproductive axes. Additionally, excessive glucocorticoid effects render target tissues resistant to sex and growth hormones.[11,22]

Blunted Immune Response. Glucocorticoids impair immunologic responsiveness. They are thought to exert their anti-inflammatory effects at least partly through inhibiting the expression of many cytokines, including tumor necrosis factor-alpha (TNF-α), IL-2, IL-3, IL-5, IL-6, and IL-8.

The glucocorticoid receptor is a nuclear hormone receptor and transcription factor that modulates the expression of a variety of genes. Gene transcription of the inflammatory cytokines appears to be decreased by the inhibitory impact that the activated steroid nuclear receptor exerts on transcription factors such as

- activating protein-1 (AP-1) and
- nuclear factor kappaB (NFκB).

The activated glucocorticoid receptor may physically associate with the p65 protein of NFκB. As a result, binding of NFκB to its recognition site on the cytokine promoter is blocked.[22]

Additionally, glucocorticoids have an inhibitory effect on the expression of adhesion molecules such as intercellular adhesion molecule-1 (ICAM-1), endothelial-selectin (E-selectin), and vascular cell adhesion molecule-1 (VCAM-1) in the vascular endothelium.[23]

Impaired Endothelial Function. Glucocorticoids impair endothelial function. Both endothelial nitric oxide synthase (eNOS) expression and NO availability are affected:

- In cultured bovine coronary artery endothelial cells, cortisol decreases the agonist-induced, calcium-mediated release of NO.
- Cortisol, via activation of glucocorticoid receptors, significantly decreases eNOS protein levels in a dose-dependent manner.[24]
- In rat vessels, glucocorticoids inhibit the expression of guanosine 5′-triphosphate (GTP) cyclohydrolase, the rate-limiting enzyme for the synthesis of tetrahydrobiopterin, an important cofactor for eNOS.

These mechanisms may contribute to the reduced endothelium-dependent vasodilation characteristic of glucocorticoid excess.[25]

Potentiation of Insulin Effect and Insulin Resistance. Glucocorticoids enhance some insulin effects in adipose tissue. However, glucocorticoids also antagonize insulin sensitivity in diverse tissues with adverse metabolic sequelae.

Potentiation of Insulin Action. Glucocorticoids potentiate insulin action in adipose tissue. With glucocorticoid excess, there is a bias toward caloric storage as fat.[26]

Visceral Adiposity. Stress-mediated glucocorticoid excess causes the development of visceral ponderosity. Several factors, including greater glucocorticoid activity and receptor density, as well as enhanced lipoprotein lipase (LPL) expression, favor the visceral accumulation of fat and abdominal adiposity, which ultimately has a negative impact on systemic insulin sensitivity.

Obese individuals have increased levels of a key enzyme of glucocorticoid metabolism, 11β-hydroxysteroid dehydrogenase type 1 (11β-HSD-1), in adipose tissue, particularly in the visceral-omental depot. In adipocytes, 11β-HSD-1 converts inactive plasma glucocorticoids to create locally elevated levels of active glucocorticoids such as

- cortisol,
- corticosterone,

which activate the glucocorticoid receptor.[22]

The glucocorticoid receptor is expressed in adipose tissue. The density of this receptor varies in different adipose depots, with higher receptor density in intra-abdominal visceral than in subcutaneous fat.[27] Correspondingly, glucocorticoid receptor mRNA levels are higher in visceral than in subcutaneous adipose tissue.[28] In hypertension and obesity, glucocorticoid receptor polymorphisms may also be associated with adipocyte hypersensitivity to glucocorticoids.[19]

In the presence of insulin, the glucocorticoid receptor in adipose tissue activates gene transcription and expression of LPL. This enzyme hydrolyzes triacylglycerols in plasma with release of free fatty acids into tissue, where they can be taken up and reassembled into triacylglycerols for storage.[28]

Insulin Resistance. Stress-induced glucocorticoid excess is implicated in the generation of insulin resistance and the metabolic syndrome (Fig. 4-2). Clinically, glucocorticoid use decreases insulin sensitivity. In 92 consecutive patients with rheumatoid arthritis receiving lipid-lowering or antidiabetic medications, previous exposure to oral prednisone or high doses of pulsed glucocorticoids was associated with decreased insulin sensitivity.[29]

Glucocorticoids counteract insulin's action in nonadipose tissue via direct and indirect mechanisms.

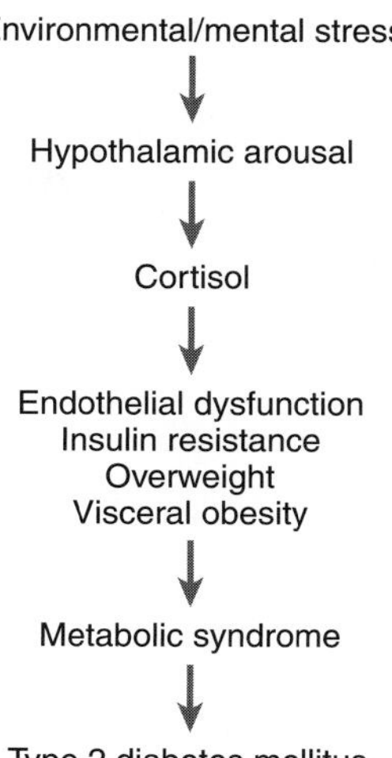

Figure 4–2.
Mental stress, activation of the hypothalamic-pituitary-adrenal axis, and the metabolic syndrome.

Direct Mechanisms. Glucocorticoids adversely affect insulin signaling at the level of the insulin receptor, the insulin receptor substrate-1 (IRS-1), and phosphatidylinositol 3-kinase (PI3K).

In liver and muscle, glucocorticoids significantly decrease the amount of mRNA for the insulin receptor and IRS-1. They lower specific insulin binding to the insulin receptor and the amount of IRS-1 and the p85 regulatory subunit of PI3K. As a result, there is reduced

- tyrosine phosphorylation of the insulin receptor,
- tyrosine phosphorylation of IRS-1,
- PI3K activity,[30]

with impairment of the PI3K insulin signaling pathway. A consequence of the effect of glucocorticoids on the liver is stimulation of hepatic gluconeogenesis. Glucocorticoids have strong gluconeogenic actions on the liver.[31,32]

Indirect Mechanisms. Glucocorticoids cause insulin resistance indirectly via numerous mechanisms. They initiate peripheral insulin insensitivity and may mediate a number of the metabolic changes associated with the metabolic syndrome.[31,32] Glucocorticoid-induced visceral adiposity plays a contributory role:

- The glucocorticoid effect on visceral fat metabolism leads to the induction of TNF-α. TNF-α is a potent inducer of insulin resistance pathways locally in adipose tissue, with potential systemic effects.[20]

- TNF-α in visceral adipose tissue engenders increased free fatty acid release. Increased plasma levels of free fatty acids are pivotal mediators of systemic insulin resistance.[33]
- By impairing endothelial function and interfering with the PI3K-insulin signaling pathway, glucocorticoids counter insulin's vasodilatory actions. As a result, insulin delivery to skeletal muscle via microcirculatory, nutritive blood flow is compromised, as is insulin action and glucose transport.
- Glucocorticoids interfere with the signaling pathway of the leptin receptor, thereby inducing leptin resistance and interfering with the central and peripheral body weight regulatory function of leptin.[20] Thus, glucocorticoids thwart leptin inhibition of the secretion of neuropeptide Y, a potent orexigenic hormone implicated in stress-mediated overeating behavior.[34]

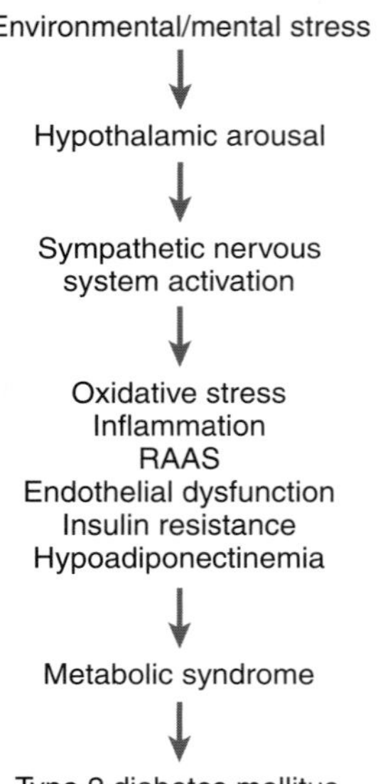

▸▸ **Figure 4–3.**
Mental stress, activation of the sympathetic nervous system, and the metabolic syndrome. RAAS, renin-angiotensin-aldosterone system.

ACTIVATION OF THE SYMPATHETIC NERVOUS SYSTEM

The stress response activates the sympatho-adrenal axis in parallel with the HPA axis. Mental stress, in particular, is associated with sympathetic activation.[35] Increased sympathetic nerve activity enhances the nerve terminal release of norepinephrine. Additionally, activation of the sympathetic nervous system increases the adrenomedullary, systemic production of epinephrine and norepinephrine with a rise in their plasma levels. Higher sympathetic activity entails an increase in heart rate and cardiac output.[1,36]

Akin to stress glucocorticoid effects, stress catecholamines may favor the development of adiposity in genetically predisposed individuals. **Catecholamines create a multiplicity of pathways that interfere with insulin signaling. They establish a metabolic milieu conducive to the development of the metabolic syndrome, arterial hypertension, and type 2 DM in susceptible persons** (Fig. 4-3).[37]

Vascular Disease. Sympathetic stress has a negative impact on vascular health. Sympathetic activation, induced by baroreceptor unloading, impairs flow-mediated brachial vasodilation.[38] Norepinephrine infusions have an atherogenic effect.[39]

Overweight. Chronic stress catecholamines, just like chronic HPA activation by stress, may favor the development of overweight. Stress increases orexigenic stimuli. It may dampen the metabolic rate and favor fat accumulation. The combination of an enhanced appetite, together with a reduction in metabolism, worsens the tendency to stress-induced ponderosity in susceptible individuals.[40]

- Chronic stress catecholamines stimulate the release of neuropeptide Y, a potent orexigenic messenger.[1]
- Cytokines decrease β_3-adrenergic receptor expression. Stress-induced β-receptor desensitization, in conjunction with stress-induced hypoadiponectinemia, has a negative effect on the metabolic rate.[40]

Insulin Resistance. Stress-induced sympathetic arousal blunts insulin sensitivity, and α- and β-adrenergic receptor mechanisms are implicated.

α-Adrenergic Effects.

- Directly, activation of the α-adrenergic receptor interferes with insulin signaling via activation of the small GTPase Rho.[41]
- α-Adrenergic receptor activation counters insulin's action via inhibition of glycogen synthase.
- Indirectly, α-adrenergic vasoconstriction attenuates the microcirculatory nutritive flow to skeletal muscle, thereby inhibiting insulin delivery and action in peripheral tissues.[42]

β-Adrenergic Effects.

- β-Adrenergic receptor activation can reduce tyrosine kinase activity. This interferes with IRS-1 phosphorylation and suppresses IRS-1 activation of PI3K activity, thereby inhibiting insulin activation of glucose transport.[43]
- Acting via β-adrenergic receptors, epinephrine attenuates glucose uptake also by inhibiting hexokinase and glucose phosphorylation.
- β-Adrenergic adenosine 3′,5′-cyclic monophosphate (cAMP) effects boost hepatic glycogenolysis and gluconeogenesis, thereby antagonizing the effect of insulin by increasing plasma glucose levels.[43]
- Catecholamines interfere with insulin-mediated lipogenesis by inhibiting LPL.
- Sympathetic hyperactivity, with elevated circulating epinephrine, enhances visceral-omental lipolysis and thus releases increased plasma levels of free fatty acids, which are implicated in mediating systemic insulin resistance.[44]
- Stress catecholamines contribute to plasma hypoadiponectinemia, thus attenuating adiponectin's
    - anti-inflammatory,
    - insulin-sensitizing,
    - thermogenic, and
    - fatty acid oxidant

  effects.[40]

Insulin and Leptin Resistance and Increased Sympathetic Tone. As sympathetic overactivity increases insulin resistance, hyperinsulinemia supervenes. **Hyperinsulinemia, in turn, may further increase sympathetic neural outflow via central mechanisms.**[14,45,46] Insulin resistance is therefore not only the result but also the cause of early derangements in autonomic nervous tone.[37]

Hyperleptinemia has a similar central, stimulatory effect on sympathetic tone.[47] The sympathetic activation engendered by hyperinsulinemia or hyperleptinemia may actually represent a physiologic, compensatory response to facilitate thermogenesis and weight loss.[48] However, ultimately the end result is a vicious circle wherein the stress-induced, adverse metabolic sequelae reinforce each other.

THE RENIN-ANGIOTENSIN-ALDOSTERONE SYSTEM

Stress and sympathetic hyperactivity activate the renin-angiotensin-aldosterone system (RAAS). The release of renin from renal juxtaglomerular cells is enhanced with increased activation of the sympathetic nervous system. However, the **HPA axis is also closely related to the RAAS** because

- ACTH is a common stimulus not only for cortisol but also for aldosterone and
- angiotensin II releases CRH and vasopressin from the hypothalamus by stimulation of angiotensin II receptors localized in the subfornical organ of the circumventricular organs of the brain, which are unprotected by the blood-brain barrier.[49-51]

Induction of the RAAS engenders the activation of inflammatory cytokines and oxidant stress. Viscosity is increased, and pivotal mediators of inflammation, insulin resistance, and atherogenesis are brought into play[1,52]**:**

- Angiotensin II is a major stimulant of oxidative stress.
- Angiotensin II induces sympathetic activation.
- Angiotensin II down-regulates the expression of peroxisome proliferator–activated receptor-alpha (PPAR-α) and PPAR-γ, thus decreasing their anti-inflammatory influence and favoring the transcription of NFκB and proinflammatory cytokines.[53,54]
- RAAS activation increases IL-6 secretion, which induces hepatic C-reactive protein

(CRP) production. IL-6 in turn stimulates the HPA axis.[21,55]

As with the sympathetic nervous system, not only does RAAS activation favor the development of insulin resistance, but **increased levels of insulin as a result of the insulin-resistant state also activate the RAAS in a vicious circle.**[56]

EXAMPLES OF STRESS EFFECTS ON METABOLISM

Very diverse, acute and chronic stressors have an effect on a variety of metabolic and inflammatory variables in otherwise healthy individuals. **With mental/environmental stress exposure, typically aspects of both the HPA and sympathetic RAAS stress pathways are activated,** and both pathways reinforce each other. Although the immediate- and short-term manifestations of each response are quite dissimilar, their long-term adverse metabolic and vascular sequelae are additive and complement each other. **Both pathways induce endothelial dysfunction and insulin resistance, ultimately leading to hypertension and metabolic and vascular disease** (Fig. 4-4).

Stress-Induced Weight Gain versus Weight Loss. Stress causes weight gain in some individuals and weight loss in others.

Both the HPA and the sympathetic stress pathways can favor the accretion of body weight. In healthy young men, the magnitude of the sympathetic response to mental stress was associated with a higher body mass index.[42] Sleep deprivation, a prevalent stressor in present-day society, entails adverse health implications. It afflicts harried parents, professionals, night shift workers, and persons plagued by insomnia. Lack of sleep causes fatigue, a lack of focus, and ill temper. More importantly, the stress of routine sleep deprivation may induce weight gain and obesity.[57]

Stress pathways can, however, also generate a catabolic response. Different body weight outcomes may reflect diverse individual susceptibilities, stress pathways, and in particular, the severity of the stress response:

1. Increased stimulation of the HPA axis increases the expression of TNF-α, which stimulates the release of leptin and anorexigenic pathways.[58]
2. β-Adrenergic stimulation increases leptin production and anorexigenic stimuli.[58] Furthermore, with increased sympathetic activation comes stimulation of the RAAS. The inflammatory response is increased, and proinflammatory cytokines are released that have a negative impact on orexigenic stimuli, that are antiadipogenic and prolipolytic,

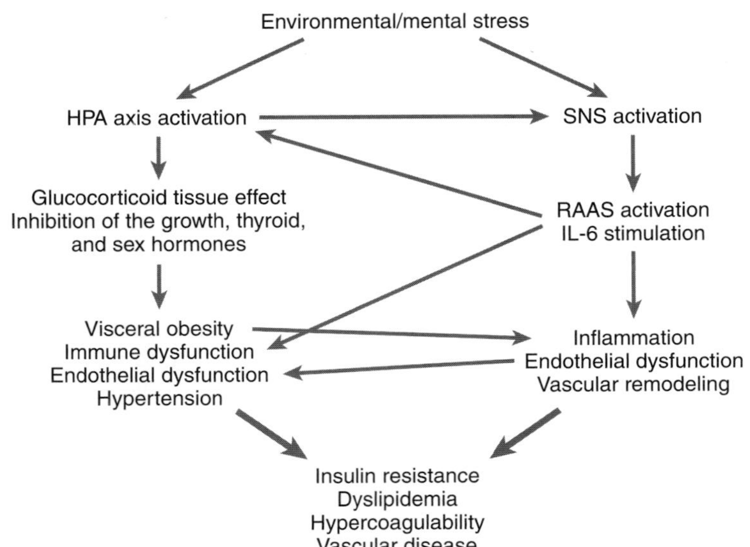

▸▸ **Figure 4–4.** Interrelationship of mental stress pathways and their metabolic and vascular sequelae. HPA, hypothalamic-pituitary-adrenal; IL-6, interleukin-6; RAAS, renin-angiotensin-aldosterone system; SNS, sympathetic nervous system.

and that establish resistance to the insulin-mediated uptake of nutrients.

Inflammatory Markers. Perceived stress may increase inflammatory markers.

The degree of perceived stress in the workforce is inversely proportional to the individual's authority and decision-making empowerment. The Whitehall II study demonstrated stress activation of inflammatory markers in white-collar workers. In that study of 283 nonindustrial, healthy nonsmoking civil servants, civil service employment grade was strongly and inversely related to circulating levels of high-sensitivity (hs)CRP and IL-6.[59] Sleep deprivation causes a rise in circulating markers of inflammation such as hsCRP.[60]

The need to care for elderly family members is increasingly commonplace for the "sandwich generation" in our society. Caregiving, despite its meritorious import, is a significant chronic stressor. Long-term caregiving, especially for those afflicted by dementia, has detrimental effects on the psychological and physical health of caregivers. It is associated with a rise in IL-6 levels.[61]

Impaired Immune Response. Chronic stress impairs the immune response. The degree of immunization achieved by chronic caregivers in response to vaccinations is attenuated.[61]

Lipoprotein Levels. Stress pathways with chronic sympathetic hyperactivity and neuroendocrine activation have an adverse impact on lipoprotein levels.

Plasma triglyceride levels were higher in public speakers and racecar drivers when active.[62,63] In healthy 19-year-old men, the magnitude of the sympathetic response to mental stress correlated positively with plasma catecholamine levels and non-HDL cholesterol and negatively with the level of HDL.[64]

Endothelial Dysfunction. Acute and chronic mental stress impairs normal endothelial function.

Psychosocial stress causes endothelial injury.[65] Even in the absence of CHD, mental stress attenuates flow-mediated brachial artery dilation.[66] Marked acute psychosocial stress, such as a verbal defense to a charge of theft on camera, acutely lowered brachial artery flow-mediated vasodilation.[67] Chronic stress for the duration of 4 weeks, as induced by sleep deprivation compounded by the pressure of term examinations, significantly compromised flow-mediated dilation in the brachial artery of young, healthy subjects.[36]

In healthy young men, the magnitude of the sympathetic response to mental stress was associated with a higher blood pressure response to stress.[42] Sleep deprivation causes endothelial dysfunction (Figs. 4-5 and 4-6)[36,68] and an increase in systolic blood pressure.[60] Sleep deprivation is a risk factor for the occurrence of myocardial infarction.[69] Stress-associated impairment of endothelial function is exacerbated by hostile affect.[66]

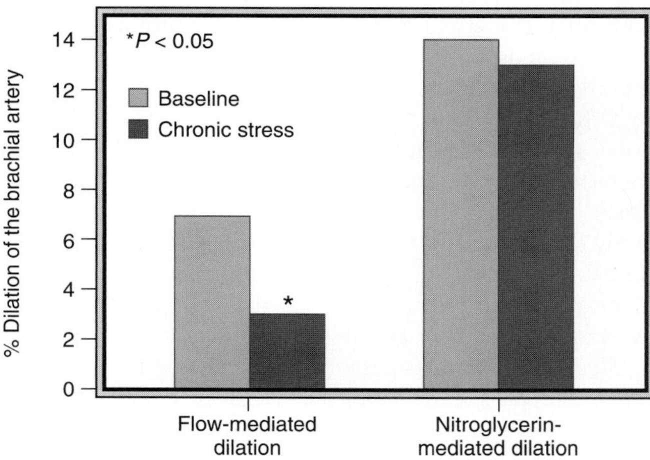

Figure 4–5.
Changes in brachial artery dilation in response to flow and nitroglycerin at baseline and after 4 weeks of chronic sleep deprivation in healthy students during examination time. *(Modified from Takase B, Akima T, Uehata A, et al. Effect of chronic stress and sleep deprivation on both flow-mediated dilation in the brachial artery and the intracellular magnesium level in humans. Clin Cardiol 2004;27:223-227.)*

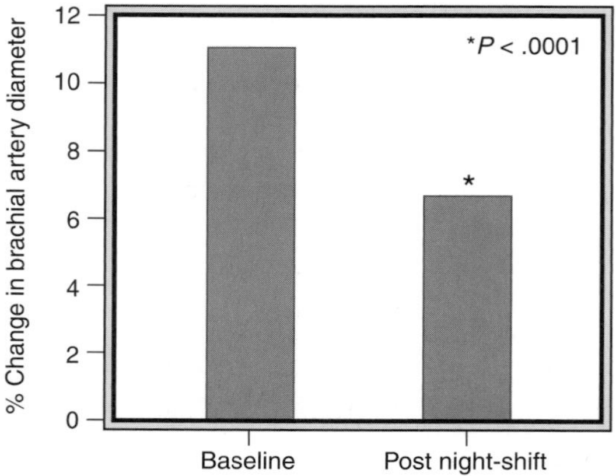

▸▸ **Figure 4–6.**
Reduction in flow-mediated brachial artery dilation after sleep deprivation because of an on-call night shift for medical residents and fellows. *(Modified from Amir O, Alroy S, Schliamser JE, et al. Brachial artery endothelial function in residents and fellows working night shifts. Am J Cardiol 2004;93:947-949.)*

Mental stress related to hostility and anger may induce myocardial ischemia.[70]

Insulin Resistance, Metabolic Syndrome, Mortality. A sustained stress response to chronic stressors may conceivably facilitate the evolution of the metabolic syndrome in susceptible individuals.

In healthy young men, the magnitude of the sympathetic response to mental stress was correlated with increasing insulin resistance.[42] Hostility, associated with increased secretion of catecholamines and glucocorticoids, is considered to be a stable personality trait over time as individuals react with hostility to perceived continual threatening and conflictual stimuli. Hostility is associated with development of the metabolic syndrome. Children who exhibited high hostility scores were likely to have metabolic syndrome in follow-up.[71] In overweight men, hostility was associated with insulin resistance and dyslipidemia.[72] In a cross-sectional study of men and women, even after adjustment for risk-related behavior, hostility was significantly associated with components of the metabolic syndrome in average- and high-risk individuals.[73]

Sleep deprivation is a risk factor for the occurrence of type 2 DM.[69] Obstructive sleep apnea (OSA) is a severe sleep disturbance that portends poor metabolic and cardiovascular health. OSA is associated with increased nocturnal sympathetic output as a result of the stress of sleep-disordered breathing, hypopnea, and apnea. Such stress promotes insulin resistance and hyperinsulinemia. In effect, OSA is an independent comorbid risk factor for hypertension and the metabolic syndrome, as well as for increased cardiovascular and cerebrovascular morbidity.[74] As contrasted to non-caregivers, there is a higher 4-year risk of total mortality in caregivers.[61]

AUTONOMIC DYSFUNCTION IN THE METABOLIC SYNDROME

The autonomic dysfunction prevalent in the metabolic syndrome can be quantitatively assessed.

Heart Rate Variability. The heart rate at rest offers a reliable index of sympathovagal balance.

Autonomic function is assessed via heart rate variability (HRV), which entails spectral and time domain analyses of harmonic components of electrocardiographic R-R intervals derived from 24-hour electrocardiographic Holter monitoring.

An index of cardiac vagal modulation is a high frequency (HF) of R-R variability (0.15 to 0.4 Hz). Sympathetic activity is reflected by a low frequency (LF) of R-R variability (0.03 to 0.15 Hz).

Sympathovagal balance may be evaluated as the ratio of low-frequency to high-frequency (LF/HF) variability. Autonomic imbalance is manifested by a shift toward sympathetic dominance demonstrated by a higher LF/HF ratio and lower HRV.[75]

Heart Rate Variability with Chronic Stress. Chronic stress activates the sympathoadrenal axis. There is increased 24-hour urinary normetanephrine excretion. HRV shows vagal withdrawal and higher cardiac sympathetic predominance.[1]

Heart Rate Variability with Overweight. Protracted stress activation may contribute to weight gain in susceptible individuals.

Obesity, even in healthy children, is associated with lower parasympathetic tone, as manifested by lower nighttime and 24-hour HF normalized units and time domain measures of vagal activity, as well as by significantly greater nighttime and 24-hour LF/HF ratios. Lower vagal tone is associated with a higher casual and ambulatory heart rate and blood pressure, in addition to metabolic disturbances such as higher fasting glucose, insulin, and triglyceride levels.[76]

Heart Rate Variability with the Metabolic Syndrome. Autonomic modulation with the metabolic syndrome is characterized by sympathetic predominance and vagal withdrawal. The central sympathetic activation and sympathetic hyperactivity may arise from chronic, physiologic, or external stressors.[45,77]

In healthy relatives of type 2 diabetics, an altered balance of parasympathetic and sympathetic nervous activity, mainly explained by attenuated parasympathetic activity, is observed and may contribute to the development of insulin resistance.[78] In healthy offspring of type 2 diabetic patients with normal glucose tolerance and normal blood pressure values, the presence of insulin resistance is associated with sympathetic activation.[37] Irrespective of body weight and blood pressure, chronic hyperinsulinemia with insulin resistance appears to be an important determinant of HRV indices reflecting enhanced sympathetic influence.[79]

CONCLUSION

Stress is a pervasive aspect of life experiences in any setting. Stress can be exciting and stimulating; it can also be enervating and soul consuming. When exposed to the same stressors, different individuals may experience vastly different emotional and physiologic responses as a function of their genetics, upbringing, environment, and training.

Stress is not solely a troublesome emotional response. Stress pathways initiate numerous major physiologic changes. From a stress-response perspective, such stress pathways are adaptive. Stress-enhanced appetite increases nutrient consumption. Increased fat deposition consolidates fuel storage. Visceral fat localization renders such fuel more labile and rapidly deployable for stress release. Endothelial dysfunction and insulin resistance target such fuel for use by immune/inflammatory organs involved in host defense.

However, if protracted or repeatedly experienced, such chronically active stress pathways turn maladaptive and elicit adverse, pathophysiologic consequences for the metabolic and cardiovascular health of susceptible individuals.

A protracted, physiologic stress response is both mentally and physiologically well entrenched.

- No person enjoys feeling stressed, yet it is difficult to extricate oneself intellectually and emotionally from the encompassing grip of stress.
- It is even harder to control the stressful responses arising from physiologic stressors such as chronic pain, chronic infection, or chronic inflammation.
- Interrupting the stress physiology may itself be a challenge because centrally and peripherally, the HPA, the RAAS, and the sympathetic stress pathways reinforce each other. With chronic stress, feedback controls are impaired or may turn into positive feedback loops. With inflammatory activation, cytokines may activate the HPA axis. Increased visceral adiposity may worsen the systemic proinflammatory state.

However, certain features of chronic stress activation may be amenable to behavioral and lifestyle intervention. A number of approaches that bear consideration are

- Modulation of the hippocampal triage function. The hippocampus may determine a stimulus not to be a threat and may inhibit activation of the HPA axis.[17] Training and familiarization with a threat situation may thus be of benefit.
- Avoidance of a passive, defeatist response to stress. Exploring likely threats with targeted offensive and defensive training may be of benefit in lessening activation of the HPA axis. This may occur in the context of martial arts, training in public speech or debate, training for emergency situations, or learning empowerment approaches to overcome physical pain or disability.
- Blunting sympathetic arousal. Meditative stress management approaches may be of benefit, whereby enhancement of parasympathetic tone may offset excessive sympathetic excitation.

Therapeutic lifestyle interventions should thus appropriately encompass behavioral approaches.

Obviously, lifestyle changes must encompass exercise, smoking cessation, a healthy diet, and weight control. In this context, however, meditative stress relaxation efforts, moving meditations such as Tai Chi or Yoga, or the relaxation of a sauna or a massage may be of particular benefit. Individuals should also devote time for the building of meaningful relationships with family and friends, for religious or philosophical introspection, for the consumption of healthy food in a peaceful relaxing milieu, for adequate sleep, for the contemplation of music and beauty, even for the time to reflect on experiences in a diary in order to blunt the chronic adverse stress responses to the repetitive and protracted stressors of present-day life.

GLOSSARY

ACTH	adrenocorticotropic hormone, or corticotropin
AP-1	activating protein-1
AVP	arginine vasopressin
cAMP	adenosine 3′,5′-cyclic monophosphate
CHD	coronary heart disease
CRH	corticotropin-releasing hormone
CRP	C-reactive protein
DM	diabetes mellitus
eNOS	endothelial nitric oxide synthase
E-selectin	endothelial-leukocyte adhesion molecule-1, or endothelial-selectin
GTP	guanosine 5′-triphosphate
HDL	high-density lipoprotein
HF	high frequency
HPA	hypothalamic-pituitary-adrenal
HRV	heart rate variability
hsCRP	high-sensitivity C-reactive protein
11β-HSD-1	11β-hydroxysteroid dehydrogenase type 1
ICAM-1	intercellular adhesion molecule-1
IL	interleukin
IRS	insulin receptor substrate
LDL	low-density lipoprotein
LF	low frequency
LPL	lipoprotein lipase
NFκB	nuclear factor kappaB
NHANES	National Health and Nutrition Examination Survey
NHES	National Health Examination Survey
NO	nitric oxide
OSA	obstructive sleep apnea
PI3K	phosphatidylinositol 3-kinase
PPAR	peroxisome proliferator–activated receptor
RAAS	renin-angiotensin-aldosterone system
TNF	tumor necrosis factor
VCAM-1	vascular cell adhesion molecule-1

REFERENCES

1. VanItallie TB. Stress: a risk factor for serious illness. Metabolism 2002;51(suppl 1):40-45
2. Kaplan JR, Manuck SB. Status, stress and atherosclerosis: the role of the environment and individual behavior. Ann N Y Acad Sci 1999;896:145-161
3. Calvert GM, Merling JW, Burnett CA. Ischemic heart disease mortality and occupation among 16- to 60-year-old males. J Occup Environ Med 1999;41:960-966
4. Castillo-Richmond A, Schneider RH, Alexander CN, et al. Effects of stress reduction on carotid atherosclerosis in hypertensive African-Americans. Stroke 2000;31:568-573
5. Rosengren A, Hawken S, Ounpuu S, et al. INTERHEART investigators. Association of psychosocial risk factors with risk of acute myocardial infarction in 11119 cases and 13648 controls from 52 countries (the INTERHEART study): case-control study. Lancet 2004;364:953-962
6. Jiang W, Babyak M, Krantz DS, et al. Mental stress–induced myocardial ischemia and cardiac events. JAMA 1996,275:1651-1656
7. Krantz DS, Kop WJ, Santiago HT, Gottdiener JS. Mental stress as a trigger for myocardial ischemia and infarction. Cardiol Clin 1996,14:271-287
8. Iso H, Date C,Yamamoto A, et al. Perceived mental stress and mortality from cardiovascular disease among Japanese men and women: the Japan Collaborative Cohort Study for Evaluation of Cancer Risk Sponsored by Monbusho (JACC Study). Circulation 2002;106:1229-1236
9. Greenwood DC, Muir KR, Packham CJ, et al. Coronary heart disease: a review of the role of psychosocial stress and social support. J Public Health Med 1996;18: 221-231
10. Vitaliano PP, Scanlan JM, Zhang J, et al. A path model of chronic stress, the metabolic syndrome, and coronary heart disease. Psychosom Med 2002;64:418-435
11. Bjoerntorp P. Abdominal obesity and the metabolic syndrome. Ann Med 1992;24:465-468
12. Bjoerntorp P. Neuroendocrine abnormalities in human obesity. Metabolism 1995;44(suppl 2):38-41

13. Hamet P, Tremblay J. Genetic determinants of the stress response in cardiovascular disease. Metabolism 2002; 51:15-24
14. Hjemdahl P. Stress and the metabolic syndrome. Circulation 2002;106:2634-2636
15. Henry JP. Biological basis of the stress response. News Physiol Sci 1993;8:69-73
16. Bjoerntorp P. Body fat distribution, insulin resistance, and metabolic diseases. Nutrition 1997;13:795-803
17. Frayn KN. Physiological regulation of macronutrient balance. Int J Obes 1995;19:4-10
18. Sapolsky R. Taming stress. Sci Am 2003;Special Issue Sept:87-95
19. Chroussos GP. The role of stress and the hypothalamic-pituitary-adrenal axis in the pathogenesis of the metabolic syndrome: neuro-endocrine and target tissue–related causes. Int J Obes 2000;24(suppl 2):S50-S55
20. Bjoerntorp P, Rosmond R. Neuroendocrine abnormalities in visceral obesity. Int J Obes 2000;24(suppl 2):S80-S85
21. Bethin KE, Vogt SK, Muglia LJ. Interleukin-6 is an essential, corticotropin-releasing hormone–independent stimulator of the adrenal axis during immune system activation. Proc Natl Acad Sci U S A 2000;97:9317-9322
22. Golub MS. The adrenal and the metabolic syndrome. Curr Hypertens Rep 2001;3:117-120
23. Xu X, Otsuki M, Saito H, et al. PPARalpha and GR differentially down-regulate the expression of nuclear factor-kappaB–responsive genes in vascular endothelial cells. Endocrinology 2001;142:3332-3339
24. Rogers KM, Bonar CA, Estrella JL, Yang S. Inhibitory effect of glucocorticoid on coronary artery endothelial function. Am J Physiol Heart Circ Physiol 2002;283:H1922-H1928
25. Johns DG, Dorrance AM, Tramontini NL, Webb RC. Glucocorticoids inhibit tetrahydrobiopterin-dependent endothelial function. Exp Biol Med 2001;226:27-31
26. Polkow B. Stress: hypothalamic functions and neuroendocrine consequences. Acta Med Scand 1988;723:61-70
27. Rebuffe-Scrive M, Lundholm K, Bjorntorp P. Glucocorticoid hormone binding to human adipose tissue. Eur J Clin Invest 1985;15:267-271
28. Cigolini M, Smith U. Human adipose tissue in culture. VIII. Studies on the insulin-antagonistic effects of glucocorticoids. Metabolism 1979;28:502-510
29. Dessein PH, Joffe BI, Stanwix AE, et al. Glucocorticoids and insulin sensitivity in rheumatoid arthritis. J Rheumatol 2004;31:867-874
30. Dupont J, Derouet M, Simon J, Taouis M. Corticosterone alters insulin signaling in chicken muscle and liver at different steps. J Endocrinol 1999;162:67-76
31. Bjorntorp P. Metabolic implications of body fat distribution. Diabetes Care 1991;14:1132-1143
32. Corry DB, Tuck ML. Selective aspects of the insulin resistance syndrome. Curr Opin Nephrol Hypertens 2001;10:507-514
33. Boden G. Interaction between free fatty acids and glucose metabolism. Curr Opin Clin Nutr Metab Care 2002;5: 545-549
34. Attoub S, Noe V, Pirola L, et al. Leptin promotes invasiveness of kidney and colonic epithelial cells via phosphoinositide 3-kinase-, rho-, and rac-dependent signaling pathways. FASEB J 2000;14:2329-2338
35. Dakak N, Quyyumi AA, Eisenhofer G, et al. Sympathetically mediated effects of mental stress on the cardiac microcirculation of patients with coronary artery disease. Am J Cardiol 1995;76:125-130
36. Takase B, Akima T, Uehata A, et al. Effect of chronic stress and sleep deprivation on both flow-mediated dilation in the brachial artery and the intracellular magnesium level in humans. Clin Cardiol 2004;27:223-227
37. Frontoni S, Bracaglia D, Baroni A, et al. Early autonomic dysfunction in glucose-tolerant but insulin-resistant offspring of type 2 diabetic patients. Hypertension 2003; 41:1223-1227
38. Hijmering ML, Stroes ES, Olijhoek J, et al. Sympathetic activation markedly reduces endothelium-dependent, flow-mediated vasodilation. J Am Coll Cardiol 2002; 39:683-688
39. Helin P, Lorenzen I, Garbarsch C, Matthiessen ME. Arteriosclerosis in rabbit aorta induced by noradrenalin: the importance of the duration of the noradrenalin action. Atherosclerosis 1970;12:125-132
40. Delporte M-L, Funahashi T, Takahashi M, et al. Pre- and post-translational negative effect of beta-adrenoceptor agonists on adiponectin secretion: in vitro and in vivo studies. Biochem J 2002;367:677-685
41. Begum N, Sandu OA, Ito M, et al. Active Rho kinase (ROK) associates with insulin receptor substrate-1 and inhibits insulin signaling in vascular smooth muscle cells J Biol Chem 2002;277:6214-6222
42. Moan A, Eide IK, Kjeldsen SE. Metabolic and adrenergic characteristics of young men with insulin resistance. Blood Pressure 1996;5(suppl 1):30-37
43. Hunt DG, Ivy JL. Epinephrine inhibits insulin-stimulated muscle glucose transport. J Appl Physiol 2002;93: 1638-1643
44. Jequier E. Pathways to obesity. Int J Obes Relat Metab Disord 2002;26(suppl):S12-S17
45. Emdin M, Gastaldelli A, Muscelli E, et al. Hyperinsulinemia and autonomic nervous system dysfunction in obesity: effects of weight loss. Circulation 2001;103:513-519
46. Scherrer U, Sartori C. Insulin as a vascular and sympathoexcitatory hormone: implications for blood pressure regulation, insulin sensitivity, and cardiovascular morbidity. Circulation 1997;96:4104-4113
47. Haynes WG. Interaction between leptin and sympathetic nervous system in hypertension. Curr Hypertens Rep 2000;2:311-318
48. Landsberg L. Insulin-mediated sympathetic stimulation: role in the pathogenesis of obesity-related hypertension (or, how insulin affects blood pressure and why). J Hypertens 2001;19:523-528
49. Dessi-Fulgheri P, Alagna S, Madeddu P, et al. Blunted adrenocorticotrophic hormone release during captopril treatment. J Hypertens Suppl 1985;3:S125-S127
50. Murck H, Held K, Ziegenbein M, et al. The renin-angiotensin-aldosterone system in patients with depression compared to controls—a sleep endocrine study. BMC Psychiatry 2003;3:15
51. Brandes RP. And what about the endothelium? On the predominance of cerebral superoxide formation for angiotensin II–induced systemic hypertension. Circ Res 2004;95:122-124
52. Middlekauff HR, Mark AL. The treatment of heart failure: the role of neurohumoral activation. Int Med 1998;37: 112-122
53. Tham DM, Martin-McNulty B, Wang Y-X, et al. Angiotensin II is associated with activation of NF kappaB–mediated genes and downregulation of PPARs. Physiol Genomics 2002;11:21-30
54. Schieffer B, Drexler H. Role of 3-hydroxy-3-methylglutaryl coenzyme A reductase inhibitors, angiotensin-converting enzyme inhibitors, cyclooxygenase-2 inhibitors, and aspirin in antiinflammatory and immunomodulatory treatment of cardiovascular disease. Am J Cardiol 2003;91(suppl):12H-18H
55. Papanikolaou DA, Wilder RL, Manolagas SC, et al. The pathophysiologic roles of interleukin-6 in humans. Ann Intern Med 1998;128:127-137

56. Deedwania PC. The deadly quartet revised. Am J Med 1998;105(suppl 1A):1S-3S
57. Hasler G, Buysse DJ, Klaghofer R, et al. The association between short sleep duration and obesity in young adults: a 13-year prospective study. Sleep 2004;27:661-666
58. Mora S, Pessin JE. An adipocentric view of signaling and intracellular trafficking. Diabetes Metab Res Rev 2002; 18:345-356
59. Hemingway H, Shipley M, Mullen MJ, et al. Social and psychosocial influences on inflammatory markers and vascular function in civil servants (the Whitehall II Study). Am J Cardiol 2003;92:984-987
60. Meier-Ewert HK, Ridker PM, Rifai N, et al. Effect of sleep loss on C-reactive protein, an inflammatory marker of cardiovascular risk. J Am Coll Cardiol 2004;43:678-683
61. Windham C. Elderly caregivers face stress toll. Wall St J 2003;July 1:D4
62. Taggart P, Carruthers M. Endogenous hyperlipidemia induced by emotional stress of racing driving. Lancet 1971;1:363-366
63. Taggart P, Carruthers M, Somerville W. Electrocardiogram, plasma catecholamines and lipids, and their modification by oxprenolol when speaking before an audience. Lancet 1973;2:341-346
64. Rostrup M, Westheim A, Kjeldsen SE, Eide I. Cardiovascular reactivity, coronary risk factors, and sympathetic activity in young men. Hypertension 1993;22:891-899
65. Bjoerk-Skantze H, Kaplan J, Pettersson K, et al. Psychosocial stress causes endothelial injury in cynomolgus monkeys via beta1-adrenoceptor activation. Atherosclerosis 1998;136:153-161
66. Gottdiener JS, Kop WJ, Hausner E, et al. Effects of mental stress on flow-mediated brachial arterial dilation and influence of behavioral factors and hypercholesterolemia in subjects without cardiovascular disease. Am J Cardiol 2003;92:687-691
67. Ghiadoni L, Donald AE, Cropley M, et al. Mental stress induces transient endothelial function in humans. Circulation 2000;102:2473-2478
68. Amir O, Alroy S, Schliamser JE, et al. Brachial artery endothelial function in residents and fellows working night shifts. Am J Cardiol 2004;93:947-949
69. Spencer J. The quest to banish fatigue. Wall St J 2003, July 1:D1
70. Burg MM, Jain D, Soufer R, et al. Role of behavioral and psychological factors in mental stress–induced silent left ventricular dysfunction in coronary artery disease. J Am Coll Cardiol 1993;22:444-448
71. Raikkonen K, Matthews KA, Salomon K. Hostility predicts metabolic syndrome risk factors in children and adolescents. Health Psychol 2003;22:279-286
72. Niaura R, Banks SM, Ward KD, et al. Hostility and the metabolic syndrome in older males: the Normative Aging Study. Psychosom Med 2000;62:7-16
73. Knox SS, Weidner G, Adelman A, et al; for the investigators of the Heart Lung, and Blood Institute Family Heart Study. Hostility and physiological risk in the Heart Lung, and Blood Institute Family Heart Study. Arch Intern Med 2004;164:2442-2448
74. Ip MSM, Lam B, Ng MMT, et al. Obstructive sleep apnea is independently associated with insulin resistance. Am J Respir Crit Care Med 2002;165:670-676
75. Pagani M, Lombardi F, Guzzetti S, et al. Power spectral analysis of heart rate and arterial pressure variabilities as a marker of sympathovagal interaction in man and conscious dog. Circ Res 1986;59:178-193
76. Martini G, Riva P, Rabbia F, et al. Heart rate variability in childhood obesity. Clin Auton Res 2001;11: 87-91
77. Liao D, Sloan RP, Cascio WE, et al. Multiple metabolic syndrome is associated with lower heart rate variability. The Atherosclerosis Risk in Community Study. Diabetes Care 1998;21:2116-2122
78. Lindmark S, Wiklund U, Bjerle P, Eriksson JW. Does the autonomic nervous system play a role in the development of insulin resistance? A study on heart rate variability in first-degree relatives of type 2 diabetes patients and control subjects. Diabet Med 2003;20: 399-405
79. Galinier M, Fourcade J, Ley N, et al. Hyperinsulinism, heart rate variability and circadian variation of arterial pressure in obese hypertensive patients. Arch Mal Coeur Vaiss 1999;92:1105-1109

Adipose Tissue and Overweight

5

The incidence of obesity is increasing at an alarming rate in the United States and the Western world. The serious pathologic states associated with obesity render it a significant threat to public health. Obesity is frequently seen as a risk factor and precursor to insulin resistance and the metabolic syndrome.

OVERWEIGHT AND OBESITY

Definition. Overweight represents a body weight exceeding the norm for a person's gender, age, height, and build. Obesity signifies an excessive accumulation of adipose tissue. An upward deviation in weight from the physiologic norm reflects an imbalance in the body's energy equation.

The Energy Equation. Energy intake via consumption of food leads to caloric storage if the intake of energy exceeds its expenditure.

Specifically, the energy balance equation for body weight is

Energy intake = Energy expenditure ± Energy storage (→Adipose tissue)

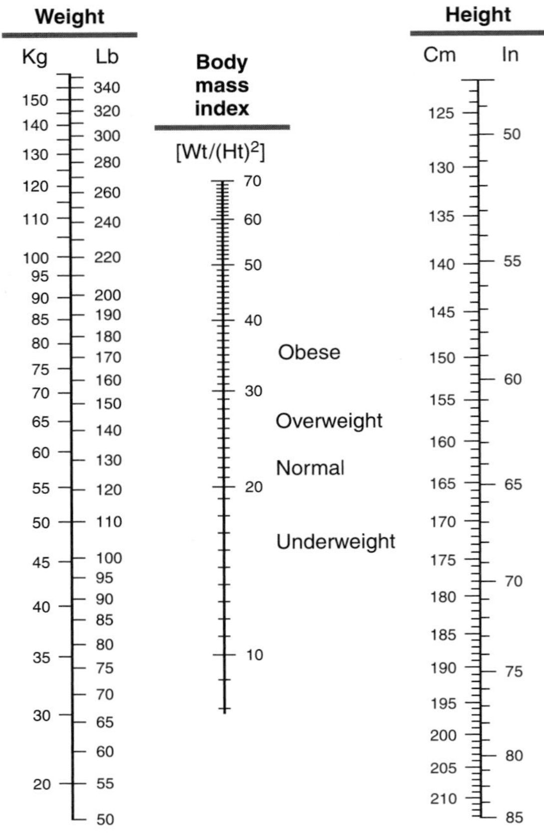

▸▸ **Figure 5–1.**
Nomogram for the calculation of body mass index (BMI). The point at which a straight line connecting an individual's weight in kilograms or pounds to height in centimeters or inches intersects the BMI scale indicates an individual's BMI. *(Modified from Bray GA. Classification and evaluation of the obesities. Med Clin North Am 1989;73:161-184.)*

Energy intake depends on

- food availability,
- opportunities for food consumption,
- appetite,
- gastrointestinal nutrient absorption, and
- an anabolic hormonal milieu for cellular nutrient uptake.

Energy expenditure depends on body heat production, or thermogenesis, and external muscular work. Specifically,

- diet-induced thermogenesis accounts for 10% to 12% of energy expenditure,
- the basal metabolic rate for 65%, and
- physical exercise, immune defense, and other processes for variable caloric expenditure.

Any imbalance between energy intake and expenditure will have an impact on energy storage. When caloric intake is less than caloric expenditure, the body mobilizes energy stores to make up the deficit. Conversely, when caloric intake exceeds expenditure, the body builds up energy stores, and the caloric surplus is stored as adipose tissue. **A chronic, positive metabolic energy balance generates an excess of adipose tissue.**

Classification of Weight. Body weight is classified via body mass index (BMI). BMI can be calculated as

Weight in kilograms/Square of height in meters

or as

Weight in pounds × 703/Square of height in inches.[1]

BMI can also be determined from a nomogram (Fig. 5-1).

Based on BMI, body weight ranges in adults are defined as follows[2]:

CLASSIFICATION	BMI (kg/m²)
Underweight	<18.5
Normal range	18.5-24.9
Overweight	25.0-29.9
Obese, class I	30.0-34.9
Obese, class II	35.0-39.9
Obese, class III	≥40.0

Adapted from National Institutes of Health, National Heart, Lung, and Blood Institute. Clinical Guidelines on the Identification, Evaluation, and Treatment of Overweight and Obesity in Adults (National Institutes of Health Publication No. 98-4083). Rockville, MD, U.S. Department of Health and Human Services, Public Health Service, 1998.

In general, **obesity is defined as BMI greater than 30 kg/m².**

Factors Having an Impact on Societal Overweight. Although ultimately, excessive caloric intake exceeding energy expenditure always underlies overweight, causes of overweight in society are manifold and complex; they affect both sides of the energy equation and span

- genetic,
- physiologic,
- psychological,

- nutritional,
- environmental, and
- societal

factors.

The genetic architecture of body fat content and adipose tissue distribution is complex. Obesity is a heterogeneous, polygenic disorder. More than 40 genes are likely to play a role in determining body composition. **Genetic factors are major contributors to overweight.**[3] **Fifty percent to 90% of the variation in body mass is inherited.**[4]

Obesity may be due to genetic variants that allow individuals to store energy when available and thus to successfully adapt to an environment of privation, of jeopardized, unpredictable food supplies. Societies of hunter-gatherers, with sporadically available food, would benefit from storage genes that predispose to obesity in an era of plenty.[3,5]

However, genetic, physiologic, and psychological factors have not dramatically changed over the centuries. Thus, **the obesity epidemic of the last 3 decades most likely reflects the interplay of nutritional, environmental, and societal changes in the consumption and expenditure of energy with the other factors.**

The current environment in industrialized societies favors energy consumption and discourages energy expenditure. Food has become easily available, inexpensive, energy dense, attractive, delicious, served in large portions, ready-made, and convenient.

On the other hand, the physical activities of daily life have decreased. Suburban life with the absence of sidewalks, bicycle paths, or even acceptable public transportation has rendered every outing and errand dependent on door-to-door automobile transport. The scarcity of accessible and safe outdoor venues such as woods, parks, and playgrounds confines recreational activities for children, teenagers, and adults to an indoor setting, with a focus on sedentary pursuits such as television, Internet surfing, and video games. Increased automation has dramatically decreased the physical effort required for jobs or chores at work and around the home.

No matter what an individual's genetic predisposition, a protracted mismatch of energy consumption exceeding expenditure tips the energy equation in favor of energy storage for every individual. Excessive food translates into body fat, and this contributes to the societal epidemic of obesity.

Prevalence of Overweight and Obesity. Overweight and obesity are inherently preventable and reversible. However, since the 1950s, overweight in America has continuously increased (Fig. 5-2).

According to the Surgeon General's Report on Overweight and Obesity, in 1999, 61% of the U.S. population was overweight.[6] According to the National Health and Nutrition Examination Survey (NHANES), **between 2001 and 2002, 65.7% of the U.S. population was overweight,** 30.6% were obese, and 5.1% were extremely obese, the latter figure up from 0.9% in 1991.[6,7] A total of 31.5% of all Americans younger than 19 years were at risk for overweight or obesity, and 16% were overweight, a figure that has doubled since the mid 1970s. The prevalence of

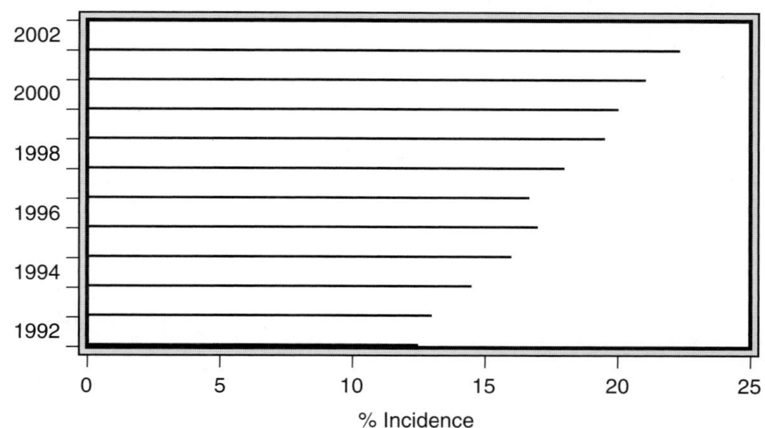

Figure 5-2. Median percentage of adults reporting a body mass index greater than 30 kg/m² to the Behavioral Risk Factor Surveillance System from 1992 to 2002. *(Adapted from MacNeil JS. Gastric bypass surgery can erase metabolic syndrome. Cardiol News 2004;April:p. 11.)*

obesity varies by age, sex, and ethnic group; it ranges from 22.9% in non-Hispanic white men aged 20 to 39 years to 50.6% in non-Hispanic black women aged 40 to 59 years. In the group older than 60 years, the prevalence of overweight is 70.8%, and the prevalence of obesity is 33.0%.[6] As of 2002 there were 44.3 million obese Americans encompassing 21.4 million men and 22.9 million women.[7] **Globally, a billion people are now overweight.**

Health Implications of Overweight. The concern about obesity constitutes not merely an inconvenience or an idle anxiety about appearance, vanity, and fashion. As stated by John Kenneth Galbraith in 1984 in *The Affluent Society,* "More die in the United States of too much food than too little."[8]

Obesity is a major predisposing factor for adverse health outcomes. The health risks associated with obesity rise with increasing overweight.

CLASSIFICATION	BMI (kg/m²)	RISK FOR COMORBID CONDITIONS
Underweight	<18.5	Increased
Normal range	18.5-24.9	Average
Overweight	25.0-29.9	Mildly increased
Obese, class I	30.0-34.9	Moderate
Obese, class II	35.0-39.9	Severe
Obese, class III	≥40.0	Very severe

Adapted from National Institutes of Health, National Heart, Lung, and Blood Institute. Clinical Guidelines on the Identification, Evaluation, and Treatment of Overweight and Obesity in Adults (National Institutes of Health Publication No. 98-4083). Rockville, MD, U.S. Department of Health and Human Services, Public Health Service, 1998.

Comorbid Conditions Linked to Obesity. The list of comorbid conditions associated with obesity is extensive. Not only cardiovascular, but all-cause morbidity and mortality are also increased with obesity.[9] Comorbid conditions include

- cardiovascular disease, including hypertension, coronary heart disease (CHD), cardiomyopathy, peripheral and cerebrovascular diseases, and atrial fibrillation;
- insulin resistance;
- the metabolic syndrome;
- dyslipidemia;
- nonalcoholic fatty liver disease and steatohepatitis;
- type 2 diabetes mellitus (DM);
- cancer of the cervix/endometrium, ovaries, prostate, breast, esophagus, liver, gallbladder, pancreas, kidney, and colon/rectum;
- lymphoma and multiple myeloma;
- gallbladder disease;
- arthritis;
- respiratory disease;
- varicosities;
- infertility;
- pregnancy complications;
- lower extremity and back weightbearing degenerative problems;
- psychological and socioeconomic difficulties; and
- dementia and Alzheimer's disease.[10-13]

Overweight is associated with increases in CHD mortality of 4% to 6% for every BMI unit increase exceeding 20 to 24 kg/m².[14] **Consistent with the societal rise in obesity is an 8.2% increase in the prevalence of type 2 DM.** A total of 16.7 million adults, 7.9% of the population, now carry the diagnosis of type 2 DM,[15] which has is own devastating comorbid conditions, including diabetic renal, ophthalmologic, neurologic, and cardiovascular disease.[16] In the United States, obesity accounts for 280,000 deaths annually.[17] **The odds for survival are significantly lower with obesity.** For a 25-year-old, morbidly obese man, a 22% decrement in life expectancy represents a loss of approximately 12 years of life.[18]

Health Sector Impact of Overweight. The public health impact of obesity may eventually rival and supplant that of smoking. Obesity has been classified by the American Heart Association as a major, modifiable risk factor for CHD.[19] Obesity and diseases related to it have joined the World Health Organization's top 10 global health risks.[20]

Health Care Costs. Obesity significantly raises direct and indirect health care costs.

In 2000, a report of the U.S. Surgeon General estimated that obesity-related health services cost the nation an estimated $117 billion a year.[21]

Overweight and obese individuals have an average of $1500 more in medical expenditures per year than normal-weight individuals do, and medical costs rise with increasing weight.[22] In men 45 to 54 years old, the lifetime cost of treating hypertension, hyperlipidemia, type 2 DM, CHD, and stroke was $29,600 and $36,500, with BMI values of 32.5 and 37.5 kg/m^2, respectively, and only $19,600 with a BMI of 22.5 kg/m^2, even taking into account the relationship between obesity and reduced longevity.[23] Obesity has been estimated to consume 5.5% to 7.8% of all health care expenditures.[22]

Correspondingly, the annual revenue of the dieting industry is estimated to exceed $33 billion. At any given time, approximately 45% of women and 30% of men in the United States are trying to lose weight. About 60,000 morbidly obese Americans undergo a surgical gastrointestinal bypass procedure to achieve weight loss in a year.[24]

Impact on Quality of Life and the Workforce. Obesity has an impact on disability and morbidity and increases unhealthy life years.

The health costs of obesity may effectively serve as proxies for pain, suffering, and medication dependence, all reflecting a poor quality of life. Obesity may lead to 39.2 million lost workdays each year.[22] In a 15-year prospective study of 19,518 Finnish men and women aged 20 to 92 years, obese men with a BMI greater than 30 kg/m^2 had 0.63 more years of work disability, 0.36 more years of CHD, and 1.68 more years of long-term medication use than normal-weight male counterparts did, with similar figures applying to obese women. The excess risk for disability, morbidity, and mortality was highest in the youngest age groups.[25]

ADIPOSE TISSUE DEVELOPMENT

Adipocytes are highly specialized cells with a critical complement of receptors and the ability to produce and secrete numerous substances. Preadipocytes derive from mesenchymal cells. Their multiplication and differentiation are in part an aspect of normal development, as well as long-term adaptation. Adipocyte hyperplasia and hypertrophy occur normally late in fetal life, in childhood, and in adolescence. Adipose tissue can increase in mass by

1. hypertrophy of existing adipocytes and/or by
2. hyperplasia with adipogenic differentiation of preadipocytes.

Two nuclear receptors,

1. the glucocorticoid receptor and
2. the peroxisome proliferator–activated receptor-gamma (PPAR-γ),

and their ligands play important roles in adipocyte differentiation and metabolism.

Normal Adipocyte Hypertrophy and Hyperplasia. Adipocyte hypertrophy precedes adipocyte hyperplasia.

Adipocyte Hypertrophy. Adipocyte hypertrophy is the normal, first response to increased caloric intake and growth.

In rats, after 1 week of consuming a 60% fat diet, the expression of 96 genes is up-regulated by greater than 50% over control. Twenty-five of these genes are involved in the modulation of

- mitochondrial respiration,
- carbohydrate/protein metabolism,
- thermogenesis, and
- ion transport.

Sixteen genes encode secretory peptides associated with critical signals for

- cell growth,
- cell differentiation,
- cell proliferation,
- cell cycle control,
- angiogenesis,
- leptin,
- adipocyte complement-related protein of 30 kDa (ACRP30), and
- resistin.[26]

The target of numerous other genes is unknown. Expression of growth factors implicated in the cell growth and development of adipocytes and stromal vascular elements is increased. Growth factors are modulated by both neural input and serum factors. This process occurs before hyperplasia.[26]

Adipocyte Hyperplasia. When hypertrophied adipocytes reach a "critical" volume,

hyperplasia occurs. The number and size of adipocytes increase with growth from approximately 5 billion measuring 45 to 75 μm at birth to 28 and 36 billion measuring 100 to 120 μm for adult men and women, respectively. Once established, adipocytes are there to stay,[26] thus rendering childhood obesity a significant predisposing risk factor for obesity in adult life.

Hyperplastic Obesity. Hyperplastic obesity occurs as growth factors induce the recruitment and proliferative response of preadipocytes, as well as a supporting infrastructure. In fact, the supporting stromal-vascular fraction, which includes fibroblasts and macrophages, accounts for at least half the total cell number. Morbid obesity is due to massive expansion of white adipose tissue.[27] **Humans can increase their adipose tissue weight by more than twice their lean body weight.**[26]

Lipogenesis. Excess caloric intake is stored as fat in a process involving lipogenesis.

Lipid accumulation at the level of the adipocyte is achieved by the activity of local, endothelially bound lipoprotein lipase (LPL). Upon the ingestion of nutrients, the secondary rise in insulin causes enhanced glucose transport into adipocytes, where glucose is metabolized to glycerol. Free fatty acid uptake by adipocytes is facilitated by increasing LPL activity. Glycerol and free fatty acids serve as substrates for esterification and the formation of storage triacylglycerols.

Insulin activation of acetyl coenzyme A (CoA) carboxylase and fatty acid synthase additionally facilitates fatty acid synthesis from glucose. However, de novo fatty acid synthesis from carbohydrate substrates is of quantitatively lesser significance.[28]

Lipolysis. Lipid mobilization, or lipolysis, is the reverse of lipogenesis. Lipolysis is the process of breakdown and release of triacylglycerol. Lipolysis occurs in the setting of increased energy expenditure, as with exercise, or in the context of starvation, in order to mobilize adipose tissue fuel for consumption by other tissues.

Activated hormone-sensitive lipase (HSL), the rate-limiting step for lipolysis, breaks triacylglycerols down to diacylglycerol (DAG) and monoacylglycerol. Monoacylglycerol lipase, in turn, hydrolyzes DAG to fatty acid and glycerol. In short, lipolysis of triacylglycerols proceeds as follows:

One triacylglycerol → three molecules of fatty acids + one of glycerol

Glycerol passively diffuses through the cell membrane into the extracellular fluid and bloodstream. The fatty acids may be re-esterified back to triacylglycerol within the same or a surrounding cell or be transferred across the cell membrane by a transport protein into the extracellular fluid and bloodstream to be used as fuel by other target tissues such as skeletal muscle.

Lipid mobilization is regulated by the activity of intracellular HSL. **Lipolysis is intensely regulated in adipocytes via modulation of the activity of HSL, which is principally controlled by insulin and the catecholamines**[29]:

1. Insulin is the major antilipolytic hormone.
2. β-Adrenergic catecholamines are major stimulators of lipolysis.

Additionally, prostaglandins, adenosine, growth hormone, testosterone, and cortisol have permissive regulatory effects.[28]

Lipolysis is increasingly stimulated as cytoplasmic cyclic adenosine monophosphate (cAMP) rises in concentration. Lipolysis occurs with fasting as a result of a fall in insulin and a rise in glucagon and catecholamine stimulation. Similarly, lipolysis with exercise derives from a decline in insulin and greater sympathetic activation. Conversely, in the sated state, the upsurge of insulin inhibits lipolysis. The rate of lipolysis declines with age as sympathetic nervous activity wanes.[28]

HORMONAL REGULATION OF APPETITE

An organism's energy balance is under complex neurohormonal regulation. In the course of a decade a person may consume approximately 10 million calories, yet experience only a modest change in weight, thus suggesting that on the whole, energy intake is largely matched to energy output.[3] In effect, **food intake is normally controlled by homeostatic mechanisms whereby hormonal signals from the digestive tract and adipose tissue provide feedback to the central nervous system and the hypothalamus to regulate appetite.**[30]

However, human evolution has occurred against the backdrop of starvation and food deprivation. Given human evolutionary history and the need to survive against the prevalent odds of a scarcity in food supplies, the body's homeostatic systems are designed primarily to protect against weight loss and starvation rather than weight gain. In this evolutionary context, the ability, in times of abundance, to ingest plentifully and establish fat reserves has constituted a survival advantage.[30]

The Enteric and Hypothalamic Appetite Control Centers. The gastrointestinal tract, via the enteric nervous system, and the central nervous system are involved in two-way communication. The neuronal linkage is effected by means of afferent sensory fibers as well as parasympathetic and sympathetic nerves composed of efferent cholinergic and noradrenergic fibers, respectively. Afferent nerves have numerous mechanoreceptor, nocireceptor, and chemoreceptor sensors at their visceral terminals in the gut, whose excitation triggers a variety of visceral reflexes regulating gastrointestinal functions, as well as food-seeking behavior.[31]

The hypothalamus is the key central regulator of food intake and energy balance, and it coordinates body adiposity and nutritional state.

Hypothalamic AMP-Activated Protein Kinase. In the hypothalamus, malonyl CoA and 5′-adenosine monophosphate–activated protein kinase (AMPK) take part in fuel-sensing and signaling mechanisms that direct food intake and energy expenditure.[32] AMPK, an intracellular energy sensor maintaining the energy balance within a cell, is controlled in the hypothalamus by hormones such as leptin and ghrelin, which regulate food intake. Activation of AMPK in the hypothalamus increases food intake.[33]

Hypothalamic Appetite Control Pathways. The hypothalamic appetite control centers integrate neural, hormonal, and nutrient messages. The hypothalamic region communicates with higher central nervous system centers within the hypothalamus that regulate feelings of hunger and satiety and thus control both short- and long-term weight regulatory systems. Such central nervous system centers are

- the arcuate nucleus,

with neurons in the arcuate nucleus projecting to

- the paraventricular nucleus,
- the lateral hypothalamic area, and
- the hypothalamic parafornical area.[30]

A large number of neurotransmitters participate in the control of appetite and energy balance. **Hypothalamic centers control energy expenditure via the autonomic nervous system and pituitary hormones.**[30]

Anorexigenic and Orexigenic Pathways. There are two major types of hypothalamic neuronal pathways with opposing actions:

1. **anorexigenic pathways** inhibit food intake with an increase in the metabolic rate, and
2. **orexigenic pathways** increase appetite and food intake and reduce metabolism.

Thus, whereas anorexigenic peptideYY3-36 (PYY) and leptin discourage feeding behavior, orexigenic ghrelin and neuropeptideY (NPY) stimulate food intake.[30,34]

The balance and interaction between anorexigenic and orexigenic factors appear to play an important role in the regulation of food intake and growth hormone release. An impairment in this balance may result in disorders of feeding behavior, weight gain, or weight loss.[31]

Short- and Long-Term Feeding Regulation. Neurotransmitters may have short- and long-term effects on feeding behavior:

1. Short-term feeding behavior appears to be modulated by hormones produced by the digestive tract, such as

   - cholecystokinin,
   - ghrelin,
   - PYY, and
   - vagal afferent neurons from the digestive tract,

   which respond to mechanical deformation, macronutrients, pH, tonicity, and hormones.

2. Long-term feeding behavior may be linked to the hormones
   - leptin and
   - insulin,

   which modulate the short-term signals.[30,34]

Anorexigenic Pathways. Anorexigenic stimuli blunt feeding behavior. They enhance sympathetic nervous system activity and thermogenesis.[30]

α-Melanocyte–Stimulating Hormone. Anorexigenic proopiomelanocortin (POMC)/cocaine-and-amphetamine–regulated transcript (CART) neurons express POMC. POMC is cleaved by prohormone convertases to yield α-melanocyte–stimulating hormone, an anorexigenic peptide.[35] **Although α-melanocyte–stimulating hormone modulates skin pigmentation via interaction with the melanocortin 1 receptor (MC1R), it is also a potent agonist of the hypothalamic receptor MC4R and causes a reduction in food intake and an increase in energy expenditure.** Another hypothalamic and limbic system receptor, MC3R, similarly mediates an increase in energy expenditure, without affecting food intake.[34,35]

Leptin. Leptin takes part in the long-term, anorexigenic regulation of food intake whereby body energy stores have an impact on signaling from the central nervous system.

An increase in fat stores enhances the expression and release of leptin, the product of the *Ob* gene, from adipocytes in proportion to the amount of fat stored. **Leptin provides an important feedback signal from fat to the central nervous system.** It acts through Ob receptors present in afferent visceral nerves, as well as in the hypothalamic arcuate nucleus, whose neurons are responsive to leptin and capable of expressing and releasing NPY and agouti-related protein, both of which activate food-seeking behavior through the paraventricular nucleus.[31] Specifically,

- leptin stimulates neurons that express POMC,
- leptin inhibits orexigenic pathways by blocking the expression of an agouti-related protein that is an MC4R antagonist,[4]
- leptin receptor activation may reduce the secretion of orexigenic NPY in the mediobasal hypothalamus,[36] and
- leptin decreases hypothalamic AMPK activity, thereby leading to a reduction in food intake.[33]

Adipose tissue in obesity engenders hyperleptinemia. However, most obese humans are leptin resistant, and the anorexigenic pathways of leptin are therefore ineffectual. In practical terms, hyperleptinemia provides little protection against weight gain in times of plenty. Low plasma levels of leptin may have greater physiologic impact than high levels by protecting the organism against weight loss during times of deprivation (Fig. 5-3).[30]

Insulin. Food intake stimulates the release of insulin. Insulin exerts long-term, central

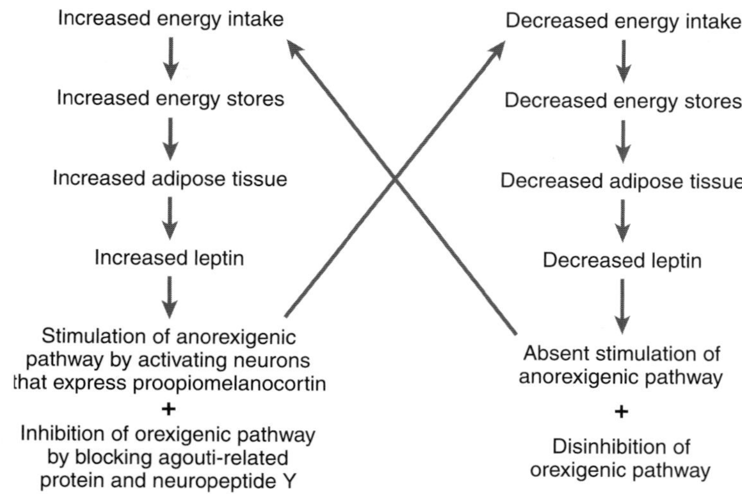

Figure 5–3. Interrelationship of adipose tissue production of leptin and central mediation of orexigenic and anorexigenic pathways.

effects to control body weight. Insulin receptors are present throughout the brain, but the appetite-suppressing actions of insulin appear to be centered in the arcuate nucleus area of the hypothalamus. Insulin has stimulatory effects on the insulin and leptin receptors of the arcuate nucleus, which

- stimulate POMC-expressing neurons and
- suppress the production of appetite-stimulating NPY.

Knockout of such central insulin receptors in a mouse model causes overeating and overweight.[34] **Insulin resistance may also affect the central insulin receptors. Conceivably, resistance of the central insulin receptors to insulin may have similarly adverse effects on body weight as the murine receptor knockout model.**

Cholecystokinin, Peptide YY3-36, and Oxyntomodulin. Cholecystokinin, PYY, and oxyntomodulin are peptides released into the blood stream from endocrine intestinal cells as anorexigenic "satiety hormones" for short-term regulation, on a meal-to-meal basis.

Hormone elaboration occurs with satiety in proportion to the amount of calories ingested, and food intake consequently decreases. These peptides act via G (guanine nucleotide regulatory) protein–coupled receptors either on afferent nerves or directly on neurons within the arcuate nucleus, which in turn inhibit the expression and the release of orexigenic NPY and agouti-related protein, thereby inducing satiety through inhibition of the paraventricular nucleus.[31]

Cholecystokinin, a meal-related signaling peptide, is secreted from the intestine in response to specific nutrients in the gut. Cholecystokinin can potently reduce the size of individual meals, but not body weight.[31]

PYY is released by the distal portion of the small intestine and the colon. When stimulated via neural mechanisms, levels rise within 15 minutes of food intake. PYY levels peak at around 60 minutes, stimulated by luminal carbohydrates and lipids, and remain elevated for a duration of about 6 hours. PYY has several mechanisms of action:

- PYY lowers ghrelin levels.[34,37]
- PYY acts on the same hypothalamic neural circuits as leptin does, via the arcuate nucleus, and inhibits the appetite-stimulating NPY/agouti-related protein pathway.
- PYY is actually related to NPY and appears to compete for the same hypothalamic receptor.[30,38]

Fasting and postprandial PYY levels are lower in obese than in lean subjects, and fasting PYY levels are inversely correlated with BMI (Fig. 5-4). Although it is unclear whether lower PYY plasma levels are a cause or the consequence of obesity, **a deficiency in circulating PYY may play a role in perpetuating established overweight.**[37]

Serotonin. Serotonin (5-hydroxytryptamine [5HT]) is a neurotransmitter formed by the hydroxylation and decarboxylation of tryptophan. The greatest concentration of serotonin (90%) is found in the enterochromaffin cells of the gastrointestinal tract. Most of the remainder

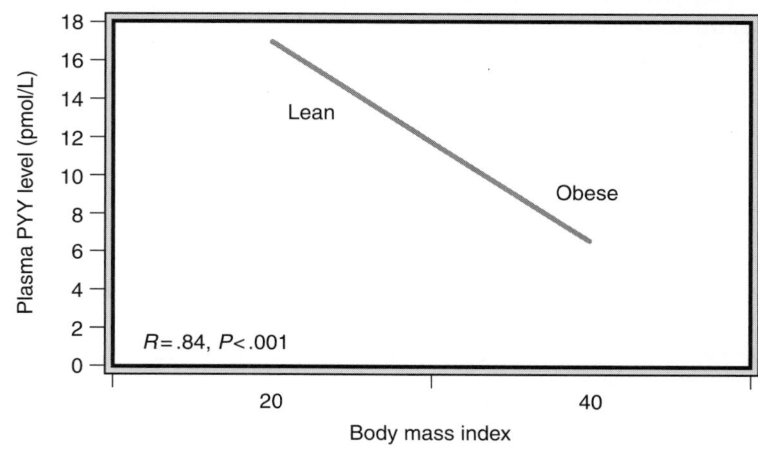

Figure 5–4. Inverse correlation between fasting plasma peptide YY (PYY) levels and body mass index. *(Modified from Batterham RL, Cohen MA, Ellis SM, et al. Inhibition of food intake in obese subjects by peptide YY3-36. N Engl J Med 2003;349:941-948.)*

of the body's serotonin is found in platelets and the central nervous system. Neurons that secrete 5HT are termed serotonergic. After the release of serotonin, a portion of serotonin is taken back up by the presynaptic, serotonergic neurons in a manner analogous to the reuptake of norepinephrine.[39,40]

Diverse serotonin receptors have been identified, such as 5HT1, 5HT2, 5HT3, 5HT4, 5HT5, 5HT6, and 5HT7. Additionally, there are receptor subtypes for the 5HT1, 5HT2, and 5HT5 receptors. The 5HT6 and 5HT7 receptors are distributed throughout the limbic system of the brain, and 5HT6 receptors have a high affinity for antidepressant drugs. Most of these receptors are coupled to G proteins that affect the activities of either adenylate cyclase or phospholipase C.[40]

In the central nervous system, serotonin decreases appetite and modulates food constituent selection. The 5HT2C receptors are thought to control food intake because mice lacking this gene become obese as a result of increased feeding. Increased plasma levels of the essential amino acid tryptophan because of protein consumption may promote brain uptake of this amino acid and promote its conversion to serotonin, thereby inducing a sated feeling. High local levels of serotonin in the central nervous system will result in a dietary preference for proteins; low levels of serotonin will have the opposite effect. **Stress-related depression, which may be associated with low central serotonin levels, in fact causes the preferential consumption of high-carbohydrate, low-protein comfort foods. Carbohydrate ingestion, by increasing insulin levels, will assist the uptake of tryptophan into the brain for conversion to serotonin, thus effectively raising hypothalamic, extracellular serotonin levels.**[39]

ANOREXIGENIC HORMONES

NAME	SITE OF ORIGIN
α-Melanocyte–stimulating hormone	Central nervous system
Leptin	Adipose tissue
Insulin	Pancreas
Cholecystokinin	Intestines
Peptide YY3-36	Intestines
Serotonin	Central nervous system

Serotonin has been a constituent of previously prescribed anorectic drugs. Its impact on food intake may underlie the weight control effects seen with some of the antidepressant selective serotonin reuptake inhibitors.[40,41]

Orexigenic Pathways. Orexigenic stimuli increase feeding behavior. They suppress sympathetic nervous system activity and thermogenesis.[30]

Orexigenic pathways produce

- agouti-related protein and
- NPY,

which are coexpressed by a subgroup of hypothalamic neurons. These orexigenic peptides antagonize the anorexigenic melanocortin signals.

Agouti-Related Protein. Agouti-related protein antagonizes the interaction between α-melanocyte–stimulating hormone and MC4R.[34]

Neuropeptide Y. NPY is a 36–amino acid neurotransmitter with complex effects on feeding, anxiety, circadian rhythms, reproduction, pituitary-adrenocortical function, and thermoregulation. It acts through at least six receptors, Y1 through Y6. Acting via the Y5 receptor, NPY inhibits thermogenesis.[42] It decreases the synthesis of thyrotropin-releasing hormone.[34]

NPY is the most powerful appetite stimulant known. NPY potently stimulates food intake through the Y5 receptor[42]:

- NPY increases the synthesis of melanin-concentrating hormone, an orexigenic peptide.
- NPY decreases expression of the gene encoding for POMC.[34]

NPY may also be involved in stress-mediated overconsumption.

Ghrelin. During fasting, the oxyntic mucosa of the gastrointestinal tract expresses and releases appetite-stimulating, orexigenic factors for short-term regulation, such as

- ghrelin,
- the orexins OX-A and OX-B, and
- cannabinoid CB1 agonist.[31]

Orexigenic ghrelin is a 28–amino acid, acylated peptide produced by oxyntic cells in the stomach fundus. Ghrelin is an endogenous ligand for and acts on growth hormone secretagogue receptors in the pituitary and hypothalamus to increase the release of growth hormone from the pituitary. It thereby derives its acronymic name.

More importantly, ghrelin modulates energy homeostasis and has a role in the central regulation of feeding behavior. **Ghrelin potently arouses appetite to stimulate the periodic intake of meals during the course of the day.** Its levels rise 1 to 2 hours preprandially and reach a nadir postprandially. Ghrelin appears to act centrally and stimulates growth hormone secretagogue receptors on hypothalamic arcuate nucleus neurons and on vagal afferents to promote the expression and release of hypothalamic NPY and agouti-related protein, thereby stimulating the paraventricular nucleus and driving ingestive behavior.[31,34] Ghrelin in vivo stimulates AMPK activity in the hypothalamus, which also increases food intake.[33]

Overproduction of ghrelin may lead to obesity, but that condition is rare. Obese humans actually have lower ghrelin levels than controls do; however, **diet-induced weight loss causes a rebound in ghrelin levels, which may undermine weight loss efforts.**[30]

OREXIGENIC HORMONES

NAME	SITE OF ORIGIN
Agouti-related protein	Central nervous system
Neuropeptide Y	Central nervous system
OX-A and OX-B	Intestines
Cannabinoid CB1 agonist	Intestines
Ghrelin	Intestines

HORMONAL REGULATORS OF ADIPOCYTE METABOLISM

Fat mass is highly variable, with significant short- and long-term plasticity determined by genetic and environmental factors.[43] Adipose tissue has a good blood supply, as well as rich sympathetic and parasympathetic nervous tissue innervation. Catecholamines, insulin, adenosine, and glucocorticoids all modulate adipocyte metabolism.[29]

Catecholamines. The sympathetic nervous system stimulates energy mobilization and energy utilization in numerous tissues. Catecholamines are the primary regulators and the most potent activators of lipolysis. Catecholamine effects are mediated through stimulation of adipocyte adrenergic receptors. Adrenergic receptors are actually the major receptors in adipocyte plasma membranes.

Adrenergic Receptors in Adipose Tissue. Adipose tissue has a mixture of adrenergic receptors:

- α_2-adrenergic receptors and
- subtypes of β-adrenergic receptors:
  - β_1,
  - β_2, and
  - β_3.

α_2-Adrenergic and β-adrenergic receptors have opposite effects on lipid mobilization:

- α_2-Adrenergic receptor stimulation inhibits lipolysis.
- β-Adrenergic receptor stimulation induces lipolysis.[28]

With sustained sympathetic activity, β_1- and β_2-adrenergic receptors are rapidly down-regulated and desensitized, whereas β_3-adrenergic receptor activity remains stable. The β_3-adrenergic receptor, which mediates negative inotropy in the myocardium, is a major regulator of the resting metabolic rate and lipolysis.[28,44]

Adrenergic Receptor Distribution in Adipose Tissue. The number and density of adrenergic receptor subtypes varies among different deposits of adipose tissue. The relative proportion of receptor subtypes in each tissue determines that tissue's metabolic activity and lipolytic versus antilipolytic tendencies. In general, the receptor density distribution in adipose tissue, in decreasing order, is as follows:

- β-adrenergic receptors: visceral-omental > abdominal subcutaneous > peripheral subcutaneous;
- α_2-adrenergic receptors: peripheral subcutaneous > abdominal subcutaneous > visceral-omental.[28,45]

The peripheral subcutaneous adipose tissue category includes gluteofemoral adipose deposits.

Adrenergic Receptor G Proteins. All adrenergic receptors are members of the G protein family. The receptors feature a long polypeptide chain that loops back and forth through the membrane seven times. On the cytoplasmic surface of the membrane, the receptor polypeptide is linked to the G protein. G proteins consist of three subunits, the G protein effector system, with different binding and functional effects. Upon catecholamine binding to the adrenergic receptor, a conformational shift activates one or more of the G protein subunits. As the activated subunits couple to different signaling molecules within the cell, a specific physiologic response is ultimately evoked.[28]

The two families of G proteins that are involved in control of lipolysis are

1. G_s protein and
2. G_i protein.

The β-adrenergic receptor, coupled to a stimulatory G_s protein, stimulates cAMP and lipolysis. The α-receptor, coupled to an inhibitory G_i protein, inhibits cAMP formation and lipolysis.[28]

G_s Protein. G_s activates adenylate cyclase to produce cAMP. Increased availability of cAMP enhances triglyceride hydrolysis.

cAMP increases the activity of protein kinase A, which, in turn, phosphorylates and activates HSL. Activated HSL translocates to the triacylglycerol storage sites, where triacylglycerol hydrolysis and lipolysis proceed.[28]

At least part of the weight loss effect of adrenergic agonists may also be mediated by the activation of AMPK in peripheral tissues.[32]

G_i Protein. In contrast to G_s effects, **the G_i protein complex attenuates the production of cAMP, thus decreasing the rate of triglyceride hydrolysis.**

Upon receptor stimulation, the G_i protein subunits may dissociate, thereby inhibiting further signal transduction to adenylate cyclase. Because of its antilipolytic effect, α_2-adrenergic stimulation is associated with larger adipocyte size, which may affect cell metabolism.[28]

Impact of Age and Adiposity on Catecholamine-Mediated Lipolysis. Adrenergic receptor distribution in adipose tissue is also a function of

- age and
- body weight.

An increase in adipocyte size and number, as seen with obesity and aging, increases the density of antilipolytic α_2-adrenergic receptors. As a result, **with increasing age and overweight, there is a reduction in lipolytic activity, thus thwarting weight loss attempts.**[28]

Impact of Sympathetic Tone on Lipolysis. Adrenergic receptors are stimulated with differential affinity by

- norepinephrine as a neurotransmitter and
- circulating epinephrine.

Because α-adrenergic receptors have the highest affinity for catecholamines, a low resting sympathetic tone, with low ambient levels of norepinephrine, would be associated with low cAMP levels and little lipolysis. In contrast, **sympathetic hyperactivity, with elevated circulating epinephrine, increases cAMP levels and enhances lipolysis to provide energy substrate to tissues during stress.**

Correspondingly, catecholamines also interfere with lipogenesis by inhibiting LPL.[28]

Parasympathetic Innervation. Adipose tissue is innervated by the parasympathetic nervous system. **Whereas the sympathoadrenal system is implicated in lipolysis, the parasympathetics mediate lipogenesis.** Parasympathetic nerves originating from different parts of the central nervous system supply the intra-abdominal visceral-omental and the subcutaneous fat depots.[46]

Parasympathetic Impact on Lipogenesis. Parasympathetic nervous system activity

- increases insulin sensitivity,
- increases triglyceride synthesis,
- increases the deposition of fat stores, and
- decreases the activity of HSL.

Rates of fat synthesis differ in diverse anatomic locations, in part as a function of the density of parasympathetic innervation. Visceral intra-abdominal fat is more heavily innervated than subcutaneous fat. Thus, **with enhanced parasympathetic tone, greater parasympathetic nervous system activity in visceral adipose tissue may lead to the preferential accumulation of visceral-abdominal rather than subcutaneous fat.**[46] This may account for the abdominal ponderosity in depictions of a restful, meditating Buddha.

Lower parasympathetic activity reduces the insulin-stimulated uptake of glucose and free fatty acids and increases the activity of HSL, the fat-degrading enzyme. **There is a reduction in parasympathetic nervous system activity and an increase in sympathetic tone with obesity and the metabolic syndrome. As a result, lipolysis is increased and plasma free fatty acid levels are raised, which contributes to systemic insulin resistance in skeletal muscle and the liver.**[46]

Insulin. Insulin is the major anabolic regulator of fat metabolism. It combines both antilipolytic and lipogenic effects.

Antilipolytic Effects. Insulin interferes with lipolysis via several mechanisms:

- Insulin may promote the internal translocation of β-adrenergic receptors and thereby blunt catecholamine action.
- Upon activation of the insulin receptor, postreceptor insulin signaling in adipocytes entails activation of phosphodiesterase, which breaks down cAMP and decreases lipolysis.
- Another action of insulin involves the dephosphorylation, or deactivation, of HSL, which inhibits the rate-limiting step of intracellular triglyceride hydrolysis.[28]

Lipogenic Effects. Insulin enhances lipogenesis in adipose tissue via a number of mechanisms:

- Insulin increases the synthesis and activity of adipose tissue LPL, thereby promoting the uptake of free fatty acids into adipocytes.
- Insulin increases glucose uptake by adipocytes to be metabolized to glycerol, the structural backbone for triacylglycerols.
- Insulin phosphorylates and activates acetyl CoA carboxylase and fatty acid synthase, thereby catalyzing the de novo formation of free fatty acids.
- Insulin stimulates the esterification process within adipocytes whereby three fatty acid chains attach to glycerol to form triacylglycerol for storage.[28]

Adenosine. Adenosine is produced by adipocytes. Adipocytes have A1 adenosine receptors, which are coupled with G_i proteins. Local autocrine/paracrine adenosine-receptor interaction would thus be expected to limit lipolysis, acting in concert with insulin.

Glucocorticoids. Glucocorticoids are lipogenic and have a significant impact on adipocyte development. Extraneous administration of glucocorticoids, or their pathologic overproduction, may cause overweight with a cushingoid phenotype. However, even stress-induced, lower levels of glucocorticoids, elaborated by activation of the hypothalamic-pituitary-adrenal axis, have an effect.[47]

11β-Hydroxysteroid Dehydrogenase. Glucocorticoids regulate body fat distribution at the local tissue level via metabolic processing of glucocorticoids within adipose tissue itself. Tissue corticosteroid activity is regulated, in part, by the enzyme 11β-hydroxysteroid dehydrogenase (11β-HSD), which exists as two isozymes,

1. 11β-HSD-1, with predominant reductase activity, and
2. 11β-HSD-2, with predominant dehydrogenase activity.

11β-HSD-1 is predominantly expressed in

- adipose,
- liver,
- gonadal, and
- central nervous system

tissues, where it serves as a reductase and converts inactive cortisone to the active glucocorticoid receptor agonists

- cortisol and
- corticosterone.

This process creates locally elevated, active steroid tissue levels. **Visceral-omental adipose tissue contains significantly more 11β-HSD-1 activity than subcutaneous adipose tissue does.** Furthermore, 11β-HSD-1 activity increases with cell maturation and with obesity.

11β-HSD-2 is expressed primarily in aldosterone target cells such as in the kidney and the colon, where it inactivates cortisol via its dehydrogenase activity. It thereby prevents excessive activation of the mineralocorticoid receptor and sequelae such as hypertension.[48]

The Glucocorticoid Receptor. The glucocorticoid receptor is a nuclear hormone receptor.

It functions as a transcription factor that modulates the expression of a variety of genes in adipose tissue. For example,

- the glucocorticoid receptor activates the gene transcription of LPL and serves to stabilize it post-translationally. Endothelially bound LPL hydrolyzes triglycerides in plasma, with release of free fatty acids into tissue for uptake and reassembly into triacylglycerols for fat storage[49];
- glucocorticoids also promote the differentiation of preadipocytes to mature adipocytes.[49]

The glucocorticoid receptor has a variable tissue density distribution in a ranking order of

Visceral > Abdominal subcutaneous > Femoral subcutaneous adipocytes.[49]

Glucocorticoid Interaction with Insulin and Sex Hormones. The presence of insulin compounds the powerful lipid-accumulating effects of glucocorticoids, and **steroid effects to increase fat storage are particularly marked in the presence of hyperinsulinemia.** Glucocorticoids may affect the free plasma concentration of sex hormones by modulating sex hormone–binding globulins.[29]

Glucocorticoids and Abdominal Obesity. The combination of the highest level of 11β-HSD-1 and the highest density of glucocorticoid receptors renders visceral-omental tissue exquisitely responsive to local activated glucocorticoids. As a result, upon steroid exposure as with stress, preadipocytes from the visceral-omental depot can more readily differentiate into adipocytes than can preadipocytes from subcutaneous tissue, and the glucocorticoid-driven overexpression of LPL will favor increased visceral fat accumulation.[29,50]

The increased expression of 11β-HSD-1 in mature adipocytes and in obesity effectively constitutes a positive feedback cycle whereby stress-associated elevation of glucocorticoids will continue to sustain visceral ponderosity in an overweight, hyperinsulinemic individual.[48,51]

Other Agents. Adipocytes are also affected by a variety of other agents, such as prostaglandins and fatty acids acting via fatty acid binding proteins. Additionally, postreceptor events in adipocytes are subject to external modulation, as are key enzymes in adipocyte metabolism, such as LPL, HSL, adenylyl cyclase, and phosphodiesterase.

Adipose tissue is itself a source for growth factors such as

- insulin-like growth factor-I (IGF-I),
- IGF binding protein,
- tumor necrosis factor-alpha (TNF-α),
- angiotensin II, and
- macrophage colony-stimulating factor (M-CSF).

These autocrine/paracrine factors are capable of stimulating cell proliferation in fat tissue.

NEUROHORMONAL IMPACT ON ADIPOSE TISSUE

FACTOR	IMPACT ON LIPOLYSIS	IMPACT ON LIPOGENESIS
β_3-Adrenergic agonist	+	–
α_2-Adrenergic agonist	–	0
Muscarinic agonist	–	+
Insulin	–	+
Adenosine	–	0
Glucocorticoids	0	+
Androgens	+	–

+, increase; –, decrease; 0, neutral.

GENDER DIFFERENCES IN ADIPOSE TISSUE

The environment and the genetic makeup of an individual influence the deposition of adipose tissue. Adipose tissue changes with age, and sex hormones induce complex, sexual dimorphisms of adipose tissue. There are sex-related differences in LPL activity and adrenergic receptor distribution that cause men and women to have regional differences in lipogenesis and lipolysis.[28]

Sex Hormone Effects on Adipose Tissue

Men. Adipose tissue in men has characteristics that on the one hand favor visceral-omental fat deposition and, on the other hand, encourage lipolysis of those tissues.

Factors Favoring Abdominal Fat Deposition. Men are particularly prone to abdominal fat storage, and visceral adipose tissue in men is less subject to lipolysis:

- In men, adrenergic receptors in visceral-abdominal adipocytes are predominantly α_2.
- Visceral-abdominal adipose tissue in men has more LPL activity than subcutaneous tissue does.[28]

Factors Favoring Lipolysis of Abdominal Fat. The androgen receptor appears to counter the very factors that render men prone to abdominal ponderosity:

- Testosterone affects adrenergic receptor gene expression. The hormonal effects may be indirect rather than direct. Testosterone appears to increase β-adrenergic receptor and adenylate cyclase activity, especially in the abdominal region, thereby favoring abdominal lipolysis.
- In men, androgen receptor density is richer in visceral than in subcutaneous fat depots. Testosterone inhibits LPL and is implicated in lipid mobilization, even in the presence of cortisol.[28,29]

Women. Women are more prone to gluteofemoral lipogenesis and fat deposition, and these tissues are less subject to lipolysis:

- In women, gluteofemoral adipocytes have more LPL activity than visceral adipocytes do. Even LPL activity in breast tissue is lower than that in gluteofemoral fat tissue.
- Progesterone and estrogen appear to further stimulate gluteofemoral LPL activity.[52]
- Additionally, gluteofemoral adipocytes in women preferentially have antilipolytic α_2-adrenergic receptors.[28]

There do not appear to be any specific estrogen or progesterone receptors on adipocytes. Estrogen may exert some paracrine control on adipocytes. In women, the androgen receptor effects may be down-regulated by estrogen. Progesterone may, however, compete with the glucocorticoid receptor and mitigate excessive glucocorticoid tissue effects.[52]

Android and Gynoid Adipose Tissue. The typical adult male and female fat distribution is termed android and gynoid, respectively. The difference obviously affects looks, but it has implications beyond appearance, with effects on morbidity.[53,54]

Android Adiposity. Men, when compared with women, have an abundance of abdominal and visceral fat that increases with age. Whereas for women at 20 years of age, 10% of abdominal fat is visceral-omental, for men it is significantly higher and increases with age[55,56]:

AGE—MEN (YR)	ABDOMINAL FAT THAT IS VISCERAL-OMENTAL (%)
20	20
46	38
67	47

Android adiposity, also termed

- male pattern,
- "apple-shaped," and
- visceral

adiposity, is characterized by subcutaneous abdominal and, more importantly, excessive visceral-omental fat tissue deposition (panniculus adiposus). This distribution is associated with a tendency to endocrinologic imbalances such as

- increased activity of the hypothalamic-pituitary-adrenal axis,
- higher glucocorticoid activity, and
- greater expression of glucocorticoid receptors in visceral adipocytes.

Such disturbances may lead to

- hyperandrogenicity in women and
- relative hypogonadism in men.[55,56]

Gynoid Adiposity. Gynoid adiposity is characterized by excessive subcutaneous fat distribution in the lower part of the abdomen and the gluteofemoral region. It is also termed

- female pattern,
- "pear-shaped," and
- peripheral

adiposity. Although women may, on average, have 50% more fat than men do, in women the proportion of android fat is less than in men. Premenopausal women with significant gynoid adiposity may be prone to mechanical disorders such as arthritis and varicosities. However, the incidence of endocrinologic imbalances and metabolic derangements associated with gynoid adiposity is significantly lower than that associated with android adiposity.[54,57]

With rising age, android or visceral adiposity increases in both sexes, especially in men. In the absence of estrogen replacement therapy, the sexual dimorphisms of adipose tissue increasingly disappear after menopause.

VISCERAL-OMENTAL ADIPOSITY: ASSESSMENT AND METABOLISM

Visceral adipose tissue is made up of the panniculus adiposus, which is composed of omental and mesenteric fat surrounding the stomach and intestines. It also includes other visceral fat depots such as the pericardial fat pad.[58]

Assessment of Visceral Adiposity. An assessment of the amount of visceral fat is helpful in risk-stratifying individuals and in research studies.

Waist Circumference. Waist circumference reflects both abdominal subcutaneous and visceral-omental adipose tissue. It thus reflects the central, truncal fat mass. Waist circumference is measured just above the iliac crest. Excess abdominal fat is clinically defined as a waist circumference exceeding

- 102 cm, or 40 inches, for men and
- 88 cm, or 35 inches, for women.[2]

This measurement is often used as an inexpensive, simple index of visceral adipose tissue.

Waist-Hip Ratio. The waist-hip ratio (WHR) is the ratio between the waist circumference and the hip circumference. Although this ratio is clearly influenced by other body tissues and the accuracy of the WHR in distinguishing abdominal visceral adipose tissue from subcutaneous tissue has not been defined, it is a useful measure in adults. The utility of the WHR is not established for children. In obese individuals, changes in visceral adiposity after weight loss are poorly related to changes in WHR.[59]

Computer-Assisted Tomography. Computer-assisted tomographic scanning has been used as a quantitative, accurate measure of the surface area and volume of subcutaneous and visceral fat at the level of the umbilicus. Based on the ratio of the visceral to the subcutaneous fat area, obesity can be more quantitatively classified into visceral fat and subcutaneous fat obesity.[60]

Lipogenic and Lipolytic Forces in Visceral Adipocytes. Excessive visceral-omental ponderosity contributes to metabolic disturbances. Visceral adipose tissue is significantly more metabolically active than subcutaneous fat tissue. There are unique metabolic aspects of visceral tissue that strongly favor abdominal fat deposition. Other metabolic features render that tissue particularly labile and prone to lipolysis with adverse metabolic sequelae. In fact, **metabolic and lipolytic activity is higher in the visceral region than in other fat depots.**

Visceral Adipocyte Features That Favor Fat Deposition. Genetic factors, as well as a unique hormonal and neuronal milieu, play a contributory role in visceral ponderosity.

Genetics. There is a strong, 30% to 50% genetic component to the increase in visceral fat with overfeeding, which correlates with insulin levels.[61]

Glucocorticoids. The lipogenic effect of steroids is optimized in visceral fat. Visceral-omental adipose tissue contains significantly more 11β-HSD-1 activity than subcutaneous adipose tissue does for conversion of inactive cortisone to active glucocorticoids.[48,49] Visceral adipocytes also have a higher glucocorticoid receptor number than do cells in other depots.[49]

Insulin. Visceral adipocytes have a greater number of insulin receptors than subcutaneous cells do.[28]

Parasympathetic Innervation. The visceral fat depot has denser parasympathetic innervation than fat tissue at other sites does, which favors visceral lipogenesis.[46]

Leptin. There is lower expression of leptin by visceral adipose tissue, thus exerting a lesser central, anorexigenic effect.[4]

Visceral Adipocyte Features That Favor Lipolysis. The visceral fat depot rapidly mobilizes free fatty acids. The high sympathetic activity and lower efficacy of insulin play a role.

Insulin and Glucose Uptake. Insulin receptor affinity and insulin signal transduction are decreased in visceral adipocytes. Visceral adipocytes have lower expression of the glucose transporter GLUT4 and less glycogen synthase, and the antilipolytic actions of insulin are less effica-cious in visceral adipocytes than in subcutaneous sites.[62]

Adrenergic Receptors. Sympathetic activity is high in visceral adipose tissue. Visceral fat is richly innervated by the sympathetic nervous system, particularly in men. Because of the decreased α_2-, but increased β-adrenergic receptor density, visceral tissue is metabolically very active and labile. Thus, **catecholamines are most active in the visceral area, and catecholamine-induced lipolysis is highest in visceral adipocytes.** With sympathetic activation, as occurs during physical exercise, triacylglycerols can be readily mobilized from the visceral depot for the rapid supply of energy substrates to other tissues.[28,63]

Miscellaneous Factors. When compared with subcutaneous tissue, visceral adipocytes have lower expression of

- adenosine receptors and
- PPAR-γ,

which results in less suppression of lipolysis and decreased adipocyte differentiation.[62]

FACTORS THAT ARE PREFERENTIALLY EXPRESSED IN VISCERAL ADIPOSE TISSUE AND METABOLIC CONSEQUENCES

FACTOR	IMPACT	CONSEQUENCE
Parasympathetic tone	Fat storage	Visceral obesity
11β-HSD-1	Fat storage	Visceral obesity
Glucocorticoid receptor	Fat storage	Visceral obesity
β-Adrenergic receptor	Lipolysis	Increased plasma free fatty acids Hypertriglyceridemia Insulin resistance

Visceral Adiposity and Insulin Resistance. The unique anatomy and physiology of visceral fat render it a powerful immune and endocrine organ. Visceral ponderosity contributes to the genesis of insulin resistance. Albeit controversial, visceral adiposity has been proposed as one of the major determinants of the metabolic syndrome with its attendant metabolic and cardiovascular complications.[64] A number of factors play a contributory role.

Free Fatty Acids. The greater the visceral adipose tissue depot, the greater the quantity of free fatty acids released by lipolytic stimuli. Elevated plasma free fatty acids, particularly as derived from active lipolysis of an enlarged visceral depot, if not consumed as fuel by working muscle become pivotal mediators of systemic insulin resistance.[65]

Adipokines. Visceral adipose tissue is an active endocrine and immune organ, and it releases proinflammatory cytokines termed adipocytokines. The production of adipocytokines, or adipokines, from visceral fat exceeds that derived from subcutaneous adipose tissue. Adipokines exert autocrine/paracrine/endocrine effects on local and peripheral tissues, thereby engendering insulin resistance.[66,67]

Hyperinsulinemia and Sympathetic Activity. The endocrine pancreas releases insulin directly into the portal venous circulation, where it is first presented to the liver. The liver clears about 50% of the insulin in the first pass. With growing resistance to insulin and compensatory hyperinsulinemia, total and relative hepatic extraction of insulin is reduced. More insulin enters the systemic circulation, and systemic hyperinsulinemia supervenes.[68]

Hyperinsulinemia may itself further raise sympathetic neural outflow via central mechanisms.[68,69] Sympathetic hyperactivity will activate the renin-angiotensin-aldosterone system (RAAS) and inflammatory pathways and further increase visceral lipolytic activity, free fatty acid generation, and adipokine release, thus increasing local and peripheral insulin resistance in a vicious circle.[68]

The Metabolic Syndrome. Significant derangements in glucose and lipid metabolism, as well as vascular function, are seen primarily with visceral obesity.[60] Increased visceral-omental fat is ultimately linked with

- decreased insulin sensitivity,
- higher fasting insulin levels,[70]

- increased glucose levels,[71]
- type 2 DM,[72] and
- CHD.[73,74]

Visceral Free Fatty Acid Production and Dyslipidemia. Visceral ponderosity is linked to atherogenic dyslipidemia.

Triglycerides. Lipolysis of visceral fat, in the absence of oxidative consumption of such fat as fuel, plays a role in the development of hypertriglyceridemia.

Visceral fat is the adipose depot with the highest potential for free fatty acid turnover. The venous effluent from visceral-omental fat drains directly into the portal vein, with all lipolysis products delivered directly and exclusively to the liver.

The hepatic metabolic pathway for increased free fatty acid levels involves either

1. fatty acid oxidation for energy or
2. fatty acid esterification for lipogenesis.

In the absence of starvation or the metabolic need to consume fatty acids in order to satisfy energy demands, hepatic de novo lipogenesis is up-regulated. Free fatty acids in the liver are esterified to form triacylglycerols.

As hepatic triacylglycerol production increases, triacylglycerols are stored in cytosolic pools, and a smaller portion is secreted in the form of very-low-density lipoprotein (VLDL). Cytosolic pool size correlates with VLDL secretion. Elevation of plasma free fatty acids thus stimulates both the production and the secretion of VLDL.[75,76]

With increasing insulin resistance and chronic hyperinsulinemia, apolipoprotein (apo) B stability in the liver is enhanced. Increased availability of apo B facilitates the increased synthesis, assembly, and secretion of triglyceride-rich VLDL particles and other apo B lipoproteins.[77] **Hepatic overproduction plus oversecretion of VLDL is a crucial consequence of visceral fat and insulin resistance.**[75,76]

Dyslipidemia. Increased visceral fat is associated with atherogenic dyslipidemia. As lipolysis from visceral adipose tissue induces elevated apo B levels and hypertriglyceridemia, these changes secondarily generate small, dense low-density lipoprotein (LDL) and lower high-density lipoprotein (HDL) levels.[67,71]

FUNCTIONS OF ADIPOSE TISSUE

Adipose tissue has long been known as a storage depot for fuel. It serves many other functions (Table 5-1).

Energy Storage. Under conditions of positive energy balance, energy is stored in the form of fatty acids and triacylglycerol. Adipose tissue is the primary and largest site for body energy storage, and more than 95% of the body's triacylglycerol is stored in adipocytes. Adipocytes are approximately 80% triacylglycerol by weight. Each adipocyte contains about 0.04 to 0.06 μg of fat, and a young, nonobese adult has 10 to 15 kg of adipose tissue, corresponding to 135,000 kcal of energy storage.[28] Fat storage is effected via insulin, which stimulates cellular glucose and long-chain fatty acid uptake, as well as lipogenesis.[78]

Adipose tissue serves as a dynamic energy storage depot from which free fatty acids are released via lipolysis when fuel is required during periods of increased energy requirement, energy shortage, and fasting. Plasma free fatty acids, released from adipose tissue, are present in micromolar concentrations and constitute the major circulating lipid fuel.

Adipose Tissue as Protection, Insulation, and Buffer. Adipose tissue plays a role in the mechanical support and protection of tissues and organs, as well as providing thermal insulation for organs.[27] Lipid-soluble substances, such as drugs, are stored in adipose tissue. Fat tissue is needed for normal glucose and lipid homeostasis. It removes and takes up circulating lipoproteins, triglyceride, and cholesterol.

Table 5-1. Functions of White Adipose Tissue

Functions
Fuel storage and provision
Thermal insulation
Mechanical protection
Glucose homeostasis
Immunity
Inflammatory response
Endocrine signaling
Secretory proteins

Modified from Trayhurn P, Beattie JH. Physiological role of adipose tissue: white adipose tissue as an endocrine and secretory organ. Proc Nutr Soc 2001:60:329-339.

Adipose Tissue Endocrine Function. The notion that adipose tissue is but a storage site for fat has undergone dramatic revision since the mid 1990s. **White fat functions as a major secretory organ. It serves as an endocrine organ when located in the viscera and as a paracrine/autocrine organ when situated intramuscularly.[66] The secretory function actually exceeds fat storage in importance.** However, quantitatively, fatty acids do remain the major secretory product of white adipose tissue.[27]

Fat depots are not all similar, and adipocytes in diverse depots secrete a differing array of substances. Thus, there are significant depot-specific variances in adipocyte gene expression, which may contribute to the specific functional properties of visceral versus subcutaneous adipocytes.

Steroid Hormone Metabolism. White adipose tissue expresses enzymes involved in the metabolism of steroid hormones. Inactive cortisone is converted to active cortisol or corticosterone in fat.[48] Estrone is converted to estradiol, androstenedione is converted to testosterone, and androgens can be aromatized to estrogens in adipose tissue.[27]

Adipokines. Adipose tissue secretes signaling molecules and hormones. These substances often have the structural properties of cytokines and are referred to as adipocytokines, or adipokines. Adipocytes express receptors for several proinflammatory molecules. Adipokines have endocrine in addition to autocrine and paracrine functions and are secreted in response to stressors such as diet and exercise, as well as in response to acute or chronic changes in the metabolic and inflammatory milieu.

Adipokine Action. **Adipokines function as inflammatory cytokines** and have a role in

- feeding behavior,
- endothelial function,
- insulin sensitivity and action,
- lipid and glucose metabolism,
- energy and fat homeostasis and adipocyte maturation,
- host defense,
- modulation of the complement system,
- vascular homeostasis, and
- reproduction.

Adipokine Source. **Cytokines are generated from adipocytes, preadipocytes, and other cell types such as stromal vascular cells,[79,80] which generate the mRNA for these factors. Because the macrophage content of adipose tissue correlates positively with BMI and adipocyte size, macrophages may in fact be the primary generators of proinflammatory molecules in adipose tissue.**

These stromal macrophages, attracted by monocyte chemotactic protein-1 (MCP-1), derive from the vasculature via infiltration and extravasation. As in the case of atherosclerosis, endothelial dysfunction, incurred as a result of stress pathways, may serve as a primary stimulus to induce such macrophage recruitment to adipose tissue.[81] Macrophages are also generated through preadipocyte conversion.[82,83]

In fact, in obesity, the nuclear fraction of circulating mononuclear cells, the presumptive precursors of adipose tissue macrophages, is associated with an increase in nuclear factor kappaB (NFκB) binding activity and p65 expression, with a decrease in the inhibitory protein IκB-β. The magnitude of NFκB binding is related to BMI and measures of insulin resistance, as is the resultant increase in the expression of NFκB-modulated genes, such as TNF-α, interleukin-6 (IL-6), and matrix metalloproteinase-9.[84]

Stimuli for Adipokine Release. **Selected stimuli for adipokine generation are**

- **lipopolysaccharide,**
- **increased fat cell size,**
- **catecholamines, and**
- **possibly insulin and cortisol.**

The mass of adipose tissue partly determines the circulating level of some adipokines.[66]

Visceral Adipocyte Activity. **Visceral adipocytes, in particular, are active secretors of adipokines.[66]** Visceral fat and subcutaneous fat are biologically distinct. Visceral fat cells, for example, produce more angiotensinogen, IL-6, leptin, plasminogen activator inhibitor-1 (PAI-1), and resistin than subcutaneous fat does. Although visceral adipocytes produce more adiponectin than subcutaneous cells do, **there is a strong, negative correlation of visceral adiponectin production with BMI.**[85]

Specific Adipokines. The following is a partial list of known adipokines[27,86-97]:

ACRP30 or adiponectin
acylation-stimulating protein
adipsin
angiotensinogen and all elements of the RAAS
apo E
cholesterol ester transfer protein
colony-stimulating factor-1
complement system products
C-reactive protein
factor VII
fasting-induced adipose factor
free fatty acids
fibrinogen-angiopoietin–related protein
inducible nitric oxide synthase (iNOS)
intercellular adhesion molecule-1
IL-1β, IL-6, IL-8
leptin
LPL
M-CSF
macrophage inflammatory protein-1α
metallothionein
MCP-1
PAI-1
resistin-like molecules
retinol binding protein
tissue factor
transforming growth factor-β
TNF-α
vascular endothelial growth factor

Actions of Selected Adipokines. Adipokines produce an effect on adipocytes via at least seven different chemokine receptors. **The proinflammatory cytokines and the RAAS components elaborated by adipose tissue are antiadipogenic and antilipogenic, thus favoring lipolysis.** They

- decrease the mRNA expression of PPAR-γ,
- lower adipocyte lipid content,
- impair preadipocyte recruitment and adipocyte differentiation, and
- positively control the post-transcriptional control of leptin.

Adipokines directly and indirectly cause and exacerbate insulin resistance and are implicated in obesity-related cardiovascular and metabolic health complications.

Free fatty acids, PAI-1, components of the RAAS, and TNF-α are most abundantly released from adipose tissue.

Free Fatty Acids. Increased free fatty acid fluxes derived from adipocyte lipolysis constitute the major circulating lipid fuel. However, free fatty acids potently

- impair insulin signaling and
- affect vascular reactivity and are linked to endothelial dysfunction.[66]

Plasminogen Activator Inhibitor-1. Insulin stimulates the production of PAI-1 from adipose tissue. Levels of PAI-1 and factor VII are elevated in obesity, and obesity is associated with hypercoagulability. PAI-1 inhibits plasmin, thereby preventing plasmin-mediated breakdown of fibrin clots. PAI-1

- is implicated in thrombogenesis[66] and
- has profibrotic properties.[98]

Angiotensin II. White adipocytes are an important source of angiotensinogen, second only to the liver, with levels rising as adiposity increases. Adipocytes also express genes encoding angiotensin-converting enzyme and angiotensin II type 1 receptors, consistent with the presence of a local adipose tissue RAAS.[27] Angiotensin II

- impairs insulin signaling,
- is antiadipogenic and prolipolytic, and
- is implicated in vascular oxidative stress and inflammation.[66]

Tumor Necrosis Factor-α. Adipose tissue expresses TNF-α constitutively. Adipose tissue in obesity has increased expression of TNF-α mRNA, with increased elaboration of TNF-α protein in obese humans.[97] Obesity may, in fact, be considered a state of TNF-α overexpression. The concentration of TNF-α is inversely proportional to HDL and proportional to BMI, fasting glucose, and insulin resistance.[99] TNF-α

- directly suppresses insulin signaling, thereby inducing insulin resistance,
- is antiadipogenic and prolipolytic, and
- causes vascular inflammation.[66]

Adipose Tissue as Part of the Immune System. There appears to be a linkage between adipose tissue and the immune system:

- Adipocyte precursors have phagocytic capability and can be transformed into macrophage-like cells in response to appropriate stimuli.[100]
- Adipocytes share with macrophages the expression of genes encoding for transcription factors, cytokines, inflammatory molecules, fatty acid transporters, and scavenger receptors.[81]
- Adipocytes share pathways such as complement activation and inflammatory cytokine production with T cells and macrophages.[97]

The adipose tissue–immune system linkage may be based on a common developmental background. Principal metabolic and immune functions appear to have evolved from a mutual source. Mammalian adipose tissue may derive from a site analogous to the *Drosophila* fat body, which contains the mammalian homologues of the liver, hematopoietic system, and other immune components.[101] As these systems evolved into differentiated and subspecialized organs, they maintained their functional capabilities with shared key regulatory molecules and pathways that mediate both metabolic and immune functions.[81]

The close relationship between adipocytes and immune cells and between metabolic and immune responses may constitute a teleologic rationale for adipokine secretion and action. Extremely malnourished individuals have an impaired immune response. Conversely, obesity appears to be an inflammatory state. Adipose tissue plays a nutritive and supportive role in inflammatory processes. The immune system uses 15% of the basal metabolic energy consumption, and fuel consumption increases with activation of the immune system. With this high level of energy utilization, the immune system needs to be linked to energy stores. **When stressed, the immune system requires the ability to mobilize fuel from energy stores and from the host in general, thus explaining the anti-adipogenic and insulin-resistant properties of proinflammatory cytokines.**[102]

Adipose tissue secretes leptin and IL-6, both of which have cytokine structures, are variably immunologically active, but also function as hypothalamic regulators. As such they may serve as messengers to

- report centrally on the status of energy stores,
- modulate immunologic preparedness,
- regulate energy expenditure, and
- control feeding behavior.[102]

OBESITY, INSULIN RESISTANCE, AND CORONARY HEART DISEASE

Insulin resistance has been thought to be the common denominator linking obesity to

1. **cardiovascular disease** with
   - endothelial dysfunction,
   - hypertension,
   - CHD risk,
   - atherosclerosis, and
   - acute ischemic syndromes and events,

as well as to

2. **metabolic diseases** of carbohydrate intolerance and dyslipidemia with
   - the metabolic syndrome,
   - glucose intolerance, and
   - type 2 DM.[103]

The progression of the severity of insulin resistance parallels the progression of the vascular and metabolic diseases.[66]

In fact, the "emerging risk factors" associated with the metabolic manifestations of insulin resistance, such as dyslipidemia, a proinflammatory and prothrombotic state, underlie the macrovascular complications of the metabolic syndrome and type 2 DM.[104] What is the link between obesity, insulin resistance, and metabolic and vascular disease?

Obesity and Insulin Resistance. Obesity can be manifested as a proinflammatory state and as such is a major determinant of the metabolic syndrome with its attendant metabolic and cardiovascular complications.[64]

Mechanism of Insulin Resistance with Obesity. Hyperplastic adipose tissue can be an active endocrine and immune organ that releases proinflammatory adipokines. Via autocrine/paracrine effects, these adipokines engender insulin resistance within adipose and neighboring tissues. The endocrine effects of such adipokines have a negative impact on the insulin sensitivity of peripheral tissues.[66,67]

The increased amounts of iNOS and TNF-α produced by skeletal muscle in obese versus lean rodents and humans[88,105] may arise from macrophages in the adipose tissue that surrounds and infiltrates muscle in the obese and thereby contribute to the decreased insulin sensitivity of muscle in obesity.[82]

Additionally, proinflammatory adipokines trigger lipolysis of adipose tissue in an autocrine/paracrine fashion. The ensuing elevated levels of plasma free fatty acids, if not beta-oxidized by working muscle, become pivotal mediators of systemic insulin resistance.[65] These same proinflammatory adipokines, acting as circulating hormones, may initiate insulin resistance mechanisms in distal target organs such as skeletal muscle or the liver.

Body Mass Index and Insulin Resistance. As a general rule, the greater the BMI, the more insulin resistant an individual will be.[106,107]

However, although obesity has been considered a risk factor for insulin resistance and cardiovascular disease across populations, there is substantial heterogeneity in the relationship between metabolic and cardiovascular abnormalities and the degree of obesity.[108] Of 1146 healthy obese individuals (BMI > 29.0 kg/m^2), the European Group for the Study of Insulin Resistance (EGIR) found only 26% to be insulin resistant, a finding similar to that seen in a more recent U.S. study that found only 25% of healthy obese individuals (BMI >30.0 kg/m^2) to have insulin resistance.[109,110] Because only healthy individuals were considered, these numbers are likely to be underestimates.

Waist-Hip Ratio and Insulin Resistance. BMI is not a perfect measure of adiposity. Beyond total-body fat mass, increased waist circumference and WHR have been thought to better reflect central fat deposition and visceral obesity, the latter being considered a contributor to insulin resistance.[111] However, there is some controversy about the importance of visceral obesity.[112] Furthermore, the EGIR study did not detect an independent correlation of WHR with insulin resistance.[109]

Obesity and Coronary Heart Disease. The relationship between obesity and CHD has also been controversial.

The Framingham Heart Study has consistently shown that increasing degrees of obesity are associated with higher CHD rates.[113] The Pathological Determinants of Atherosclerosis in Youth autopsy study of 3000 individuals aged 15 to 34 years who died of noncardiac causes showed BMI and a thick panniculus adiposus (visceral fat) to be positively correlated with early atheromatous disease (fatty streaks and raised atherosclerotic lesions) in men (Fig. 5-5). The relationship did not pertain to women except in the presence of significant visceral obesity. Conventional risk factors appeared to account for only 15% of the disease process.[114]

In contrast, the Seven Countries Study revealed little correlation between body weight and CHD.[115] Similar results were obtained in the Geographic Pathology of Atherosclerosis autopsy study.[116]

It appears to be the metabolic syndrome, rather than BMI, that actually predicts future cardiovascular risk, at least in women. In the Women's Ischemia Syndrome Evaluation study of 780 women who were referred for coronary angiography to evaluate suspected myocardial ischemia, BMI and the metabolic syndrome were strongly associated, but only the metabolic syndrome was associated with significant CHD. Similarly, increases in BMI (normal to overweight to obese) were not associated with a 3-year risk for death or major adverse cardiovascular events, whereas metabolic status (normal to metabolic syndrome to type 2 DM) conferred an approximately twofold adjusted risk for death (hazard ratio, 2.01) and major adverse cardiovascular events (hazard ratio, 1.88).[117]

Metabolic Obesity. There are many exceptions to the association of obesity with the metabolic syndrome. Thin individuals may have insulin resistance; obese individuals can be insulin sensitive,[108] **and in fact, the majority of obese individuals are insulin sensitive.**[109,110]

A more pertinent question, with greater relevance to insulin resistance, may therefore

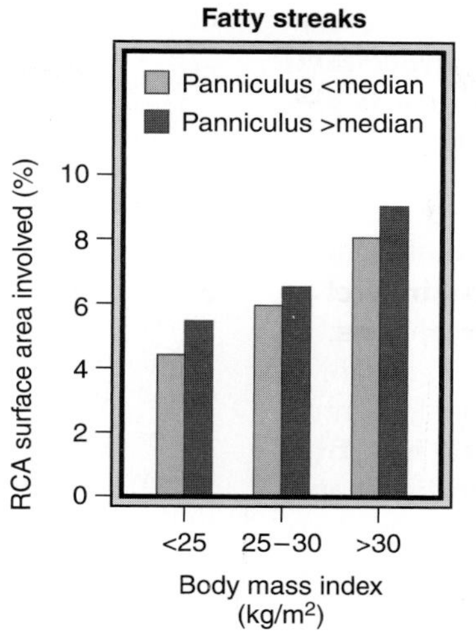

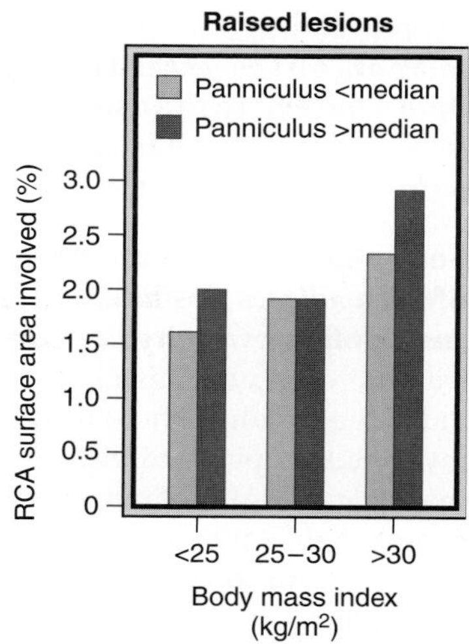

Figure 5–5. The Pathological Determinants of Atherosclerosis in Youth autopsy study of 3000 individuals aged 15 to 34 years who died of noncardiac causes showed body mass index and a thick panniculus adiposus (visceral fat) to be positively correlated with early coronary atheromatous fatty streaks and raised lesions. RCA, right coronary artery. *(Modified from McGill HC, McMahan A, Herderick EE, et al. Obesity accelerates the progression of coronary atherosclerosis in young men. Circulation 2002;105: 2712-2718.)*

be whether an individual is "metabolically obese," regardless of BMI, as defined by the presence of significant ectopic fat storage or intramyocellular lipid.[118] The metabolic syndrome reflects the failure of intracellular lipid homeostasis in overnourished individuals to confine the lipid overload to cells specifically designed to store large quantities of surplus calories, the white adipocytes. This failure allows for the ectopic accumulation of intracellular triacylglycerol, which may be a determinant of insulin resistance.[119]

Ectopic Fat Storage and Intramyocellular Lipid. A proinflammatory state is antiadipogenic and, in fact, lipolytic. The inhibition of preadipocyte recruitment and failure of adipocyte differentiation render fat tissue incapable of additional fat storage. As a result, excess plasma triglycerides are distributed to ectopic, nonfat tissues such as the

- liver,
- pancreas, and
- skeletal and cardiac muscle.

The deposition of excess calories in tissues not meant to store fat, such as intramyocellular lipid within myocytes, is termed ectopic fat storage.[118]

Intramyocellular Lipid and Insulin Resistance. In skeletal muscle, increased intramyocellular lipid is associated with insulin resistance. Cytosolic metabolites resulting from an increase in intracellular fatty acid metabolism interfere with insulin signaling pathways. The mechanisms involved are complex, and many pathways are involved.[65]

There is circumstantial evidence that the presence of ectopic intracellular lipid correlates with insulin resistance in humans.

1. Lipodystrophy, a failure of adipose tissue development, is associated with ectopic fat storage. Despite the extreme paucity of discrete adipose tissue, there is severe insulin resistance and a high incidence of DM.[120]
2. In obese persons, large fat cells may arise because of failure of adipocyte proliferation and differentiation. With the inability of fat tissue to expand, further energy intake by adipose tissue is curtailed. As a result, excess dietary fat is shunted to skeletal muscle and the liver, tissues not designed for fat storage. The degree of insulin resistance correlates closely with the extent of lipid infiltration in these tissues.
3. Thiazolidinediones, which are PPAR-γ activators, promote the differentiation and proliferation of fat cells. By increasing the lipid storage capacity of adipose tissue, thiazolidinediones diminish ectopic fat deposition and improve insulin sensitivity.[118,121]

There is considerable evidence that intramyocellular lipid in particular, as measured by nuclear magnetic resonance imaging, may be a critical determinant of insulin resistance.[119] In young individuals with prediabetes, intramyocellular and intra-abdominal lipid accumulations are closely linked to the development of severe peripheral insulin resistance.[122] In fact, **the correlation of the severity of intramyocellular lipid content with insulin resistance is significantly higher than the correlation of BMI with insulin resistance.**[123]

Body Mass Index and Intramyocellular Lipid. BMI correlates positively with intramyocellular lipid. However, there are exceptions: as was the case with insulin resistance and BMI, individuals with high BMI may have low intramyocellular lipid; **individuals with low BMI may have high intramyocellular lipid and, despite being thin, may be metabolically obese with insulin resistance and adverse metabolic consequences.**[118]

Obesity, Inflammation, Intramyocellular Lipid, and Insulin Resistance. Ultimately, the culprit underlying insulin resistance would appear to be inflammation rather than obesity. Inflammatory pathways render thin individuals metabolically obese and insulin resistant. Obesity may just serve to amplify an inflammatory stimulus.

Obesity, when stimulated to produce proinflammatory adipokines, may turn into a proinflammatory state. In that proinflammatory milieu, inflammatory mediators and their sequelae impair the local metabolic and vascular insulin sensitivity within adipose tissue. Systemic insulin sensitivity may secondarily supervene as adipokines and free fatty acids, released by adipose tissue, exert their metabolic and vascular effects systemically.

Additionally, proinflammatory adipokines are antiadipogenic and prolipolytic. They are consequently implicated in the generation of ectopic, intracellular lipid stores and the evolution of insulin resistance in affected tissues, thereby further aggravating systemic insulin resistance and the detrimental sequelae of the metabolic syndrome.

Finally, **reduced secretion of adiponectin with "inflamed" obesity may be a major factor contributing to the development of insulin resistance, thus providing a pivotal link between adiposity, inflammation, type 2 DM, and atherosclerosis.** Adiponectin is a vasculoprotective, anti-inflammatory adipokine that powerfully enhances insulin sensitivity and endothelial function. These protective effects are forfeited with its loss.[124]

CONCLUSION

Having evolved against a backdrop of uncertain food supplies and deprivation, physiologic mechanisms truly conspire to preserve the fuel stores that an organism may have laboriously accumulated. These mechanisms are geared to protect against times of scarcity, the physiologic equivalent of the food storage during the 7 fat years in order to survive the ensuing 7 lean years. In fact, being overweight restructures physiology to impede weight loss as it generates its own lack of restraint and positive feedback loops. For example,

- leptin resistance renders central leptin and insulin pathways ineffectual, thereby leading to overeating,
- PYY levels are deficient in overweight individuals,
- increased α_2-adrenergic receptor density in obesity is antilipolytic, and
- 11β-HSD-1 activity increases with obesity.

It is also understandable that some stress responses engender weight gain. Such responses would appropriately increase fuel storage to ready the organism for the anticipated increased physical demands and potential scarcity of time or opportunity for food intake. In this respect,

- NPY is involved in stress-mediated overeating behavior,
- stress engenders the consumption of high-carbohydrate comfort foods that stimulate the release of insulin and the effective storage of calories, and
- glucocorticoid effects on fat tissue are enhanced with stress.

Visceral-omental adipose tissue, in particular, is very stress responsive, is highly sensitive to the metabolic needs of the organism, and serves a very useful purpose under normal circumstances. With physically demanding stress, it serves as a rapid and ready storage depot for fat, which can then be very expeditiously mobilized for energy consumption when called upon. In essence, it serves as a rapid deployment fuel source. Specifically,

- its proximity to the intestine may facilitate fuel storage;

- its rich innervation renders it sensitive to autonomic neuronal regulation;
- in its central location it is readily perfused and thus affected by circulating neurohormonal and proinflammatory mediators;
- sympathetic stress will initiate lipolysis, and
- conceivably, higher levels of stress, with the elaboration of products from the RAAS and inflammatory cytokines, will consolidate a lipolytic, antiadipogenic milieu engendering local and ultimately systemic insulin resistance to support the higher energy requirements of an activated immune response.

Obesity is increasingly prevalent in our society, largely because of nutritional, societal, and environmental factors. Obesity can, at times, be benign. We all know obese individuals who are free of insulin resistance, abnormal hemodynamics, and adverse metabolic sequelae. However, is the detrimental aspect of obesity a function of time? With the passage of time, do healthy, obese individuals incur metabolic derangements?

Life is stressful, be it due to psychological, interpersonal, job-related, and societal stress or due to trauma, infections, deprivations, chronic pain, and so on. Stress of any source is translated into inflammatory and oxidative stress pathways. By themselves, these pathways mediate endothelial dysfunction, as well as insulin resistance. In fact, as in the case of atherosclerosis, the endothelial and microvascular dysfunction incurred as a result of stress pathways may serve as a primary stimulus for the inflammatory response in fat by inducing monocyte/macrophage recruitment to adipose tissue.[81]

The association of excessive energy intake and inadequate energy utilization together with exposure to stressful stimuli and stress pathways renders obesity and, in particular, the visceral rapid deployment fat depot deleterious:

1. Excessive, long-term caloric intake, necessitating excessive storage, enlarges the central fat depot, thus effectively amplifying the potential free fatty acid and adipokine release in response to neurohormonal and proinflammatory stimuli.
2. In the absence of adequate physical activity, the excessive stress-mediated mobilization of free fatty acids is not consumed as fuel but contributes to insulin resistance via ectopic storage in an antiadipogenic, inflammatory milieu.

In today's sedentary lifestyle, with much of our stress being psychological or mental in nature, the deleterious effect of excessive visceral fat mobilization is further augmented by the lack of a corresponding physical outlet for its consumption.

In particular, excessive visceral fat is effectively poised to promote inflammatory pathologic states. Any inflammatory process with systemic manifestations may thus be vastly augmented through the activation of visceral adipose tissue to produce an amplified inflammatory response with increased cytokine production and a resultant disturbance in insulin action (Fig. 5-6).

Peaceful obesity, aside from mechanical, weight-bearing–related injuries, may not be unhealthy, as seen with serene, meditating, peaceful, uninfected, pain-free, presumably healthy Buddha

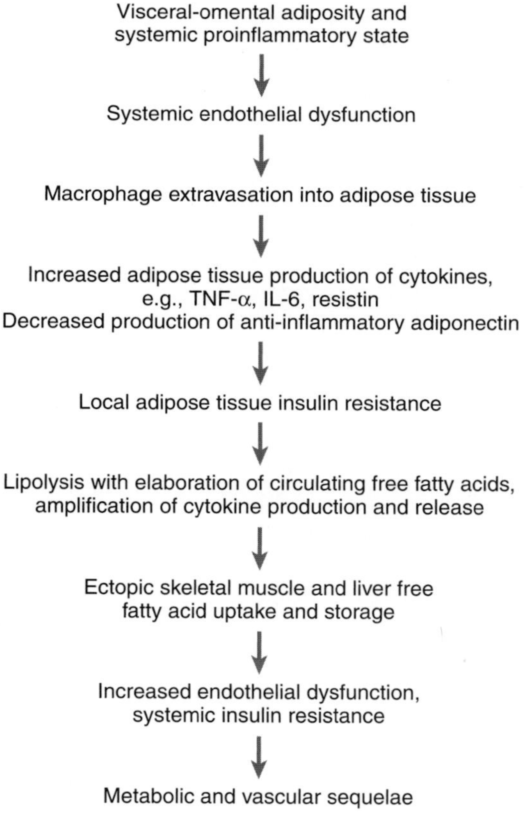

Visceral-omental adiposity and systemic proinflammatory state

↓

Systemic endothelial dysfunction

↓

Macrophage extravasation into adipose tissue

↓

Increased adipose tissue production of cytokines, e.g., TNF-α, IL-6, resistin
Decreased production of anti-inflammatory adiponectin

↓

Local adipose tissue insulin resistance

↓

Lipolysis with elaboration of circulating free fatty acids, amplification of cytokine production and release

↓

Ectopic skeletal muscle and liver free fatty acid uptake and storage

↓

Increased endothelial dysfunction, systemic insulin resistance

↓

Metabolic and vascular sequelae

Figure 5–6.
Pathophysiologic effects of visceral adiposity: the impact of cytokine and free fatty acid release on local adipose insulin insensitivity and the progression to systemic insulin resistance. IL, interleukin; TNF, tumor necrosis factor.

figures, theoretically low in sympathetic tone and stress and high in parasympathetic tone. For any normal person engulfed in the stresses of life, obesity serves to amplify the harmful, metabolic impact of stress-related inflammatory pathways, and therein may lie the potentially deleterious effects of obesity. It is in this respect that infection avoidance behavior (e.g., dental hygiene) and stress relaxation techniques may be of benefit and that exercise and physical fitness, by providing an appropriate metabolic outlet for consumption of the released lipids, become so important in the preservation of health in obesity.

GLOSSARY

ACRP30	adipocyte complement-related protein of 30 kDa
AMPK	5′-adenosine monophosphate–activated protein kinase
apo	apolipoprotein
BMI	body mass index
cAMP	cyclic adenosine monophosphate
CART	cocaine-and-amphetamine–regulated transcript
CB	cannabinoid
CoA	coenzyme A
CHD	coronary heart disease
DM	diabetes mellitus
DAG	diacylglycerol
EGIR	European Group for the Study of Insulin Resistance
G protein	guanine nucleotide regulatory protein
GLUT	glucose transporter
HDL	high-density lipoprotein
11β-HSD	11β-hydroxysteroid dehydrogenase
HSL	hormone-sensitive lipase
5HT	5-hydroxytryptamine
IGF-I	insulin-like growth factor-I
IκB	inhibitory protein kappaB
IL	interleukin
iNOS	Inducible nitric oxide synthase
LDL	low-density lipoprotein
LPL	lipoprotein lipase
MC1R	melanocortin 1 receptor
MCP-1	monocyte chemotactic protein-1
M-CSF	macrophage colony-stimulating factor
NFκB	nuclear factor kappaB
NHANES	National Health and Nutrition Examination Survey
NPY	neuropeptide Y
OX	orexin
PAI-1	plasminogen activator inhibitor-1
POMC	proopiomelanocortin
PPAR	peroxisome proliferator–activated receptor
PYY	peptide YY3-36
RAAS	renin-angiotensin-aldosterone system
TNF	tumor necrosis factor
VLDL	very-low-density lipoprotein
WHR	waist-hip ratio

REFERENCES

1. Bray GA. Classification and evaluation of the obesities. Med Clin North Am 1989;73:161-184
2. National Institutes of Health, National Heart, Lung, and Blood Institute. Clinical Guidelines on the Identification, Evaluation, and Treatment of Overweight and Obesity in Adults (National Institutes of Health Publication No. 98-4083). Rockville, MD, U.S. Department of Health and Human Services, Public Health Service, 1998
3. Friedman JM. A war on obesity, not the obese. Science 2003;299:856-858
4. List JF, Habener JF. Defective melanocortin 4 receptors in hyperphagia and morbid obesity. N Engl J Med 2003;348:1160-1163
5. Diamond J. Guns, Germs, and Steel: The Fates of Human Societies. New York, Norton, 1999
6. Hedley AA, Ogden CL, Johnson CL, et al. Prevalence of overweight and obesity among US children, adolescents, and adults, 1999-2002. JAMA 2004;291:2847-2850
7. Ford ES, Giles WH, Dietz WH. Prevalence of the metabolic syndrome among US adults. JAMA 2002;287:356-359
8. Galbraith JK. The Affluent Society, 4th ed. Boston, Houghton Mifflin, 1984
9. Havlik RJ, Hubert HB, Fabsitz RR, Feinleib M. Weight and hypertension. Ann Intern Med 1983;98:855-859
10. Dvorak R, Starling RD, Calles-Escandon J, et al. Drug therapy for obesity in the elderly. Drugs Aging 1997;11:338-351
11. Calle EE, Rodriguez C, Walker-Thurmond K, Thun MJ. Overweight, obesity, and mortality from cancer in a prospectively studied cohort of U.S. adults. N Engl J Med 2003;348:1625-1638
12. Yaffe K, Kanaya A, Lindquist K, et al. The metabolic syndrome, inflammation, and risk of cognitive decline. JAMA 2004;292:2237-2242
13. Wang TJ, Parise H, Levy D, et al. Obesity and the risk of new-onset atrial fibrillation. JAMA 2004;292: 2471-2477
14. Jousilahti P, Tuomilehto J, Vartiainen E, et al. Body weight, cardiovascular risk factors, and coronary mortality. 15-Year follow-up of middle-aged men and women in eastern Finland. Circulation 1996;93:1372-1379
15. Mokdad AH, Ford ES, Bowman BA, et al. Prevalence of obesity, diabetes, and obesity-related health risk factors, 2001. JAMA 2003;289;76-79

16. West KM, Kalbfleisch JM. Influence of nutritional factors on prevalence of diabetes. Diabetes 1971;20: 99-108
17. Peeters A, Barendregt JJ, Willekens F, et al. Obesity in adulthood and its consequences for life expectancy: a life-table analysis. Ann Intern Med 2003;138:24-32
18. Fontaine KR, Redden DT, Wang C, et al. Years of life lost due to obesity. JAMA 2003;289:187-193
19. Eckel RH, Krauss RM. American Heart Association call to action: obesity as a major risk factor for coronary heart disease. Circulation 1998;97:2099-2100
20. Consultation on Obesity. Geneva, World Health Organization, June 3-5, 1997
21. http://www.surgeongeneral.gov/topics/obesity/calltoaction/foreward.htm
22. Hill JO, Wyatt HR, Reed GW, Peters JC. Obesity and the environment: Where do we go from here? Science 2003;299:853-855
23. Thompson D, Edelsberg J, Colditz JA, et al. Lifetime health and economic consequences of obesity. Arch Intern Med 1999;159:2177-2183
24. Serdula MK, Mokdad AH, Williamson DF, et al. Prevalence of attempting weight loss and strategies for controlling weight. JAMA 1999;282:1353-1358
25. Visscher TLS, Rissanen A, Seidell JC, et al. Obesity and unhealthy life-years in adult Finns. An empirical approach. Arch Intern Med 2004;164:1413-1420
26. Li J, Yu X, Pan W, Unger RH. Gene expression profile of rat adipose tissue at the onset of high-fat-diet obesity. Am J Physiol Metab 2002;282:E1334-E1341
27. Trayhurn P, Beattie JH. Physiological role of adipose tissue: white adipose tissue as an endocrine and secretory organ. Proc Nutr Soc 2001:60:329-339
28. Jequier E. Pathways to obesity. Int J Obes Relat Metab Disord 2002;26(suppl):S12-S17
29. Bjoerntorp P. Hormonal control of regional fat distribution. Hum Reprod 1997;12:21-25
30. Marx J. Cellular warriors at the Battle of the Bulge. Science 2003;299:846-849
31. Konturek SJ, Konturek JW, Pawlik T, Brzozowski T. Brain-gut axis and its role in the control of food intake. J Physiol Pharmacol 2004;55:137-154
32. Ruderman NB, Saha AK, Kraegen EW. Minireview: malonyl CoA, AMP-activated protein kinase, and adiposity. Endocrinology 2003;144:5166-5171
33. Andersson U, Filipsson K, Abbott CR, et al. AMP-activated protein kinase plays a role in the control of food intake. J Biol Chem 2004;279:12005-12008
34. Korner J, Leibel RL. To eat or not to eat—how the gut talks to the brain. N Engl J Med 2003;349:926-928
35. Yeo GS, Farooqi IS, Challis BG, et al. The role of melanocortin signaling in the control of body weight: evidence from human and murine genetic models. QJM 2000;93:7-14
36. Attoub S, Noe V, Pirola L, et al. Leptin promotes invasiveness of kidney and colonic epithelial cells via phosphoinositide 3-kinase–, rho-, and rac-dependent signaling pathways. FASEB J 2000;14:2329-2338
37. Batterham RL, Cohen MA, Ellis SM, et al. Inhibition of food intake in obese subjects by peptide YY3-36. N Engl J Med 2003;349:941-948
38. Gura T. Obesity drug pipeline not so fat. Science 2003; 299:849-852
39. Rouch C, Meile MJ, Orosco M. Extracellular hypothalamic serotonin and plasma amino acids in response to sequential carbohydrate and protein meals. Nutr Neurosci 2003;6:117-124
40. http://www.indstate.edu/thcme/mwking/nerves.html#5ht
41. Curzon G, Gibson EL, Oluyomi AO. Appetite suppression by commonly used drugs depends on 5-HT availability. TIPS 1197;18:21-25
42. Inui A. Neuropeptide Y feeding receptors: are multiple subtypes involved? Trends Pharmacol Sci 1999;20:43-46
43. Xu H, Hirosumi J, Uysal T, et al. Exclusive action of transmembrane TNFalpha in adipose tissue leads to reduced adipose mass and local but not systemic insulin resistance. Endocrinology 2002;143:1502-1511
44. De Matteis R, Arch JR, Petroni ML, et al. Immunochemical identification of the beta(3)-adrenoceptor in intact human adipocytes and ventricular myocardium: effect of obesity and treatment with ephedrine and caffeine. Int J Obes Relat Metab Disord 2002;26: 1442-1450
45. Imbeault P, Couillard C, Tremblay A, et al. Reduced alpha2-adrenergic sensitivity of subcutaneous abdominal adipocytes as a modulator of fasting and postprandial triglyceride levels in men. J Lipid Res 2000;41: 1367-1375
46. Boden G, Hoeldtke RD. Nerves, fat, and insulin resistance. N Engl J Med 2003;349:1966-1967
47. Rask E, Olsson T, Soderberg S, et al. Tissue-specific dysregulation of cortisol metabolism in human obesity. J Clin Endocrinol Metab 2001;86:1418-1421
48. Berger J, Tanen M, Elbrecht A, et al. Peroxisome proliferator–activated receptor-gamma ligands inhibit adipocyte 11beta-hydroxysteroid dehydrogenase type 1 expression and activity. J Biol Chem 2001;276:12629-12635
49. Cigolini M, Smith U. Human adipose tissue in culture. VIII. Studies on the insulin-antagonistic effects of glucocorticoids. Metabolism 1979;28:502-510
50. Rebuffe-Scrive M, Lundholm K, Bjorntorp P. Glucocorticoid hormone binding to human adipose tissue. Eur J Clin Invest 1985;15:267-271
51. Golub MS. The adrenal and the metabolic syndrome. Curr Hypertens Rep 2001;3:117-120
52. Rebuffe-Scrive M, Enk L, Crona N, et al. Fat cell metabolism in different regions in women: effect of menstrual cycle, pregnancy, and lactation. J Clin Invest 1985;75: 1973-1976
53. Vague J. La differentiation sexuelle facteur determinant des formes de l'obesitie. Presse Med 1947;55:339-340
54. Kiessebah AH, Krakower GR. Regional adiposity and morbidity. Physiol Rev 1994;74:775-811
55. Bouchard C, Despres JP, Mauriege P. Genetic and nongenetic determinants of regional fat distribution. Endocr Rev 1993;14:72-93
56. Mauriege P, Prud'homme D, Lemieux S, et al. Regional differences in adipose tissue lipolysis from lean and obese women: existence of postreceptor alterations. Am J Physiol 1995;269:E341-E350
57. Yamashita S, Kazuaki K, Tadashi N, et al. Insulin resistance and body fat distribution. Diabetes Care 1996; 19:346-350
58. Iacobellis G, Ribaudo MC, Zappaterreno A, et al. Relation between epicardial adipose tissue and left ventricular mass. Am J Cardiol 2004;94:1084-1087
59. van der Kooy K, Leenen R, Seidell JC, et al. Waist-hip ratio is a poor predictor of changes in visceral fat. Am J Clin Nutr 1993;57:327-333
60. Matsuzawa Y, Shimomura I, Nakamura T, et al. Pathophysiology and pathogenesis of visceral fat obesity. Ann N Y Acad Sci 1993;676:270-278
61. Levine JA, Eberhardt NL, Jensen MD. Role of nonexercise activity thermogenesis in resistance to fat gain in humans. Science 1999;283:212-214
62. Vidal H. Gene expression in visceral and subcutaneous adipose tissues. Ann Med 2001;33:547-555

63. Goldstein BJ. Insulin resistance as the core defect in type 2 diabetes mellitus. Am J Cardiol 2002;90(suppl):3G-10G
64. Nieves DJ, Cnop M, Retzlaff B, et al. The atherogenic lipoprotein profile associated with obesity and insulin resistance is largely attributable to intra-abdominal fat. Diabetes 2003;52:172-179
65. Boden G. Interaction between free fatty acids and glucose metabolism. Curr Opin Clin Nutr Metab Care 2002;5:545-549
66. Hsueh WA, Law R. The central role of fat and effect of peroxisome proliferator–activated receptor-gamma on progression of insulin resistance and cardiovascular disease. Am J Cardiol 2003;92(suppl):3J-9J
67. Despres JP, Moorjani S, Ferland M, et al. Adipose tissue distribution and plasma lipoprotein levels in obese women: importance of intraabdominal fat. Arteriosclerosis 1989;9:203-210
68. Emdin M, Gastaldelli A, Muscelli E, et al. Hyperinsulinemia and autonomic nervous system dysfunction in obesity: effects of weight loss. Circulation 2001;103:513-519
69. Hjemdahl P. Stress and the metabolic syndrome. Circulation 2002;106:2634-2636
70. Carey DG, Jenkins AB, Campbell LV, et al. Abdominal fat and insulin resistance in normal and overweight women: direct measurements reveal a strong relationship in subjects at low and high risk of NIDDM. Diabetes 1996;45:633-638
71. Fujoka S, Matsuzawa Y, Tokunaga K, Tarui S. Contribution of intra-abdominal fat accumulation to the impairment of glucose and lipid metabolism in human obesity. Metabolism 1987;36:54-59
72. Shuman WP, Morris LL, Leonetti DL, et al. Abnormal body fat distribution detected by computed tomography in diabetic men. Invest Radiol 1986;21:483-487
73. Carr MC, Hokanson JE, Zambon A, et al. The contribution of intraabdominal fat to gender differences in hepatic lipase activity and low/high density lipoprotein heterogeneity. J Clin Endocrinol Metab 2001;86:2831-2837
74. Lemieux S, Despres JP, Moorjani S, et al. Are gender differences in cardiovascular disease risk factors explained by the level of visceral adipose tissue? Diabetologia 1994;37:757-764
75. Adeli K, Taghibiglou C, Van Iderstine SC, Lewis GF. Mechanisms of hepatic very low-density lipoprotein overproduction in insulin resistance. Trends Cardiovasc Med 2001;11:170-176
76. Ruotolo G, Howard BV. Dyslipidemia of the metabolic syndrome. Curr Cardiol Rep 2002;4:494-500
77. Ayyobi AF, Brunzell JD. Lipoprotein distribution in the metabolic syndrome, type 2 diabetes mellitus, and familial combined hyperlipidemia. Am J Cardiol 2003;92 (suppl):27J-33J
78. Stahl A, Evans JG, Pattel S, et al. Insulin causes fatty acid transport protein translocation and enhanced fatty acid uptake in adipocytes. Dev Cell 2002;2:477-488
79. Ross SE, Erickson RL, Gerin I, et al. Microarray analyses during adipogenesis: understanding the effects of Wnt signaling on adipogenesis and the roles of liver X receptor alpha in adipocyte metabolism. Mol Cell Biol 2002;22: 5989-5999
80. Fain JN, Cheema PS, Bahouth SW, Lloyd Hiler M. Resistin release by human adipose tissue explants in primary culture. Biochem Biophys Res Commun 2003;300:674-678
81. Wellen KE, Hotamisligil GS. Obesity-induced inflammatory changes in adipose tissue. J Clin Invest 2003; 112:1785-1788
82. Weisberg SP, McCann D, Desai M. Obesity is associated with macrophage accumulation in adipose tissue. J Clin Invest 2003;112:1796-1808
83. Xu H, Barnes GT, Yang Q, et al. Chronic inflammation in fat plays a crucial role in the development of obesity-related insulin resistance. J Clin Invest 2003;112:1821-1830
84. Ghanim H, Aljada A, Hofmeyer D, et al. Circulating mononuclear cells in the obese are in a proinflammatory state. Circulation 2004;110:1564-1571
85. Atzmon G, Yang XM, Muzumdar R, et al. Differential gene expression between visceral and subcutaneous fat depots. Horm Metab Res 2002;34:622-628
86. Fried, SK, Bunkin DA, Greenberg AS. Omental and subcutaneous adipose tissues of obese subjects release interleukin-6: depot difference and regulation by glucocorticoid. J Clin Endocrinol Metab 1998;83:847-850
87. Vgontzas AN. Elevation of plasma cytokines in disorders of excessive daytime sleepiness: role of sleep disturbance and obesity. J Clin Endocrinol Metab 1997;82:1313-1316
88. Perreault M, Marette A. Targeted disruption of inducible nitric oxide synthase protects against obesity-linked insulin resistance in muscle. Nat Med 2001;7:1138-1143
89. Samad F, Yamamoto K, Pandey M, Loskutoff DJ. Elevated expression of transforming growth factor-beta in adipose tissue from obese mice. Mol Med 1997;3:37-48
90. Visser M, Bouter LM, McQuillan GM, et al. Elevated C-reactive protein levels in overweight and obese adults. JAMA 1999;282:2131-2135
91. Weyer C, Yudkin JS, Stehouwer CD, et al. Humoral markers of inflammation and endothelial dysfunction in relation to adiposity and in vivo insulin action in Pima Indians. Atherosclerosis 2002;161:233-242
92. Sartipy P, Loskutoff DJ. Monocyte chemoattractant protein 1 in obesity and insulin resistance. Proc Natl Acad Sci U S A 2003;100:7265-7270
93. Samad F, Yamamoto K, Loskutoff DJ. Distribution and regulation of plasminogen activator inhibitor-1 in murine adipose tissue in vivo. Induction by tumor necrosis factor-alpha and lipopolysaccharide. J Clin Invest 1996;97:37-46
94. Samad F, Pandey M, Loskutoff DJ. Tissue factor gene expression in the adipose tissues of obese mice. Proc Natl Acad Sci U S A 1998;95:7591-7596
95. De Pergola G, Pannacciulli N. Coagulation and fibrinolysis abnormalities in obesity. J Endocrinol Invest 2002;25: 899-904
96. Levine JA, Jensen MD, Eberhardt NL, O'Brien T. Adipocyte macrophage colony-stimulating factor is a mediator of adipose tissue growth. J Clin Invest 1998; 101:1557-1564
97. Hotamisligil GS, Shargill NS, Spiegelman BM. Adipose expression of tumor necrosis factor-alpha: direct role in obesity-linked insulin resistance. Science 1993;259:87-91
98. Hsueh WA, Quinones MJ. Role of endothelial dysfunction in insulin resistance. Am J Cardiol 2003;92(suppl):10J-17J
99. Hotamisligil GS, Arner P, Caro JF, et al. Increased adipose tissue expression of tumor necrosis factor-alpha in human obesity and insulin resistance. J Clin Invest 2995;95:2409-2415
100. Charriere G, Cousin B, Arnaud E, et al. Preadipocyte conversion to macrophage. Evidence of plasticity. J Biol Chem 2003;278:9850-9855
101. Tong Q, Dalgin G, Xu H, et al. Function of GATA transcription factors in preadipocyte-adipocyte transition. Science 2000;290:134-138
102. Coppack SW. Pro-inflammatory cytokines and inflammatory tissue. Proc Nutr Soc 2001;60:349-356
103. Laws A, Reaven GM. Insulin resistance and risk factors for coronary heart disease. Baillieres Clin Endocrinol Metab 1993;7:1063-1078
104. Grundy SM. Obesity, metabolic syndrome, and coronary atherosclerosis. Circulation 2003;105:2696-2698

105. Saghizadeh M, Ong JM, Garvey WT, et al. The expression of TNF alpha by human muscle. Relationship to insulin resistance. J Clin Invest 1996;97:1111-1116
106. Rabinowitz D, Zierler KL. Forearm metabolism in obesity and its response to intraarterial insulin: characterization of insulin resistance and evidence for adaptive hyperinsulinism. J Clin Invest 1962;12:2173-2181
107. Bogardus C, Lilioja S, Mott D, et al. Relationship between obesity and maximal insulin stimulated glucose uptake in vivo and in vitro in Pima Indians. J Clin Invest 1984;73:800-805
108. Reaven GM. Banting lecture 1988. Role of insulin resistance in human disease. Diabetes 1988;37: 1595-1607
109. Ferrannini E, Natali A, Bell P, et al, on behalf of the European Group for the Study of Insulin Resistance (EGIR). Insulin resistance and hypersecretion in obesity. J Clin Invest 1997;100:1166-1173
110. Abbasi F, Brown BW, Lamendola C, et al. Relationship between obesity, insulin resistance, and coronary heart disease. J Am Coll Cardiol 2002;40:937-943
111. Stern MP, Haffner SM. Body fat distribution and hyperinsulinemia as risk factors for diabetes and cardiovascular disease. Atherosclerosis 1986;6:123-130
112. Frayn KN. Visceral fat and insulin resistance—causative or correlative? Br J Nutr 2000;83(suppl 1):S71-S77
113. Hubert HB, Feinleib M, McNamara PM, Castelli WP. Obesity as an independent risk factor for cardiovascular disease: a 26-year follow-up of participants in the Framingham Heart Study. Circulation 1983;67:968-977
114. McGill HC, McMahan A, Herderick EE, et al. Obesity accelerates the progression of coronary atherosclerosis in young men. Circulation 2002;105:2712-2718
115. Keys A, Menotti A, Aravanis C, et al. The seven countries study: 2289 deaths in 15 years. Prev Med 1984;13:141-154
116. McGill HC Jr. Geographic Pathology of Atherosclerosis. Baltimore, Williams & Wilkins, 1986
117. Kip KE, Marroquin OC, Kelley DE, et al. Clinical importance of obesity versus the metabolic syndrome in cardiovascular risk in women: a report from the Women's Ischemia Syndrome Evaluation (WISE) study. Circulation 2004;109:706-713
118. Colhoun HM. The big picture on obesity and insulin resistance. J Am Coll Cardiol 2002;40:944-945
119. Sinha R, Dufour S, Petersen KF, et al. Assessment of skeletal muscle triglyceride content by ^{1}H nuclear magnetic resonance spectroscopy in lean and obese adolescents: relationships to insulin insensitivity, total body fat, and central adiposity. Diabetes 2002;51:1022-1027
120. Frayn KN. Adipose tissue and the insulin resistance syndrome. Proc Nutr Soc 2001;60:375-380
121. Krssak M, Falk Petersen K, Dresner A, et al. Intramyocellular lipid concentrations are correlated with insulin sensitivity in humans: a ^{1}H NMR spectroscopy study. Diabetologia 1999;42:1-2
122. Weiss R, Dufour S, Taksali SE, et al. Prediabetes in obese youth: a syndrome of impaired glucose tolerance, severe insulin resistance, and altered myocellular and abdominal fat partitioning. Lancet 2003;362:951-957
123. McGarry JD. Banting lecture 2001: dysregulation of fatty acid metabolism in the etiology of type 2 diabetes. Diabetes 2002;51:7-18
124. Yamauchi T, Kamon J, Waki H, et al. The fat-derived hormone adiponectin reverses insulin resistance associated with both lipoatrophy and obesity. Nat Med 2001;7:941-946

Adipokines of Adipose Tissue

6

Adipose tissue is an active secretory organ that elaborates a variety of messenger molecules (Table 6-1) that exert potent autocrine/paracrine effects on adipose tissue. There is mounting evidence that adipocyte-derived hormones play a key role in adipose tissue metabolism and in the development of insulin resistance.[1] Because adipocytes are interspersed throughout diverse tissues and major target receptors for these messengers are also found in other tissues such as the hypothalamus, skeletal muscle, and liver, adipocyte-derived messengers may also exert endocrine effects and participate in a complex interplay between several tissues.[2] Adipocyte-derived hormones have structural homology to cytokines. They are thus collectively referred to as adipocytokines, or adipokines.[3]

Selected adipokines that have an impact on insulin sensitivity are discussed in this chapter.

ADIPOKINES WITH BENEFICIAL METABOLIC EFFECT

Leptin. Leptin is a 16-kDa protein hormone.[4] Its name is derived from *leptos,* meaning "thin" in Greek. The hormone plays an important role in the control of feeding behavior and energy expenditure. **Leptin modulates body weight, energy balance, metabolism, and reproductive function** (Table 6-2).[5] Leptin appears to have evolved as a signal to counter starvation rather than adiposity. In fact, **the primary biologic role of leptin appears to be adaptation to low energy intake rather than prevention of overconsumption and obesity.** The leptin pathway thus appears to be more suitably

Table 6-1. Protein Factors and Adipokines Secreted from White Adipose Tissue

ACRP30 (adipocyte complement–related protein of 30 kDa), or adiponectin
Acylation-stimulating protein
Adipsin
Angiotensinogen, all element of the renin-angiotensin-aldosterone system
Apolipoprotein E
Cholesteryl ester transfer protein
Complement system products
Fasting-induced adipose factor
Fibrinogen-angiopoietin–related protein
Interleukin-1β, IL-6, IL-8
Leptin
Lipoprotein lipase
Macrophage colony-stimulating factor
Macrophage inflammatory protein-1α
Metallothionein
Monocyte chemotactic protein-1
Plasminogen activator inhibitor
Resistin-like molecules
Retinol binding protein
Tissue factor
Transforming growth factor-β
Tumor necrosis factor-α
Vascular endothelial growth factor

Modified from Trayhurn P, Beattie JH. Physiological role of adipose tissue: White adipose tissue as an endocrine and secretory organ. Proc Nutr Soc 2001;60:329-339.

Table 6-2. Leptin Action and Target Tissues

ACTION	TARGET
Reduced hyperphagia	Hypothalamus
Increased glucose metabolism	Whole body
Decreased glycogen content	Liver
Stimulation of fatty acid oxidation	Skeletal muscle
Inhibition of insulin secretion	Pancreas
Proliferation of CD4+ lymphocytes	T lymphocytes
Accelerated maturation	Reproductive organs

Modified from Mora S, Pessin JE. An adipocentric view of signaling and intracellular trafficking. Diabetes Metab Res Rev 2002;18:345-356

designed for physiologic adaptation to eras of nutritional deficiency than to periods of caloric excess.[5]

Leptin Production. Leptin is an adipokine that is predominantly derived from adipose tissue. **Leptin levels reflect an organism's total adipocyte mass and its nutritional status** (Fig. 6-1). In its hormonal function, leptin appears to report on the state of adipose tissue throughout the body.[6]

Adipocytes. The obesity (*ob*) gene encodes leptin. Leptin is produced predominantly by white fat adipocytes, although small amounts may be produced by epithelial cells of the stomach, as well as the liver, skeletal muscle, and placenta.

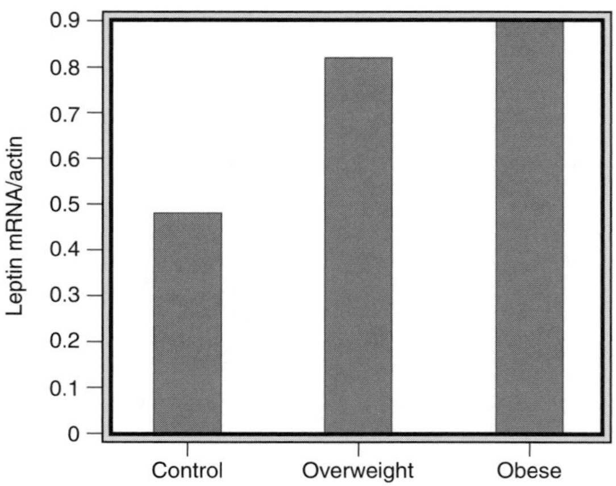

▸▸ **Figure 6–1.**
Levels of adipose tissue leptin in relation to adiposity. *(Modified from Bullo M, Garcia-Lorda P, Peinado-Onsurbe J, et al. TNF-alpha expression of subcutaneous adipose tissue in obese and morbid obese females: relationship to adipocyte LPL activity and leptin synthesis. Int J Obes 2002;26:652-658.)*

The amount of leptin expressed by adipocytes correlates well with the lipid content of the cells; specifically, as adipocytes increase in size as a result of the accumulation of triacylglycerol, they synthesize more leptin.[6]

Positive Determinants of Leptin Production. Determinants of leptin expression and secretion, other than adipocyte size, are

- increased cytoplasmic levels of glucosamine in adipocytes and skeletal myocytes because of increased glucose consumption,
- refeeding,
- insulin,
- glucocorticoids,
- endothelin-1, and
- inflammatory mediators such as tumor necrosis factor-alpha (TNF-α) and interleukin-1 (IL-1).

Accordingly, **the anorexia and loss of body mass commonly associated with severe acute or chronic inflammation may derive from cytokine-induced leptin production.**[6]

Once synthesized, leptin is not stored. The majority of leptin is secreted via a constitutive pathway, with only a small amount able to undergo regulated exocytosis.[2]

Negative Determinants of Leptin Production. Circulating leptin levels are down-regulated by

- fasting,
- β-adrenergic receptor agonists,
- receptor agonists that increase cytoplasmic adenosine 3′,5′-cyclic phosphate (cAMP),
- peroxisome proliferator–activated receptor-gamma (PPAR-γ) activators,
- thyroid hormone,
- androgens, and
- phorbol esters.[2]

The Leptin Receptor

Structure. The functional form of membrane-associated leptin receptors, Ob-Rb, is structurally related to the class II cytokine group receptors that bind IL-2, interferon, and growth hormone. It is also closely related to the gp130 signal-transducing component of the IL-6 receptor and the granulocyte colony-stimulating factor (C-CSF) receptor.[6,7]

Distribution. The leptin receptor has a widespread receptor tissue distribution suggestive of diverse biologic actions for leptin. It is highly expressed in

- areas of the hypothalamus that are involved in body weight regulation,[8]
- the intestine,
- the liver,
- the kidney,
- the lungs,
- cardiac muscle,
- skeletal muscle,
- inflammatory blood cells and T lymphocytes,
- vascular endothelial cells, and
- insulin-secreting pancreatic beta cells.[9-11]

Leptin Receptor Signaling. Leptin signaling is multifaceted. Leptin can act through some of the components of the insulin signaling cascade, such as insulin receptor substrate-1 (IRS-1) and IRS-2, phosphatidylinositol 3-kinase (PI3K), and mitogen-activated protein kinase (MAPK).[12]

The leptin receptor oligomerizes with itself and also signals via Janus kinase (JAK)/signal transducers and activators of transcription (STAT) elements with crosstalk from PI3K pathways. Upon leptin stimulation, the receptor activates JAK-2 via transphosphorylation. Activated JAKs phosphorylate tyrosine residues on STAT. Phosphorylated STAT proteins dimerize and translocate to the nucleus to activate the transcription of target genes.[6,7]

The leptin signaling pathway, which depends on activation of trimeric G proteins and PI3K also entails activation of the Rho and Rac family of small guanosine 5′-triphosphatases (GTPases).[6,13]

Leptin and Body Weight Loss. Leptin's effect on body weight is mediated largely through its interaction with hypothalamic receptors that control body temperature and energy expenditure, hunger, and eating behavior.[14] It also appears to have some peripheral effects.

Energy Expenditure—Central. Leptin causes thermogenesis via hypothalamic signaling and activation of the sympathoadrenal axis.

Energy expenditure is increased with a measurable rise in oxygen consumption and a higher body temperature. The promotion of lipolysis results in a selective loss of adipose tissue mass with no apparent effect on lean body mass, which may actually increase.[14]

Metabolism and Energy Expenditure—Peripheral. Leptin enhances glucose metabolism in peripheral tissues such as skeletal muscle and brown adipose tissue, but not in white adipose tissue.

Leptin enhances the bradykinin or the nitric oxide (NO) system, or both, by increasing local NO release. Leptin may thus directly or indirectly contribute to enhanced glucose uptake in skeletal muscles by increasing NO-mediated glucose uptake or by favoring nutritive blood perfusion.[15,16]

Leptin may also have direct tissue effects in modulating energy expenditure in the liver, in skeletal and cardiac muscle, and in the pancreas by partitioning fatty acids to oxidation rather than triacylglycerol storage.[11] In skeletal muscle, leptin activates 5′-adenosine monophosphate–activated protein kinase (AMPK) to stimulate fatty acid oxidation. Concurrently, it stimulates a kinase that inhibits acetyl coenzyme A (CoA) carboxylase, a key enzyme in lipid synthesis. In the liver, leptin inhibits stearyl CoA desaturase-1 in similar fashion and decreases hepatic glycogen content. Although leptin activates fatty acid oxidation in the heart, the effects of leptin in the heart are independent of changes in the AMPK–acetyl CoA carboxylase–malonyl CoA axis.[11] As a result, fatty acid energy substrate is shunted from fat synthesis to fat oxidation and energy expenditure, and the cellular triacylglycerol content in nonfatty tissue is decreased.[2,17]

Feeding Behavior. Leptin is an anorexigenic hormone that decreases food intake.

- In the mediobasal hypothalamic centers, leptin inhibits the synthesis of neuropeptide Y, a potent stimulator of feeding behavior, thus decreasing hunger and food intake.
- Proopiomelanocortin expression is upregulated by leptin. Proopiomelanocortin is cleaved by prohormone convertases to yield α-melanocyte–stimulating hormone, which upon interaction with the melanocortin 4 receptor, causes a reduction in food intake.[18]

- In vivo administration of leptin decreases hypothalamic AMPK activity, which also leads to a reduction in food intake.[19]

In contrast, nonoccupancy of the hypothalamic leptin receptor disinhibits or activates a number of orexigenic adiposity signals and causes increased food intake and decreased energy expenditure.

Leptin and Insulin. There are complex interactions between the leptin and insulin signaling pathways.

Leptin can potentially lead to differential modification of the metabolic and mitotic effects of insulin exerted through IRS-1 and IRS-2 and the downstream kinases that they activate. Leptin can modulate insulin-induced changes in gene expression in vitro and in vivo.[12]

Leptin increases energy expenditure and thermogenesis. As a result, leptin not only induces weight loss and adipose tissue lipolysis, but it also lowers the triacylglycerol content in insulin-sensitive muscle and hepatic tissues via increased fat oxidation and as such may improve insulin signaling in these tissues.[11]

Leptin and Obesity. The obesity (*ob*) gene encodes leptin. The ob–/ob– mouse, deficient in the *ob* gene product leptin, is a classic murine model of obesity and insulin resistance, and leptin deficiency accounts for the obesity of ob–/ob– mice.[20] Administration of leptin to such mice markedly reduces food intake. It increases thermogenesis and physical activity and thus causes a reduction in body weight.[2]

Mutations in the *ob* or *db* genes inducing leptin deficiency are a very rare cause of morbid obesity in humans, as are defects in the leptin receptor.[21]

Rather than suffering from leptin deficiency, overweight individuals have elevated plasma leptin concentrations. There is a higher concentration of ob mRNA in adipose tissue from obese than from lean individuals. Plasma leptin concentrations correlate positively with adipose tissue mass and with the percentage of body fat.[6]

Leptin Resistance and Insulin Resistance. Instead of suffering from a deficiency of leptin, **obese individuals with hyperleptinemia suffer from "leptin resistance,"** akin to insulin resistance, a desensitization of the leptin receptor to its ligand.[22]

Mechanism of Leptin Resistance. Leptin receptor insensitivity and leptin resistance in the setting of caloric excess and obesity are common. Resistance to leptin can be explained, at least partly, by

- leptin-induced expression of suppressor of cytokine signaling-3 (SOCS-3) mRNA in regions of the hypothalamus that express the long form of the leptin receptor[6] and
- phosphorylation of the leptin receptor leading to decreased leptin signaling.[23]

Concurrent Insulin Resistance. Leptin resistance is most often associated with impaired insulin signaling or insulin resistance. The usual clinical setting for leptin resistance is, in fact, concurrent insulin resistance as seen in

- obesity,
- hypertension,
- type 2 diabetes mellitus (DM),
- heart failure, and
- after myocardial infarction.[24,25]

In fact, leptin resistance and the resultant hyperleptinemia may play a crucial role in the development of insulin resistance.[26]

Implications of Leptin Resistance. Leptin resistance creates the physiology of effective, tissue-level leptin deficiency. This has implications on body metabolism and cardiovascular physiology.

Body Weight. A leptin-resistant organism is unable to "read" leptin's "thermogenesis" signals.[27,28] In obese individuals, leptin thus fails to reduce appetite and induce energy expenditure.[23] In fact, **akin to primary leptin deficiency, the relative leptin deficiency induced by leptin resistance paradoxically produces orexigenic adiposity signals that engender a state of hyperphagia and decreased energy expenditure.** In this setting, crosstalk between the leptin and insulin signaling systems leads to increased food intake and further obesity.[29]

The Metabolic Syndrome. **Both hyperleptinemia and leptin resistance contribute to insulin resistance and the metabolic syndrome.**

Hyperleptinemia contributes to a proinflammatory milieu, which may participate in the genesis of insulin resistance. Leptin and its receptors structurally resemble proinflammatory cytokines and their receptors. Leptin levels increase acutely during inflammation, and leptin is itself proinflammatory and has immunomodulatory function. Leptin may lead to transcriptional induction of the IL-6 gene.[30] It modulates T-cell responses.[31,32] Via activation of the Rho and Rac family of small GTPases, leptin may have an adverse impact on oxidative stress, endothelial function, and insulin resistance.[6,13]

Leptin resistance contributes to the failure of intracellular lipid homeostasis in overnourished individuals, which also plays a role in genesis of the metabolic syndrome. Instead of confining large quantities of surplus calories to adipocytes specifically designed to store lipid overload, the inability, in leptin resistance, to read leptin signaling permits the storage of excess fat ectopically in nonadipose tissue. In the liver, skeletal and cardiac muscle, and pancreas, leptin resistance has an adverse effect on energy expenditure by diverting fatty acids in these tissues to ectopic triacylglycerol storage rather than oxidative consumption.[11] The ensuing ectopic accumulation of intracellular triacylglycerol contributes to the dysfunction of these organs and is a critical determinant of insulin resistance.[33]

Cardiovascular Impact. **Leptin resistance has adverse effects on the cardiovascular system via central and peripheral receptors, with a negative impact on the vasculature and myocardium.**

Elevated serum leptin levels are independent predictors of cardiovascular morbidity and mortality.[34] High plasma leptin levels are predictive of cardiovascular events, independent of traditional risk factors, body mass index (BMI), and C-reactive protein (CRP) levels.[35]

- Leptin receptors in brain regions implicated in cardiovascular control may exert a stimulatory effect on sympathetic activation that results in autonomic hyperactivity.[8,36] Leptin induces the synthesis of endothelin-1 and exerts a pressor effect.[37,38]
- Leptin is a proinflammatory adipokine with immunomodulatory functions.[31,32] Via activation of the Rho and Rac family of small GTPases, leptin may have an adverse impact on oxidative stress and engender endothelial dysfunction.[6,13] Leptin signaling is also implicated in platelet aggregation and the pathogenesis of arterial thrombosis.[39,40]
- Leptin impairs arterial distensibility and promotes angiogenesis.[41,42]
- Leptin receptors, which are present in the myocardium, may affect ventricular remodeling. Primary leptin deficiency in ob–/ob– mice induces ventricular hypertrophy. The degree of myocardial hypertrophy is independent of body mass, and exogenous administration of leptin rapidly reduces ventricular hypertrophy.[43] Clinically, with relative leptin deficiency as a result of leptin resistance, plasma leptin levels are correlated with increased myocardial wall thickness, independent of body weight composition and blood pressure levels.[44]

The underlying mechanism may derive from self-preservation during periods of starvation with low leptin levels. In the interest of self-protection, there may be a redistribution of lean muscle mass directed to preserve central organs at the expense of peripheral muscle bulk. A similar mechanism may inappropriately pertain to the relative leptin deficiency caused by receptor insensitivity. Deficient leptin signaling in this setting will lead to the myocardial hypertrophy seen with obesity, type 2 DM, or hypertension.[7,44]

Adiponectin. Adiponectin, or adipocyte complement-related protein of 30 kDa (ACRP30, AdipoQ, apM1, or GBP28), is a 30-kDa, 247–amino acid, collagen-like protein consisting of an amino-terminal collagenous domain and a carboxy-terminal globular domain. The carboxy-terminal domain has significant homology with the TNF family and with the globular domain of the complement factor C1q. **Adiponectin enhances skeletal muscle insulin sensitivity,[2] and adiponectin expression and secretion appear to correlate with systemic insulin sensitivity.[45,46]**

Adiponectin Synthesis. Adiponectin is exclusively derived from adipose tissue.

Adipose Tissue. The adiponectin gene, on chromosome 3q27, is expressed predominantly by differentiated adipocytes within adipose tissue after activation by PPAR-γ. Adipose tissue is thus the only source for the circulating hormone. Secretion of adiponectin by visceral-omental adipocytes is higher than that by subcutaneous adipocytes.[46,47]

In contrast to leptin and TNF-α, however, **adiponectin's tissue expression and plasma concentration are decreased in obesity, in type 2 DM, and with cardiovascular disease.**[48,49] Specifically, there is a strong, negative correlation of visceral fat adiponectin production with BMI. In contrast, secretion from subcutaneous fat cells is unrelated to BMI. The reduced secretion from the visceral-omental adipose depot may account for the decline in plasma adiponectin observed in obesity,[47] and impaired depot-specific expression of adiponectin may be a contributing factor for the development of insulin resistance.[50]

Adiponectin tissue expression is higher in lean individuals, and higher levels of adiponectin are associated with greater degrees of insulin sensitivity.[51] Not surprisingly, plasma adiponectin levels are 30% higher, or almost double, in anorexia nervosa patients than in control subjects, with a reverse pattern pertaining for leptin concentration.[52]

Determinants of Adiponectin Production. Whereas in mice high-fat feeding reduces circulating levels of adiponectin and caloric restriction increases its plasma level, adiponectin levels are relatively constant in humans. Adiponectin expression from adipose tissue is higher in women than in men.[51]

Both insulin and PPAR-γ activators increase adiponectin elaboration, as do moderate alcohol consumption and blockade of both the renin-angiotensin system and the cannabinoid CB1 receptor.[2,53-55]

β-Adrenergic stimulation has both pretranslational and post-translational effects that down-regulate adiponectin.[49] Chronic endothelin-1 exposure, as in obesity and DM, decreases adiponectin levels.[56] Corticosteroid metabolism also down-regulates expression of adiponectin and induces TNF-α.[57] TNF-α and IL-6 suppress mRNA levels of the gene encoding adiponectin.[58] Angiotensin II and leptin, as well as ghrelin acutely, may also down-regulate its expression (Table 6-3).[45,53,59]

Table 6-3. Determinants of Adiponectin Secretion

Factors Favoring Adiponectin Secretion
Insulin
High-density lipoprotein
Peroxisome proliferator–activated receptor-γ
Moderate alcohol consumption
Blockade of the renin-angiotensin-aldosterone system
Blockade of the cannabinoid CB1 receptor
Factors Antagonizing Adiponectin Secretion
β-Adrenergic stimulation
Angiotensin II
Endothelin-1
Corticosteroids
Leptin
Ghrelin
Interleukin-6
Tumor necrosis factor-α

The Adiponectin Receptor. Identification of the adiponectin receptor is still ongoing. However, given the homology of adiponectin's globular domain with complement factor C1q, it is conceivable that the C1q receptor may be the receptor, or one of the receptors, for adiponectin. The adiponectin receptor is highly expressed in endothelium, in smooth and skeletal muscle, and in hepatocytes.[49,60] Adiponectin receptors may be present in the central nervous system as well.[61]

Body Weight Loss. Adiponectin plays a role in the control of body weight and fuel homeostasis[62] **via phosphorylation and activation of AMPK.**[63] As a result, there is stimulation of fatty acid oxidation and weight loss in murine models of diet-induced obesity. Injection of adiponectin increases skeletal muscle fatty acid metabolism and energy dissipation. Adiponectin injection achieves a large and sustainable reduction in weight.[2,64]

Adiponectin may have an impact on fuel homeostasis via central effects as well. In mice, intravenous injection of adiponectin also caused the appearance of adiponectin in cerebrospinal fluid, consistent with brain transport. Intracerebroventricular administration of adiponectin decreases body weight mainly by stimulating energy expenditure, possibly via the melanocortin pathway.[61]

Impact on Plasma Lipids. As a result of enhanced fatty acid oxidation, **high adiponectin**

levels are associated with lower plasma triglyceride levels and correspondingly higher high-density lipoprotein (HDL) levels. Injection of adiponectin causes a transient decline in plasma free fatty acids.[2,64] Lower free fatty acid fluxes, with the effects of adiponectin on liver and muscle metabolism, are probable underlying causes.

Anti-inflammatory and Vasculoprotective Effects. Adiponectin has anti-inflammatory effects.

It negatively regulates hematopoiesis and immune functions[45] and inhibits the nuclear factor kappaB (NFκB) signaling pathway. Adiponectin antagonizes the actions of proinflammatory cytokines such as TNF-α and some of the interleukins. It may lower levels of TNF-α, CRP, IL-6, and other proinflammatory cytokines.[46]

Endothelial Function. Adiponectin enhances endothelial production of NO.

In cultured bovine aortic endothelial cells, adiponectin activates endothelial nitric oxide synthase (eNOS) NO production through a PI3K-dependent pathway. This occurs via AMPK phosphorylation of eNOS at Ser1179.[65]

Vascular Inflammation. Adiponectin attenuates endothelial inflammatory responses.

After arterial injury, adiponectin rapidly accumulates in the subendothelial space.[66] It suppresses endothelial adhesion molecule expression and inhibits smooth muscle cell proliferation.[67] It thwarts the transformation of macrophages into foam cells and the production of TNF-α by macrophages in vitro.[49,62] In human monocyte-derived macrophages, adiponectin selectively increases the expression of tissue inhibitor of metalloproteinase-1 (TIMP-1) through induction of the anti-inflammatory IL-10.[68]

Vasculogenesis. Adiponectin promotes new blood vessel growth.

In mouse and rabbit models of angiogenesis, adiponectin induces endothelial cell differentiation and migration with blood vessel development by promoting crosstalk between AMPK and Akt kinase signaling within endothelial cells.[69]

Antiatherogenic Impact. Adiponectin appears to prevent atherogenesis in humans.

Adiponectin is inversely associated with traditional cardiovascular risk factors such as hypertension, relative tachycardia, and hyperlipidemia. It is positively related to levels of HDL. High plasma adiponectin levels are associated with a lower risk for coronary heart disease (CHD) in American Indians with type 2 DM and a lower risk for myocardial infarction in men.[46,70] A mutation of the adiponectin gene is a common genetic background associated with CHD in the Japanese population,[71] and in general, adiponectin levels are decreased with CHD.[51]

Insulin-Sensitizing Effects. Adiponectin improves insulin sensitivity. The anti-inflammatory effects of adiponectin, as well as its metabolic effects on fatty acid metabolism, may play contributory roles.

Injection of adiponectin increases skeletal muscle fatty acid metabolism and energy dissipation with an attendant transient decline in basal glucose levels.[2,64] Irrespective of body weight, insulin-sensitive subjects demonstrate a twofold higher plasma level of adiponectin than do insulin-resistant individuals (11.2 ± 1.1 versus 5.6 ± 0.6 μg/mL, respectively; $P < .0005$).[51]

Decreased expression of adiponectin is correlated with insulin resistance[67] and is predictive of the development of type 2 DM in the Pima Indian population.[72] A mutation of the adiponectin gene is a common genetic background associated with the metabolic syndrome in the Japanese population,[71] and adiponectin levels are decreased in type 2 DM.[51]

Inflammation and Insulin Resistance. Suppression of adiponectin participates in the genesis of systemic insulin resistance[45] and may constitute one of the links between adiposity, inflammation, type 2 DM, and atherosclerosis.[73]

Adiponectin is negatively correlated with markers of inflammation, and its synthesis may be suppressed by proinflammatory cytokines. Specifically, in 3T3-L1 cultured adipocyte cells, TNF-α and, especially, IL-6 reversibly down-regulated adiponectin gene expression via a p44/42 MAPK pathway.[58] In nondiabetic individuals with varying degrees of insulin resistance and obesity, there was a significant, inverse correlation between plasma adiponectin and TNF-α mRNA expression. Individuals with the lowest levels of TNF-α from their adipose tissue in vitro had the highest levels of adiponectin mRNA expression.[51] TNF-α significantly decreases the expression of PPAR-γ with a negative impact on adiponectin production.[2,45,74] In normoglycemic Pima Indians, adiponectin was negatively correlated with CRP, IL-6, soluble phospholipase A_2, and soluble endothelial-selectin.[73]

Fatty Acid Metabolism. Adiponectin's net metabolic effect, derived primarily from the peripheral actions of the adipokine, is akin to that observed with leptin, which acts primarily centrally, via hypothalamic stimulation. Specifically, **both adiponectin and leptin improve insulin signaling in part through a reduction in muscle and liver triacylglycerol content via increased fat oxidation, which ultimately restores insulin signaling** and thereby enhances insulin sensitivity and glucose metabolism in vitro and in vivo (Table 6-4).[60]

The mechanism of action appears to involve AMPK activation in skeletal muscle and the liver with an increase in the expression of genes mediating fatty acid transport, fatty acid beta oxidation, and increased energy expenditure:

- In skeletal muscle, via activation of AMPK, adiponectin stimulates phosphorylation of acetyl CoA carboxylase, fatty acid beta oxidation, reduced fatty acid synthesis, glucose uptake, and lactate production.
- In the liver, AMPK activation phosphorylates acetyl CoA carboxylase, with a reduction of molecules involved in gluconeogenesis and a reduction of glucose levels in vivo.[63]

Table 6-4. Adiponectin Action and Target Tissues

ACTION	TARGET
Improvement in endothelial function	Vasculature
Reduction of vascular inflammation	Vasculature
Decrease in plasma glucose levels	Whole body
Enhancement of insulin action	Liver
Stimulation of fatty acid oxidation	Skeletal muscle
Reduction of circulating free fatty acid levels	Plasma

Modified from Mora S, Pessin JE. An adipocentric view of signaling and intracellular trafficking. Diabetes Metab Res Rev 2002;18:345-356

The enhanced thermogenesis and fat oxidation lower both myocyte and hepatocyte ectopic triacylglycerol content, thereby contributing to normalization of organ function and systemic insulin sensitivity.

ADIPOKINES WITH DETRIMENTAL METABOLIC EFFECT

Resistin. Resistin was discovered while searching for the mechanism of action of rosiglitazone in a mouse animal model. In rodents, resistin links obesity to DM.

Resistin is an adipocyte-secreted factor and was named for "resistance to insulin." It antagonizes insulin action and impairs glucose tolerance. Its genes are expressed solely in adipocytes, during adipocyte differentiation. The magnitude of gene expression correlates with the degree of obesity. Circulating resistin levels are elevated in obese mice.

Although resistin itself appears to be limited in expression to rodents, a family of related molecules expressed in human adipose tissue may have physiologic effects similar to resistin.[75]

Tumor Necrosis Factor-α. TNF-α is a pleiotropic cytokine associated with the acute phase response of inflammation. In the acute phase, it is produced by monocytes and macrophages in response to endotoxemia, inflammation, and cancer.[76] It causes the classic trilogy of

1. necrosis,
2. shock, and
3. cachexia.

More specifically, TNF-α modulates

- apoptosis,
- cell proliferation,
- immunomodulation,
- inflammation,
- viral replication,
- allergy,
- arthritis,
- septic shock,
- autoimmune diseases,

and other pathologic conditions. **TNF-α is a potent negative inotrope and is implicated**

in causing insulin resistance via various direct and indirect mechanisms.[77]

TNF-α Production. TNF-α is produced during inflammatory processes.

Stimulants of Synthesis. Immunologic stimulants for TNF-α elaboration are

- endotoxin,
- lipopolysaccharide,
- phorbol esters,
- phosphatase inhibitors, and
- TNF-α itself.

Physiologic inducers of TNF-α expression are

- high-fat diets,
- triglycerides, and
- free fatty acids.

Other stimulants for TNF-α secretion are

- increasing age,
- hyperinsulinemia,
- obesity, and
- cancer.[32,78]

Membrane and Soluble TNF-α. TNF-α and its main receptors are part of a superfamily of related cytokines and receptors. TNF-α is synthesized as a 26-kDa transmembrane protein (mTNF-α). It may be present on the cell surface or may be processed by the TNF-α–converting enzyme (TACE) to release a 17-kDa soluble polypeptide (sTNF-α), which is active in a homotrimeric constitution.[79]

Sites of TNF-α Synthesis. TNF-α is produced principally by immune system cells such as macrophages. It is also elaborated by adipose tissue, muscle, and the myocardium. It is expressed in the muscle cells of insulin-resistant individuals at higher levels than in insulin-sensitive individuals.[80,81]

Adipose Tissue mTNF-α in Obesity. Synthesis of TNF-α may occur in adipose tissue, specifically in the adipocyte fraction.[80,81] There is TNF-α mRNA expression in adipocytes.[79] **Obesity is the only known condition wherein TNF-α is expressed at elevated levels in adipocytes** (Fig. 6-2).[82]

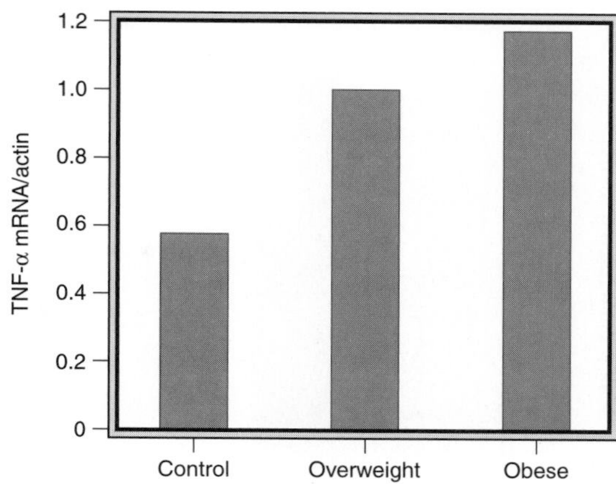

Figure 6–2.
Levels of adipose tissue tumor necrosis factor-alpha (TNF-α) expression in relation to adiposity. *(Modified from Bullo M, Garcia-Lorda P, Peinado-Onsurbe J, et al. TNF-alpha expression of subcutaneous adipose tissue in obese and morbid obese females: relationship to adipocyte LPL activity and leptin synthesis. Int J Obes 2002;26:652-658.)*

In humans, TNF-α tissue expression is proportional to the

- percentage of body fat and
- BMI.[82]

The aberrant expression of TNF-α in adipocytes has been considered by some to be a molecular compensatory mechanism for modulation of insulin action in adipose tissue to limit its expansion.[83]

Circulating levels of TNF-α are disproportionately low when compared with TNF-α tissue expression.[82] Obese humans have increased mTNF-α in adipose tissue because of higher production of TNF-α with decreased processing of the protein by TACE to the cleaved, soluble circulating state (Fig. 6-3). Transmembrane mTNF-α is capable of effecting a variety of biologic functions via cell contact–dependent signaling. Conceivably, as a result of its low plasma concentration, TNF-α, specifically mTNF-α, functions primarily locally in adipose tissue via autocrine/paracrine mechanisms.[82,84]

TNF-α Receptors. There are several TNF receptors.

Receptor Subtypes. TNF-α transduces cellular responses through two major, distinct receptors:

1. 60-kDa TNF receptor type I (TNFR1), which is expressed on all cell types, and

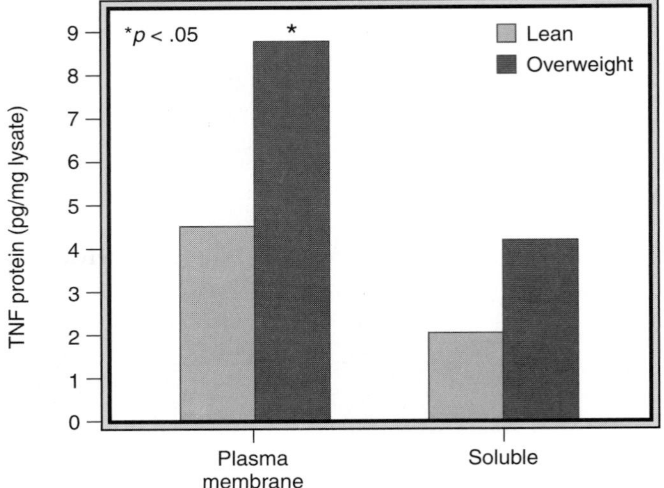

▸▸ **Figure 6–3.**
Expression of membrane versus soluble tumor necrosis factor (TNF)-α in human adipose tissue. *(Modified from Xu H, Uysai T, Becherer JA, et al. Altered tumor necrosis factor-alpha [TNF-alpha] processing in adipocytes and increased expression of transmembrane TNF-alpha in obesity. Diabetes 2002;51: 1876-1883.)*

2. 80-kDa TNF receptor type II (TNFR2), which is expressed on cells of the immune system and on endothelial cells.

Both TNF-α receptors are active in adipocytes.[85]

Soluble TNF-α Receptors. Soluble TNF receptors are derived by proteolytic cleavage from TNF cell surface receptors after their induction by TNF or other cytokines such as IL-6, IL-1β, or IL-2. Soluble TNF receptors have a longer half-life and are detected with higher sensitivity than TNF-α is.[86]

The biologic function of soluble receptors is not entirely clear. They may bind to TNF-α and attenuate its biologic activity. On the other hand, the soluble receptors also promote the formation of complexes with TNF-α, thereby preserving its active trimeric form and preventing its decay into inactive, monomeric forms. In that construct, soluble receptors may serve as a slow-release reservoir for TNF-α and thus prolong its half-life.[86]

TNFR1. TNF-α receptor stimulation results in a partial shift of its receptor to the caveolin-enriched plasma membrane fractions. TNFR1 colocalizes with the scavenger receptor CD36 in plasma membrane caveolae, which suggests that **TNF-α–initiated functions, such as apoptosis, occur from caveolae.**[87]

At the cellular level, upon ligand binding, this receptor initiates the pathways leading to

- activation of the transcription factor NFκB,
- activation of the c-Jun and c-Fos heterodimer transcription factor activator protein-1 (AP)-1,
- apoptosis,
- antiadipogenic effects and lipolysis,[88]
- activation of MAPK and mitogenic effects,
- cell proliferation, and
- induction of insulin insensitivity.[32]

These TNF-α functions occur via interactions with the TNFR1 death domain. The death domain, an 80–amino acid region, is located at the carboxy terminus of TNFR1. The TNFR1 death domain and the TNFR1-associated death domain protein (TRADD) interact with downstream effectors such as Fas-associated death domain protein (FADD), receptor interaction protein (RIP), and TNFR-associated factor 2 (TRAF2).[88] Binding of TRAF2 to TNFR1 is normally induced after TNF-α stimulation. This carrier activates one or more MAPKs, thereby leading to mitogenic effects.[32]

TNFR1 has two other regions:

1. The juxtamembrane domain (JM) produces phosphatidylinositol 4,5-biphosphate, a precursor of the second messengers phosphatidyl 1,4,5-triphosphate and 1,2-diacylglycerol.
2. The caveolin-sensitive, neutral sphingomyelinase-activating domain (NSD) activates membrane sphingomyelinase to produce the lipid signaling molecule ceramide via hydrolysis of membrane sphingomyelin.[88]

Sphingomyelin is a phospholipid that is ubiquitously present in the plasma membrane of mammalian cells. The sphingolipid ceramide, and its metabolites sphingosine and sphingosine 1-phosphate, have been recognized as important mediators of signal transduction processes leading to a variety of cellular responses, including apoptosis.[89]

TNF-α Signaling Pathways. The TNF receptors do not exhibit any enzymatic activity. They transmit their signals through the recruitment of more than a dozen different signaling proteins and signaling cascades.[85]

Nuclear Factor kappaB. TNF-α is a transcriptional regulator that activates NFκB and AP-1, followed by the increased expression of proinflammatory cytokines.[90]

Through activation of NFκB and AP-1, TNF-α regulates immune and inflammatory gene responses.[91] NFκB is an obligatory mediator of TNF-α responses. NFκB activation occurs within 15 minutes of adipocyte exposure to TNF-α. Within 4 to 24 hours of exposure to TNF-α, as assayed by a microarray of 220 genes, 142 genes are up-regulated and 78 genes are down-regulated (Fig. 6-4). The cytokine cascade is initiated and the expression of chemokines and adhesion molecules is facilitated. TNF-α induces cytokines such as

- IL-6,
- leptin,
- interferon-α,
- interferon-γ,
- cytokine-induced proteins,
- growth factors, and
- enzyme-signaling molecules.[45]

TNF-α can also stimulate its own transcription.[85]

Rho and Rac. TNF-α interaction with the TNFR1 subtype activates small GTPases of the Rho family, RhoA and Rac.[92-94]

RhoA activation of Rho kinase is implicated in mediating insulin resistance via serine phosphorylation of IRS-1.[92,93] Rho family GTPases are involved in the induction of NFκB signaling by TNF-α, and isoprenylated regulatory proteins participate in the regulation of NFκB by TNF-α.[95] Rac is activated in TNF-α–stimulated cells and plays a critical role in inciting the extracellular signal–related kinase (ERK) signaling pathway.[94]

TNF-α Actions. As part of its proinflammatory repertory of actions, TNF-α is implicated in mediating endothelial dysfunction, antiadipogenic effects, and insulin resistance.

Endothelial Dysfunction. TNF-α inhibits eNOS in a dose-dependent fashion as measured by Western blotting.[90]

TNF-α impairs insulin-stimulated vasodilation. Because the proximal insulin signaling pathway in vascular endothelium resembles the steps of the metabolic insulin cascade in other

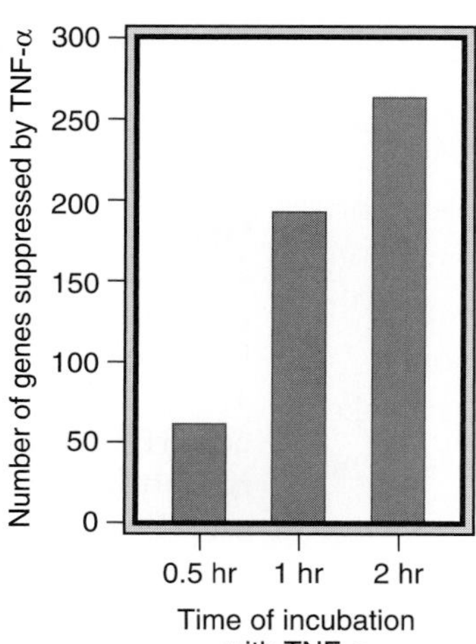

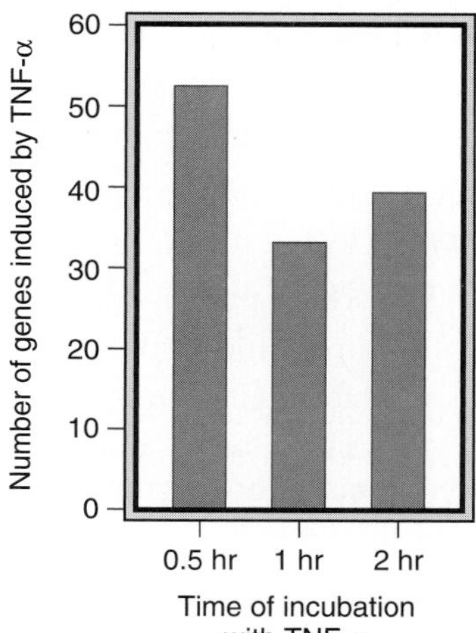

Figure 6–4. Tumor necrosis factor-alpha (TNF-α)-induced changes in the expression of adipocyte genes. *(Modified from Ruan H, Hacohen N, Golub TR, et al. Tumor necrosis factor-alpha suppresses adipocyte-specific genes and activates expression of preadipocyte genes in 3T3-L1 adipocytes. Diabetes 2002;51:1319-1336.)*

insulin-responsive tissues, TNF-α impairs the insulin-mediated production of NO. In humans, TNF-α inhibits insulin-stimulated glucose uptake coincident with an inhibitory effect on insulin-stimulated endothelial function.[96,97]

Antiadipogenic Effects. TNF-α has pronounced autocrine/paracrine effects on adipose tissue. **TNF-α functions as an adipostat and is thus antiadipogenic.**

The potent antiadipogenic effects of secreted and transmembrane TNF-α are mediated solely via the TNFR1 receptor.[88] In the process, TNF-α inhibits the expression of major regulators of adipose tissue differentiation, such as

- the nuclear receptor PPAR-γ2,
- the nuclear retinoid X receptor-α, and
- the transcription factor C/EBPα.[45]

These TNF-α–induced changes devolve into the subsequent down-regulation of numerous developmental and metabolic markers of adipocyte differentiation, as well as down-regulation of the adipocyte-abundant gene products. Some of these down-regulated proteins participate in insulin signaling and include

- the insulin receptor,
- IRS-1,
- protein kinase B (Akt),
- the glucose transporter GLUT4,
- lipoprotein lipase (LPL),
- glycerol-3-phosphate dehydrogenase (GPDH),
- fatty acid binding protein,
- acetyl CoA carboxylase,
- long-chain fatty acyl CoA synthase,
- adiponectin,[78] and
- fatty acid transport proteins 1 and 4.[79]

As a result, TNF-α interferes with adipose functioning by

- blocking preadipocyte gene expression,[45]
- suppressing adipocyte differentiation,
- inhibiting insulin-stimulated glucose uptake,
- blocking basal and insulin-induced long-chain fatty acid uptake, and
- thwarting lipogenesis.[78,79]

TNF-α in adipose tissue thereby effectively limits the expansion of fat tissue and is a potent inhibitor of the differentiation of fat cell precursors into adipocytes.[78]

TNF-α may also have central effects on body weight by decreasing energy intake or by inducing thermogenesis.[83]

Lipolytic Effects. TNF-α modulates gene expression in adipocytes to the effect of stimulating lipolysis.[78] **Chronic exposure of adipocytes to TNF-α ultimately causes the reversion of adipocytes to a preadipocyte phenotype of fibroblast morphology.**[32,78]

Specific TNF-α actions that have an impact on adipocyte catabolism are

- Stimulation of hormone-sensitive lipase. On TNF-α exposure, mature adipocytes are actually stimulated to mobilize lipids, possibly via stimulation of hormone-sensitive lipase.[78] The early intracellular signals entailed in TNF-α–mediated lipolysis may involve members of the MAPK family. Specifically, p44/42 and c-Jun NH_2-terminal kinase (JNK) appear to be involved.[98]
- Phosphorylation of perilipin. Another mechanism for TNF-α–induced lipolysis is as follows: TNF-α activates MAPK kinase (MAPKK), and MAPKK activates ERK. ERK ultimately decreases the expression of cyclic nucleotide phosphodiesterase 3B by 50%, which causes an increase in cytoplasmic cAMP. Activated cAMP-dependent protein kinase A (PKA) causes perilipin hyperphosphorylation. Perilipins are phosphoproteins located at the surface of lipid droplets in adipocytes that bar lipase access to the intracellular lipids. Perilipin phosphorylation modifies the lipid surface and allows lipase access. Lipase access to lipids increases lipolysis.[99]

Hypertriglyceridemia. Suppression of LPL is a central action of TNF-α that has an impact on lipogenesis. In human adipocytes, TNF-α is inversely proportional to LPL activity, and TNF-α blocks fat deposition by decreasing LPL activity. **TNF-α lipolytic effects, together with inhibition of LPL expression, lead to an elevation in plasma free fatty acids, increased triglycerides, and a reduction in HDL.**[79]

In humans, TNF-α tissue expression is proportional to serum triglyceride levels.[82]

Table 6-5. Tumor Necrosis Factor-α Production and Actions in Adipose Tissue

Fatty acids
Endothelial dysfunction
Inflammation
Macrophages
Other factors

↓

Increased adipocyte production of
TNF-α
TNFR p60
TNFR p80

Adipose tissue local autocrine/paracrine effects:
Impairment of insulin signaling
Reduction in adiponectin expression
Stimulation of lipolysis/delipidation
Inhibition of adipocyte differentiation and growth
Dedifferentiation of adipocytes
Promotion of apoptosis

TNF, tumor necrosis factor; TNFR, TNF receptor.
Adapted from Hube F, Hauner H. The role of TNF-alpha in human adipose tissue: prevention of weight gain at the expense of insulin resistance? Horm Metab Res 1999;31:626-631.

Not surprisingly, TNF-α levels are also inversely related to HDL cholesterol levels.[78,81]

Insulin Resistance. The TNF-α–induced changes in adipocyte gene expression contribute to insulin resistance within adipose tissue (Table 6-5). There are numerous direct and indirect mechanisms whereby TNF-α may induce insulin resistance not only locally but also systemically.

In humans, TNF-α tissue expression is proportional to measures of insulin resistance, such as

- fasting glucose levels,
- fasting insulin levels, and
- leptin expression.[82]

Directly, TNF-α interferes in the proximal steps of the insulin signaling cascade:

- TNF-α induces serine phosphorylation of IRS-1, which impairs the tyrosine kinase activity of the insulin receptor.[100]
- TNF-α also causes sustained induction of SOCS-3, which lowers insulin-induced IRS-1 tyrosine phosphorylation and IRS-1 association with p85, the regulatory subunit of PI3K, thus interfering with insulin signaling at the level of proximal receptor substrates.[101]

Indirectly, TNF-α causes insulin resistance through several mechanisms:

- TNF-α stimulates the production of proinflammatory cytokines, which induce insulin resistance.
- TNF-α increases the expression of inducible NO synthase (iNOS) and oxidative stress.[102]
- TNF-α acts as a negative regulator of PPAR-γ by lowering PPAR-γ mRNA levels, thus leading to insulin resistance.[45]
- TNF-α increases plasma levels of free fatty acids through increased lipolysis of adipose tissue, thereby indirectly effecting systemic insulin resistance.[98]
- TNF-α may activate p38 MAPK, which is situated downstream of MAPKK6 and MAPKK3. Activation of p38 MAPK leads to a marked down-regulation of insulin-induced glucose uptake via GLUT4.[103]
- TNF-α inhibits the synthesis of adiponectin, thereby relinquishing its insulin-sensitizing propensities.[104]

Although all these pathways implement insulin resistance locally in adipose tissue, a number of mechanisms have a systemic reach that contributes to systemic insulin resistance via

- circulation of released humoral mediators, such as cytokines and free fatty acids;
- reduction of circulating adiponectin levels; and
- ectopic fat storage. In overnourished individuals, TNF-α's antiadipogenic and lipolytic effects contribute to the failure of adipocyte metabolism to appropriately confine the lipid overload to fat cells, instead diverting fatty acids to ectopic storage in muscle, liver, and the pancreas.[11] Ectopic lipid storage is a critical determinant of insulin resistance.[33]

Interleukin-6. IL-6 is a circulating, multifunction cytokine produced by numerous tissues, including mononuclear cells, endothelial cells, and adipocytes. Circulating IL-6 concentrations display a high-amplitude circadian rhythm with peak nocturnal values. IL-6 acts on the liver and the hypothalamus.

Insulin Resistance. IL-6 has a negative impact on insulin resistance in a variety of ways:

- IL-6 stimulates the hypothalamic-pituitary adrenal (HPA) axis[105];
- via a p44/42 MAPK pathway, IL-6 reversibly down-regulates expression of the adiponectin gene[58]; and
- IL-6 inhibits LPL.

The Renin-Angiotensin-Aldosterone System. Expression of the renin-angiotensin-aldosterone system (RAAS) genes for

- renin,
- angiotensinogen,
- angiotensin-converting enzyme,
- angiotensin II, and
- the angiotensin II type 1 receptor

is increased during adipogenesis. Angiotensinogen secretion and angiotensin II generation are characteristic features of adipogenesis. **The RAAS is established within human adipose tissue and is richly expressed, particularly in visceral-omental fat.**[106]

The adipose RAAS is regulated by hormonal and nutritional factors. Its activity correlates with the degree of obesity. Angiotensin II may modulate adipose tissue blood flow, growth, and metabolism. **An up-regulated adipose RAAS produces deleterious local and systemic effects in obese individuals by contributing to inflammation, insulin resistance, and hypertension.**[102]

RAAS activation increases IL-6 secretion and oxidative stress. It reduces adiponectin elaboration.[53,107]

The local RAAS system is antiadipogenic. It functions as a paracrine, negative feedback loop for adipogenesis. Mature adipocytes can inhibit preadipocyte differentiation via the angiotensin II type 1 receptor. Stimulation of the angiotensin II type 1 receptor by angiotensin II reduces adipose conversion and adipogenesis,[108] an effect that facilitates the ectopic storage of excess fat and contributes to insulin resistance.[109]

CONCLUSION

Adipose tissue plays a critical role as an endocrine gland by secreting a variety of endocrine hormones. These adipokines exert potent autocrine/paracrine effects on the metabolism of adipose tissue and endocrine effects on distant tissues (Fig. 6-5).

Increased adipose tissue mass alters adipokine production in adipose tissue. TNF-α, IL-6, leptin, components of the RAAS, and other adipokines are overexpressed, whereas adiponectin is underexpressed. The proinflammatory state generated by these changes provides a potential link between two major potential causes for the evolution of insulin resistance: the autocrine/paracrine/endocrine paradigm and the ectopic fat storage paradigm.

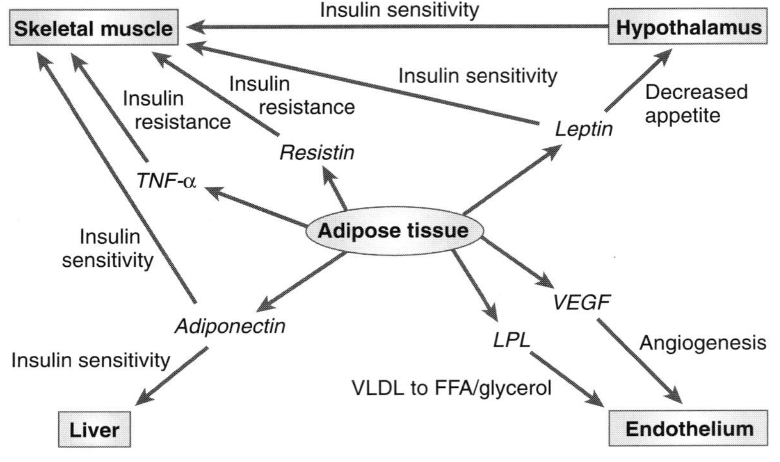

▸▸ **Figure 6–5.** Endocrine signals of adipokines. FFA, free fatty acid; LPL, lipoprotein lipase; TNF, tumor necrosis factor; VEGF, vascular endothelial growth factor; VLDL, very-low-density lipoprotein. *(Modified from Mora S, Pessin JE. An adipocentric view of signaling and intracellular trafficking. Diabetes Metab Res Rev 2002;18:345-356.)*

Table 6-6. Progression of Insulin Resistance Localized to Adipose Tissue to a Systemic Phenomenon

Adipose tissue expansion + proinflammatory milieu
↓
Increased production of insulin resistance factors, e.g., TNF-α, resistin Decreased production of insulin sensitizers, e.g., adiponectin
↓
Adipose tissue insulin resistance
↓
Lipolysis, circulating free fatty acids and cytokines, ectopic skeletal muscle and liver free fatty acid uptake and storage
↓
Endothelial dysfunction Systemic insulin resistance
↓
Metabolic and vascular sequelae

TNF, tumor necrosis factor.

Hormonal Paradigm. TNF-α, IL-6, and the RAAS activate the small GTPases of the Rho family. The Rho signaling pathway constitutes one of the molecular mechanisms by which these adipokines may mediate insulin resistance. Adipokines may at first confine the impairment of insulin signaling to adipose tissue. Distant tissue effects may derive from the endocrine impact of circulating adipokines or, secondarily, as a result of the release of free fatty acids engendered by lipolysis (Table 6-6).

Importantly, several agents, such as TNF-α, angiotensin II, and IL-6, also impair systemic insulin metabolism through a reduction of adiponectin levels. In autocrine/paracrine fashion, these proinflammatory adipokines block adiponectin secretion from adipocytes. The loss of adiponectin signaling may play a critical role in the genesis of systemic insulin resistance. In this context, the increased elaboration of leptin with evolving leptin resistance leads to a de facto deficiency of this adipokine, which also contributes to the systemic insulin resistance pathophysiology.

Ectopic Fat Paradigm. TNF-α, IL-6, and angiotensin II are all antiadipogenic and lipolytic. They compromise and undermine the ability of adipose tissue to act as the principal capacitor designed to store large quantities of surplus calories in overnourished individuals, thus forcing the storage of excess fat in ectopic, nonadipose loci.

Antiadipogenic adipokine effects complement the metabolic impact of adiponectin deficiency and de facto leptin deficiency secondary to leptin resistance. A lack of these two insulin-sensitizing adipokines undercuts the central and peripheral regulation of energy metabolism and thermogenesis by metabolically facilitating the ectopic storage of excess fat in skeletal and cardiac muscle, the liver, and the pancreas and implementing the additional insulin resistance mechanisms derived from that pathophysiology.

Modulation of the Adipokine Axis. Modulation of the adipokine axis may offer promise in the treatment of insulin resistance. Although obesity is considered an inflammatory state, the proinflammatory adipokine output from fat tissue may be sensitive to the ambient activation of systemic stress pathways and become increased in a proinflammatory and decreased in a noninflammatory, antioxidant milieu. Lifestyle measures that decrease stress and inflammatory activation, such as smoking cessation, moderate weight loss, moderate aerobic exercise training, stress relaxation, and the consumption of an anti-inflammatory diet, would be expected to be of benefit. Interestingly, moderate wine consumption may increase adiponectin levels and play a protective role. Beyond lifestyle modifications, anti-inflammatory interventions as with statins, RAAS antagonists, and PPAR-γ ligands have been shown to lower levels of proinflammatory cytokines. RAAS antagonists and PPAR-γ activators increase adiponectin levels. Ultimately, there may be the potential for adiponectin, or a homologue of adiponectin, to serve as a therapeutic agent for individuals suffering from insulin resistance and its adverse metabolic and vascular sequelae.

GLOSSARY

ACRP30 adipocyte complement-related protein of 30 kDa
AMPK 5′-adenosine monophosphate–activated protein kinase
AP-1 activator protein-1
BMI body mass index
cAMP adenosine 3′,5′-cyclic phosphate
CB cannabinoid
CHD coronary heart disease
CoA coenzyme A
CRP C-reactive protein
DM diabetes mellitus
eNOS endothelial nitric oxide synthase
ERK extracellular signal–related kinase
FADD Fas-associated death domain protein
G-CSF granulocyte-colony-stimulating factor
GLUT glucose transporter
GPDH glycerol-3-phosphate dehydrogenase
GTP guanosine 5′-triphosphate
HDL high-density lipoprotein
HPA hypothalamic-pituitary-adrenal
IL interleukin
iNOS inducible NO synthase
IRS insulin receptor substrate
JAK Janus kinase
JM juxtamembrane domain
JNK c-Jun NH_2-terminal kinase
LPL lipoprotein lipase
MAPK mitogen-activated protein kinase
MAPKK MAPK kinase
NFκB nuclear factor kappaB
NO nitric oxide
NSD neutral sphingomyelinase-activating domain
PI3K phosphatidylinositol 3-kinase
PKA protein kinase A
PPAR peroxisome proliferator–activated receptor
RAAS renin-angiotensin-aldosterone system
RIP receptor interaction protein
SOCS suppressor of cytokine signaling
STAT signal transducers and activators of transcription
TACE TNF-α–converting enzyme
TIMP-1 tissue inhibitor of metalloproteinase-1
TNF tumor necrosis factor
TNFR TNF receptor
TRADD TNFR1-associated death domain protein
TRAF2 TNFR-associated factor 2

REFERENCES

1. Matsuzawa Y, Funahashi T, Nakamura T. Molecular mechanism of metabolic syndrome X: contribution of adipocytokines. Ann NY Acad Sci 1999;892:146-154
2. Mora S, Pessin JE. An adipocentric view of signaling and intracellular trafficking. Diabetes Metab Res Rev 2002; 18:345-356
3. Saltiel AR. You are what you secrete. Nat Med 2001; 7:887-888
4. Halaas TL, Gajiwala KS, Koivisto VA. Exercise and the metabolic syndrome. Diabetologia 1997;40:115-125
5. Attoub S, Noe V, Pirola L, et al. Leptin promotes invasiveness of kidney and colonic epithelial cells via phosphoinositide 3-kinase–, rho-, and rac-dependent signaling pathways. FASEB J 2000;14:2329-2338
6. Hofbauer KG. Molecular pathways to obesity. Int J Obes Relat Metab Disord 2002;26:S18-S27
7. Sader S, Nian M, Liu P. Leptin: a novel link between obesity, diabetes, cardiovascular risk, and ventricular hypertrophy. Circulation 2003;108:644-646
8. Tartaglia LA, Dembski M, Weng X, et al. Identification and expression cloning of a leptin receptor, OB-R. Cell 1995;83:1263-1271
9. Chen SC, Kochan JP, Campfield LA, et al. Splice variants of the OB receptor gene are differentially expressed in brain and peripheral tissues of mice. J Recept Signal Transduct Res 1999;19:245-266
10. Van Heek M, Mullins DE, Wirth MA, et al. The relationship of tissue localization, distribution and turnover to feeding after intraperitoneal ^{125}I-leptin administration to ob/ob and db/db mice. Horm Metab Res 1996;28:653-658
11. Atkinson LL, Fischer MA, Lopaschuk GD. Leptin activates cardiac fatty acid oxidation independent of changes in the AMP-activated protein kinase–acetyl-CoA carboxylase–malonyl-CoA axis. J Biol Chem 2002;277:29424-29430
12. Szanto I, Kahn CR. Selective interaction between leptin and insulin signaling pathways in a hepatic cell line. Proc Natl Acad Sci U S A 2000;97:2355-2360
13. Mareel M, Leroy A. Clinical, cellular, and molecular aspects of cancer invasion. Physiol Rev 2003;83:337-376
14. Halaas TL, Gajiwala KS, Maffei M, et al. Weight-reducing effects of the plasma protein encoded by the obese gene. Science 1995;269:543-546
15. Fruhbeck G. Pivotal role of nitric oxide in the control of blood pressure after leptin administration. Diabetes 1999;48:903-908
16. Shiuchi T, Nakagami H, Iwai M, et al. Involvement of bradykinin and nitric oxide in leptin-mediated glucose uptake in skeletal muscle. Endocrinology 2001;142: 608-612
17. Steinberg GR, Rush JW, Dyck DJ. AMPK expression and phosphorylation are increased in rodent muscle after chronic leptin treatment. Am J Physiol Endocrinol Metab 2003;284:E648-E654
18. Yeo GS, Farooqi IS, Challis BG, et al. The role of melanocortin signaling in the control of body weight: evidence from human and murine genetic models. QJM 2000;93:7-14
19. Andersson U, Filipsson K, Abbott CR, et al. AMP-activated protein kinase plays a role in the control of food intake. J Biol Chem 2004;279:12005-12008

20. Zhang Y, Proenca R, Maffei M, et al. Positional cloning of the mouse obese gene and its human homologue. Nature 1994;372:425-432
21. List JF, Habener JF. Defective melanocortin 4 receptors in hyperphagia and morbid obesity. N Engl J Med 2003;348:1160-1163
22. Marx J. Cellular warriors at the Battle of the Bulge. Science 2003;299:846-849
23. Frederich RC, Hamann A, Anderson S, et al. Leptin levels reflect body lipid content in mice: evidence for diet-induced resistance to leptin action. Nat Med 1995; 1:1311-1314
24. Reaven GM. Pathophysiology of insulin resistance in human disease. Physiol Rev 1995;75:473-486
25. Leyva F, Godsland IF, Ghatei M, et al. Hyperleptinemia as a component of a metabolic syndrome of cardiovascular risk. Arterioscler Thromb Vasc Biol 1998;18:928-933
26. Zimmet P, Boyko EJ, Collier GR, de Courten M. Etiology of the metabolic syndrome: potential role of insulin resistance, leptin resistance, and other players. Ann NY Acad Sci 1999;892:25-44
27. Diamond J. Guns, Germs, and Steel: The Fates of Human Societies. New York, Norton, 1999
28. Friedman JM. A war on obesity, not the obese. Science 2003;299:856-858
29. Cohen B, Novick D, Rubinstein M. Modulation of insulin activities by leptin. Science 1996;274:1185-1188
30. Faruqi TR, Gomez D, Bustelo XR, et al. Rac1 mediates STAT3 activation by autocrine IL-6. Proc Natl Acad Sci U S A 2001;98:9014-9019
31. Fantuzzi G, Faggioni R. Leptin in the regulation of immunity, inflammation, and hematopoiesis. J Leukoc Biol 2000;68:437-446
32. Coppack SW. Pro-inflammatory cytokines and inflammatory tissue. Proc Nutr Soc 2001;60:349-356
33. Sinha R, Dufour S, Petersen KF, et al. Assessment of skeletal muscle triglyceride content by ^{1}H nuclear magnetic resonance spectroscopy in lean and obese adolescents: relationships to insulin insensitivity, total body fat, and central adiposity. Diabetes 2002; 51:1022-1027
34. Soderberg S, Ahren B, Jansson JH, et al. Leptin is associated with increased risk of myocardial infarction. J Intern Med 1999;246:409-418
35. Wallace AM, McMahon AD, Packard CJ, et al. Plasma leptin and the risk of cardiovascular disease in the West of Scotland Coronary Prevention Study (WOSCOPS). Circulation 2001;104:3052-3056
36. Haynes WG, Morgan DA, Walsh SA, et al. Receptor-mediated regional sympathetic nerve activation by leptin. J Clin Invest 1997;100:270-278
37. Quehenberger P, Exner M, Sunder-Plassmann R, et al. Leptin induces endothelin-1 in endothelial cells in vitro. Circ Res 2002;90:711-718
38. Shek EW, Brands WM, Hall JE. Chronic leptin infusion increases arterial pressure. Hypertension 1998;312: 409-414
39. Konstantinides S, Schafer K, Koschnick S, Loskutoff JD. Leptin-dependent platelet aggregation and arterial thrombosis suggests a mechanism for atherothrombotic disease in obesity. J Clin Invest 2001;108:1533-1540
40. Bodary PF, Westrick RJ, Wickenheiser KJ, et al. Effect of leptin on arterial thrombosis following vascular injury in mice. JAMA 2002;287:1706-1709
41. Singhal A, Farooqi IS, Cole TJ, et al. Influence of leptin on arterial distensibility: a novel link between obesity and cardiovascular disease? Circulation 2002;106:1919-1924
42. Bouloumie A, Drexler HC, Lafontan M, Busse R. Leptin, the product of Ob gene, promotes angiogenesis. Circ Res 1998;83:1059-1066
43. Barouch LA, Berkowitz DE, Harrison RW, et al. Disruption of leptin signaling contributes to cardiac hypertrophy independently of body weight in mice. Circulation 2003;108:754-759
44. Paolisso G, Tagliamonte MR, Galderisi M, et al. Plasma leptin level is associated with myocardial wall thickness in hypertensive insulin-resistant men. Hypertension 1999;34:1047-1052
45. Ruan H, Hacohen N, Golub TR, et al. Tumor necrosis factor-alpha suppresses adipocyte-specific genes and activates expression of preadipocyte genes in 3T3-L1 adipocytes. Diabetes 2002;51:1319-1336
46. Pischon T, Girman CJ, Hotamisgilil GS, et al. Plasma adiponectin levels and risk of myocardial infarction in men. JAMA 2004;291:1730-1737
47. Motoshima H, Wu X, Sinha MK, et al. Differential regulation of adiponectin secretion from cultured human omental and subcutaneous adipocytes: effects of insulin and rosiglitazone. J Clin Endocrinol Metab 2002;87:5662-5667
48. Hotta K, Funahashi T, Arita Y, et al. Plasma concentrations of a novel, adipose-specific protein, adiponectin, in type 2 diabetic patients. Arterioscler Thromb Vasc Biol 2000;20:1595-1599
49. Delporte ML, Funahashi T, Takahashi M, et al. Pre- and post-translational negative effect of beta-adrenoceptor agonists on adiponectin secretion: in vitro and in vivo studies. Biochem J 2002;367:677-685
50. Altomonte J, Harbaran S, Richter A, Dong H. Fat depot–specific expression of adiponectin is impaired in Zucker fatty rats. Metabolism 2003;52:958-963
51. Kern PA, Di Gregorio GB, Lu T, et al. Adiponectin expression from human adipose tissue: relation to obesity, insulin resistance, and tumor necrosis factor-alpha expression. Diabetes 2003;52:1779-1785
52. Delporte ML, Brichard SM, Hermans MP, et al. Hyperadiponectinaemia in anorexia nervosa. Clin Endocrinol (Oxf) 2003;58:22-29
53. Furuhashi M, Ura N, Higashiura K, et al. Blockade of the renin-angiotensin system increases adiponectin concentrations in patients with essential hypertension. Hypertension 2003;42:76-81
54. Sierksma A, Patel H, Ouchi N, et al. Effect of moderate alcohol consumption on adiponectin, tumor necrosis factor-alpha, and insulin sensitivity. Diabetes Care 2004;27:184-189
55. Despres J-P, Golay A, Sjostrom L, for the Rimonabant in Obesity-Lipids Study Group. Effects of rimonabant on metabolic risk factors in overweight patients with dyslipidemia. N Engl J Med 2005; 353:2121-2134
56. Clarke KJ, Zhong Q, Schwartz DD, et al. Regulation of adiponectin secretion by endothelin-1. Biochem Biophys Res Commun 2003;312:945-949
57. Rask E, Olsson T, Soderberg S, et al. Tissue-specific dysregulation of cortisol metabolism in human obesity. J Clin Endocrinol Metab 2001;86:1418-1421
58. Fasshauer M, Kralisch S, Klier M, et al. Adiponectin gene expression and secretion is inhibited by interleukin-6 in 3T3-L1 adipocytes. Biochem Biophys Res Commun 2003;301:1045-1050
59. Ott V, Fasshauer M, Dalski A, et al. Direct peripheral effects of ghrelin include suppression of adiponectin expression. Horm Metab Res 2002;34:640-645
60. Yamauchi T, Kamon J, Waki H, et al. The fat-derived hormone adiponectin reverses insulin resistance associated with both lipoatrophy and obesity. Nat Med 2001;7: 941-946
61. Qi Y, Takahashi N, Hileman SM, et al. Adiponectin acts in the brain to decrease body weight. Nat Med 2004; 10:524-529

62. Ouchi N, Kihara S, Arita Y, et al. Novel modulator for endothelial adhesion molecules: adipocyte-derived plasma protein adiponectin. Circulation 1999;100: 2473-2476
63. Yamauchi T, Kamon J, Minokoshi Y, et al. Adiponectin stimulates glucose utilization and fatty-acid oxidation by activating AMP-activated protein kinase. Nat Med 2002;8:1288-1295
64. Heilbronn LK, Smith SR, Ravussin E. The insulin-sensitizing role of the fat derived hormone adiponectin. Curr Pharm Des 2003;9:1411-1418
65. Chen H, Montagnani M, Funahashi T, et al. Adiponectin stimulates production of nitric oxide in vascular endothelial cells. J Biol Chem 2003;278:45021-45026
66. Okamoto Y, Arita Y, Nishida M, et al. An adipocyte-derived plasma protein, adiponectin, adheres to injured vascular walls. Horm Metab Res 2000;32:47-50
67. Ukkola O, Santaniemi M. Adiponectin: a link between excess adiposity and associated comorbidities? J Mol Med 2002;80:696-702.
68. Kumada M, Kihara S, Ouchi N, et al. Adiponectin specifically increased tissue inhibitor of metalloproteinase-1 through interleukin-10 expression in human macrophages. Circulation 2004;109:2046-2049
69 Ouchi N, Kobayashi H, Kihara S, et al. Adiponectin stimulates angiogenesis by promoting cross-talk between AMP-activated protein kinase and Akt signaling in endothelial cells. J Biol Chem 2004;279:1304-1309
70. Lindsay R, Resnick H, Ruotolo G, et al. Adiponectin, relationship to proteinuria but not coronary heart disease: the Strong Heart Study. Diabetes 2003;52(suppl 1):A161
71. Ohashi K, Ouchi N, Kihara S, et al. Adiponectin I164T mutation is associated with the metabolic syndrome and coronary artery disease. J Am Coll Cardiol 2004; 43:1195-1200
72. Lindsay RS, Funahashi T, Hanson RL, et al. Adiponectin and development of type 2 diabetes mellitus in the Pima Indian population. Lancet 2002;360:57-58
73. Krakoff J, Funahashi T, Stehouwer CD, et al. Inflammatory markers, adiponectin, and risk of type 2 diabetes in the Pima Indian. Diabetes Care 2003;26:1745-1751
74. Sewter C, Blows F, Considine R, et al. Differential effects of adiposity on peroxisomal proliferator-activated receptor gamma1 and gamma2 messenger ribonucleic acid expression in human adipocytes. J Clin Endocrinol Metab 2002;87:4203-4207
75. Steppan CM, Brown EJ, Wright CM, et al. A family of tissue-specific resistin-like molecules. Proc Natl Acad Sci U S A 2001;98:502-506
76. Hotamisligil GS, Spiegelman BM. Through thick and thin: wasting, obesity and TNF-alpha. Cell 1993;73:625-627
77. Hotamisligil GS, Murray DL, Choy LN. Tumour necrosis factor alpha inhibits signaling from the insulin receptor. Proc Natl Acad Sci U S A 1994;91:4854-4858
78. Hube F, Hauner H. The role of TNF-alpha in human adipose tissue: prevention of weight gain at the expense of insulin resistance? Horm Metab Res 1999;31:626-631
79. Hotamisligil GS, Arner P, Caro JF. Increased adipose tissue expression of tumor necrosis factor alpha in human obesity and insulin resistance. J Clin Invest 1995;95:2409-2415
80. Gurevitch J, Frolkis I, Yuhas Y, et al. Tumor necrosis factor-alpha is released from the isolated heart undergoing ischemia and reperfusion. J Am Coll Cardiol 1996;28:247-252
81. Nilsson J, Jovinge S, Niemann A, et al. Relation between plasma tumor necrosis factor-alpha and insulin sensitivity in elderly men with non–insulin-dependent diabetes mellitus. Arterioscler Thromb Vasc Biol 1998;18:1199-1202
82. Xu H, Uysai T, Becherer JA, et al. Altered tumor necrosis factor-alpha (TNF-alpha) processing in adipocytes and increased expression of transmembrane TNF-alpha in obesity. Diabetes 2002;51:1876-1883
83. Bullo M, Garcia-Lorda P, Peinado-Onsurbe J, et al. TNF-alpha expression of subcutaneous adipose tissue in obese and morbid obese females: relationship to adipocyte LPL activity and leptin synthesis. Int J Obes 2002;26:652-658
84. Kern PA, Saghizad M, Ong JM. The expression of TNF factor in human adipose tissue: regulation by obesity, weight loss and relationship to lipoprotein lipase. J Clin Invest 1995;95:2111-2119
85. Aggarwal BB. Tumour necrosis factors receptor associated signaling molecules and their role in activation of apoptosis, JNK and NF-kappaB. Ann Rheum Dis 2000;59(suppl 1):i6-i16
86. Pischon T, Hankinson SE, Hotamisligil GS, et al. Habitual dietary intake of n-3 and n-6 fatty acids in relation to inflammatory markers among US men and women. Circulation 2003;108:155-160
87. Ko YG, Lee JS, Kang YS, et al. TNF-alpha–mediated apoptosis is initiated in caveolae-like domains. J Immunol 1999;162:7217-7223
88. Xu H, Hotamisligil GS. Signaling pathways utilized by tumor necrosis factor receptor 1 in adipocytes to suppress differentiation. FEBS Lett 2001;506:97-102
89. Veldman RJ, Maestre N, Aduib OM, et al. A neutral sphingomyelinase resides in sphingolipid-enriched microdomains and is inhibited by the caveolin-scaffolding domain: potential implications in tumour necrosis factor signaling. Biochem J 2001;355:859-868
90. Aljada A, Ghanim H, Assian E, Dandona P. Tumor necrosis factor-alpha inhibits insulin-induced increase in endothelial nitric oxide synthase and reduces insulin receptor content and phosphorylation in human aortic endothelial cells. Metabolism 2002;51:487-491
91. Hippenstiel S, Schmeck B, Seybold J, et al. Reduction of TNF-alpha related nuclear factor-kappaB (NF-kappaB) translocation but not inhibitor kappa-B (Ikappa-B)-degradation by Rho protein inhibition in human endothelial cells. Biochem Pharmacol 2002;64:971-977
92. Begum N, Sandu OA, Ito M, et al. Active Rho kinase (ROK-α) associates with insulin receptor substrate-1 and inhibits insulin signaling in vascular smooth muscle cells. J Biol Chem 2002;277:6214-6222
93. Hunter I, Cobban HJ, Vandenabeele P, et al. Tumor necrosis factor-alpha–induced activation of RhoA in airway smooth muscle cells: role in the Ca^{2+} sensitization of myosin light chain 20 phosphorylation. Mol Pharmacol 2003;63:714-721
94. Nosaka Y, Arai A, Kanda E, et al. Rac is activated by tumor necrosis factor alpha and is involved in activation of Erk. Biochem Biophys Res Commun 2001;285:675-679
95. Gnad R, Kaina B, Fritz G. Rho GTPases are involved in the regulation of NF-kappaB by genotoxic stress. Exp Cell Res 2001;264:244-249
96. Kim F, Gallis B, Corson MA. TNF-alpha inhibits flow and insulin signaling leading to NO production in aortic endothelial cells. Am J Physiol Cell Physiol 2001;280: C1057-C1065
97. Rask-Madsen C, Dominguez H, Ihlemann N, et al. Tumor necrosis factor-alpha inhibits insulin's stimulating effect on glucose uptake and endothelium-dependent vasodilation in humans. Circulation 2003; 108:1815-1821
98. Ryden M, Dicker A, van Harmelen V, et al. Mapping of early signaling events in tumor necrosis factor-alpha–mediated lipolysis in human fat cells. J Biol Chem 2002;2772:1085-1091

99. Zhang HH, Halbleib M, Faiyaz A, et al. Tumor necrosis factor-alpha stimulates lipolysis in differentiated human adipocytes through activation of extracellular signal–related kinase and elevation of intracellular cAMP. Diabetes 2002;51:2929-2935
100. Hotamisligil GS, Spiegelman BM. Tumor necrosis factor alpha: a key component in the obesity-diabetes link. Diabetes 1994;43:1271-1278
101. Emanuelli B, Peraldi P, Filloux C, et al. SOCS-3 inhibits insulin signaling and is up-regulated in response to tumor necrosis factor-alpha in the adipose tissue of obese mice. J Biol Chem 2001;276:47944-47949
102. Prasad A, Quyyumi AA. Renin-angiotensin system and angiotensin receptor blockers in the metabolic syndrome. Circulation 2004;110:1507-1512
103. Fujishiro M, Gotoh Y, Katagiri H, et al. MKK6/3 and p38 MAPK pathway activation is not necessary for insulin-induced glucose uptake but regulates glucose transporter expression. J Biol Chem 2001;276:19800-19806
104. Ruan H, Lodish HF. Insulin resistance in adipose tissue: direct and indirect effects of tumor necrosis factor-alpha. Cytokine Growth Factor Rev 2003;14:447-455
105. Bethin KE, Vogt SK, Muglia LJ. Interleukin-6 is an essential, corticotropin-releasing hormone–independent stimulator of the adrenal axis during immune system activation. Proc Natl Acad Sci U S A 2000;97:9317-9322
106. Giacchetti G, Faloia E, Mariniello B, et al. Overexpression of the renin-angiotensin system in human visceral adipose tissue in normal and overweight subjects. Am J Hypertens 2002;15:381-388
107. Papanikolaou DA, Wilder RL, Manolagas SC, et al. The pathophysiologic roles of interleukin-6 in humans. Ann Intern Med 1998;128:127-137
108. Janke J, Engeli S, Gorzelniak K, et al. Mature adipocytes inhibit in vitro differentiation of human preadipocytes via angiotensin type 1 receptors. Diabetes 2002;51:1699-1707
109. Engeli S, Schling P, Gorzelniak K, et al. The adipose-tissue renin-angiotensin-aldosterone system: role in the metabolic syndrome? Int J Biochem Cell Biol 2003;35:807-825

Insulin Resistance and the Metabolic Syndrome

7

Features of the metabolic syndrome have been described for many years. In the early 1920s, the Swedish clinical investigator Dr. Eskil Kylin described a disorder characterized by the constellation of hypertension, hyperglycemia, and hyperuricemia.[1] Clustering of cardiovascular risk factors, specifically, hypertension, diabetes mellitus (DM), dyslipidemia, and obesity, was further described in the 1960s and 1970s, albeit without elucidation of possible causes for the syndrome.[2,3] In 1988, Reaven termed this constellation of cardiovascular risk factors syndrome X and posited insulin resistance as its underlying cause.[4] The metabolic syndrome is also known as the

- cardiometabolic syndrome,
- dysmetabolic syndrome,
- deadly quartet,
- insulin resistance syndrome,
- metabolic syndrome X,
- syndrome X, and
- Reaven's syndrome.

DIAGNOSTIC CRITERIA FOR THE METABOLIC SYNDROME

The metabolic syndrome is a multifactorial disease with considerable heterogeneity. Many aspects of the metabolic syndrome are yet to be delimited, and the interrelationships of all the pathophysiologic derangements, particularly with insulin resistance, are not fully understood. Not surprisingly, diagnostic criteria for the metabolic syndrome are not clearly defined, and several standardized criteria are used for its diagnosis.

The metabolic syndrome has been defined by the World Health Organization (WHO),[5,6] by the

National Cholesterol Education Program (NCEP),[7] and by the American Association of Clinical Endocrinology.[8] Clinical diagnosis of the syndrome is based on the following criteria:

	DEFINING ENTITY		
RISK FACTOR	**World Health Organization**	**National Cholesterol Education Program**	**American Association of Clinical Endocrinology**
BMI	BMI >30 kg/m² *or*		
Waist/hip ratio			
Men	>0.90		
Women	>0.85		
Waist circumference			
Men		>40 in (102 cm)	>102 cm (40 in)
Women		>35 in (88 cm)	>88 cm (35 in)
Triglycerides	>150 mg/dL	≥150 mg/dL	≥150 mg/dL
HDL Men	<35 mg/dL	<40 mg/dL	<35 mg/dL
HDL Women	<40 mg/dL	<50 mg/dL	<45 mg/dL
Blood pressure	Current antihypertensive therapy *or* BP ≥140/90 mm Hg	Current antihypertensive therapy *or* BP ≥135/85 mm Hg	Hypertension
Glucose	Type 2 DM *or* Impaired glucose tolerance	Fasting glucose ≥110 mg/dL	Fasting glucose ≥110 mg/dL *or* Type 2 DM
Other	Microalbuminuria		Insulin resistance *or* Acanthosis nigricans
Requirement for diagnosis	Confirmed type 2 DM *or* Impaired glucose tolerance *and* Any other 2 of the above criteria	Any 3 of the above criteria	Consider also minor criteria such as polycystic ovary syndrome, hypercoagulability, endothelial dysfunction, microalbuminuria, and CHD

BMI, body mass index; CHD, coronary heart disease; DM, diabetes mellitus; HDL, high-density lipoprotein.

A panel of the American Heart Association, the National Heart, Lung, and Blood Institute, and the American Diabetes Association has replaced the fasting glucose criterion to a value greater than 100 mg/dL. The panel's recommendations also allow an alternative to impaired fasting glucose, specifically, impaired glucose tolerance 2 hours after a 75-g oral glucose tolerance test with glucose values ranging between 140 and 200 mg/dL.[9]

Although the definitions of metabolic syndrome vary slightly between the different organizations, **the stated criteria basically define the same group of individuals with abdominal obesity, impaired glucose homeostasis, dyslipidemia, and hypertension. The NCEP definition is easier to use in clinical practice** because testing of glucose tolerance, insulin resistance, and microalbuminuria is not required. Importantly, not all the clinical features of the syndrome or all their sequelae will develop in all individuals with the metabolic syndrome. Furthermore, the abnormalities or clinical sequelae can develop in any chronologic order.

Other biomarkers that may contribute to the clinical diagnosis of metabolic syndrome are

- insulin resistance with
  elevated fasting insulin and a high insulin-glucose ratio and
  impaired glucose tolerance or an abnormal 2-hour postprandial glucose;
- dyslipidemia with
  elevated triglycerides,
  small, dense low-density lipoprotein (LDL) particles, and
  decreased HDL;

- prothrombotic state with impaired fibrinolysis as a result of
  elevated serum plasminogen activator inhibitor-1 (PAI-1) and
  elevated fibrinogen;
- proinflammatory state and mitogenic effects with
  elevated high sensitivity (hs) C-reactive protein (CRP),
  elevated insulin-like growth factor type I, and
  elevated tissue angiotensin II levels;
- vascular dysfunction with
  microalbuminuria,
  hypertension, and
  heightened risk for atherosclerotic disease; and
- elevated serum uric acid.[10]

The metabolic syndrome may have as associated history or clinical findings

- a history of gestational diabetes,
- nonalcoholic fatty liver disease and steatohepatitis,
- a cardiomyopathic process,
- polycystic ovaries, and
- acanthosis nigricans.

PREVALENCE OF THE METABOLIC SYNDROME

The metabolic syndrome is being diagnosed with increasing frequency worldwide. In many individuals, it is associated with obesity and a sedentary lifestyle. Based on the NCEP Adult Treatment Panel (ATP) III guidelines, the prevalence of the metabolic syndrome in adults in the United States older than 20 years is estimated to be 23.7%, which corresponds to 22% of men and 24% of women. This figure implies that as many as 47 million adult U.S. residents may have the syndrome based on current census data.[7]

The prevalence of metabolic syndrome varies among ethnic groups. In the United States, its prevalence is highest in Hispanics. For Mexican Americans, the age-adjusted prevalence of the syndrome is 31.9%. Aboriginal people of North America and people who originate from the Indian subcontinent also have an increased susceptibility for the development of metabolic syndrome. The prevalence is lower in the non-Hispanic white population and African Americans and lowest in individuals of Chinese origin.[7]

The age-specific incidence of metabolic syndrome increases steeply with age. The prevalence in 50-year-olds is higher than 30% and rises to 40% in individuals 60 years and older. The incidence is higher for women than for men of African American, Mexican American, South Asian, and Native Indian extraction.[7,11,12]

INSULIN RESISTANCE

With any glucose challenge, three coordinated events preserve glucose homeostasis, specifically

1. insulin secretion by pancreatic beta cells,
2. suppression of hepatic glucose production by blocking glycogenolysis and gluconeogenesis, and
3. stimulation of glucose uptake by the liver, skeletal muscle, and adipose tissue.

With insulin resistance, the second and third steps are dysfunctional. In overt type 2 DM, all three steps are imbalanced.[13]

Insulin Resistance and Hyperinsulinemia. Insulin resistance is a key feature and a hallmark of the metabolic syndrome.[4] Impaired insulin action occurs when target tissues are unable to respond to normal circulating concentrations of insulin.

In a compensatory response, the beta cells of the pancreas secrete increased amounts of insulin. In the initial stages, insulin secretion and hyperinsulinemia remain adequate to maintain euglycemia.

The term *insulin resistance* is defined as impaired insulin-stimulated glucose disposal manifested by

- a steady-state plasma glucose level that is in excess of what should be seen with the prevailing plasma insulin level and
- a plasma insulin level that is in excess of the norm for fasting or for 2-hour post–glucose challenge plasma glucose levels.

Insulin Resistance and Type 2 Diabetes Mellitus. Insulin resistance is the primary feature and the most important predictor of type 2 DM and precedes overt hyperglycemia and type 2 DM by 10 to 20 years.

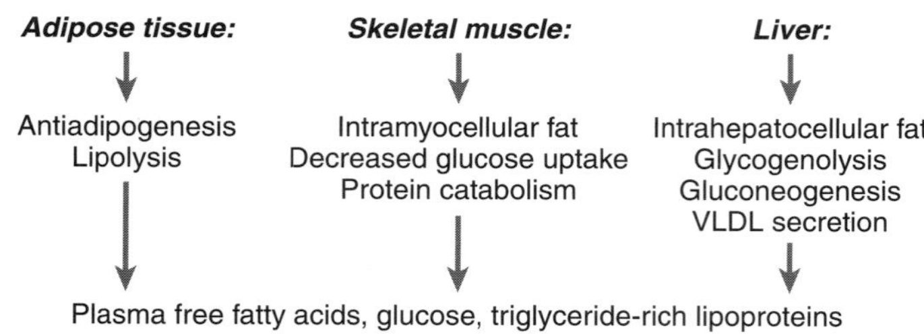

▸▸ **Figure 7–1.** Organ manifestations of systemic insulin resistance in adipose tissue, skeletal muscle, and the liver and their metabolic sequelae. VLDL, very-low-density lipoprotein.

In a significant number of individuals, functional defects in insulin secretion arise with the passage of time. Compensatory hyperinsulinemia fails, and type 2 DM supervenes.[14,15] Conversely, 60% to 85% of diabetic patients have documented insulin resistance.[16]

Multiorgan Manifestations of Insulin Resistance. Insulin resistance engenders impaired insulin action in a variety of insulin-sensitive tissues. The state of insulin resistance thus causes a constellation of multiple metabolic disturbances that ultimately produce the metabolic syndrome.

In a detailed study of the metabolic syndrome in 119 nondiabetic offspring of diabetic probands, insulin resistance was seen not only in skeletal muscle but also in adipose tissue and led to multiple defects in glucose and energy metabolism. Hypoadiponectinemia, as well as high levels of cytokines and adhesion molecules indicative of low-grade inflammation and endothelial dysfunction, were found to be essential findings in subjects with the metabolic syndrome.[17]

Manifestations of insulin resistance in some of the affected tissues are

- disturbances in blood vessel endothelial function, increased vascular inflammation, and changes in key regulators of thrombosis in the vascular endothelium and vascular smooth muscle cells;
- abnormalities in glucose and fatty acid metabolism, reduced disposal of glucose, and decreased oxidation of fatty acids in skeletal muscle and myocardium;
- decreased adipogenesis and increased lipolysis causing the release of free fatty acids (FFAs) in adipose tissue;
- decreased glucokinase activity and products of enhanced lipolysis stimulating hepatic gluconeogenesis in the liver. There is decreased hepatic extraction of insulin, abnormalities in lipid metabolism, and dyslipidemia with enhanced very-low-density lipoprotein (VLDL) synthesis and secretion (Fig. 7-1); and
- loss of the central weight control functions of insulin in the central nervous system.

Insulin resistance also affects the intestines.

Selective Insulin Resistance. The same insulin receptor controls diverse cellular response pathways such as

- metabolic signaling,
- the vascular cascade, and
- the mitogenic pathway.

Activation of the phosphatidylinositol 3-kinase (PI3K) pathway is associated with the glucose and lipid metabolic as well as with the nitric oxide synthase (NOS) regulatory effects of insulin. Mitogen-activated protein kinase (MAPK) activation is associated with mitogenic effects such as cell growth and proliferation.

Although insulin resistance affects many tissues, some insulin-mediated processes remain sensitive to insulin. Insulin resistance differentially affects the PI3K and the MAPK signaling pathways. **Specifically, in the setting of insulin resistance, insulin has reduced effects on the PI3K pathways, whereas insulin sensitivity to MAPK signaling is preserved.**[18]

The concept of "selective insulin resistance" entails

1. **insulin signaling in residual insulin-sensitive, mitogenic pathways and**
2. **defective insulin signaling in insulin-resistant, metabolic and vascular pathways.**[19]

In fact, MAPK signaling may actually be enhanced with insulin resistance. Insulin activation of PI3K negatively regulates Raf-1, the upstream activator for MAPK. With impaired PI3K activation as a result of insulin insensitivity, insulin-mediated MAPK activity may be enhanced, thus promoting MAPK-mediated mitogenic effects.[20] Compensatory hyperinsulinemia will further increase mitogenic stimulation.

Hyperinsulinemia-induced activation of MAPK can greatly stimulate vascular and nonvascular cell growth with vascular remodeling, increase vascular inflammation, and contribute to the pathogenesis of macrovascular complications.[21] Additionally, hyperinsulinemia stimulates the sympathetic nervous system, enhances renal sodium absorption, and contributes to hypertension.[22,23] Hyperinsulinemia also increases ovarian androgen production, the integral hormonal imbalance observed with polycystic ovary syndrome, which affects 1 in 10 U.S. women of childbearing age.[24]

The multiorgan impact of selective insulin resistance, in concert with mitogenic hyperactivity, engenders dyslipidemia, hypertension, hypercoagulation, impaired fibrinolysis, and vascular disease.[19] **Together, the multisystem metabolic and vascular sequelae of these derangements constitute the metabolic syndrome.**

Diagnosis of Insulin Resistance. **The criteria used in the clinical diagnosis of metabolic syndrome have low sensitivity for detecting the presence of insulin resistance.**

Metabolic Syndrome Criteria. Of the risk factors listed in the WHO or NCEP ATP III guidelines for the metabolic syndrome, hypertriglyceridemia and low HDL levels are most closely associated with insulin resistance.[25] Fasting and 2-hour post–glucose challenge plasma glucose, albeit necessary to diagnose DM, are of limited utility for the diagnosis of insulin resistance in nondiabetic individuals. Many individuals with insulin resistance have preserved glucose levels.[4] In fact, application of the NCEP ATP III criteria to subjects studied at the third National Health and Nutrition Examination Survey (NHANES III) showed that impaired fasting glucose criteria were met by only 10% of individuals with the metabolic syndrome, consistent with a significant underestimation of insulin resistance with the use of this approach, particularly in ethnic minorities.[26] Similarly, in a study of 119 nondiabetic offspring of diabetic probands, the NCEP ATP III criteria were found to be quite specific for insulin resistance, but with rather low sensitivity.[17]

Alternative Diagnoses of Insulin Resistance. Various approaches are used to refine the diagnosis of insulin resistance.

- **The hyperinsulinemic-euglycemic clamp technique is considered the gold standard** but is cumbersome. It requires a prolonged insulin infusion to maintain a constant plasma insulin level and repeated blood sampling. Glucose is then infused, and as the plasma level of glucose falls because of the action of insulin, more glucose is added to maintain a steady level. The amount of glucose infused over time provides a measure of insulin resistance.
- A glucose-insulin tolerance testing–based approach is inconvenient because it requires repeated blood sampling. **The 2-hour post–glucose challenge glucose and insulin levels are considered a clinically sensitive and simple available test.**
- **Surrogate measures of insulin sensitivity, including the Homeostasis Model Assessment (HOMA)** (insulin resistance = fasting plasma glucose [mmol/L] × fasting insulin [μU/mL]/22.5 or fasting plasma glucose [mg/dL] × fasting plasma insulin [μU/mL]/405) **and the Quantitative Insulin Sensitivity Check Index (QUICKI), have been developed and can be applied to single measurements of fasting insulin and glucose. These surrogates have been shown to correlate well with the direct, gold standard glucose clamp measure.**[27-30]

Clearly, measurement of the plasma insulin concentration is required for a more sensitive means of identifying insulin resistance, and the development of standardized insulin assays, or alternative biomarkers of insulin resistance, will facilitate the prediction of CHD risk in patients with the metabolic syndrome.

In general, fasting blood levels of insulin are usually less than 10 mU/L. Fasting insulinemia, greater than 15 mU/L, defines hyperinsulinemia and correlates highly with the euglycemic clamp study. The 2-hour post–glucose challenge insulin value may be of even greater utility. At present, analytic methods for insulin measurement are not yet standardized, and absolute values, in the absence of frequency distributions and norms, are difficult to correlate between different assays.[31]

THE METABOLIC SYNDROME—CARDIOVASCULAR RISK

Insulin resistance and the confluence of conventional and novel risk factors that encompass the metabolic syndrome have a synergistic, negative impact on cardiovascular prognosis (Table 7-1). The NCEP ATP III guidelines establish the importance of the metabolic syndrome as a major cardiovascular risk factor.[8] The metabolic syndrome is associated with some of the most common diseases afflicting modern societies, such as

- hypertension,
- CHD,
- type 2 DM,

and their end-organ sequelae, and as such it is a major public health concern.

Insulin resistance is the pathophysiology underlying the clustering of lipid and nonlipid, conventional and unconventional cardiovascular risk factors in the metabolic syndrome.[4] These same cardiovascular risk factors prevail not only in prediabetic and diabetic individuals but also in insulin-resistant individuals without clinical glucose intolerance.[32] **Indices of insulin resistance predict atherosclerosis, cardiovascular events, and mortality independent of other risk factors, including fasting glucose and lipid levels.**[33,34] However, it is unclear whether insulin resistance underlies all cardiovascular risk factors.[35]

As estimated by Framingham algorithms, most individuals with the metabolic syndrome are at intermediate risk (10% to 20%) for CHD. However, 20% of men are at high risk (>20%) over a follow-up of 10 years.[36,37]

Table 7-1. Cardiovascular Risk Factors Associated with the Metabolic Syndrome

Hypertension
Reduced vascular compliance
Absent nocturnal dipping of blood pressure
Increased high-sensitivity C-reactive protein levels and inflammatory markers
Endothelial dysfunction
Insulin resistance
Low high-density lipoprotein cholesterol levels
High triglyceride levels
Small, dense, oxidized low-density lipoprotein cholesterol
Increased apolipoprotein B particles
Increased fibrinogen levels
Increased plasminogen activator inhibitor-1 levels
Hyperuricemia

Modified from McFarlane SI, Kumar A, Sowers JR. Mechanisms by which angiotensin-converting enzyme inhibitors prevent diabetes and cardiovascular disease. Am J Cardiol 2003;91:30H-37H.

Vascular Disease. The metabolic syndrome increases the incidence of atherosclerotic cardiovascular disease.

In 471 participants in the Baltimore Longitudinal Study on Aging, the presence of metabolic syndrome was associated with increased arterial stiffness and carotid intimal-medial thickness, independent of cardiovascular risk covariates, including each of the components of the metabolic syndrome.[38] There is a higher incidence of coronary artery calcification in individuals with the metabolic syndrome.[39] In 840 asymptomatic, nondiabetic individuals with a family history of premature CHD, the metabolic syndrome, as defined by NCEP criteria, was associated with the presence of coronary artery calcification (odds ratio, 1.93; $P < .001$), even after controlling for multiple established CHD risk factors and plasma levels of CRP. HOMA measures of insulin resistance, but not plasma CRP levels, provided independent and additive value to the NCEP definition of metabolic syndrome in predicting coronary calcification scores.[40] For patients with normal glucose tolerance, indices of insulin resistance such as post–glucose load insulin, fasting insulin, and HOMA are independently correlated with the number of diseased coronary arteries as determined by coronary angiography.[41] In nondiabetic patients, insulin resistance evaluated by HOMA predicts restenosis after coronary stent placement.[42]

Cardiovascular Events. The metabolic syndrome increases the incidence of acute ischemic events.

In the Women's Ischemia Syndrome Evaluation study, for women with angiographically significant CHD, the presence of metabolic syndrome resulted in a significantly higher risk for cardiovascular events than did normal metabolic status (hazard ratio, 4.93; $P = .05$). Every 1-mg/L increase in the blood level of the acute phase reactant serum amyloid A corresponded to a greater than 3% increase in the 3-year risk for cardiovascular events.[43] A total of 10,357 NHANES III subjects were evaluated for a history of myocardial infarction (MI), stroke, and either MI or stroke (MI/stroke). After applying NCEP ATP III criteria, in multivariate analysis the metabolic syndrome was significantly related to MI (odds ratio, 2.01), stroke (odds ratio, 2.16), and MI/stroke (odds ratio, 2.05) in both women and men.[44] In the Atherosclerosis Risk in Communities study of a community-based cohort of 14,502 middle-aged African American and white men and women from 1987 to 1989, the prevalence of ATP III–defined metabolic syndrome was 30%. Subjects with the metabolic syndrome, relative too those without the metabolic syndrome, were twice as likely to have a history of MI or revascularization (7.4% versus 3.6%, $P < .0001$). Metabolic syndrome subjects free of known CHD or stroke, versus those without the syndrome, had significantly greater carotid intimal-medial wall thickness (747 versus 704 μm, $P < .0001$).[45]

Mortality. Insulin resistance increases total mortality.

The presence of metabolic syndrome is associated with not only an odds ratio of 3 for CHD and stroke but also a fivefold greater risk for cardiovascular mortality. The occurrence of microalbuminuria further increases the risk for mortality.[46] In the Malmö Preventive Project, fasting hyperinsulinemia and insulin resistance with the associated cluster of risk factors were predictors of total mortality and CHD in nondiabetic men. Two-hour post–glucose challenge hyperinsulinemia appeared to be a strong and independent predictor of mortality over long-term follow-up.[47] The prospective Kuopio Ischemic Heart Disease Risk Factor Study of 2700 Finnish men 42 years and older over a median follow-up of 11.6 years (9.1 to 13.7 years) actually found CHD mortality to be 2.4 to 3.4 times higher in men with the metabolic syndrome than in controls, with reduced Kaplan-Meier estimates of overall survival at 79% versus 90%.[48] The prospective Diabetes Epidemiology: Collaborative Analysis of Diagnostic Criteria in Europe study monitored 6156 adult men and 5356 women without DM for 8.8 years. Individuals with hyperinsulinemia and two modified WHO criteria for the metabolic syndrome had an increased risk for all-cause death and death from cardiovascular disease with hazard ratios of 1.44 and 2.26, respectively, for men and 1.38 and 2.78, respectively, for women.[49] In a prospective cohort study of 6255 subjects 30 to 75 years of age (54% female) from NHANES II monitored for 13.3 ± 3.8 years, the presence of metabolic syndrome as defined by modified NCEP criteria, when compared with a cohort free of metabolic syndrome and established cardiovascular disease and adjusted for age, gender, and risk factors, was associated with a hazard ratio for CHD mortality of 2.02. The metabolic syndrome cluster more strongly predicted CHD, cardiovascular, and total mortality than its individual components did.[50]

GENETIC AND ENVIRONMENTAL FACTORS UNDERLYING THE METABOLIC SYNDROME

A multiplicity of genetic and environmental factors underlie insulin resistance (Fig. 7-2).

Genetics. Insulin resistance develops in individuals with a genetic predisposition, as determined by family history or population group.[51] However, the genetic underpinning for insulin resistance is not absolute. Environmental factors clearly play a role.

Family studies suggest a complex, but significant genetic basis for the individual constituents of the metabolic syndrome. A "thrifty genotype

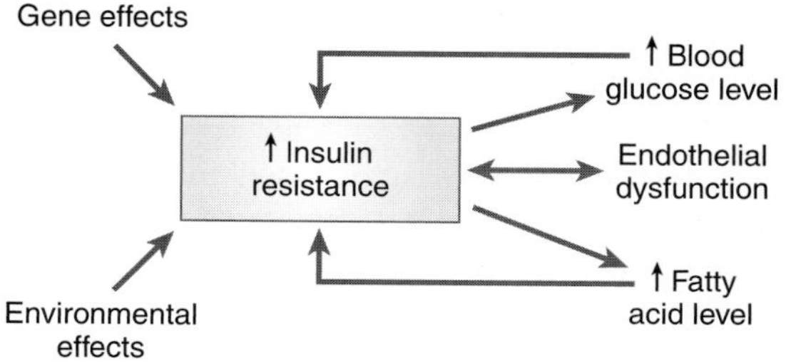

Figure 7–2.
Genetic, environmental, and metabolic effects on insulin resistance. *(Modified from McIntyre EA, Walker M. Genetics of type 2 diabetes and insulin resistance: knowledge from human studies. Clin Endocrinol 2002;57:303-311.)*

hypothesis" implicates the evolutionary selection of metabolic genes that allow individuals in hunter-gatherer societies, accustomed to long periods of deprivation punctuated by brief periods of abundance, to efficiently deposit and conserve energy stores. The expression of such genes, in the current setting of physical inactivity and dietary excess, may devolve into the metabolic syndrome.[26]

Stress and Inflammation. Sensitivity to insulin signaling is decreased by a multiplicity of conditions that are stressful to normal physiology, such as

- psychological and mental stress,
- infection,
- injury,
- sepsis,
- inflammatory diseases,
- starvation,
- pregnancy,

and other conditions of glucocorticoid excess, sympathetic hyperactivity, and neurohormonal activation that divert energy substrate to immune tissues. The insulin-resistant state is well recognized in hypertension and heart failure and after MI.[52]

The metabolic syndrome is also associated with the presence of elevated iron stores. High iron stores may contribute to insulin resistance via inflammatory pathways deriving from oxidative free radical damage.

Low Birth Weight. Children born prematurely have a reduction in insulin sensitivity when compared with controls.[53]

Low birth weight is associated with hyperactivity of the hypothalamic-pituitary-adrenal (HPA) axis and the metabolic syndrome. Adult plasma cortisol levels, albeit in the normal range, decrease with increasing birth weight and correlate with adult systolic blood pressure, glucose levels, triglyceride, waist-hip ratios, and insulin resistance.[54]

Physical Inactivity. Physical inactivity plays a central role in the development of insulin resistance.

Insulin insensitivity develops with inactivity, as may occur even after several days of bed rest. The reduced insulin sensitivity of aging is also in part due to physical inactivity.[55] With inactivity, type II fast-twitch, glycolytic, insulin-insensitive muscle fibers are increasingly expressed with a diminution in skeletal muscle blood flow and impaired insulin-mediated capillary recruitment.[56]

Federal statistics show that 7 of 10 adults get too little exercise and 4 of 10 get none. Insulin sensitivity correlates with cardiovascular fitness and is inversely associated with the degree of obesity.[57,58]

Obesity. Insulin resistance is strongly linked to obesity.[59]

In particular, increased ponderosity in the visceral compartment is negatively correlated with insulin sensitivity.[60] Visceral fat is metabolically very active. It is a major factor in the enhanced elaboration of inflammatory cytokines such as tumor necrosis factor-alpha (TNF-α) and PAI-1 and in the reduced production of adiponectin. It is instrumental in mediating the systemic release of FFAs.

Insulin Resistance as a (Mal)Adaptive Mechanism to Obesity. The hypothesis has been advanced that adipocyte insulin resistance arises as a compensatory measure in response to excessive obesity.

In adipose tissue, insulin resistance limits further adipogenesis and adipocyte differentiation, instead leading to lipolysis. There is an inverse relationship between the severity of adiposity and the degree of insulin resistance. Furthermore, insulin-sensitizing pharmacologic agents, irrespective of their mechanism of action, do enhance weight gain. Obesity is the only known condition in which TNF-α is expressed at elevated levels in adipocytes, and TNF-α may be a major mediator of local adipose tissue insulin resistance.[61,62]

Local and Systemic Insulin Resistance. Insulin resistance may, in certain instances, be initiated in adipocytes as a local process.[61] **With increasing local expression, it may, secondarily, encompass other target tissues, such as skeletal muscle, the liver, and the brain, via the systemic effects of adipose tissue adipokines and FFAs.**

Medications. Medications may contribute to insulin resistance.

Protease inhibitors for the treatment of human immunodeficiency viral infection directly affect insulin sensitivity. Other medications such as antidepressants, antihistamines, antipsychotics, antihypertensive α- or β-adrenergic blockers, and certain protein pump inhibitors are conducive to adipose tissue weight gain and indirectly increase the risk for insulin resistance. Glucocorticoids induce resistance to insulin via both direct and indirect mechanisms.[63]

Aging. Insulin resistance is associated with aging, particularly in sedentary individuals, and is in part due to physical inactivity.[55]

As lean body mass is lost and replaced by adipose tissue, there is less muscle tissue available for glucose disposal. This process, together with the secondary metabolic changes, leads to insulin resistance.

MOLECULAR MECHANISMS UNDERLYING INSULIN RESISTANCE

A single common denominator for insulin resistance has been difficult to discern. Given the array of genetic variations, combined with external factors, that play a role in causing insulin resistance, it seems unlikely that there would be only one primary defect in signaling. In fact, **multiple biochemical mechanisms have been found to account for the impaired tissue response to insulin.** In some individuals, the insulin receptor is abnormal; in others, certain aspects of insulin signaling become dysfunctional,[64] such as the following:

1. The autophosphorylation capacity of the insulin receptor is diminished.[65]
2. The normal insulin receptor–mediated tyrosine phosphorylation of insulin receptor substrate (IRS) proteins is prevented by the phosphorylation of IRS serine or threonine residues.
3. Tyrosine phosphatases dephosphorylate the insulin receptor and its substrates and terminate the signal generated via tyrosine kinases.[66] Increased expression of several protein tyrosine phosphatases may be seen in obesity.[67]
4. Reduced expression of IRS-1 is observed in the myocytes and adipocytes of obese, insulin-resistant persons.[68]
5. PI3K activity is impaired.
6. Worsening insulin resistance in primates progressively compromises insulin-stimulated activation of the serine-threonine kinase Akt/protein kinase B (PKB) and the atypical protein kinase C (PKC) molecular switches needed for inducing glucose transport responses.[69,70]
7. In the liver, activated Akt kinase inhibits hepatic glucose output when glucose is available. With insulin resistance, overexpression of TRB3, a mammalian homologue of *Drosophila* tribbles, causes TRB3 to bind to inactive and unphosphorylated Akt, thereby preventing its activation and blocking action.[71]

It is not clear whether these or other defects are primary lesions of insulin resistance or arise secondarily in response to other biochemical disturbances.

PRIMARY MEDIATORS OF INSULIN RESISTANCE

A multiplicity of pathways engender insulin resistance (Fig. 7-3). **Resistance to anabolic insulin signaling is elicited as the metabolic response to basically any adversity that challenges an organism's physiologic and psychological soundness, be it via oxidative stress, inflammation, proinflammatory cytokines/neurohormones, or pathways elicited in response to stressors.** The mechanisms leading to impaired metabolic insulin signaling are manifold, multitiered, and redundant, with positive feedback loops, thus effectively securing the establishment of insulin resistance.

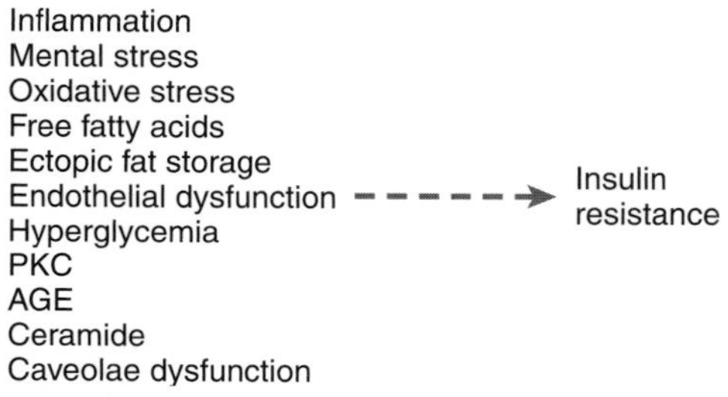

Inflammation
Mental stress
Oxidative stress
Free fatty acids
Ectopic fat storage
Endothelial dysfunction ------→ Insulin resistance
Hyperglycemia
PKC
AGE
Ceramide
Caveolae dysfunction

Figure 7–3.
A multiplicity of causes of insulin resistance. AGE, advanced glycosylation end product; PKC, protein kinase C.

Oxidative Stress. Reactive oxygen species play a role in the generation of insulin resistance, in its deterioration, and in DM-related sequelae. Reactive oxygen and nitrogen species directly oxidize and damage DNA, proteins, and lipids.

Oxidant stress interferes with insulin signaling at various levels. For example, IRS-1 tyrosine residues may be nitrated by nitric oxide (NO)-derived reactive nitrogen species and rendered inaccessible for phosphorylation. In addition to their ability to directly inflict damage on macromolecules, reactive oxygen and nitrogen species indirectly induce damage to the microvasculature by activating cellular stress-sensitive pathways. Oxidant stress may stimulate aldose reductase and diacylglycerol and activate common stress-activated signaling pathways such as

- nuclear factor kappaB (NFκB),
- p38 MAPK,
- c-Jun NH_2-terminal kinase (JNK)/stress-activated protein kinases (SAPKs),
- PKC,
- sorbitol/hexosamine, and
- advanced glycosylation end product (AGE) interaction with AGE receptors (RAGEs),

all of which underlie the development of both insulin resistance and impaired insulin secretion.[72]

p38 MAPK, which is situated downstream of MAPK kinase 6 (MAPKK6) and MAPKK3, is activated by mitogenic stimuli or by oxidative stress. Activation of p38 MAPK interferes at a point downstream of Akt/PKB and leads to a marked down-regulation of insulin-induced glucose uptake via the glucose transporter GLUT4.[73] MAPKK appears to interfere with insulin signaling by inducing serine phosphorylation of IRS-1. JNK, also stimulated by oxidant stress, appears to impair insulin signaling via Ser307 phosphorylation of IRS-1.[64,74,75]

Inflammation. Inflammation, dyslipidemia, and insulin resistance are intimately interrelated. In general, **acute inflammation and chronic inflammation are triggers for insulin resistance, and insulin resistance begets further inflammation.**

Serine Phosphorylation of Insulin Receptor Substrate. Inflammatory signal transduction pathways mediating insulin resistance converge at the level of IRS-1.

These pathways increase IRS-1 serine phosphorylation, in particular, the phosphorylation of Ser307 on IRS-1. The Ser307 residue is located near the phosphotyrosine binding domain in IRS-1. Its phosphorylation disrupts the interaction between the catalytic domain of the insulin receptor and the phosphotyrosine binding domain of IRS-1.[74]

Serine-phosphorylated IRS-1 and IRS-2, in fact, function as inhibitors of tyrosine kinase activity of the insulin receptor. They consequently inhibit tyrosine phosphorylation of both the insulin receptor and IRS, thereby inhibiting IRS-1 activation and suppressing downstream insulin effectors. Inflammatory pathways thus counter-regulate the insulin response (Table 7-2).[74,76]

Rho/Rho Kinase. From a molecular perspective, the Rho family of small guanosine 5′-triphosphatases (GTPases) may be playing a central role in implementing inflammation-mediated insulin resistance. RhoA is activated by

- growth factors;
- inflammatory cytokines;
- vasoconstrictors such as angiotensin II, endothelin-1, and α_1-adrenergic agonists; and
- cardiovascular risk factors such as hypertension and DM.

Activation of RhoA inhibits insulin action via stimulation of a Rho-dependent, serine/threonine protein kinase. Activated Rho-dependent kinase associates with IRS-1 and induces the IRS-1 serine phosphorylation seen with inflammatory pathways, thus blocking insulin-mediated IRS-1 tyrosine phosphorylation. As a consequence, the association of the regulatory subunit p85 of PI3K with IRS-1 is thwarted, as is insulin stimulation of PI3K enzymatic activity and glucose uptake. **Activated RhoA also up-regulates MAPKs by enhancing the activity of Ras.**[77]

Long-term up-regulation of RhoA/Rho kinase activity, as may occur in the metabolic syndrome,

Table 7-2. Inflammatory Pathways and Serine Phosphorylation of Insulin Receptor Substrate

Inflammatory stimulus
↓
Increased serine/threonine kinase cascade
↓
Increased IRS-1/IRS-2 serine/threonine phosphorylation with decreased IRS-1/IRS-2 tyrosine phosphorylation
↓
Decreased phosphatidylinositol 3-kinase activation
↓
Decreased GLUT4 translocation and glucose transport

GLUT4, glucose transporter 4; IRS, insulin receptor substrate.

causes an increased Rho kinase/IRS-1 association. This would be expected to inhibit insulin signaling via the PI3K pathway and chronically interfere with insulin metabolic and vascular NO/cyclic guanosine 3′,5′-monophosphate (cGMP) signaling.[77]

Furthermore, activated RhoA diminishes insulin's protective effects. With intact insulin signaling, insulin normally inactivates Rho/Rho kinase, thereby preventing the Rho kinase/IRS-1 association, in order to preserve the downstream metabolic and vascular pathways. With chronically up-regulated RhoA activity, the metabolic syndrome impairs this negative regulatory feedback mechanism.[77]

Tumor Necrosis Factor-α and Inflammatory Cytokines. TNF-α is a proinflammatory cytokine that is primarily produced by macrophages and is involved in host defense by stimulating inflammatory responses. TNF-α is also released by adipocytes.

TNF-α interferes with insulin signaling in fat, muscle, and the liver. It has been implicated in mediating both endothelial dysfunction and insulin resistance. Indirect and direct mechanisms are implicated.

Indirect Mediation of Insulin Resistance by TNF-α. TNF-α disruption of normal endothelial and adipose function impairs insulin sensitivity.

Vasoconstrictors and Endothelial Dysfunction. TNF-α impairs the perfusion of insulin target tissues.

It is implicated in the development of endothelial dysfunction. In endothelial cells, TNF-α decreases the number and function of insulin receptors.[78] It stimulates vascular smooth muscle endothelin-1 and angiotensin II production.[79,80]

The constrictive or mitogenic vascular remodeling effects (or both) attenuate the microcirculatory vasodilatory responses and nutritive flow to skeletal muscle, thereby engendering episodic, relative hypoperfusion. **Impaired glucose and insulin delivery inhibits insulin action in skeletal muscle and results in diminished glucose transport, uptake, and utilization, with insulin resistance as its metabolic consequence.**

Antiadipogenesis and Lipolysis. TNF-α is instrumental in increasing FFA release from adipose tissue.

TNF-α negatively modulates peroxisome proliferator–activated receptor-gamma (PPAR-γ) expression and exerts autocrine/paracrine effects on adipose tissue itself. It inhibits the differentiation of adipocytes and stimulates their apoptosis (Fig. 7-4). An elevation in TNF-α decreases lipoprotein lipase (LPL) activity in white adipocytes. It suppresses adipocyte gene expression of key enzymes involved in fatty acid uptake and lipogenesis. In fact, TNF-α increases hepatic and

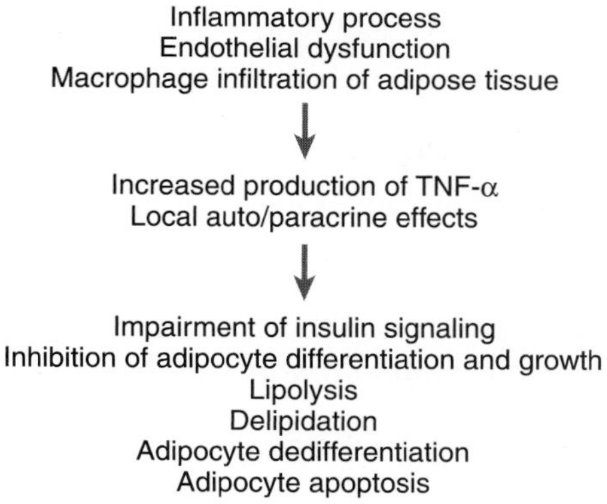

Inflammatory process
Endothelial dysfunction
Macrophage infiltration of adipose tissue

↓

Increased production of TNF-α
Local auto/paracrine effects

↓

Impairment of insulin signaling
Inhibition of adipocyte differentiation and growth
Lipolysis
Delipidation
Adipocyte dedifferentiation
Adipocyte apoptosis

Figure 7–4.
Tumor necrosis factor-α (TNF-α) production and actions in adipose tissue. *(Adapted from Hube F, Hauner H. The role of TNF-alpha in human adipose tissue: prevention of weight gain at the expense of insulin resistance? Horm Metab Res 1999;31:626-631.)*

adipocyte lipolysis. **Antiadipogenesis and TNF-α–stimulated lipolysis increase plasma FFAs.** FFAs impair endothelial function and are implicated in mediating insulin resistance systemically.[81]

Direct Mediation of Insulin Resistance by TNF-α. TNF-α directly interferes with insulin signaling. It decreases insulin receptor and IRS-1 protein expression. TNF-α may induce serine phosphorylation of IRS-1 and IRS-2, consequently inhibiting tyrosine phosphorylation of both the insulin receptor and IRS. TNF-α inhibits Akt/PKB phosphorylation and causes lower expression of the GLUT4 transporter.[74]

Gangliosides. Gangliosides may play a role in TNF-α–mediated insulin desensitization.

Gangliosides are glycosphingolipids present in receptor-rich membrane microdomains and caveolae. TNF-α increases the expression of ganglioside GM_3 and GM_2. GM_3 causes insulin resistance in adipocytes via IRS-1 serine phosphorylation. GM_2 excess in microdomains appears to suppress insulin action by excluding the ligand-bound insulin receptor from the microdomain.[74]

Ceramide. TNF-α–induced ceramide may suppress insulin signaling.

Ceramide is a sphingolipid. As TNF-α binds to its p55 TNF receptor type 1, it activates sphingomyelinase to promote release of the sphingolipid metabolite ceramide. Ceramide increases IRS-1 serine phosphorylation and interferes with the catalytic activity of downstream targets such as Akt/PKB by inhibiting Akt translocation to the plasma membrane.[74] Ceramide is increased in the muscle of diabetic mice, and exogenous ceramide inhibits insulin-stimulated Akt/PKB phosphorylation and GLUT4 translocation in adipocytes.[82]

Insulin Resistance Pathways Shared by TNF-α and Other Proinflammatory Mediators

RhoA/Rho Kinase. TNF-α interaction with the TNF receptor type 1 subtype activates RhoA and Rho kinase. RhoA activation of Rho kinase effects the serine phosphorylation of IRS-1. This is a common pathway for inflammatory cytokines and vasoconstrictors to mediate insulin resistance.[77,83]

IkappaB Kinase. TNF-α and other NFκB-activating cytokines may interfere with insulin signaling by inducing NFκB and stress hormone production via IkappaB (IκB) kinase (IKK). IKK appears to be a point of convergence for most NFκB-activating cytokines and another potential link between TNF-α, proinflammatory cytokines, and obesity-linked insulin resistance.[74,84]

IκBs are a superfamily of inhibitory proteins that inhibit NFκB activation. Stimulated by TNF-α and other factors, IKK phosphorylates IκB. Phosphorylated IκB disinhibits NFκB, thereby allowing it to translocate to the nucleus to activate a large number of genes in response to inflammation.[74,84]

Suppressors of Cytokine Signaling. Suppressors of cytokine signaling (SOCS) may participate in cytokine-mediated insulin resistance.

TNF-α, interleukin-1 (IL-1), IL-6, and interferon-γ cause sustained induction of SOCS-3, which should provide negative feedback for cytokine pathways and thus mitigate insulin resistance. However, SOCS-3, as well as SOCS-1 and SOCS-6, decrease insulin-induced IRS-1 tyrosine phosphorylation and its association with the p85 regulatory subunit of PI3K. SOCS-3 also impairs insulin activation of Akt/PKB and extracellular signal–regulated kinases (ERK1/ERK2). Its effects are most marked in adipose tissue.[74]

Stress Pathways. TNF-α and other inflammatory cytokines are implicated in causing insulin resistance by stimulating stress pathways, the MAPK cascades. TNF-α activates

- ERK1/ERK2 (p42/p44 MAPK),
- p38 MAPK, and
- JNK.

Inducible Nitric Oxide Synthase. TNF-α and inflammatory cytokines may interfere with insulin sensitivity by stimulating the expression and activity of inducible nitric oxide synthase (iNOS).

iNOS is the calcium-independent, high-output NO pathway. It is expressed not only in macrophages but also in skeletal muscle, myocardium, adipose tissue, and the liver.

Induction of iNOS causes marked impairment of insulin signaling, specifically in skeletal muscle, and it appears to play a major role in rodent models of insulin resistance. Although the specific mechanisms are unclear, oxidative protein modifications via reactive nitrogen species may be involved.[74]

In pancreatic beta cells, TNF-α induces iNOS, which is in part responsible for TNF-α's inhibitory effect on insulin secretion.[78]

Adiponectin. Suppression of insulin-sensitizing adiponectin by the autocrine/paracrine effects of TNF-α and IL-6 in adipose tissue may be a critical contributory factor for the generation of insulin resistance.[84]

Obesity, TNF-α Expression, and Insulin Resistance. TNF-α is considered to be a mediator primarily of obesity-linked insulin resistance.

TNF-α is overexpressed in the adipose tissue of obese, insulin-resistant persons and is released by adipose tissue. In obese humans, elevated expression of TNF-α in adipose and muscle tissue is correlated with fasting hyperinsulinemia.[85,86] There is a positive correlation between the TNF-α concentration and insulin resistance over a wide range of adiposity.[87] TNF-α is responsible for a variety of catabolic effects in adipose tissue that mediate local insulin resistance.[88]

There are more animal than human data, however, to support the role of TNF-α in insulin resistance. Furthermore, it is not clear whether adipose tissue overexpression of TNF-α induces insulin resistance in nonadipose, distant organs. Neutralization of TNF-α improves insulin sensitivity in rats, but not in humans.[88] Intravenously administered TNF-neutralizing antibody to patients with type 2 DM fails to improve measures of insulin sensitivity.[89] Coculture of human myocytes and human adipocytes blocks insulin-induced tyrosine phosphorylation of IRS-1 in myocytes with changes in IRS-1 and markedly reduces insulin-regulated activation of Akt kinase, akin to the effect of TNF-α. However, in that setting, TNF-α is undetectable in the culture medium. Despite a wealth of supportive data in animal models, such observations raise questions about the role of TNF-α as a mediator of insulin resistance in humans and as a mediator of systemic insulin resistance in nonadipose tissue.[90]

It is conceivable, however, that **autocrine/paracrine mechanisms for TNF-α action may be operative in humans.**[88] The high levels of TNF-α expression in adipose tissue are present primarily in the uncleaved, transmembrane form, mTNF-α, with disproportionately low circulating levels. Circulating levels of TNF-α in obese people or patients with type 2 DM are elevated, but rarely more than approximately threefold when compared with lean, healthy control subjects.[91] Transmembrane mTNF-α is biologically active, thus suggesting primarily autocrine/paracrine effects with insulin resistance expressed at the local adipose tissue level.[92]

Insulin resistance, however, does not remain confined to adipose tissue. In fact, adipose tissue interstitial levels of TNF-α and circulating FFA levels are positively correlated.[92] **Circulating FFAs or cytokines induced by TNF-α, such as IL-6 or interferon-α and interferon-γ, may be the secondary, hormonal factors antagonizing the systemic action of insulin.** Additionally or alternatively, it is likely that **several proinflammatory agents, such as TNF-α or IL-6, may mediate their systemic effects on insulin metabolism indirectly via autocrine/paracrine induction of systemic hypoadiponectinemia** (Fig. 7-5).[93]

The Renin-Angiotensin-Aldosterone System. The beneficial effects of angiotensin-converting enzyme (ACE) inhibition and angiotensin receptor blockade on the development of type 2 DM in large clinical trials suggest a pathophysiologic role of the adipose tissue renin-angiotensin system in metabolic syndrome.[94,95]

The renin-angiotensin-aldosterone system (RAAS) is stimulated by sympathetic activation and by inflammatory cytokines such as TNF-α. Additionally, insulin, via the mitogenic pathway, activates the RAAS by increasing the expression of angiotensinogen, angiotensin II, and the angiotensin II type 1 (AT_1) receptor. The hepatic production of angiotensinogen remains insulin sensitive in the face of insulin resistance. As a result, **there is accelerated activation of the RAAS and increased responsiveness to angiotensin II with hyperinsulinemia.**[96,97]

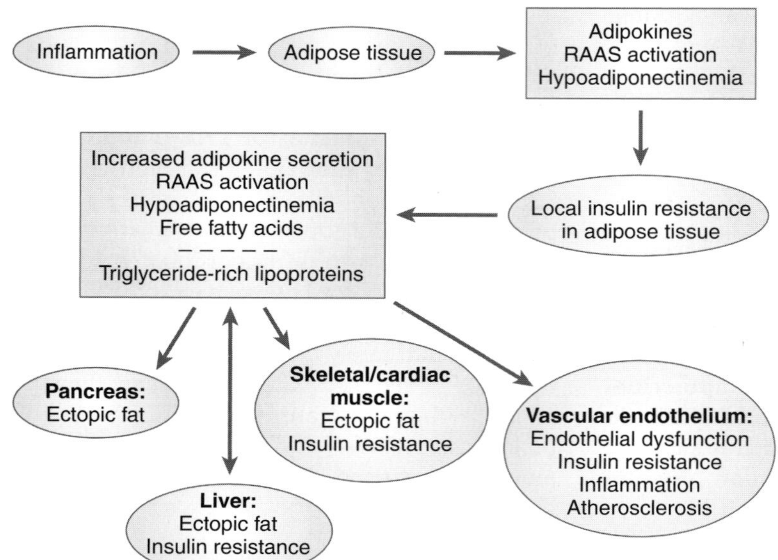

▸▸ **Figure 7–5.** Pathophysiologic effect of adipokines released from adipose tissue: progression from local adipose to systemic insulin resistance. RAAS, renin-angiotensin-aldosterone system.

Angiotensin II. Angiotensin II is associated with insulin resistance and the metabolic syndrome both at the local tissue level and systemically. Angiotensin II has an adverse impact on the metabolism of the vasculature, adipose tissue, skeletal muscle, and the liver. It disrupts glucose homeostasis by inducing hepatic gluconeogenesis.[98] Angiotensin II is a pluripotential hormone that stimulates multiple signaling pathways, including the

- Src family kinases,
- MAPKs, and
- Akt/PKB.[99]

Insulin Signaling. Angiotensin II inhibits insulin signaling at multiple levels.

Angiotensin II increases serine phosphorylation of the insulin receptor and IRS-1, thus inhibiting tyrosine phosphorylation of the insulin receptor and IRS-1, as well as PI3K activation.[100]

Via the AT_1 receptor, angiotensin II activates RhoA/Rho kinase, which serine-phosphorylates IRS-1. In human umbilical vein endothelial cells, angiotensin II, acting via the AT_1 receptor, increases IRS-1 phosphorylation at Ser312 and Ser616 via JNK and ERK1/ERK2 activation, respectively. These changes are associated with a concomitant reduction in IRS-1 phosphorylation at Tyr612 and Tyr632, which is essential for engaging the p85 regulatory subunit of PI3K. As a result, activation of IRS-1–associated PI3K is impaired.[101]

Acting via this pathway, angiotensin II exerts an inhibitory effect on the vascular insulin signaling pathway that thwarts the sequential activation of Akt/endothelial nitric oxide synthase (eNOS) and the production of NO.[101] Endogenous angiotensin II suppresses insulin signaling in spontaneously hypertensive rats, in part by activating ERK.[102]

Oxidative Stress. Angiotensin II contributes to insulin resistance by increasing oxidative stress.

It is one of the most potent endogenous stimuli for the generation of superoxide by activation of the nicotinamide adenine dinucleotide phosphate (NADH/NADPH) oxidase enzyme. Angiotensin II–induced oxidative stress may impair insulin signaling downstream from PI3K activation.[103]

Peroxisome Proliferator–Activated Receptors. Angiotensin II down-regulates the expression of PPAR-α and PPAR-γ.

In mice, angiotensin II decreases elaboration of the respective mRNAs and protein precursors. Down-regulation of PPAR-α and PPAR-γ decreases the anti-inflammatory impact of the PPARs and thereby leads to increased transcription of NFκB. NFκB in turn induces proinflammatory genes and increases the transcription of proinflammatory cytokines with adverse effects on insulin signaling.

Down-regulation of PPAR-γ decreases the production of adiponectin.

Antiadipogenesis. **Angiotensin II inhibits preadipocyte differentiation.**

The increased production of angiotensin II by adipocytes has an antiadipogenic impact in human adipose tissue. This increases fatty acid fluxes and causes the redistribution of storage triacylglycerols to ectopic storage in the liver, pancreas, and skeletal muscle, with adverse metabolic sequelae.[104]

Vasoconstriction. **Angiotensin II compromises nutritive skeletal muscle perfusion.** Because of its vasoconstrictive and vascular remodeling effects, angiotensin II impairs microcirculatory skeletal muscle blood flow.

Aldosterone. Another product of the locally expressed RAAS is the mineralocorticoid hormone aldosterone. Physiologically excessive levels of aldosterone in the rat can induce severe inflammatory lesions.[105,106]

Alterations in aldosterone metabolism may be linked to insulin resistance and the metabolic syndrome.[107,108] Plasma aldosterone correlates with plasma cortisol in men and women and correlates with measures of visceral obesity and insulin resistance.[107] Visceral adipocytes may produce a fatty acid adrenal secretagogue to stimulate adrenal aldosterone production.[109]

Interestingly, aldosterone excess, as seen in aldosterone-producing adenomas, is associated with insulin resistance and may lead to type 2 DM.[110] After surgical removal of such adenomas, with normalization of plasma aldosterone levels, blood pressure and plasma potassium concentrations return to normal values, and insulin action is significantly improved.[111]

Stress, the Hypothalamic-Pituitary-Adrenal Axis, and the Sympathetic Nervous System.

External mental or physical stressors activate the

1. HPA axis and
2. sympathetic nervous system.

Both systems are implicated in mediating insulin resistance (Fig. 7-6).

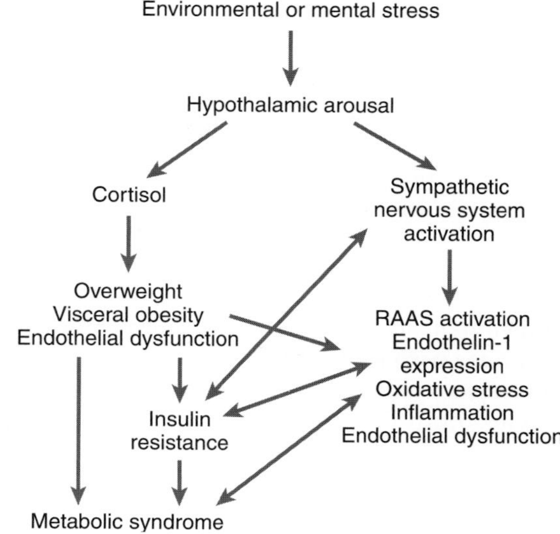

Figure 7–6.
Mental and emotional stress pathways and their relationship to insulin resistance. RAAS, renin-angiotensin-aldosterone system.

Hypothalamic-Pituitary-Adrenal Hyperactivity. Glucocorticoids are implicated in mediating insulin resistance.

With hyperactivity of the HPA axis as a result of any stressor, the normal hormonal milieu is deranged. Cortisol levels are effectively elevated with chronic stress, and there is enhanced peripheral conversion of inactive to active glucocorticoids. Protracted stress leads to positive feedback stimulation of the HPA axis. Furthermore, there are enhanced pituitary responses to vasopressin and corticotropin-releasing hormone, which further stimulate the HPA axis. As part of the activated HPA axis, dihydroepiandrostenedione and aldosterone also play a role in worsening insulin sensitivity.

Interference with Insulin Signaling. **Glucocorticoids interfere with insulin signaling at the level of the insulin receptor and IRS.**

In 3T3-L1 adipocytes, corticosteroids reduce IRS-1 protein content by inhibiting the synthesis of IRS-1 mRNA.[112] In rat skeletal muscle[113] and in a chicken model of insulin resistance, glucocorticoids significantly decrease insulin receptor and IRS-1 mRNA. As a result, there is reduced insulin binding to its receptor, with lower amounts of IRS-1 and the p85 regulatory subunit of PI3K in the liver and muscle. Tyrosine phosphorylation and activation of the insulin receptor, IRS-1, and PI3K are decreased.[114]

Glucocorticoids inhibit glucose transport in muscle also beyond changes in early insulin signaling events. In rats, corticosteroids reduce basal and maximal glucose transport in skeletal muscle in response to insulin and non–insulin-related stimuli, conceivably by affecting GLUT4 subcellular trafficking.[115]

Impairment of Nutritive Blood Flow. Steroids interfere with nutritive blood flow to insulin-sensitive tissues such as skeletal muscle.

Glucocorticoids counter insulin's vasodilatory actions and consequently compromise microcirculatory perfusion and the delivery of insulin and fuel to peripheral tissues.[116,117]

Free Fatty Acids. Glucocorticoids worsen insulin sensitivity of the liver and muscle indirectly via an FFA mechanism.

Glucocorticoids modulate the lipolytic effects of other hormones. They interfere with the re-esterification of FFAs in adipocytes. Their net effect is one of lipid mobilization resulting in marked increases in circulating plasma FFAs.[116,118,119]

In a rat model, high circulating levels of FFAs activate, rather than inhibit the HPA axis in a positive feedback loop.[120]

Impact on Human Growth Hormone and Sex Hormones. Although normally, human growth hormone (HGH) and sex hormones antagonize the effects of cortisol, corticotropin-releasing hormone may, via central effects, actually reduce HGH and sex hormone levels.[116]

IL-6, TNF-α, and Adiponectin. IL-6 may stimulate the HPA axis and thus secondarily worsen insulin sensitivity.[121] **Corticosteroid metabolism down-regulates the adipocyte expression of adiponectin but induces elaboration of TNF-α with adverse effects on insulin sensitivity.**[122]

The Sympathetic Nervous System. The sympathetic nervous system directly and indirectly deranges glucose and lipid metabolism.

Directly, there is crosstalk between the insulin and catecholamine signaling pathways that has an effect on glucose transport and uptake.[123]

α_1-Adrenergic Receptors. α_1-Adrenergic activation has direct effects on insulin signaling:

1. Rho GTPases. α_1-Adrenergic receptor stimulation leads to activation of the Rho family of small GTPases.[124] Specifically, α_1-adrenoceptor–Gq signaling activates the RhoA/Rho kinase pathway rather than the PKC pathway in a calcium-dependent manner.[125,126] Rho kinase is implicated in insulin receptor desensitization.[77]
2. Glycogen synthase. α-Adrenergic receptor activation counters insulin action by inhibition of glycogen synthase.

β-Adrenergic Receptors. There are several direct mechanisms whereby β-adrenergic stimulation counteracts insulin.

1. Adenosine 3′,5′-cyclic monophosphate (cAMP). Acting via β-adrenergic receptors, epinephrine induces adenylate cyclase activity and consequently increases cAMP. **Agonists that increase cAMP reduce tyrosine kinase activity and thus decrease IRS-1 tyrosine phosphorylation** with resultant suppression of IRS-1–associated PI3K activation, thereby inhibiting insulin activation of glucose transport at moderate insulin concentrations.

   β-Adrenergic activation attenuates glucose uptake by inhibiting hexokinase and glucose phosphorylation.

   β-Agonists counter the effects of insulin in the liver and in peripheral tissues via cAMP activation of protein kinase A (PKA), akin to the action of glucagon. This induces glycogenolysis and gluconeogenesis and as a result increases plasma glucose levels.[123]

   Epinephrine diminishes insulin secretion via a cAMP-coupled mechanism.
2. Adiponectin. **Stress effects via activation of the β-receptor lower adiponectin production, thus decreasing insulin sensitivity.**

   The effects are both pretranslational and post-translational. β-Adrenergic agonists, via cAMP, inhibit the gene expression of adiponectin in visceral adipocytes and decrease adiponectin mRNA. Less adiponectin is released, and there is a qualitative change in adiponectin secretion, such as elaboration of immature adiponectin species.[127]

Indirect Effects. Catecholamines have potent indirect means of impairing insulin sensitivity.

1. FFAs. **Catecholamines stimulate adipocytes to mobilize FFAs and to elaborate inflammatory cytokines.** The sympathetic nervous system is the major mediator for triacylglycerol lipolysis from white adipose tissue.[128,129]
2. Nutritive blood flow. **Chronic elevation of sympathetic tone may, via constrictive or mitogenic vascular remodeling effects (or via both), attenuate the microcirculatory vasodilatory responses and nutritive flow to skeletal muscle.**[130]

Accessory Adipokines. Other factors secreted by adipose tissue also affect insulin sensitivity. Adipocytokines, or adipokines, other than TNF-α and the interleukins, that are elaborated by visceral adipocytes contribute to insulin resistance.[131]

Leptin. Leptin is an adipocyte-specific hormone. It contributes to appetite regulation and affects energy balance. Plasma levels of leptin increase with increasing body fat mass. With the development of hyperleptinemia, however, leptin resistance supervenes.

Hyperleptinemia and leptin resistance may play a crucial role in the development of insulin resistance. Leptin interferes with insulin signaling and insulin action in cell models.[88,132]

With intact leptin signaling in the periphery, leptin partitions metabolic fuel toward utilization and away from storage. Leptin also has a direct thermogenic effect in skeletal muscle. By increasing fatty acid oxidation, leptin reduces the triacylglycerol content of skeletal muscle, thereby dramatically increasing insulin sensitivity. **With resistance to leptin signaling and loss of its lipopenic effect, intramyocellular lipid accumulation and insulin resistance pathways are facilitated.**[133,134]

Resistin. Resistin, named for "resistance to insulin," antagonizes insulin action and impairs glucose tolerance. Although resistin expression appears to be limited to rodents, a family of related molecules secreted by human adipose tissue may have physiologic effects resembling those of resistin.[135]

Adiponectin. The adiponectin gene is expressed exclusively in adipose tissue. With a plasma concentration normally around 5 μg/mL, adiponectin is one the most abundant circulating proteins.[88]

Adiponectin improves insulin sensitivity in both skeletal muscle and the liver. Specifically, the hormone improves insulin-mediated glucose uptake in skeletal muscle while suppressing hepatic glycogenolysis and gluconeogenesis.[136] **The mechanism by which adiponectin improves insulin signaling may involve a reduction in the ectopic storage of lipid.** In rodent skeletal muscle, adiponectin effects a transient activation of 5′-AMP–activated protein kinase (AMPK), followed by sustained inhibition of acetyl coenzyme A (CoA) carboxylase and reduction of malonyl CoA levels.[137] As a result, fatty acid oxidation is enhanced, the ectopic triacylglycerol content of muscle and liver decreases, and sensitivity to insulin signaling is restored.[136] **Adiponectin also has anti-inflammatory effects via inhibition of the NFκB signaling pathway.**

Adiponectin's plasma concentration decreases in obesity, possibly via autocrine/paracrine effects of adipokines such as TNF-α or IL-6. **Loss of its insulin-sensitizing and anti-inflammatory effects may play a significant role in the genesis of systemic insulin resistance and metabolic syndrome.**[138]

Plasma Membrane Caveolae and Caveolin. Beyond the direct molecular interactions of signaling molecules with the insulin pathway, there are other factors that affect sensitivity to insulin. The situation of the insulin receptor within the signaling microdomain of the plasma membrane has an impact on its signal transmission.

Caveolar dysfunction may play a role in the pathogenesis of insulin resistance. The plasma membranes of adipocytes, skeletal and smooth muscle cells, and vascular endothelial cells contain numerous caveolae, which are sphingolipid- and cholesterol-enriched microdomains. Upon receptor stimulation, the insulin receptor appears to be situated in caveolae.

Selective transduction pathways of receptor signals are critically dependent on caveolar integrity.

Caveolar destruction, as per cholesterol depletion, leaves the insulin receptor itself unaffected. **With loss of caveolar integrity, insulin's mitogenic control via ERK1, ERK2, and MAPK signaling remains intact, whereas the metabolic control by insulin is inhibited.** Specifically, adequate caveolar membrane cholesterol is required for insulin stimulation of

- IRS-1 binding to the insulin receptor,
- IRS-1 phosphorylation, and
- Akt/PKB phosphorylation

and is thus necessary for the transactions of the metabolic/vascular pathway.[139]

Dysfunctional or Absent Caveolae and Insulin Resistance. The structural integrity of caveolae is critical for metabolic/vascular insulin signaling to occur.

Enlarged Adipocytes. Large, hypertrophied fat cells, as seen with inadequate adipose tissue expansion, are associated with marked insulin resistance. They exhibit a relative decrease in membrane cholesterol content. Cholesterol depletion of plasma membranes induces the internalization of caveolins, the main structural proteins of caveolae and strong activators of insulin signaling. **The resultant disorganization of caveolae with adipocyte hypertrophy may disrupt metabolic and vascular insulin signaling.**[140]

On the other hand, disruption of caveolae via cholesterol depletion of the adipocyte membrane up-regulates the expression of genes encoding secreted products such as TNF-α, angiotensinogen, and IL-6, which may further impair metabolic insulin signaling.[140]

Absent Caveolae. In cell types with few or no intact caveolae, insulin signaling proceeds mainly via the MAPK pathway. **Caveolae may thus have a critical role in sorting insulin signaling for metabolic versus mitogenic control.**[139]

Caveolin and Insulin Resistance. Proper insulin signaling requires intact interaction of the insulin receptor with caveolin.

Defective Caveolin-1 Binding. Caveolin-1, an integral protein component of caveolae, has an effect on insulin receptor activation. The scaffolding domain of caveolin-1 (residues 82 to 101) binds to a specific motif within the kinase domain of the insulin receptor (residues 1193 to 1200). Mutations within the caveolin-binding motif of the human insulin receptor (W1193L and W1200S) destabilize the location of the insulin receptor within the caveolae and result in a syndrome of severe insulin resistance.[141]

Excessive Scaffolding Proteins. Expression of caveolin and flotillin is markedly elevated in skeletal muscle from the insulin-resistant, stroke-prone, spontaneously hypertensive rat when compared with normotensive controls. It is unclear whether overexpression of caveola-associated structural proteins can result in the sequestration of important insulin signaling components in an inactive environment or act as an inhibitor of downstream effects. However, they appear to blunt the ability of insulin receptors to signal to proximal molecules in the insulin signaling cascade.[142]

Deficient Caveolin-1. A mouse model lacking caveolin-1 with loss of caveolae demonstrates metabolic sequelae consistent with an insulin-resistant state. Although this model has overt resistance to diet-induced obesity, caveolin-1 null mice have severely elevated

- triglyceride,
- FFA,
- chylomicron, and
- VLDL

levels, as well as severe perturbations in endothelial cell function.[143]

Caveolae and Autocrine/Paracrine Adipokine Effects. Lipid rafts and caveolae may function in the negative regulation of insulin signaling via autocrine/paracrine effectors. Caveolae may be important sites for crosstalk between tyrosine kinase and sphingolipid signaling pathways.

TNF-α signaling may be initiated in caveolar-like domains via stimulation of sphingomyelinase activity with the generation of ceramide from sphingomyelin. Ceramide is implicated as a mediator of insulin resistance induced by TNF-α in adipocytes. Because of the proximity of insulin signaling molecules in adipocyte caveolae/rafts, local production of ceramide in these structures may affect insulin signal transmission.[82]

In fact, inhibition of TNF-α–induced caveolar ceramide production reverses the decrease in insulin receptor tyrosine phosphorylation in response to TNF-α. In conjunction with other TNF-α–dependent signals, caveolar pools of ceramide may be critical components for autocrine/paracrine modulation of insulin sensitivity by TNF-α.[144]

SECONDARY MEDIATORS OF INSULIN RESISTANCE

In a vicious circle, insulin resistance begets more insulin resistance. Numerous metabolic sequelae of cellular resistance to insulin actively interfere with insulin signaling pathways and are themselves major mediators of resistance to insulin. Such factors are listed as secondary mediators inasmuch as they derive from "primary" stimuli. Cytokines induced by TNF-α may serve as secondary hormonal factors that antagonize the systemic action of insulin, abetted by the autocrine/paracrine induction of systemic hypoadiponectinemia. **Increased release of circulating FFAs, ectopic fat storage, and the vascular dysfunction associated with insulin resistance are critical factors, with systemic reach compounding the loss of metabolic and vascular insulin action.**

Free Fatty Acids. FFAs are an important link between obesity and systemic insulin resistance, and they are potentially the major cause of peripheral and hepatic insulin resistance. FFAs account for 50% of insulin resistance in the obese.[145]

There is, in fact, an inverse correlation between high fasting plasma FFA concentrations and decreased insulin sensitivity.[146] Acute elevations of FFAs produce a dose-dependent decline in insulin-stimulated glucose uptake. Chronically elevated FFAs cause insulin resistance. Conversely, a reduction in plasma FFA levels restores insulin sensitivity. Increased plasma levels of fatty acids are a characteristic finding in insulin resistance.[145]

Adipose Tissue Insulin Resistance and Free Fatty Acids. Excess fat, as an energy reservoir, is normally stored in adipose tissue. The inflammatory stress pathways of insulin resistance are antiadipogenic and prolipolytic. They inhibit the preadipocyte recruitment and adipocyte differentiation necessary to accommodate the storage of excess calories.

Fat deposition, as opposed to lipolysis, the breakdown of triacylglycerols and release of fatty acids, is implemented through insulin action.[147] With the loss of adipose tissue sensitivity to insulin, stress pathways interfere with the normal repression of lipolysis by insulin in adipocytes. Lipolysis of triacylglycerols proceeds, and fatty acids are released into the bloodstream.

Disruption of normal adipose storage of surplus calories, together with rapid mobilization of lipid from adipose tissue via lipolysis, causes circulating FFA levels to rise.[147]

Visceral Fat and Free Fatty Acid Elevation. In particular, visceral-omental fat plays a major role in releasing FFAs.

Visceral fat is more resistant to insulin than subcutaneous fat is and is thus less sensitive to suppression of lipolysis by insulin. Because of its receptor complement and active sympathetic nervous system innervation, particularly in men, visceral adipose tissue is metabolically very active and labile and is, in fact, the adipose depot with the highest FFA turnover.[147]

Free Fatty Acid Insulin Resistance Pathways. Acute FFA-induced insulin resistance is associated with activation of NFκB. The attendant inflammatory processes play a pivotal role in the pathogenesis of FFA-induced peripheral insulin resistance, endothelial dysfunction, and vascular disease.[145]

Elevated FFAs levels increase oxidative stress. By having an adverse impact on mitochondrial function, FFA metabolites uncouple oxidative phosphorylation and generate reactive oxygen species such as superoxide. Specifically, high intracellular concentrations of long-chain acyl CoA esters inhibit mitochondrial adenine nucleotide translocators and thereby lead to intramitochondrial deficiency of adenosine diphosphate, a major factor predisposing to increased mitochondrial production of reactive oxygen species.[148] Oxidative stress results in the expression of gene products implicated in impaired insulin sensitivity.[72]

The FFA-associated rise in oxidative stress is exacerbated by FFA-mediated reduction of antioxidant defenses. Glutathione is a major endogenous antioxidant. Fasting plasma FFA levels are inversely correlated with the ratio of reduced to oxidized glutathione. With low antioxidant levels, toxic byproducts of lipid oxidation are created, such as malondialdehyde.[72]

Free Fatty Acid Impact on the Liver. The venous effluent from visceral-omental fat drains into the portal vein and delivers visceral FFAs directly and exclusively to the liver.[147] **In the liver, elevated plasma levels of FFAs, occurring as a result of uncontrolled lipolysis of adipose tissue, impair hepatic insulin extraction, metabolism, and action.** FFA-induced insulin resistance is a result of increased acetyl CoA production and inhibition of glucose oxidation by FFA. In fact, FFAs enhance glucose output from the liver. They

- interfere with insulin suppression of hepatic glycogenolysis,
- activate pyruvate carboxylase and enhance hepatic gluconeogenesis, and
- increase hepatic synthesis of triglyceride-rich VLDLs.[83]

Free Fatty Acid Impact on the Vasculature. Increased FFA fluxes impair vascular reactivity and are linked to endothelial dysfunction.[149] Oxidative stress elicited by FFAs, with subsequent activation of stress-sensitive pathways, causes premature NO degradation to peroxynitrite with endothelial dysfunction.[72] Infusions of Intralipid in healthy subjects induce vascular dysfunction. FFAs are implicated among the substances that cause the postprandial endothelial dysfunction associated with a high-fat meal.[150]

Free Fatty Acid Impact on Pancreatic Beta Cells and Hyperinsulinemia. In pancreatic beta cells, FFAs potentiate glucose-stimulated insulin secretion. As a result, the onset of type 2 DM is delayed or prevented in 80% of individuals with insulin resistance.[145] Higher pancreatic output of insulin, together with decreased hepatic extraction of insulin, engenders systemic hyperinsulinemia.

Higher secretion of insulin cannot be sustained in the long run because of lipotoxicity and other factors. Ultimately, FFA exposure leads to an impairment in glucose-stimulated insulin release, apoptosis, and progressive loss of beta cell function.[150]

Free Fatty Acid Impact on Muscle Tissue. Acute and chronic elevations in plasma FFA levels generate insulin resistance in muscle. They reduce glucose and fatty acid oxidative disposal. **In muscle, FFAs must first be re-esterified and accumulate as intramyocellular triacylglycerol before they induce insulin resistance.** Specifically, it is the metabolites involved in the synthesis of triacylglycerols that impair insulin signaling.[145]

Ectopic Fat Storage. Antiadipogenic factors contribute to ectopic fat.

Impaired preadipocyte differentiation and adipocyte apoptosis, compounded by uncontrolled lipolysis, drastically curtail normal adipose storage of excess calories. **These antiadipogenic forces not only raise the level of plasma FFAs but also effect the redistribution of lipid to storage in peripheral, nonadipose tissues.** As a result, excess calories are consigned as ectopic fat to sites not meant to store lipids, specifically to

- skeletal muscle,
- myocardium,
- liver,
- pancreas,
- blood,[151]
- endothelium, and
- vascular smooth muscle cells.[152]

Mechanisms Leading to Ectopic Lipid Accumulation. Although increased fatty acid fluxes into nonadipose tissues importantly contribute to ectopic cytosolic lipid, reduced fatty acid oxidation plays a pivotal role in the process.

Reduced fatty acid beta-oxidative capacity in affected organs may underlie the ectopic accumulation of lipid. Biopsy studies in patients with type 2 DM demonstrated diminished mitochondrial size at only 55% of normal with impaired mitochondrial oxidative capacity.[153] Correspondingly, in young, lean, insulin-resistant offspring of parents with type 2 DM, the rate of mitochondrial adenosine triphosphate synthesis in skeletal muscle was 30% lower than in a group

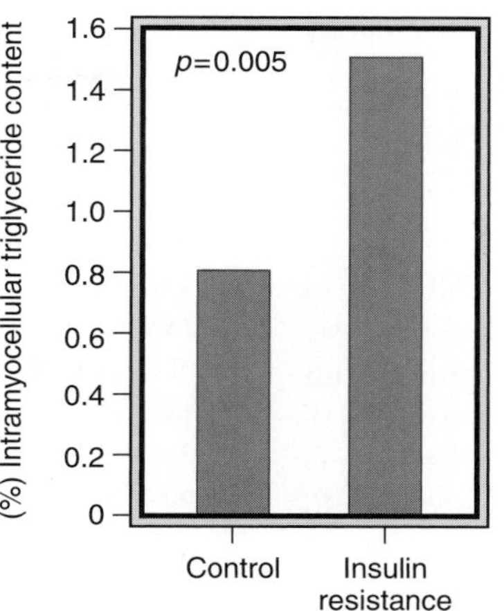

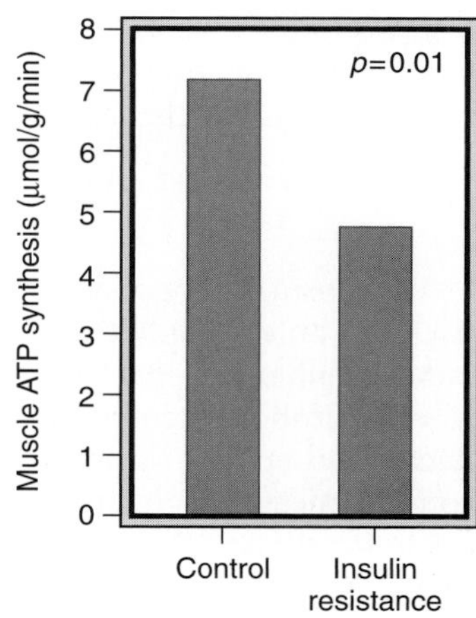

Figure 7–7. Intramyocellular fat and impaired mitochondrial adenosine triphosphate (ATP) synthesis in the skeletal muscle of young, lean, healthy, insulin-resistant offspring of type 2 diabetics when compared with a group of control subjects with normal insulin sensitivity and matched for physical activity. *(Modified from Petersen KF, Dufour S, Befroy D, et al. Impaired mitochondrial activity in the insulin-resistant offspring of patients with type 2 diabetes. N Engl J Med 2004;350:664-671.)*

of control subjects with normal insulin sensitivity and matched for physical activity (Fig. 7-7).[154]

Carnitine Palmitoyl Transferase-I. Reduced levels of intracellular carnitine palmitoyl transferase I (CPT-I) are implicated in the reduction of fatty acid oxidation.

CPT-I is the enzyme that controls the transfer of long-chain fatty acyl CoA from the cytosol into mitochondria for oxidation.[155] Specifically, CPT-I catalyzes the rate-limiting step in the translocation of activated fatty acids into the inner membrane of mitochondria to be oxidized. CPT-I levels may be up to 50% lower in overweight individuals than in lean subjects, inversely correlating with insulin resistance.[156]

Malonyl CoA. Increased intracellular levels of malonyl CoA are implicated in ectopic fat storage.

Malonyl CoA is an intermediary in fatty acid biosynthesis. It is a potent, allosteric inhibitor of CPT-I and thus plays a key role regulating the biosynthesis versus the oxidation of fatty acids.

A rise in cytoplasmic malonyl CoA levels

- inhibits CPT-I,
- diminishes long-chain fatty acid oxidation, and
- shunts long-chain fatty acids toward esterification and the biosynthesis of diacylglycerols and triacylglycerols, which results in increased ectopic intracellular fatty acid storage.[72]

Mechanisms of Impaired Fatty Acid Beta Oxidation. Abnormalities in muscle fatty acid metabolism are strongly associated with the development of insulin resistance. Reasons for the reduction of fatty acid beta-oxidative capacity are unclear.

Several factors associated with ectopic lipid deposition are implicated in lowering fatty acid beta oxidation.

5′-AMP–Activated Protein Kinase. A decrease in AMPK may be playing a role. AMPK activation increases the oxidation of fatty acids and inhibits the synthesis of triacylglycerols. This AMPK action is brought about by two mechanisms:

1. AMPK lowers malonyl CoA levels by effects on enzymes that govern the synthesis and degradation of malonyl CoA;
2. AMPK increases the expression of uncoupling proteins and the transcriptional regulator PPAR-γ coactivator-1alpha (PGC-1α), a master regulator of mitochondrial biogenesis that may increase energy expenditure.[155] PGC-1 has also been implicated in the development of oxidative type I skeletal muscle fibers.[157]

A reduction in AMPK activity lowers metabolic activity.

Inflammation. Inflammatory pathways may partition fatty acid metabolism toward synthesis rather than oxidative consumption, thus contributing to the accumulation of intramyocellular and intrahepatocellular triacylglycerol.

Lower CPT-I levels, suggestive of decreased lipid beta oxidation, may be seen with

- systemic inflammatory responses,
- oxidative stress, and
- sepsis.[158]

Endotoxin, or lipopolysaccharide, TNF-α, and IL-1 not only stimulate adipose tissue lipolysis but also enhance hepatic fatty acid synthesis and re-esterification, thereby contributing to dyslipidemia and ectopic fat in the liver, with serious consequences for hepatic energy levels and organ function.[159] Cytokines induce an inappropriate switch from fatty acid oxidation to fatty acid synthesis in an vitro rat hepatocyte model. The inhibitory effects of TNF-α on fatty acid oxidation are enhanced by either IL-1 or IL-6 and are associated with increased production of malonyl CoA.[160]

Correspondingly, these **proinflammatory mediators also suppress fatty acid oxidation in the heart and muscle, which allows the accumulation of ectopic fat in these tissues.**[159,161] During inflammatory processes in skeletal muscle, principally four proinflammatory cytokines, IL-1, IL-6, TNF-α, and interferon-γ, induce metabolic alterations that include lower fatty acid oxidation and resistance to insulin signaling.[162]

Complement C3 is also involved in the pathogenesis of insulin resistance and may provide another missing link between inflammation, FFA metabolism, and insulin resistance.[163]

The loss of adiponectin with inflammation may increase the storage of ectopic lipid. Adiponectin promotes fatty acid beta oxidation in humans and thus results in lower circulating fatty acid levels and reduced intramyocellular and intrahepatocellular triacylglycerol content. High circulating levels of adiponectin are associated with lower intracellular fat and improved insulin action in humans.[164,165] Adiponectin levels are reduced with inflammation, directly and as a result of reduced PPAR-γ activity. With loss of adiponectin's physiologic actions, there is a rise in ectopic intracellular lipid and insulin resistance.

Physical Inactivity. Lack of exercise lowers fatty acid oxidative capacity.

During exercise, when the need for fatty acid oxidation is increased, malonyl CoA levels fall. **Exercise activates AMPK,** which phosphorylates and inhibits acetyl CoA carboxylase. As a result, the concentration of malonyl CoA decreases.[166]

Obesity. The changes in adipokine elaboration occurring with obesity may affect oxidative capacity.

With leptin resistance and adiponectin deficiency compounding proinflammatory adipokine effects, AMPK stimulation is lost. The metabolic sequelae are particularly adverse for muscle and hepatic tissues. Ironically, **diminished oxidative capacity will contribute to obesity in a positive feedback loop.**

Excessive Glucose. Hyperglycemia or prolonged elevations of plasma glucose contribute to decreased fatty acid oxidation.

Malonyl CoA levels are elevated when the supply of glucose and insulin to muscle is increased, in keeping with a decreased need for fatty acid oxidation. Changes in glucose supply regulate malonyl CoA by directly modulating the concentration of cytosolic citrate. Citrate functions as an allosteric activator of acetyl CoA carboxylase, the rate-limiting enzyme for malonyl CoA formation.[166]

Gene Expression. PGC-1 is a transcriptional regulator of genes responsible for mitochondrial biogenesis, the development of oxidative type I muscle fibers, and synthesis of the mitochondrial enzymes involved in fatty acid beta oxidation.[157] Polymorphisms, decreased expression of PGC-1, or both occur in populations with type 2 DM or in overweight individuals with a family history of type 2 DM.[153]

Role of Ectopic Fat Storage in Insulin Resistance. Ectopic storage of fat in nonadipose tissues not only compromises their function but also promotes insulin resistance and the metabolic syndrome.

Ectopic lipid concentrations correlate with insulin resistance in humans.[167] With nutritional excess, inadequate adipose tissue expansion leads to the ectopic deposition of dietary fat. In obese persons, the degree of insulin resistance correlates closely with lipid infiltration of skeletal muscle and the liver. Adipocyte hypertrophy reflects inadequate adipose expansion and is predictive of the development of type 2 DM.[168] Correspondingly, lipodystrophy, a failure of adipose tissue development, necessitates nonadipose storage of fat and results in severe insulin resistance and DM.[169] In contrast, pharmacologic PPAR-γ activators promote adipogenesis by increasing the lipid storage capacity of adipose tissue. In the process, they diminish ectopic fat deposition with an improvement in insulin sensitivity.

Intramyocellular Lipid. There is considerable evidence that in particular, intramyocellular lipid, measured by nuclear magnetic resonance imaging, may be a critical determinant of insulin resistance.[170]

Intramyocellular lipid content, measured by ^{1}H magnetic resonance spectroscopy, was 80% higher in lean, healthy, but insulin-resistant offspring of type 2 diabetics than in insulin-sensitive control subjects.[154] In young individuals with prediabetes, intramyocellular and intra-abdominal lipid accumulations were closely linked to the development of significant peripheral insulin resistance.[171] In fact, the correlation of the severity of intramyocellular lipid content with insulin resistance was significant and greater than the correlation of BMI and insulin resistance.[172]

Although BMI itself correlates positively with intramyocellular lipid, there are exceptions:

- high-BMI individuals may have low intramyocellular lipid;
- thin, low-BMI individuals may have high intramyocellular lipid and, despite being thin, be metabolically obese.[173]

Mechanisms of Insulin Resistance with Intramyocellular Lipid. In skeletal muscle, increased intramyocellular triglyceride is only a marker for insulin resistance. It appears to be the cytosolic metabolites resulting from altered intracellular fatty acid metabolism that interfere with insulin signal transduction.

The mechanisms involved are complex, and many pathways are implicated. In muscle, cytosolic accumulation of the metabolically active long-chain fatty acyl CoAs leads to impaired insulin signaling and impaired enzyme activity (e.g., of glycogen synthase or hexokinase) either directly or via chronic translocation/activation of mediators such as PKC. Ceramides and diacylglycerols are also implicated in ectopic lipid–induced insulin resistance (Fig. 7-8).[174]

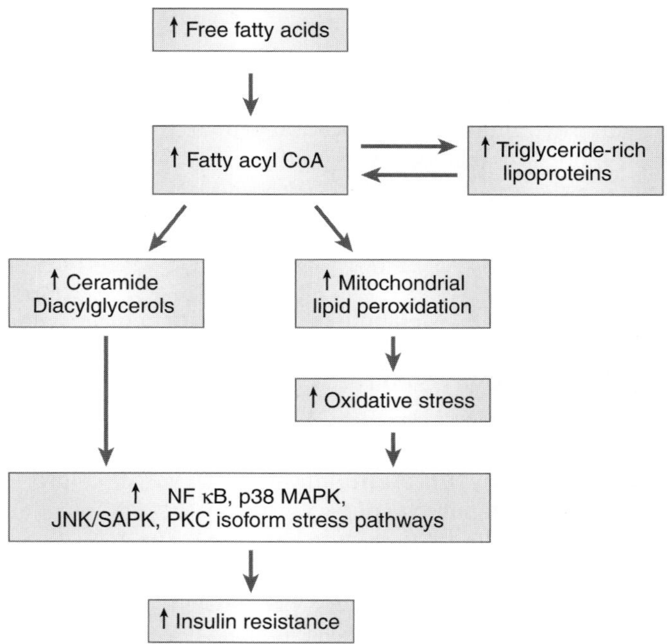

▶▶ **Figure 7–8.**
Intramyocellular lipids and insulin resistance. CoA, coenzyme A; JNK, c-Jun NH_2-terminal kinase; MAPK, mitogen-activated protein kinase; NF, nuclear factor; PKC, protein kinase C; SAPK, stress-activated protein kinase. *(Modified from Petersen KF, Shulman GI. Pathogenesis of skeletal muscle insulin resistance in type 2 diabetes mellitus. Am J Cardiol 2002;90:11G-18G.)*

PKC–IRS-1 Serine Phosphorylation. In muscle, metabolically active, long-chain fatty acyl CoAs can convert FFA metabolites into intracellular signaling molecules, which can be further processed to

- ceramide and
- diacylglycerol.

Ceramide or diacylglycerol allosterically activates several isoforms of PKC, including

- PKC-β (vasculature),
- PKC-β/δ (human skeletal muscle),
- PKC-θ (rat skeletal muscle),[145,175] and
- PKC-ε.[174]

Novel PKC-θ isoforms are abundant in skeletal muscle. When activated, PKC-θ isoforms inhibit insulin receptor function through activation of a serine/threonine phosphorylation cascade that results in increased serine phosphorylation of IRS-1 and IRS-2. As noted previously, this step decreases insulin-activated IRS-1 tyrosine phosphorylation, PI3K/Akt kinase activation, and metabolic and vascular insulin signaling.[69,176]

PKC Stress Pathways. Tissue elevation of FFA-derived signaling molecules and activation of PKC-θ provide a unique ability to activate

- NFκB,[72]
- NFκB-activating kinases,
- p38 MAPK, and
- JNK/SAPK.[177,178]

Such activation results in the stimulation of serine/threonine kinase cascades, which leads to the phosphorylation of serine/threonine sites on IRS-1 and IRS-2, thus interrupting the cellular mechanisms of metabolic and vascular insulin signaling.[177,178]

Free Fatty Acid Metabolites and Oxidative Stress. FFAs and their metabolites also impair insulin sensitivity indirectly by increasing oxidative stress.[72,148]

Endothelial Dysfunction. Physiologic, vasomotive considerations determine the actual delivery of insulin to its cell surface receptor and delivery of glucose and fatty acids to their target cells. Endothelial dysfunction is present in insulin resistance[150,179] and is related to the severity of insulin resistance.[180] Endothelial dysfunction is a link between insulin resistance and cardiovascular disease.

However, endothelial dysfunction may not only be caused by insulin resistance. **Endothelial dysfunction may be implicated in the pathogenesis of insulin resistance and type 2 DM.** Dysfunctional eNOS or deficient NO availability, or both, may directly and indirectly contribute to insulin insensitivity.

Directly, the NO/cGMP signaling pathway thwarts RhoA inhibition of insulin action via the Rho kinase association with and serine phosphorylation of IRS-1.[77] With endothelial dysfunction, these protective effects of NO/cGMP on insulin signaling are lost. Furthermore, eNOS participates directly in glucose and lipid homeostasis. It is expressed in skeletal muscle, where it appears to govern metabolic processes.[181] This metabolic function is lost with dysfunctional eNOS.

Insulin's vasodilatory efficacy is correlated with insulin sensitivity. The vasorelaxant effects of insulin are mediated via eNOS-derived NO. The parallels between the metabolic and vascular insulin signaling pathways suggest a coupling of insulin's metabolic and hemodynamic actions.[182] Insulin resistance thus affects both metabolic and vascular signaling.

Indirectly, eNOS controls microvascular nutritive perfusion in peripheral target organs. Endothelial dysfunction, plus the loss of insulin's vasodilatory actions, compromises regional blood flow. By interfering with the distribution and disposal of glucose and fatty acids, endothelial dysfunction further exacerbates tissue resistance to insulin.[183]

Hyperglycemia. Hyperglycemia supervening on worsening insulin resistance further impairs insulin signaling.

Hyperglycemia itself decreases insulin-stimulated glucose utilization and glycogen synthesis in skeletal muscle, adipocytes, and endothelial cells. Hyperglycemia impairs the functional properties of cytosolic and nuclear proteins through O-linked glycosylation modification. Via involvement of the hexosamine pathway, the metabolic and vascular branch of insulin signaling is impaired, with decreased insulin receptor activation of the IRS/PI3K cascade.

CONCLUSION

The rising popularity of low-carbohydrate diets has given insulin a "bad name." However, insulin has diverse beneficial anti-inflammatory and vasculoprotective effects that are implemented by a signaling pathway that shares numerous initial steps with its anabolic pathway.

Whereas the anabolic and vascular effects of insulin are compromised by insulin resistance mechanisms, insulin's mitogenic signaling appears to be immune to such constraints and is, in fact, enhanced. The selective nature of insulin insensitivity has significant, adverse effects that contribute to the multiplicity of detrimental cardiovascular and metabolic sequelae of insulin resistance.

There is a profusion of pathways that lead to insulin resistance. For any individual, a diverse set of genetic, environmental, and nutritional factors apply, and different aspects may assume primary versus secondary importance. In some, the process may be initiated locally, later to become systemic. In others, it may occur systemically.

The redundancy of mechanisms that impair anabolic insulin signaling suggests a potential physiologic benefit of insulin resistance. Insulin resistance occurs in response to adverse physiologic or psychological challenges. Aspects of inflammatory and oxidative stress pathways appear to underlie most, if not all mechanisms of insulin resistance. Insulin resistance is effectively a part of the inflammatory response, in effect its metabolic adaptation. In the course of human development, humans have had to weather innumerable hardships such as repetitive starvation, deprivation, injury, infection, illness, and other stresses. With insulin resistance, the ensuing stress inflammatory responses terminate anabolic pathways and engender a catabolic state to secure a ready supply of fuel to immune system cells and the brain during the periods of stress. For survival in a hostile environment, insulin resistance pathways may provide an organism with the capacity to effectively overcome and survive repetitive insults.

As with most aspects of physiology, the survival benefit of insulin resistance pathways is lost when what should be a temporary, compensatory response is, in fact, sustained over the long term. Once insulin resistance is established chronically, its redundant, complementary, and mutually reinforcing mechanisms, compounded by current nutritional and lifestyle challenges, engender pathophysiologic vicious circles. In the absence of a reversal of precipitating factors or effective intervention, insulin resistance, once established, begets further insulin resistance and the metabolic syndrome, devastating vascular disease, and type 2 DM.

In view of the redundant mechanisms of insulin resistance, it is not surprising that a multifaceted approach is needed for its prevention or reversal. Antioxidant, anti-inflammatory, stress-relieving interventions consisting of lifestyle, nutritional, and pharmacologic measures will be of benefit. Additionally, fatty acid effects need to be contained by focusing on an improved balance between energy intake and expenditure.

GLOSSARY

ACE	angiotensin-converting enzyme
AGE	advanced glycosylated end product
AMPK	5′-AMP–activated protein kinase
AT_1	angiotensin II type 1
ATP	Adult Treatment Panel
BMI	body mass index
BP	blood pressure
cAMP	cyclic adenosine 3′,5′-monophosphate
cGMP	cyclic guanosine 3′,5′-monophosphate
CHD	coronary heart disease
CoA	coenzyme A
CPT	carnitine palmitoyl transferase
DM	diabetes mellitus
eNOS	endothelial nitric oxide synthase
ERK	extracellular signal–regulated kinase
FFA	free fatty acid
GLUT	glucose transporter
GTP	guanosine 5′-triphosphate
HDL	high-density lipoprotein
HGH	human growth hormone
HOMA	Homeostasis Model Assessment
HPA	hypothalamic-pituitary-adrenal
hsCRP	high-sensitivity C-reactive protein
IKK	IκB kinase
IκB	I kappa B
IL	interleukin
iNOS	inducible nitric oxide synthase
IRS	insulin receptor substrate

JNK	c-Jun NH_2-terminal kinase
LDL	low-density lipoprotein
LPL	lipoprotein lipase
MAPK	mitogen-activated protein kinase
MAPKK	MAPK kinase
MI	myocardial infarction
NADH/NADPH	nicotinamide adenine dinucleotide phosphate oxidase
NCEP	National Cholesterol Education Program
NFκB	nuclear factor kappaB
NHANES	National Health and Nutrition Examination Survey
NO	nitric oxide
NOS	nitric oxide synthase
PAI-1	plasminogen activator inhibitor-1
PGC-1	PPAR-γ coactivator-1
PI3K	phosphatidylinositol 3-kinase
PKA	protein kinase A
PKB	protein kinase B
PKC	protein kinase C
PPAR	peroxisome proliferator–activated receptor
QUICKI	Quantitative Insulin Sensitivity Check Index
RAAS	renin-angiotensin-aldosterone system
RAGE	receptor for advanced glycosylation end products
SAPK	stress-activated protein kinase
SOCS	suppressor of cytokine signaling
TNF	tumor necrosis factor
VLDL	very-low-density lipoprotein
WHO	World Health Organization

REFERENCES

1. Nilsson S. Research contributions of Eskil Kylin. Sven Med Tidskr 2001;5:15-28
2. Avogaro P, Crepaldi G, Enzi G, et al. Associazione di iperlipidemia, diabete mellito e obesita di medio grado. Acta Diabetol Lat 1967;4:36-41
3. Haller H. Epidemiologie und assoziierte Risikofaktoren der Hyperlipoproteinaemie. Z Gesammte Inn Med 1977;32:124-128
4. Reaven G. Banting Lecture 1988. Role of insulin resistance in human disease. Diabetes 1988;37:1595-1607
5. Definition, Diagnosis and Classification of Diabetes Mellitus and Its Complications: Report of a WHO Consultation. Geneva, Department of Noncommunicable Disease Surveillance, World Health Organization, 1999
6. Alberti KG, Zimmet PZ. Definition, diagnosis and classification of diabetes mellitus and its complications, part 1: diagnosis and classification of diabetes mellitus provisional report of a WHO consultation. Diabet Med 1998;15:539-553
7. Ford ES, Giles WH, Dietz WH. Prevalence of the metabolic syndrome among US adults: findings from the Third National Health and Nutrition Examination survey. JAMA 2002;287:356-359
8. Expert Panel on Detection, Evaluation, and Treatment of High Blood Cholesterol in Adults. Executive Summary of the Third Report of the National Cholesterol Education Program (NCEP) Expert Panel on Detection, and Treatment of High Blood Cholesterol in Adults (Adult Treatment Panel III). JAMA 2001;285:2486-2497
9. Grundy SM, Brewer HB Jr, Cleeman JI, et al. Definition of metabolic syndrome: report of the National Heart, Lung, and Blood Institute/American Heart Association conference on scientific issues related to definition. Arterioscler Thromb Vasc Biol 2004;24:e13-e18
10. Fagan DC, Deedwania PC. The cardiovascular dysmetabolic syndrome. Am J Med 1998;105(suppl 1):77S-82S
11. Anand SS, Yi Q, Gerstein H, et al, for the Study of Health Assessment and Risk in Ethnic groups (SHARE) and Study of Health Assessment and Risk Evaluation in Aboriginal Peoples (SHARE-AP) Investigators. Relationship of metabolic syndrome and fibrinolytic dysfunction to cardiovascular disease. Circulation 2003;108:420-425
12. Park YW, Zhu S, Palaniappan L, et al. The metabolic syndrome: prevalence and associated risk factor findings in the US population from the Third National Health and Nutrition Examination Survey, 1988-1994. Arch Intern Med 2003;163:427-436
13. DeFronzo RA, Bonadonna RC, Ferrannini E. Pathogenesis of NIDDM: a balanced overview. Diabetes Care 1992;15:318-368
14. Warram JH, Martin BC, Krolewski AS, et al. Slow glucose removal rate and hyperinsulinemia precede the development of type II diabetes in the offspring of diabetic parents. Ann Intern Med 1990;113:909-915
15. Haffner SM, Mykkanen L, Festa A, et al. Insulin-resistant prediabetic subjects have more atherogenic risk factors than insulin-sensitive prediabetic subjects: implications for preventing coronary heart disease during the prediabetic state. Circulation 2000;101:975-980
16. Haffner SM, Howard G, Mayer E, et al. Insulin sensitivity and acute insulin response in African-Americans, non-Hispanic whites, and Hispanics with NIDDM: the Insulin Resistance Atherosclerosis Study. Diabetes 1997;46:63-69
17. Salmenniemi U, Ruotsalainen E, Pihlajamäki J, et al. Multiple abnormalities in glucose and energy metabolism and coordinated changes in levels of adiponectin, cytokines, and adhesion molecules in subjects with metabolic syndrome. Circulation 2004;110:3842-3848
18. Cusi K, Maezono K, Osman A, et al. Insulin resistance differentially affects the PI 3-kinase– and MAP kinase–mediated signaling in human muscle. J Clin Invest 2000;105:311-320
19. Goldstein BJ. Insulin resistance as the core defect in type 2 diabetes mellitus. Am J Cardiol 2002;90(suppl): 3G-10G
20. Federici M, Menghini R, Mauriello A, et al. Insulin-dependent activation of endothelial nitric oxide synthase is impaired by O-linked glycosylation modification of signaling proteins in human coronary endothelial cells. Circulation 2002;106:466-472
21. Montagnani M, Golovchenko I, Kim I, et al. Inhibition of phosphatidylinositol 3-kinase enhances mitogenic actions of insulin in endothelial cells. J Biol Chem 2002;277:1794-1799

22. Reaven GM, Lithell H, Landsberg L. Mechanisms of disease: hypertension and associated metabolic abnormalities. The role of insulin resistance and the sympathoadrenal system. N Engl J Med 1996;334: 374-381
23. Ginsberg HN. Insulin resistance and cardiovascular disease. J Clin Invest 2000;106:453-458
24. Dunaif A, Thomas A. Current concepts in the polycystic ovary syndrome. Annu Rev Med 2001;52:401-419
25. Abbasi F, Brown BW, Lamendola C, et al. Relationship between obesity, insulin resistance, and coronary heart disease risk. J Am Coll Cardiol 2002;40:937-943
26. Reilley MP, Rader DJ. The metabolic syndrome. More than the sum of its parts? Circulation 2003;108:1546-1551
27. Howard G, Bergman R, Wagenknecht LE, et al. Ability of alternative indices of insulin sensitivity to predict cardiovascular risk: comparison with the "minimal model." Insulin Resistance Atherosclerosis Study (IRAS) Investigators. Ann Epidemiol 1998;8:358-369
28. Laakso M. How good a marker is insulin level for insulin resistance? Am J Epidemiol 1993;137:959-965
29. Matthews DR, Hosker JP, Rudenski AS, et al. Homeostasis model assessment: insulin resistance and β-cell function from fasting plasma glucose and insulin concentrations in man. Diabetologia 1985;28:412-419
30. Hanley AJ, Karter AJ, Festa A, et al. Factor analysis of metabolic syndrome using directly measured insulin sensitivity: the Insulin Resistance Atherosclerosis Study. Diabetes 2002;51:2642-2647
31. Tuan C-Y, Abbasi F, Lamendola C, et al. Usefulness of plasma glucose and insulin concentrations in identifying patients with insulin resistance. Am J Cardiol 2003; 92:606-610
32. Festa A, Hanley AJ, Tracy RP, et al. Inflammation in the prediabetic state is related to increased insulin resistance rather than decreased insulin secretion. Circulation 2003;108:1822-1830
33. Despres J, Lamarche B, Mauriege P, et al. Hyperinsulinemia as an independent risk factor for ischemic heart disease. N Engl J Med 1996;334:952-957
34. Hanley AJ, Williams K, Stern MP, et al. Homeostasis model assessment of insulin resistance in relation to the incidence of cardiovascular disease: the San Antonio Heart Study. Diabetes Care 2002;25:1177-1184
35. Haffner S, Taegtmeyer H. Epidemic obesity and the metabolic syndrome. Circulation 2003;108:1541-1545
36. Wilson PWF, D'Agostino RB, Levy D, et al. Prediction of coronary heart disease using risk factor categories. Circulation 1998;97:1837-1847
37. Wong ND, Pio JR, Franklin SS, et al. Preventing coronary events by optimal control of blood pressure and lipids in patients with the metabolic syndrome. Am J Cardiol 2003;91:1421-1426
38. Scuteri A, Najjar SS, Muller DC, et al. Metabolic syndrome amplifies the age-associated increases in vascular thickness and stiffness. J Am Coll Cardiol 2004;43:1388-1395
39. Wong ND, Sciammarella MG, Pol D, et al. The metabolic syndrome, diabetes, and subclinical atherosclerosis assessed by coronary calcium. J Am Coll Cardiol 2003; 41:1547-1553
40. Reilly MP, Wolfe ML, Rhodes T, et al. Measures of insulin resistance add incremental value to the clinical diagnosis of metabolic syndrome in association with coronary atherosclerosis. Circulation 2004;110:803-809
41. Sasso FC, Carbonara O, Nasti R, et al. Glucose metabolism and coronary heart disease in patients with normal glucose tolerance. JAMA 2004;291:1857-1863
42. Sekiguchi M, Kurabayashi M, Adachi H, et al. Usefulness of the insulin resistance measured by homeostasis model assessment in predicting restenosis after coronary stent placement in nondiabetic patients. Am J Cardiol 2004;93:920-922
43. Marroquin OC, Kip KE, Kelley DE, et al. Women's Ischemia Syndrome Evaluation Investigators. Metabolic syndrome modifies the cardiovascular risk associated with angiographic coronary artery disease in women: a report from the Women's Ischemia Syndrome Evaluation. Circulation 2004;109:714-721
44. Ninomiya JK, L'Italien G, Criqui MH, et al. Association of the metabolic syndrome with history of myocardial infarction and stroke in the Third National Health and Nutrition Examination Survey. Circulation 2004; 109:42-46
45. McNeill AM, Rosamond WD, Girman CJ, et al. Prevalence of coronary heart disease and carotid arterial thickening in patients with the metabolic syndrome (the ARIC Study). Am J Cardiol 2004;94:1249-1254
46. Isomaa B, Almgren P, Tuomi T, et al. Cardiovascular morbidity and mortality associated with the metabolic syndrome. Diabetes Care 2001;24:683-689
47. Nilsson P, Nilsson JA, Hedblod B, et al. Hyperinsulinaemia as long-term predictor of death and ischaemic heart disease in nondiabetic men: the Malmö Preventive Project. J Intern Med 2003;253:136-145
48. Lakka HM, Laaksonen D, Lakka T, et al. The metabolic syndrome and total and cardiovascular disease mortality in middle-aged men. JAMA 2002;288:2709-2716
49. Hu G, Qiao Q, Tuomilehto J, et al, for the DECODE Study Group. Prevalence of the metabolic syndrome and its relation to all-cause and cardiovascular mortality in nondiabetic European men and women. Arch Intern Med 2004;164;1066-1076
50. Malik S, Wong ND, Franklin SS, et al. Impact of the metabolic syndrome on mortality from coronary heart disease, cardiovascular disease, and all causes in United States adults. Circulation 2004;110:1245-1250
51. Kahn CR. Banting lecture: insulin action, diabetogenes, and the cause of type II diabetes. Diabetes 1994;43: 1066-1084
52. Reaven GM. Pathophysiology of insulin resistance in human disease. Physiol Rev 1995;75:473-486
53. Hofman PL, Regan F, Jackson WE, et al. Premature birth and later insulin resistance. N Engl J Med 2004;351: 2179-2186
54. Golub MS. The adrenal and the metabolic syndrome. Curr Hypertens Rep 2001;3:117-120
55. Winder WW. AMP-activated protein kinase: possible target for treatment of type 2 diabetes. Diabetes Technol Ther 2000;2:441-448
56. Clark MG, Wallis MG, Barrett EJ, et al. Blood flow and muscle metabolism: a focus on insulin action. Am J Physiol Endocrinol Metab 2003;284:E241-E258
57. Hollenbeck CB, Haskell W, Rosenthal M, Reaven GM. Effect of habitual physical activity on regulation of insulin-stimulated glucose disposal in older males. J Am Geriatr Soc 1984;33:273-277
58. Bogardus C, Lillioja S, Mott DM, et al. Relationship between degree of obesity and in vivo insulin action in man. Am J Physiol Endocrinol Metab 1985;248: E286-E291
59. Mokdad AH, Bowman BA, Ford ES, et al. The continuing epidemic of obesity and diabetes in the United States. JAMA 2001;286:1195-1200
60. Carey DG, Jenkins AB, Campbell AV, et al. Abdominal fat and insulin resistance in normal and overweight women: direct measurements reveal a strong relationship in subjects at both low and high risk of NIDDM. Diabetes 1996;45:633-638

61. Xu H, Hirosumi J, Uysal T, et al. Exclusive action of transmembrane TNF-alpha in adipose tissue leads to reduced adipose mass and local but not systemic insulin resistance. Endocrinology 2002;143:1502-1511
62. Bullo M, Garcia-Lorda P, Peinado-Onsurbe J, et al. TNF-alpha expression of subcutaneous adipose tissue in obese and morbid obese females: relationship to adipocyte LPL activity and leptin synthesis. Int J Obes 2002;26:652-658
63. Grundy SM, Hansen B, Smith SC Jr, et al. Clinical management of metabolic syndrome: report of the American Heart Association/National Heart, Lung, and Blood Institute/American Diabetes Association conference on scientific issues related to management. Arterioscler Thromb Vasc Biol 2004;24:e19-e24
64. Litherland GJ, Hajduch E, Hundai HS. Intracellular signaling mechanisms regulating glucose transport in insulin-sensitive tissues (review). Mol Membr Biol 2001; 18:195-204
65. Youngren JF, Keen S, Kulp JL, et al. Enhanced muscle insulin receptor autophosphorylation with short-term aerobic exercise training. Am J Physiol Endocrinol Metab 2001;280:E528-E533
66. Saltiel AR. Putting the brakes on insulin signaling. N Engl J Med 2003;349:2560-2562
67. Adeli K, Taghibiglou C, Van Iderstine SC, Lewis GF. Mechanisms of hepatic very low-density lipoprotein overproduction in insulin resistance. Trends Cardiovasc Med 2001;11:170-176
68. Zierath JR. Exercise effects of muscle insulin signaling and action. Invited review: exercise training–induced changes in insulin signaling in skeletal muscle. J Appl Physiol 2002;93:773-781
69. Farese RV. Function and dysfunction of aPKC isoforms for glucose transport in insulin-sensitive and insulin-resistant states. Am J Physiol Endocrinol Metab 2002; 283:E1-E11
70. Standaert ML, Ortmeyer HK, Sajan MP, et al. Skeletal muscle insulin resistance in obesity-associated type 2 diabetes in monkeys is linked to a defect in insulin activation of protein kinase C delta/lambda. Diabetes 2002;51:2936-2943
71. Du K, Herzig S, Kulkarni RN, Montminy M. TRB3: a tribbles homolog that inhibits Akt/PKB activation by insulin in liver. Science 2003;300:1574-1577
72. Evans JL, Goldfine ID, Maddux BA, Grodsky GM. Oxidative stress and stress-activated signaling pathways: a unifying hypothesis of type 2 diabetes. Endocrinol Rev 2002;23:599-622
73. Maddux BA, See W, Lawrence JC Jr, et al. Protection against oxidative stress–induced insulin resistance in rat L6 muscle cells by micromolar concentrations of alpha-lipoic acid. Diabetes 2001;50:404-410
74. Marette A. Mediators of cytokine-induced insulin resistance in obesity and other inflammatory settings. Curr Opin Clin Nutr Metab Care 2000;5:377-383
75. Fujishiro M, Gotoh Y, Katagiri H, et al. MKK6/3 and p38 MAPK pathway activation is not necessary for insulin-induced glucose uptake but regulates glucose transporter expression. J Biol Chem 2001;276:19800-19806
76. Grimble RF. Inflammatory status and insulin resistance. Curr Opin Clin Nutr Metab Care 2002;5:551-559
77. Begum N, Sandu OA, Ito M, et al. Active Rho kinase (ROK-β) associates with insulin receptor substrate-1 and inhibits insulin signaling in vascular smooth muscle cells. J Biol Chem 2002;277:6214-6222
78. Hotamisligil GS. Mechanisms of TNF-alpha–induced insulin resistance. Exp Clin Endocrinol Diabetes 1999;107:119-125
79. Kahaleh MB, Fan PS. Effect of cytokines on production of endothelin by endothelial cells. Clin Exp Rheumatol 1997;15:163-167
80. Brasier AR, Li J, Wimbish KA. Tumor necrosis factor activates angiotensinogen gene expression by the Rel A transactivator. Hypertension 1996;27:1009-1017
81. Pausova Z, Deslauriers B, Gaudet D, et al. Role of tumor necrosis factor-alpha gene locus in obesity and obesity-associated hypertension in French Canadians. Hypertension 2000;36:14-19
82. Bickel PE. Lipid rafts and insulin signaling. Am J Physiol Endocrinol Metab 2002;282:E1-E10
83. Hunter I, Cobban HJ, Vandenabeele P, et al. Tumor necrosis factor-alpha–induced activation of RhoA in airway smooth muscle cells: role in the Ca^{2+} sensitization of myosin light chain20 phosphorylation. Mol Pharmacol 2003;63:714-721
84. Ruan H, Hacohen N, Golub TR, et al. Tumor necrosis factor-alpha suppresses adipocyte-specific genes and activates expression of preadipocyte genes in 3T3-L1 adipocytes. Diabetes 2002;51:1319-1336
85. Hotamisligil GS, Arner P, Caro JF, et al. Increased adipose tissue expression of tumor necrosis factor-alpha in human obesity and insulin resistance. J Clin Invest 1995;95:2409-2415
86. Saghizadeh M, Ong JM, Barvey WT, et al. The expression of TNF-alpha by human muscle: relationship to insulin resistance. J Clin Invest 1996;97:1111-1116
87. Zinman B, Hanley AJG, Harris SB, et al. Circulating tumor necrosis factor-alpha concentrations in a native Canadian population with high rates of type 2 diabetes mellitus. J Clin Endocrinol Metab 1999;84:272-278
88. Stumvoll M, Haering H-U. Glitazones: clinical effects and molecular mechanisms. Ann Med 2002;34: 217-224
89. Hube F, Hauner H. The role of TNF-alpha in human adipose tissue: prevention of weight gain at the expense of insulin resistance? Horm Metab Res 1999; 31:626-631
90. Dietze P, Koenen M, Roehrig K, et al. Impairment of insulin signaling in human skeletal muscle cells by co-culture with human adipocytes. Diabetes 2002;51:2369-2376
91. Hotamisligil GS. The role of TNF and TNF receptors in obesity and insulin resistance. J Intern Med 1999;245: 621-625
92. Zhang HH, Halbleib M, Faiyaz A, et al. Tumor necrosis factor-alpha stimulates lipolysis in differentiated human adipocytes through activation of extracellular signal–related kinase and elevation of intracellular cAMP. Diabetes 2002;51:2929-2935
93. Ukkola O, Santaniemi M. Adiponectin: a link between excess adiposity and associated comorbidities? J Mol Med 2002;80:696-702
94. The Heart Outcomes Prevention Evaluation Study Investigators. Effects of an angiotensin-converting enzyme inhibitor, ramipril, on cardiovascular events in high-risk patients. N Engl J Med 2000;342:145-153
95. Lindholm LH, Ibsen H, Dahlof B, et al. Cardiovascular morbidity and mortality in patients with diabetes in the Losartan Intervention For Endpoint reduction in hypertension study (LIFE): a randomized trial against atenolol. Lancet 2002;359:1004-1010
96. Prasad A, Quyyumi AA. Renin-angiotensin system and angiotensin receptor blockers in the metabolic syndrome. Circulation 2004;110:1507-1512
97. Lim HS, MacFayen RJ, Lip GYH. Diabetes mellitus, the renin-angiotensin-aldosterone system, and the heart. Arch Intern Med 2004;164:1737-1748

98. Rao RH. Pressor doses of angiotensin II increase hepatic glucose output and decrease insulin sensitivity in rats. J Endocrinol 1996;148:311-318
99. Ushio-Fukai M, Hilenski L, Santanam N, et al. Cholesterol depletion inhibits epidermal growth factor receptor transactivation by angiotensin II in vascular smooth muscle cells: role of cholesterol-rich microdomains and focal adhesions in angiotensin II signaling. J Biol Chem 2001;276:48269-48275
100. Rakugi H, Kamide K, Ogihara T. Vascular signaling pathways in the metabolic syndrome. Curr Hypertens Rep 2002;4;105-111
101. Andreozzi F, Laratta E, Sciacqua A, et al. Angiotensin II impairs the insulin signaling pathway promoting production of nitric oxide by inducing phosphorylation of insulin receptor substrate-1 on Ser312 and Ser616 in human umbilical vein endothelial cells. Circ Res 2004;94:1211-1218
102. Fukuda N, Satoh C, Hu WY, et al. Endogenous angiotensin II suppresses insulin signaling in vascular smooth muscle cells from spontaneously hypertensive rats. J Hypertens 2001;19:1651-1658
103. Ogihara T, Asano T, Ando K, et al. Angiotensin II–induced insulin resistance is associated with enhanced insulin signaling. Hypertension 2002;40:872-879
104. Engeli S, Schling P, Gorzelniak K, et al. The adipose-tissue renin-angiotensin-aldosterone system: role in the metabolic syndrome? Int J Biochem Cell Biol 2003;35:807-825
105. Rocha R, Funder JW. The pathophysiology of aldosterone in the cardiovascular system. Ann N Y Acad Sci 2002;970:89-100
106. Rocha R, Rudolph AE, Frierdich GE, et al. Aldosterone induces a vascular inflammatory phenotype in the rat heart. Am J Physiol Heart Circ Physiol 2002;283: H1802-1810
107. Goodfriend TL, Egan BM, Kelley DE. Plasma aldosterone, plasma lipoproteins, obesity and insulin resistance in humans. Prostaglandins Leukot Essent Fatty Acids 1999;60:401-405
108. Haenni A, Reneland R, Lind L, Lithell H. Serum aldosterone changes during hyperinsulinemia are correlated to body mass index and insulin sensitivity in patients with essential hypertension. J Hypertens 2001;19:107-112
109. Goodfriend TL, Kelley DE, Goodpaster DH, et al. Visceral obesity and insulin resistance are associated with plasma aldosterone levels in women. Obes Res 1999;7:355-362
110. Widimsky J Jr, Strauch B, Sindelka G, Skrha J. Can primary hyperaldosteronism be considered as a specific form of diabetes mellitus? Physiol Res 2001;50:603-607
111. Sindelka G, Widimsky J, Haas T, et al. Insulin action in primary hyperaldosteronism before and after surgical or pharmacological treatment. Exp Clin Endocrinol Diabetes 2000;108:21-25
112. Turnbow MA, Keller SR, Rice KM, Garner CW. Dexamethasone down-regulation of insulin receptor substrate-1 in 3T3-L1 adipocytes. J Biol Chem 1994; 269:2516-2520
113. Giorgino F, Almahfouz A, Goodyear LJ, Smith RJ. Glucocorticoid regulation of insulin receptor and substrate IRS-1 tyrosine phosphorylation in rat skeletal muscle in vivo. J Clin Invest 1993;91:2020-2030
114. Dupont J, Derouet M, Simon J, Taouis M. Corticosterone alters insulin signaling in chicken muscle and liver at different steps. J Endocrinol 1999;162:67-76
115. Weinstein SP, Paquin T, Pritsker A, Haber RS. Glucocorticoid-induced insulin resistance: dexamethasone inhibits the activation of glucose transport in rat skeletal muscle by both insulin- and non–insulin-related stimuli. Diabetes 1995;44:441-445
116. Corry DB, Tuck ML. Selective aspects of the insulin resistance syndrome. Curr Opin Nephrol Hypertens 2001;10:507-514
117. Bjorntorp P. Metabolic implications of body fat distribution. Diabetes Care 1991;14:1132-1143
118. Divertie G, Jensen M, Miles J. Stimulation of lipolysis in humans by physiological hypercortisolemia. Diabetes 1991;40:1228-1232
119. Guillaume-Gentil C, Assimacopoulos-Jeannet F, Jeanrenaud B. Involvement of non-esterified fatty acid oxidation in glucocorticoid-induced peripheral insulin resistance in vivo in rats. Diabetologia 1993;36:899-906
120. Widmaier EP, Rosen K, Abbott B. Free fatty acids activate the hypothalamic-pituitary-adrenocortical axis in rats. Endocrinology 1992;131:2313-2318
121. Bethin KE, Vogt SK, Muglia LJ. Interleukin-6 is an essential, corticotropin-releasing hormone–independent stimulator of the adrenal axis during immune system activation. Proc Natl Acad Sci U S A 2000;97:9317-9322
122. Rask E, Olsson T, Soderberg S, et al. Tissue-specific dysregulation of cortisol metabolism in human obesity. J Clin Endocrinol Metab 2001;86:1418-1421
123. Hunt DG, Ivy JL. Epinephrine inhibits insulin-stimulated muscle glucose transport. J Appl Physiol 2002; 93:1638-1643
124. Yamauchi J, Hirasawa A, Miyamoto Y, et al. Role of Dbl's big sister in the anti-mitogenic pathway from alpha1B-adrenergic receptor to c-Jun N-terminal kinase. Biochem Biophys Res Commun 2002;296:85-92
125. Suematsu N, Satoh S, Kinugawa S, et al. Alpha1-adrenoceptor-Gq-RhoA signaling is upregulated to increase myofibrillar Ca^{2+} sensitivity in failing hearts Am J Physiol Heart Circ Physiol 2001;281: H637-H646
126. Sakurada S, Takuwa N, Sugimoto N, et al. Ca^{2+}-dependent activation of Rho and Rho kinase in membrane depolarization–induced and receptor stimulation–induced vascular smooth muscle contraction. Circ Res 2003;93:548-556
127. Delporte M-L, Funahashi T, Takahashi M, et al. Pre- and post-translational negative effect of beta-adrenoceptor agonists on adiponectin secretion: in vitro and in vivo studies. Biochem J 2002;367:677-685
128. Bjoerntorp P, Rosmond R. The metabolic syndrome—a neuroendocrine disorder? Br J Nutr 2000;83(suppl I): S49-S57
129. Trayhurn P, Beattie JH. Physiological role of adipose tissue: white adipose tissue as an endocrine and secretory organ. Proc Nutr Soc 2001:60:329-339
130. Moan A, Eide IK, Kjeldsen SE. Metabolic and adrenergic characteristics of young men with insulin resistance. Blood Pressure 1996;5(Suppl 1):30-37
131. Matsuzawa Y, Funahashi T, Nakamura T. Molecular mechanism of metabolic syndrome X: contribution of adipocytokines. Ann N Y Acad Sci 1999;892:146-154
132. Zimmet P, Boyko EJ, Collier GR, de Courten M. Etiology of the metabolic syndrome: potential role of insulin resistance, leptin resistance, and other players. Ann N Y Acad Sci 1999;892:25-44
133. Dulloo AG, Stock MJ, Solinas G, et al. Leptin directly stimulates thermogenesis in skeletal muscle. FEBS Lett 2002;515:109-113
134. Ceddia RB, William WN Jr, Curi R. The response of skeletal muscle to leptin. Front Biosci 2001;6:D90-D97
135. Steppan CM, Brown EJ, Wright CM, et al. A family of tissue-specific resistin-like molecules. Proc Natl Acad Sci U S A 2001;98:502-506

136. Yamauchi T, Kamon J, Waki H, et al. The fat-derived hormone adiponectin reverses insulin resistance associated with both lipoatrophy and obesity. Nat Med 2001;7:941-946
137. Tomas E, Tsao TS, Saha AK, et al. Enhanced muscle fat oxidation and glucose transport by ACRP30 globular domain: acetyl-CoA carboxylase inhibition and AMP-activated protein kinase activation. Proc Natl Acad Sci U S A 2002;99:16309-16313
138. Hotta K, Funahashi T, Arita Y, et al. Plasma concentrations of a novel, adipose-specific protein, adiponectin, in type 2 diabetic patients. Arterioscler Thromb Vasc Biol 2000;20:1595-1599
139. Parpal S, Karlsson M, Thorn H, Stralfors P. Cholesterol depletion disrupts caveolae and insulin receptor signaling for metabolic control via insulin receptor substrate-1, but not for mitogen-activated protein kinase control. J Biol Chem 2001;276:9670-9678
140. Le Lay S, Krief S, Farnier C, et al. Cholesterol, a cell size–dependent signal that regulates glucose metabolism and gene expression in adipocytes. J Biol Chem 2001;276:16904-16910
141. Cohen AW, Razani B, Wang XB, et al. Caveolin-1 deficient mice show post-prandial hyper-insulinemia, insulin resistance, and defective insulin receptor (IR-β) protein expression in adipose tissue. Am J Physiol Cell Physiol 2003;285:C222-C235
142. James DJ, Cairns F, Salt IP, et al. Skeletal muscle of stroke-prone spontaneously hypertensive rats exhibits reduced insulin-stimulated glucose transport and elevated levels of caveolin and flotillin. Diabetes 2001; 50:2148-2156
143. Razani B, Combs TP, Wang XB, et al. Caveolin-1–deficient mice are lean, resistant to diet-induced obesity, and show hypertriglyceridemia with adipocyte abnormalities. J Biol Chem 2002;277:8635-8647
144. Grigsby RJ, Dobrowsky RT. Inhibition of ceramide production reverses TNF-induced insulin resistance. Biochem Biophys Res Commun 2001;287:1121-1124
145. Boden G. Interaction between free fatty acids and glucose metabolism. Curr Opin Clin Nutr Metab Care 2002;5:545-549
146. Perseghin G, Ghosh S, Gerow K, Shulman GI. Metabolic defects in lean nondiabetic offspring of NIDDM parents: a cross-sectional study. Diabetes 1997;46:1001-1009
147. Zierath JR, Livingston JN, Thoerne A, et al. Regional difference in insulin inhibition of non-esterified fatty acid release from human adipocytes: relation to insulin receptor phosphorylation and intracellular signaling through the insulin receptor substrate-1 pathway. Diabetologia 1998;41:1343-1354
148. Bakker SJL, Ijzerman RG, Teerlink T, et al. Cytosolic triglycerides and oxidative stress in central obesity: the missing link between excessive atherosclerosis, endothelial dysfunction, and beta-cell failure? Atherosclerosis 2000;148:17-21
149. Sunayama S, Watanabe Y, Daida H, Yamaguchi H. Thiazolidinediones, dyslipidemia and insulin resistance syndrome. Curr Opin Lipidol 2000;11:397-402
150. Hsueh WA, Law R. The central role of fat and effect of peroxisome proliferator–activated receptor-gamma on progression of insulin resistance and cardiovascular disease. Am J Cardiol 2003;92(suppl):3J-9J
151. Petersen KF, Shulman GI. Pathogenesis of skeletal muscle insulin resistance in type 2 diabetes mellitus. Am J Cardiol 2002;90:11G-18G
152. Gielen S, Hambrecht R. The childhood obesity epidemic: impact on endothelial function. Circulation 2004;109:1911-1913
153. Taylor R. Causation of type 2 diabetes—the Gordian knot unravels. N Engl J Med 2004;350:639-641
154. Petersen KF, Dufour S, Befroy D, et al. Impaired mitochondrial activity in the insulin-resistant offspring of patients with type 2 diabetes. N Engl J Med 2004; 350:664-671
155. Ruderman NB, Saha AK, Kraegen EW. Minireview: malonyl CoA, AMP-activated protein kinase, and adiposity. Endocrinology 2003;144:5166-5171
156. Muoio DM, Way JM, Tanner CJ, et al. Peroxisome proliferator–activated receptor-alpha regulates fatty acid utilization in primary human skeletal muscle cells. Diabetes 2002;51:901-909
157. Russell AP, Feilchenfeldt J, Schreiber S, et al. Endurance training in humans leads to fiber type–specific increases in levels of peroxisome proliferator–activated receptor-gamma coactivator-1 and peroxisome proliferator–activated receptor-alpha in skeletal muscle. Diabetes 2003;52:2874-2881
158. Eaton S, Fukumoto K, Stefanutti G, et al. Myocardial carnitine palmitoyltransferase I as a target for oxidative modification in inflammation and sepsis. Biochem Soc Trans 2003;31:1133-1136
159. Memon RA, Feingold KR, Moser AH, et al. Regulation of fatty acid transport protein and fatty acid translocase mRNA levels by endotoxin and cytokines. Am J Physiol 1998;274:E210-E217
160. Nachiappan V, Curtiss D, Corkey BE, Kilpatrick L. Cytokines inhibit fatty acid oxidation in isolated rat hepatocytes: synergy among TNF, IL-6, and IL-1. Shock 1994;1:123-129
161. Memon RA, Bass NM, Moser AH, et al. Down-regulation of liver and heart specific fatty acid binding proteins by endotoxin and cytokines in vivo. Biochim Biophys Acta 1999;1440:118-126
162. Zhang Y, Pilon G, Marette A, Baracos VE. Cytokines and endotoxin induce cytokine receptors in skeletal muscle. Am J Physiol Endocrinol Metab 2000;279:E196-E205
163. Castro Cabezas M, Erkelens DW, van Dijk H. Free fatty acids: mediators of insulin resistance and atherosclerosis. Ned Tijdschr Geneeskd 2002;146:103-109
164. Thamer C, Machann J, Tschritter O, et al. Relationship between serum adiponectin concentration and intramyocellular lipid stores in humans. Horm Metab Res 2002;34:646-649
165. Havel PJ. Control of energy homeostasis and insulin action by adipocyte hormones: leptin, acylation stimulating protein, and adiponectin. Curr Opin Lipidol 2002;13:51-59
166. Ruderman NB, Dean D. Malonyl CoA, long chain fatty acyl CoA and insulin resistance in skeletal muscle. J Basic Clin Physiol Pharmacol 1998;9:295-308
167. Krssak M, Falk Petersen K, Dresner A, et al. Intramyocellular lipid concentrations are correlated with insulin sensitivity in humans: a ^{1}H NMR spectroscopy study. Diabetologia 1999;42:1-2
168. Ravussin E, Smith SR. Increased fat intake, impaired fat oxidation, and failure of fat cell proliferation result in ectopic fat storage, insulin resistance, and type 2 diabetes mellitus. Ann N Y Acad Sci 2002; 967:363-378
169. Frayn KN. Adipose tissue and the insulin resistance syndrome. Proc Nutr Soc 2001;60:375-380

170. Sinha R, Dufour S, Petersen KF, et al. Assessment of skeletal muscle triglyceride content by ^{1}H nuclear magnetic resonance spectroscopy in lean and obese adolescents: relationships to insulin insensitivity, total body fat, and central adiposity. Diabetes 2002; 51:1022-1027
171. Weiss R, Dufour S, Taksali SE, et al. Prediabetes in obese youth: a syndrome of impaired glucose tolerance, severe insulin resistance, and altered myocellular and abdominal fat partitioning. Lancet 2003;362:951-957
172. McGarry JD. Banting lecture 2001: dysregulation of fatty acid metabolism in the etiology of type 2 diabetes. Diabetes 2002;51:7-18
173. Colhoun HM. The big picture on obesity and insulin resistance. J Am Coll Cardiol 2002;40:944-945
174. Hegarty BD, Furler SM, Ye J, et al. The role of intramuscular lipid in insulin resistance. Acta Physiol Scand 2003;178:373-383
175. Pulawa LK, Eckel RH. Overexpression of muscle lipoprotein lipase and insulin sensitivity. Curr Opin Clin Nutr Metab Care 2002;5:569-574
176. Dresner A, Laurent D, Marcucci M, et al. Effects of free fatty acids on glucose transport and IRS-1–associated phosphatidylinositol 3-kinase activity. J Clin Invest 1999;103:253-259
177. Shulman GI. Cellular mechanisms of insulin resistance. J Clin Invest 2000;106:171-176
178. Griffin ME, Marcucci MJ, Cline GW, et al. Free fatty acid–induced insulin resistance is associated with activation of protein kinase C theta and alterations in the insulin signaling cascade. Diabetes 1999;48:1270-1274
179. Tooke JE, Hannemann MM. Adverse endothelial function and the insulin resistance syndrome. J Intern Med 2000;247:425-431
180. Vozarova B, Weyer C, Lindsay RS, et al. High white blood cell count is associated with a worsening of insulin sensitivity and predicts the development of type 2 diabetes. Diabetes 2002;51:455-461
181. Duplain H, Burcelin R, Sartori C, et al. Insulin resistance, hyperlipidemia, and hypertension in mice lacking endothelial nitric oxide synthase. Circulation 2001;104: 342-345
182. Zeng G, Nystrom FH, Ravichandran LV, et al. Roles for insulin receptor, PI3-kinase, and Akt in insulin-signaling pathways related to production of nitric oxide in human vascular endothelial cells. Circulation 2000;101:1539-1545
183. Schnyder B, Pittet M, Durand J, Schnyder-Candrian S. Rapid effects of glucose on the insulin signaling of endothelial NO generation and epithelial Na transport. Am J Physiol Endocrinol Metab 2001;282:E87-E94

Section III

Targets and Causes of Insulin Resistance

The Endothelium and Nitric Oxide

8

The endothelium comprises a monolayer of cells covering the basement membrane of all blood vessels. **Its strategic, anatomic position renders the endothelium an important, active barrier between circulating blood, the vessel wall, and subjacent tissues. As such, vascular endothelial cells are critical participants in the biologic reaction to stressful, infectious, or inflammatory stimuli.** As a result, they are intimately involved in the development of inflammation-mediated vascular and tissue injury.

The vascular endothelium plays a pivotal role in the regulation of blood flow, coagulation, and inflammation in the vessel wall. Dysfunction of the endothelium is the initial step in cardiovascular pathology. **Abnormal endothelial function is caused by insulin resistance and underlies**

the vascular disease of the metabolic syndrome and type 2 diabetes mellitus (DM). On the other hand, loss of endothelial functional integrity contributes to the genesis of impaired insulin signaling.

ENDOTHELIAL FUNCTION

The endothelium exerts a multiplicity of autocrine, paracrine, and endocrine functions that are critical for the maintenance of normal vascular physiology. When disturbed, the ensuing dysfunction of the endothelium contributes importantly to the vascular disease process.

Control of Vascular Structure and Function. The endothelium plays a major role in vascular biology by regulating and protecting normal vascular function and structure (Table 8-1). Specifically, the endothelium

- regulates vascular tone through a balance between its vasodilatory substances, such as
  - prostacyclin,
  - C-type natriuretic peptide,
  - endothelium-derived hyperpolarizing relaxing factor,
  - bradykinin, and
  - nitric oxide (NO),

  and vasoconstrictor substances, such as
  - endothelin-1 (ET-1),
  - angiotensin II,
  - vasoconstrictor prostaglandins, and
  - reactive oxygen species (ROS);
- balances thrombogenesis and thrombolysis by regulating
  - platelet activity,
  - the clotting cascade, and
  - the fibrinolytic system;
- modulates the inflammatory response through its capacity to produce substances that regulate and direct the inflammatory process, such as
  - cytokines and
  - adhesion molecules; and
- controls and modulates vascular remodeling by regulating
  - vascular permeability,
  - matrix protein synthesis, and
  - cell growth.[1]

Table 8-1. Endothelial Cell Functions, Action Site, and Mediators

Lumen	**Vasoconstriction** Endothelin-1 Angiotensin II Thromboxane A_2 Prostaglandin H_2	**Vasodilation** Nitric oxide Bradykinin Hyperpolarizing factor Prostacyclin
Growth	**Stimulation** Platelet-derived growth factor Fibroblast-derived growth factor Endothelin-1 Insulin-like growth factor-I Angiotensin II	**Inhibition** Nitric oxide Prostaglandin I_2 Transforming growth factor
Inflammation	**Proinflammatory** Adhesion molecules Monocyte chemotactic factor-1 Interleukins 1, 6, 18 Tumor necrosis factor-alpha	**Anti-inflammatory** Nitric oxide
Hemostasis	**Prothrombotic** Plasminogen activator inhibitor-1 Tissue factor Thrombomodulin von Willebrand factor Prostaglandins	**Antithrombotic** Prostaglandin I_2 Tissue plasminogen activator Nitric oxide Heparins Prostaglandins

Endothelial Function and Vascular Disease. Normal endothelial function entails the maintenance of normal vascular tone and blood fluidity, with minimal or no expression of proinflammatory factors, and a balance of atherogenic and antiatherogenic, thrombotic, and fibrinolytic opposing factors. **Intact vascular function, particularly at the level of the endothelium, correlates with the prevention or delay of cardiovascular disease.**[1]

FUNCTIONS OF NITRIC OXIDE

The availability of NO is a key marker of endothelial function. NO was originally termed endothelium-derived relaxing factor. It was voted the molecule of the year by *Science Magazine* in 1992.[2] A low-molecular-weight, highly lipophilic molecule, NO can rapidly diffuse into neighboring cells. NO is a potent cell-signaling effector and vasodilator molecule in the cardiovascular system. It importantly modulates vascular and autonomic neuronal tone, thrombogenesis, inflammation, oxidant stress, and metabolism in the heart and vasculature, in muscle and neuronal tissues, in the kidney, and in many other tissues.[3]

Vasodilation. NO is the most potent endogenous vasodilator known. It functions via a cyclic guanosine 3′,5′-monophosphate (cGMP)-mediated mechanism.

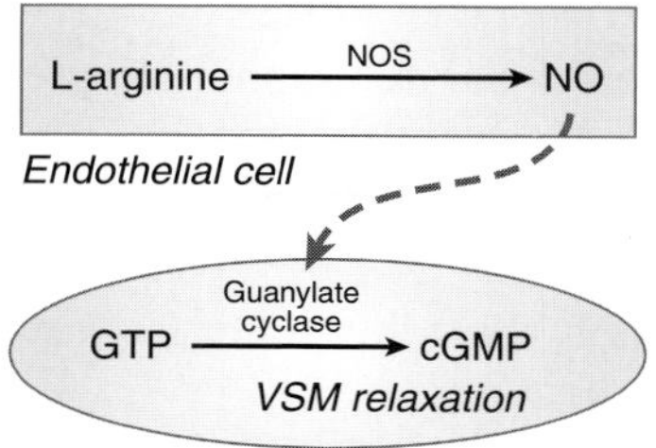

Figure 8–1.
Endothelial cell nitric oxide (NO) production as regulator of vascular smooth muscle (VSM) relaxation. c-GMP, cyclic guanosine 3′,5′-monophosphate; GTP, guanosine triphosphate; NOS, nitric oxide synthase. *(Modified from Calles-Escandon J, Cipolla M. Diabetes and endothelial dysfunction: a clinical perspective. Endocr Rev 2001:22:36-52.)*

cGMP. NO binds to and stimulates soluble guanylate cyclase in an autocrine fashion within the endothelium and in a paracrine fashion in subjacent vascular smooth muscle cells (Fig. 8-1). Activated guanylate cyclase produces cGMP from guanosine 5′-triphosphate (GTP). The amount of cGMP generated is proportional to the amount of NO. NO/cGMP activates cGMP-dependent protein kinases (cGKs) as downstream effectors.[4]

NO/cGMP/cGK pathways accomplish vasodilation by further increasing NO production and by mediating vascular smooth muscle relaxation.

Nitric Oxide Production. In endothelial cells, NO/cGMP/cGK, in positive feedback, enhances NO production via several mechanisms. cGK

- activates endothelial nitric oxide synthase (eNOS) via phosphorylation,
- may in some cases modulate the calcium (Ca^{2+}) dependence of eNOS, and
- phosphorylates and activates 6-pyruvoyltetrahydropterin synthase to produce the tetrahydrobiopterin (BH_4) needed by nitric oxide synthase (NOS) for NO synthesis.[4]

Smooth Muscle Relaxation. The NO/cGMP/cGK-induced relaxation of smooth muscle cells causes

- **dilation of blood vessels and**
- **a lowering of blood pressure.**[5]

As a result, NO is a critical modulator of blood flow and blood pressure. It plays an important role in flow-mediated vasodilation and opposes the vasoconstrictor effects of norepinephrine, ET-1, angiotensin II, and serotonin.[6]

In vascular smooth muscle cells, cGK mediates smooth muscle relaxation via two mechanisms:

1. cGK lowers cytoplasmic Ca^{2+} concentrations.[5]
2. cGK reduces myofibrillar Ca^{2+} sensitivity. The NO/cGMP cascade desensitizes smooth muscle to Ca^{2+} by enhancing myosin-bound phosphatase activity.

Increased activity of myosin phosphatase decreases the degree of myosin light chain phosphorylation, thus lessening smooth muscle contraction at any given level of cytoplasmic Ca^{2+}, consistent with Ca^{2+} desensitization of the myofilaments.

Rho kinase phosphorylates myosin light chain phosphatase, thereby inhibiting its activity. In addition, Rho kinase activates an inhibitor of myosin phosphatase.

The NO/cGMP/cGK signaling pathway inactivates RhoA by phosphorylation and impaired isoprenylation. As a result, Rho kinase activation is suppressed. cGK thus prevents the inhibition of myosin phosphatase by blocking RhoA.[4,7]

Inhibition of Platelet Activation. NO/cGMP/cGK inhibits platelet

- **activation,**
- **aggregation, and**
- **adhesion to the endothelium.**

Platelet cGK, but not endothelial or smooth muscle cGK, is essential to prevent intravascular adhesion and aggregation of platelets. NO/cGMP/cGK causes phosphorylation of the platelet substrate protein VASP, which correlates with blockade of platelet activation via inhibition of the fibrinogen receptor (integrin GPIIb/IIIa). NO/cGMP signaling through cGK also inhibits platelet G_q/G_i-coupled receptor responses and the platelet adenosine 5′-diphosphate (ADP) receptor P2Y12.[4]

Antioxidant Activities. NO may function as an antioxidant.

The decrease in ROS levels by NO attenuates the activity of extracellular signal–regulated kinase (ERK1/ERK2). NO negatively regulates the Ras/Raf/ERK signaling pathway and gene expression by inhibiting early growth response-1 (Egr-1) expression.[8]

NO increases the antioxidant potential, lowers lipoprotein oxidation, and decreases the production of ROS:

- NO increases expression of the antioxidant extracellular superoxide dismutase (SOD) in vascular smooth muscle in a cGMP-dependent fashion.[9]
- NO inhibits low-density lipoprotein (LDL) oxidation.[10]
- NO inhibits the production of ROS by decreasing the activity of Rac-dependent endothelial nicotinamide adenine dinucleotide phosphate (NADH/NADPH) oxidase. The inhibitory effect of NO is not mediated by cGMP. In the process, NO may
  - reduce superoxide production via direct interaction with NADH/NADPH oxidase,
  - inactivate NADH/NADPH oxidase by inhibiting its assembling process, or
  - reduce NADH/NADPH oxidase activity via inhibition of protein kinase C (PKC).[8]

Anti-inflammatory and Antiatherogenic Activities. Endothelial NO is a potent anti-inflammatory agent that interferes with both the early and the later stages of atherogenesis.[8]

NO protects blood vessels from endogenous injury by mediating molecular signals that prevent inflammatory cytokine activation, platelet and leukocyte interaction with the vascular wall, endothelial cell apoptosis, and vascular smooth muscle cell proliferation and migration.[11-13] NO

- inhibits the transcription of nuclear factor kappaB (NFκB);
- modulates and inhibits redox-sensitive gene expression, including cytokine-induced
  - vascular cell adhesion molecule-1 (VCAM-1),
  - intercellular adhesion molecule-1 (ICAM-1), and
  - monocyte chemoattractant protein-1 (MCP-1);[9]
- prevents the adhesion of leukocytes to the endothelium;
- interferes with leukocyte migration into the vascular wall by decreasing the expression of a multiplicity of factors, including the surface adhesion molecules
  - CD11/CD18 and
  - P-selectin;
- decreases endothelial permeability, thereby reducing the influx of oxidized lipoproteins into the vascular wall[10];

- thwarts vascular smooth muscle cell proliferation by inhibiting
  - DNA synthesis and
  - mitogenesis;
- blocks smooth muscle cell migration;
- inhibits the synthesis and secretion of extracellular matrix proteinases that degrade extracellular matrix proteins such as
  - matrix metalloproteinase-2 (MMP-2) and
  - MMP-9; and
- increases the expression of tissue inhibitor of matrix metalloproteinases (TIMP).[10]

Parasympathetic Input. Endogenous NO has been implicated in the modulation of parasympathetic input to the heart at both the presynaptic and postsynaptic levels. Defective cardiac NOS may participate in the loss of heart rate variability in the high-frequency band reflecting parasympathetic activity.[14]

Glucose Uptake. NO stimulates glucose uptake through a mechanism that is distinct from both the insulin and muscle contraction signaling pathways.[15]

Insulin Sensitivity. NO improves insulin sensitivity via direct and indirect mechanisms:

- NO indirectly improves insulin signaling by enhancing nutritive, microvascular blood flow and by its antioxidant and anti-inflammatory actions.
- The NO/cGMP/cGK signaling pathway directly improves insulin sensitivity by interfering with the small GTPase Rho/Rho kinase. Rho kinase impairs insulin signaling through its association with the insulin receptor substrate-1 (IRS-1). Specifically, cGK inactivates RhoA directly by increasing RhoA phosphorylation, and it prevents Rho kinase activation by impairing RhoA isoprenylation. By inhibiting the Rho kinase/IRS-1 association, cGK enhances insulin signaling.[7]

NITRIC OXIDE SYNTHASE

NO is produced in a variety of tissues from L-arginine by the dioxygenase enzyme NOS, which closely resembles cytochrome P-450.[16] **Three distinct isoforms of NOS elaborate NO:**

1. **neuronal NOS-1 (nNOS),**
2. **inducible NOS-2 (iNOS), and**
3. **endothelial NOS-3 (eNOS).**

The three NOS enzymes have 50% homology, indicative of a common derivation. However, each NOS isoform is transcribed from a separate gene.[3] NO is produced in a variety of tissues through the activation of different isoforms of NOS. Dimerization of the NOS isozymes is required for their activity.[17]

Endothelial Nitric Oxide Synthase. Chromosome number 7 contains the gene that encodes the transcription and synthesis of the 1203–amino acid enzyme eNOS.[3] **eNOS is the rate-limiting enzyme responsible for the production of endothelial-derived NO. It is a constitutive isoform of NOS and continuously elaborates NO.** eNOS is expressed in

- vascular endothelium,
- endocardial endothelium,
- atrial cardiac myocytes,
- ventricular myocytes,
- smooth muscle cells,
- airway epithelium,
- platelets,
- male and female reproductive tracts,
- the brain, and
- certain other cell types.[16,18,19]

eNOS plays a major role in the regulation of vascular tone.

Caveolae and eNOS. Caveolae are small invaginations of the plasma membrane expressed in many differentiated eukaryotic cells. They may occupy up to 30% of the cell surface in capillary endothelial cells and contain the scaffolding protein caveolin. Golgi-localized eNOS associates with nascent caveolae[20] such that **in endothelial cells caveolae are enriched in eNOS. Caveolin binds directly to eNOS in caveolae and maintains the enzyme in an inactive configuration.**[21,22]

eNOS Association with Caveolae. Although the mechanisms that target proteins to caveolae and organize their signaling activities are not known, the lipid environment of the caveolar membrane plays an essential role.

Many cell surface proteins associate with the exoplasmic leaflet of the caveolar membrane bilayer by means of a glycosylphosphatidylinositol (GPI) anchor. However, transmembrane and intracellular signaling proteins such as eNOS are targeted to the inner, cytoplasmic leaflet of the caveolae membrane bilayer differently, specifically by covalent acylation with fatty acyl moieties such as

- myristate,
- palmitate, and
- isoprenyl groups,

and their acylation sites are essential for the interaction.[23]

These lipophilic acyl groups, under physiologic conditions, target the acylated proteins to the lipid cytoplasmic leaflet of the caveolar membrane bilayer. The high packing order of these saturated myristoyl and palmitoyl moieties facilitates their interactions with membrane liquid-ordered subdomains. **The localization of proteins such as eNOS to the cytoplasmic aspect of caveolae is important for their appropriate function in cell signaling.**[24]

Myristoylation and Palmitoylation. Proteins such as eNOS are targeted to the cytoplasmic aspect of caveolae via covalent acylation, specifically myristoylation and palmitoylation.

Myristoylation, or fatty acyl substitution of the N-terminal amino group of proteins such as eNOS via amide bondage with myristoyl residues, occurs cotranslationally and is irreversible. However, for attachment to the plasma membrane and localization in the membrane lipid domains, proteins such as eNOS require at least a second, post-translational fatty acyl substitution on cysteines, usually with palmitoyl residues, termed palmitoylation. Protein *S*-acylation prefers, but is not restricted to, palmitoyl moieties. Therefore, other saturated and even unsaturated fatty acyl moieties may be linked to cysteine residues of proteins. This protein *S*-acylation is reversible and further regulates the subcellular localization of proteins such as eNOS.[24]

ENDOTHELIAL NITRIC OXIDE SYNTHESIS

The enzymatic production of NO from eNOS is significantly affected by basic primary considerations such as enzyme

- **abundance,**
- **subcellular localization, and**
- **substrate and cofactor availability.**

eNOS activity is also regulated by dimerization of enzyme subunits.[25,26]

eNOS Abundance. eNOS abundance is regulated via transcriptional and post-translational controls in that it is affected by gene transcription, as well as by mRNA and protein stability.[25,26] An increase in eNOS expression is probably mediated via activation of stimulus-responsive elements in the promoter region of the eNOS gene or via stabilization of eNOS mRNA.[27]

Whereas eNOS activity can be rapidly modulated by stimuli that phosphorylate the eNOS enzyme, eNOS expression is affected more slowly and chronically by signals that modify its gene transcriptional activity, such as

- transforming growth factor-β (TGF-β),
- estradiol,
- insulin,
- fluid shear stress, and
- 3-hydroxy-3-methylglutaryl (HMG) coenzyme A (CoA) reductase inhibitors.[27]

Intracellular Translocation. eNOS is preferentially membrane bound, associated with Golgi membranes or with plasmalemmal caveolae, where it is quantitatively associated with caveolin. Cotranslational and post-translational processing leads to trafficking of the enzyme to the plasma membrane.[5]

Translocation of eNOS to different subcellular sites is an important regulator of NO production. In fact, dynamic cycling of eNOS from Golgi to the plasma membrane may play a role in regulating eNOS activity.[28,29] It is determined in a dynamic fashion by multiple mechanisms:

1. cotranslational *N*-myristoylation is required for eNOS membrane association and Golgi binding,
2. post-translational palmitoylation is needed for eNOS localization to caveolae, and
3. the presence of a caveolin binding domain on eNOS allows the enzyme to interact with the caveolin scaffolding domain.

Caveolin binding, together with the dual eNOS acylation by myristate and palmitate, assists in targeting this enzyme to the caveolae. A caveolar location is necessary for eNOS activation by agonists such as carbachol.[28,29]

L-Arginine. Optimal function of eNOS is dependent on the availability of L-arginine, an essential amino acid, as natural substrate for eNOS. NO is produced by eNOS through five-electron oxidation of the guanidine nitrogen terminal of its substrate L-arginine.

In the process, there is a flow of electrons from the reductase to the oxygenase domain of eNOS. For all isoforms, an electron donor, NADH/NADPH, binds to a site at the carboxyl terminus of eNOS. Electrons are transferred from NADPH to flavins bound within the eNOS reductase domain. With enzyme activation, electrons are transferred to a heme group in the oxygenase domain. Upon heme reduction, L-arginine is catalyzed to citrulline and NO.[5]

Endothelial plasmalemmal caveolae provide a mechanism for highly efficient substrate delivery to eNOS and allow the regulation of NO production by L-arginine delivery. Within caveolae, eNOS colocalizes with caveolin-1 and is complexed with the cationic amino acid-1 (CAT-1) transporter for L-arginine.[30]

Tetrahydrobiopterin. For optimal synthetic function, eNOS also requires the availability of intracellular cofactors such as flavonoids and BH_4.

BH_4 is synthesized by the rate-limiting action of GTP cyclohydrolase.[31] It is the necessary cofactor for coupling L-arginine to the eNOS enzyme for L-arginine to be oxidized to NO and L-citrulline. BH_4 mediates the transfer of electrons from the eNOS heme group to L-arginine.[9]

REGULATION OF NITRIC OXIDE SYNTHESIS

Because of the high biologic reactivity and diffusibility of NO, there are multiple tiers of secondary regulation for NO biosynthesis that modulate the output of eNOS enzymatic activity.

Activation of eNOS enzymatic activity is brought about by two basic mechanisms:

1. the short-term, calcium-calmodulin–dependent stimulation of eNOS and
2. the prolonged, calcium-calmodulin–independent activation of eNOS.

Calcium-Mediated eNOS Activation. Classic eNOS activation occurs via the first Ca^{2+}-calmodulin–dependent pathway, in which eNOS produces NO in response to a variety of agonists[26,28] such as

- acetylcholine,
- adenosine nucleotides such as ADP,
- thrombin,
- A23187,
- histamine, and
- bradykinin,

which stimulate NO synthesis through receptor-operated mechanisms and serine phosphorylation.[32]

Ca^{2+}-Calmodulin. Cytoplasmic Ca^{2+} levels regulate eNOS activity. The inhibitory association of eNOS with caveolin, the resident, scaffolding protein of caveolae, decreases in reciprocal fashion as a function of cytoplasmic Ca^{2+} levels.

In the resting state, caveolin, complexed to eNOS, inhibits enzymatic activity. The inhibitory effect of caveolin on eNOS is reversed via receptor agonist–mediated, transient increases in cytoplasmic Ca^{2+}. Consequent to receptor activation, there is G protein–dependent activation of phospholipase C with stimulation of downstream Ca^{2+}-mobilizing pathways. As cytoplasmic Ca^{2+} levels rise, Ca^{2+} complexes with calmodulin, and the rise in the cytoplasmic Ca^{2+} transient initiates a regulatory cycle: the Ca^{2+}/calmodulin complex disrupts the heteromeric eNOS/caveolin association by displacing caveolin from eNOS. eNOS is thus disinhibited, and its enzymatic activity is stimulated to produce NO.[21,33] Thereafter, activated caveolin-free eNOS translocates from the caveolar membrane and is then probably desensitized. As cytoplasmic Ca^{2+} levels return to baseline, Ca^{2+} dissociates from calmodulin, thus releasing the Ca^{2+}/calmodulin complex from eNOS and allowing caveolin to displace calmodulin. Upon reassociation of eNOS with caveolin, the synthase is inactivated. The inhibitory, heteromeric eNOS/caveolin complex is then restored to the caveolae, a process facilitated by eNOS palmitoylation.[29]

eNOS Phosphorylation. Although eNOS activity may be coupled to changes in endothelial cell Ca^{2+} levels, eNOS activation is also dependent on enzyme phosphorylation and dephosphorylation. The phosphorylation status of two amino acid residues seems to be particularly important in regulating eNOS activity:

1. a serine residue in the reductase domain (human Ser1177 = bovine Ser1179) and
2. a threonine residue (Thr495) located within the calmodulin binding domain.

NO release from endothelial cells occurs after eNOS activation via phosphorylation of eNOS at the Ser1177 site. Increased phosphorylation of that site correlates with greater activation of eNOS and higher NO release.[3] Stimulus-induced eNOS activation by phosphorylation of Ser1177 and dephosphorylation of Thr495 is regulated by a number of kinases and phosphatases that continuously associate with and dissociate from the eNOS signaling complex.[34]

eNOS Phosphorylation Sites. There are actually at least five potential eNOS phosphorylation sites.[27] Such residues on eNOS undergo phosphorylation by kinases to activate or inactivate eNOS, and some residues may undergo phosphorylation by more than one kinase.[21] Phosphorylation of

- Ser617,
- Ser633 (bovine Ser635), and
- Ser1177(bovine Ser1179)

promotes enzyme activity. Phosphorylation of

- Ser116 and
- Thr495

inhibits eNOS enzymatic activity. Shear stress appears to phosphorylate Ser633 with a slower kinetic than is the case with Ser1177.[25]

Protein Kinases. Several protein kinases have been implicated in eNOS regulation through the phosphorylation of Ser1177 or other residues, including

- phosphatidylinositol 3-kinase (PI3K) via protein kinase B (PKB)/Akt,
- calmodulin-dependent kinase,
- 5′-adenosine monophosphate (AMP)-activated protein kinase (AMPK),
- mitogen-activated protein kinase (MAPK),
- PKC,
- cyclic AMP–dependent protein kinase, and
- cGK.[25]

A variety of stimuli regulate eNOS activity through signaling pathways involving Akt kinase or MAPK, or both.

Calcium-Independent eNOS Activation. There are calcium-independent activation pathways for eNOS that are mediated by PKB/Akt kinase or ceramide. Just as the inhibitory conformation of eNOS can be reversed by an increase in cytoplasmic Ca^{2+}, it can also be reversed, for example, by Akt-induced phosphorylation of eNOS.[20] **Calcium-independent activation of eNOS, in contrast to short-term, calcium-mediated stimulation of eNOS, has a prolonged effect.**[27]

PKB/Akt Kinase. Induction and phosphorylation of the serine/threonine kinase PKB/Akt occur via activation of PI3K. PKB/Akt, in turn, phosphorylates eNOS at the amino acid residue Ser1177 to effect enzyme activation and enhanced NO production.[27]

Endothelial PKB/Akt can be activated by

- fluid shear stress,
- insulin,
- insulin-like growth factor type I (IGF-I), and
- vascular endothelial growth factor (VEGF).

In contrast to the transient agonist-mediated Ser1177 phosphorylation, shear stress–induced phosphorylation of eNOS is sustained.[3,25]

In addition to its control of vascular tone, PKB/Akt serves as a multifunctional regulator of

- endothelial cell survival,
- angiogenesis mediated by VGEF, and
- glucose metabolism.[35]

Protein-Protein Interactions within Caveolae as Modulators of eNOS Activity. In addition to its regulation via Ca^{2+}/calmodulin and phosphorylation, eNOS activity is also controlled by protein-protein interactions.[25,26]

As a component of caveolae, eNOS may transiently interact with caveolar proteins other than caveolin. Such protein-protein interactions also affect its activity, spatial distribution, and proximity to regulatory proteins or intended targets.[17,36] **Caveola-targeted proteins may thus be implicated in modulating eNOS activity.**[21,22] The caveolar compartmentalization spatially facilitates the regulation of eNOS by vasoactive agonists:

1. the enzyme's interactions with caveolin tonically repress basal eNOS activity,
2. vasodilatory agonist stimulation efficiently activates eNOS,[37] and
3. vasoconstrictors effectively impair eNOS activity.

Specifically, several resident and recruited proteins of plasmalemmal caveolae, ranging from scaffolding proteins to membrane receptors, function as eNOS binding partners and may affect its activity. Thus,

- calmodulin,
- caveolins,
- anchoring proteins,
- the bradykinin B2 receptor,
- certain steroid hormone receptors,
- lipoprotein receptors,[21,22]
- G protein–coupled receptors such as the angiotensin II type 1 (AT_1) receptor,
- kinases,
- the CAT-1 arginine transporter,
- argininosuccinate synthase,
- argininosuccinate lyase,
- heat shock protein 90 (Hsp 90),
- Raf-1,
- PKB/Akt,
- ERK,
- eNOS interacting protein,
- eNOS traffic inducer,
- unidentified tyrosine-phosphorylated proteins, and
- molecular chaperones

all modulate the activity and trafficking of eNOS in the endothelium.[17,36,38] **Because caveola formation and eNOS subcellular localization are dynamically regulated, pathologic states may ensue upon disruption of eNOS-caveolae interactions.**

SPECIFIC ENHANCERS OF NITRIC OXIDE SYNTHESIS

Numerous specific physiologic stimuli have a positive impact on NO synthesis. Shear stress is the most important modulator of NO production. Peroxisome proliferator–activated receptor (PPAR) agonists, estrogen, muscarinic agonists, bradykinin, high-density lipoprotein (HDL), and insulin also positively affect NO elaboration.

Shear Stress. Local rheologic forces influence endothelial phenotype and ultimately atherogenesis. Arterial flow patterns, vascular compliance, and pulse pressure have complex, interacting effects on endothelial cell function.

One of the most physiologically important stimuli for NO release is laminar shear stress, the tangential dragging force exerted by fluid flow over the endothelial surface.

In the vascular bed, numerous tissue-derived physicochemical stimuli such as adenosine, acidity, higher temperature, PO_2, PCO_2, and magnesium and potassium ions cause dilation of resistance vessels. Vasodilation of resistance vessels creates a pressure gradient that stimulates increased blood flow. **Fluid shear stress is determined by blood flow and viscosity** and stimulates NO release from the vascular endothelium. As NO diffuses to the underlying vascular smooth muscle cells, it activates guanylate cyclase to produce cGMP from GTP for smooth muscle relaxation and further vasodilation.[16]

Fluid Shear Stress Sensors. Vascular endothelial caveolae, anchored by the actin cytoskeleton, may function as flow sensors

and convert external mechanical stimuli into chemical signals for the cell. Cultured endothelial cells respond to changes in the flow environment by modulating

- caveolin expression,
- caveolin distribution,
- caveolar density, and
- mechanosensitivity to subsequent changes in hemodynamic forces.

Caveolin. With laminar flow, the expression of caveolin-1 increases, and there is a greater number of caveolin-1 molecules in the cells.[39] Caveolin-1 translocates from the Golgi to the luminal plasma membrane. In cultured endothelial cells exposed to laminar flow, the highest concentration of caveolin-1 distribution was found at the upstream side of the cell body, where the hydrostatic pressure and the spatial gradient of shear stress were at a maximum.[40]

Caveolae. The number of invaginated caveolae is dynamically controlled by shear stress, and shear stress may be a major determinant of the density of invaginated caveolae. Prolonged exposure to shear stress significantly increases the number of caveolae, probably because of the increased caveolin-1 presence in the luminal plasma membrane.[41]

Caveolar-Based Mechanosensors. Potential caveolar-based mechanosensors that sense shear stress may be

- the caveolar structure itself,
- G protein–coupled receptors,
- G proteins,
- integrin interaction with the cytoskeleton, and
- ion channels,

all of which interact with caveolin-1. The shear stress–sensitive signaling molecules are assembled in caveolae by binding to the scaffolding domain of caveolin-1 in the inactive state. Changes in shear stress level trigger rapid, organized, and compartmentalized signaling cascades to activate ERK pathways.[42]

Biochemical Responses to Flow. The different shear regimens (laminar, turbulent, step, and gradual changes) induce distinct responses over differing time courses from the endothelium. Vascular endothelial cells respond to shear stress both acutely and chronically by producing autocrine and paracrine factors. Endothelial responses to shear stress encompass

- alterations in gene expression,
- activation of MAPK, and
- modulation of NO release.[41]

Gene Expression. Shear stress–induced endothelial responses control vascular tone, vessel wall remodeling, leukocyte binding to the endothelium, and hemostasis. Shear stress transiently activates NFκB, immediate early response genes, and transcription factors that are probably involved in the regulation of shear stress–dependent gene expression. A shear stress response element with the core sequence GAGACC has been identified in many shear-sensitive genes,[43] including those for

- platelet-derived growth factor B (PDGF-B),
- ICAM-1,
- tissue plasminogen activator (tPA), and
- TGF-1,

thus suggesting a significant role for shear stress–dependent gene regulation.[41]

Activation of MAPK. Some of the shear stress impact on nuclear responses and shear-stimulated gene expression appears to be mediated through regulation of MAPK. Members of the MAPK family,

- ERK1/ERK2,
- c-Jun NH_2-terminal kinase (JNK) (also known as stress-activated protein kinase [SAPK]), and
- p38 kinase,

are important signaling components linking extracellular stimuli to cellular responses such as cell growth, differentiation, metabolic regulation, and death.

Shear stress differentially regulates activation of ERK and JNK via different time constants and two separate signaling pathways that depend on different heterotrimeric G proteins.

1. ERK: Shear stress rapidly and transiently activates ERK in the cholesterol-enriched

cytoplasmic aspect of caveolae. Upstream signaling molecules for ERK are

- PKC,
- Src,
- focal adhesion kinase (FAK), and
- Ras.

ERK activation becomes blunted in shear stress–preconditioned cells.[40]

2. JNK: Shear stress slowly activates JNK. Upstream regulators for the shear-dependent activation of JNK are
   - PI3K,
   - Src,
   - FAK, and
   - Ras.

The differential activation of ERK and JNK, involving the common signaling molecules Src, FAK, and Ras, requires spatial or temporal compartmentalization of signaling (or both) within caveolar-like domains.[41]

Nitric Oxide Release. Laminar shear stress increases the production of NO. As a result,

- **acute increases in arterial flow stimulate the release of NO** and other endothelium-derived relaxing factors to dilate the blood vessel and reduce shear stress toward normal;
- **chronic increases in arterial flow enhance the expression of eNOS** and engender changes in endothelial cell shape, cell alignment, vessel structure, and vessel size, with new vessel growth via angiogenesis; and
- **repetitive short-term increases in flow exert a beneficial effect akin to chronic, sustained increases and underlie the beneficial effects of physical exercise on coronary and peripheral arteries.**[44]

Increased laminar shear stress releases NO by increasing eNOS activity and expression:

1. eNOS activity. With exposure to laminar flow, phosphorylated caveolin-1 and eNOS proteins are preferentially localized to caveolar microdomains. Activation of the shear-sensitive signaling molecule Akt is accelerated with chronic shear exposure and preconditioning. Shear stress significantly increases Ser1179 phosphorylation of eNOS over no-flow controls.[40,45]
2. eNOS expression. Shear stress enhances eNOS expression. One of the earliest signaling events in response to laminar shear in the endothelium is activation of tyrosine kinases. The tyrosine kinase c-Src is activated within seconds after the onset of shear and in turn phosphorylates the tyrosine kinase Flk-1. Shear activation of c-Src leads to increased eNOS expression in response to shear via two divergent pathways, one leading to an early, transient increased eNOS expression and a second leading to prolonged stabilization of the eNOS message:
   - c-Src activation of Ras/Raf and ERK1/ERK2 increases the eNOS transcription rate.
   - Another pathway dependent on c-Src, but independent of Ras/Raf/ERK, increases the half-life of eNOS mRNA. Enhanced eNOS mRNA stability in response to shear is critical for the sustained expression of eNOS in response to shear stress.[43]

Shear-Type Determinants of Endothelial Response. Although the entire arterial tree is exposed to identical systemic risk factors, **early atherosclerosis develops in curved and branched arterial regions, which are associated with disturbed or low shear stress conditions (or with both).**[44] **In contrast, laminar shear stress appears to exert atheroprotective effects in vivo inasmuch as vascular segments with steady laminar flow and physiologic shear stress are protected from atherosclerosis.**[44]

Different rheologic characteristics of blood flow have distinct effects on endothelial function. The physiologically most important determinants for the continuous generation of NO, and thus for the regulation of local blood flow, are fluid shear stress and pulsatile stretch.[34]

Preservation of Endothelial Function. In general, endothelial function is preserved with

- laminar shear stress with steady laminar flow at approximately 12 dyne/cm^2 on the endothelium and
- oscillatory flow that remains unidirectional,

both of which elicit multiple synergistic mechanisms to enhance NO production.[46,47] Even mechanically mediated increased fluid shear stress appears to improve endothelial function,[48] which translates into atheroprotective effects.

Perturbation of Endothelial Function. Endothelial cell function is disturbed with

- stasis,
- low net flow,
- low shear stress at approximately 0.4 dyne/cm^2,
- turbulent flow,
- local shear gradients,
- rapidly changing flow, and
- oscillatory flow with flow reversal,

all of which may increase NFκB activation and oxidative stress and promote atherogenesis.[46,47] Additionally, **decreased compliance of the arterial wall and higher pulse pressure adversely modulate the effect of flow signals on the vessel wall.**[44]

Anti-inflammatory, Antioxidant, and Vasculoprotective Effects. Physiologic laminar shear stress may have an anti-inflammatory effect because it prevents the inflammatory process of early atherosclerosis in which the endothelium is activated by proinflammatory cytokines. Shear stress may affect atherogenesis through its effect on endothelial-mediated alterations in coagulation, leukocyte and monocyte migration, smooth muscle cell growth, lipoprotein uptake and metabolism, and endothelial cell survival.[47] A number of mechanisms appear to play a role:

1. NO. The principal anti-inflammatory and atheroprotective impact of shear stress may arise from shear stress–stimulated NO production.[47]
2. Tumor necrosis factor-alpha (TNF-α). Blood flow with chronic, physiologic shear stress prevents TNF-α–mediated signal transduction through an NO-independent pathway. It prevents the TNF-α–induced expression of proinflammatory adhesion molecules in intact vessels.[47,49]

   The effects of shear stress are specific to endothelial cells and not observed in vascular smooth muscle. Chronic flow at physiologic shear stress inhibits TNF-α activation of all the MAPK pathways via NO-independent signaling, whereas NFκB cascades are not affected. Physiologic shear stress prevents a proximal event in TNF-α signaling, specifically the association of TNF receptor type 1 (TNFR1) with TNF receptor–associated factor 2 (TRAF2) as the initial step. TNF-α regulates proinflammatory gene expression (e.g., for ICAM-1 and VCAM-1) in endothelial cells, in part by stimulating JNK, which phosphorylates transcription factors. Shear stress inhibits JNK and partially blocks p38 activation through multiple mechanisms, including stimulation of counter-regulatory MAPKs such as ERK1/ERK2 and ERK5, as well as inhibition of the apoptosis signal–regulated kinase.[47,49]
3. Oxidative stress. Direct shear stress–mediated effects on endothelial function also encompass reduced NADH/NADPH oxidase activity by down-regulation of the angiotensin AT_1 receptor and enhanced antioxidative protection through the induction of endothelial cell SOD.[50]

Peroxisome Proliferator–Activated Receptors. The ligand-activated nuclear receptors PPAR-α and PPAR-γ are expressed in endothelial cells and enhance the release of NO.

PPAR-α and PPAR-γ influence vascular responses and endothelial cell biology both directly and indirectly via alteration of gene expression. The vasculoprotective, antiatherogenic effect of PPAR-γ ligands is mediated, in part, through stimulation of endothelial-derived NO and suppression of ET-1 release from multiple vascular sites in order to protect the vascular wall. PPAR-γ ligands appear to increase NO release through a transcriptional process that is unrelated to eNOS expression.[51-53]

Estrogen. Hormone replacement therapy and endothelial function have been extensively studied.[54] Whereas estrogen replacement in postmenopausal women improves endothelium-dependent vasodilation and reduces plasminogen activator inhibitor-1 (PAI-1) levels,[55] the combination of estrogen with a progesterone preparation may blunt the benefits of estrogen.[56]

Direct Effects on Nitric Oxide. Estrogens have direct effects on endothelial function and vascular reactivity as a result of the enhanced production of vasoactive compounds such as NO. Estrogen

- stimulates the expression of both eNOS and iNOS in vascular cells,
- affects the regulation of genes encoding essential cofactors, and
- enhances NO production by increasing eNOS activity.

Estrogen activates eNOS directly through a membrane-associated steroid hormone receptor. Although estrogen receptors classically serve as transcription factors, the hormone's effects on eNOS activity are nongenomic and mediated by the estrogen receptor alpha, which is located in endothelial cell caveolae. Within the caveolae, the steroid hormone receptor is coupled to eNOS as a fast-action complex.[57,58]

Estrogen binding to the estrogen receptor alpha in caveolae causes the activation of tyrosine kinase–MAPK, Akt/PKB signaling, stimulation of Hsp 90 binding to eNOS, and perturbation of the local cytoplasmic Ca^{2+} environment, all leading to eNOS phosphorylation and calmodulin-mediated eNOS stimulation.[57,58]

Indirect Effects on Nitric Oxide. Estrogen indirectly increases the bioavailability of NO.

- Estrogen has a direct antioxidant effect.
- Estrogen lowers levels of asymmetric dimethylarginine (ADMA), the endogenous competitive inhibitor of NO synthesis, by stimulating the activity of endothelial cell dimethylarginine dimethylaminohydrolase (DDAH), which metabolizes ADMA to citrulline.[58]

Clinical Impact. Despite the apparent beneficial effects of estrogen on endothelial function, clinical outcome studies have failed to demonstrate the benefit of hormone replacement therapy for the primary[59] or secondary[60] prevention of coronary heart disease (CHD) events. Explanations for the poor clinical outcomes remain uncertain. Estrogen and progesterone clearly have complex cellular effects. Conceivably,

- the benefits of estrogen may be confounded by concurrent progesterone therapy, and
- adverse prothrombotic and proinflammatory effects may outweigh the benefits of improved endothelial function.[1]

Muscarinic Agonists. Muscarinic acetylcholine receptors activate eNOS in a Ca^{2+}-dependent fashion. They belong to the superfamily of G protein–coupled receptors that link extracellular stimuli to plasmalemmal and intracellular effectors, including ion channels and enzymes such as adenylate cyclase and phospholipases. Agonist binding to muscarinic receptors leads to the targeting of stimulated receptors to plasmalemmal caveolae. Stimulation with carbachol induces Ca^{2+} mobilization, which leads to disruption of the inhibitory eNOS-caveolin complex by Ca^{2+}/calmodulin, thereby activating eNOS. The resultant NO production and generation of cGMP cause vasodilation.[61] **During physical exercise, in addition to the direct effects of shear stress, acetylcholine from the neuromuscular junctions diffuses to the vascular endothelium and activates muscarinic receptors, thereby stimulating the enzymatic activity of eNOS.**

Bradykinin. Calcium-independent activation of eNOS occurs via bradykinin, which increases cellular ceramide levels to effect enhanced NO production. The nonapeptide bradykinin is an important determinant of vascular function. Bradykinin B2 receptors in endothelial cells modulate vasodilation, vascular permeability, mitogenesis, adhesion molecule expression, and other responses. The bradykinin receptor is a G protein–coupled receptor. Upon agonist stimulation, the bradykinin B2 receptor undergoes rapid translocation and is targeted to the caveolae of endothelial cells, wherein several essential transducers of the bradykinin response, such as MAPK components and eNOS, all colocalize.[62]

High-Density Lipoprotein. Lipoproteins have potent effects on eNOS localization and function by affecting caveolar membrane cholesterol homeostasis and the level of eNOS activation.[63]

HDL has a favorable impact on vascular function. It increases prostacyclin release by endothelial cells and may inhibit the secretion of ET-1. HDL enhances endothelial NO bioavailability and vasodilation by increasing eNOS activity and expression and by antagonizing the adverse effects of LDL.[63]

Clinically, an increase in HDL levels improves flow-mediated vasodilation.[64] Some of the beneficial, atheroprotective features of HDL may be due to direct effects on signal transduction mechanisms in endothelial cells. In contrast, **low levels of HDL are associated with abnormal endothelial function and an increased risk for CHD.**[63]

High-Density Lipoprotein Impact on Caveolar Cholesterol and eNOS Function. Lipid-caveolae interactions may be critically involved in the earliest phases of atherogenesis. Because eNOS normally resides in a signaling module within cholesterol-enriched endothelial caveolae, **eNOS function is affected by caveolar cholesterol content.**[63]

Caveolae serve as acceptor membranes for newly synthesized cholesterol.[65] The class B scavenger receptor CD36 and the scavenger receptor B1 (SR-B1) are enriched in plasma membrane caveolae and colocalize with eNOS. Both receptors bind HDL as well as native and oxidized LDL. LDL depletes the cholesterol content of caveolae and negatively affects caveolar integrity and endothelial function.[63]

The adverse effects of LDL are fully prevented and reversed by HDL. In contrast to the caveolar cholesterol–depleting effects of LDL, **the caveolar cholesterol content is maintained by cholesteryl ester uptake from HDL as it binds to SR-B1. Preservation of caveolar cholesterol protects eNOS in its signaling module, which ensures efficient activation of eNOS upon agonist stimulation.**[63]

Direct High-Density Lipoprotein Effects on Nitric Oxide Availability. Aside from its favorable impact on eNOS signaling by preserving the integrity of caveolae, **HDL directly enhances NO bioavailability.**

eNOS Activation. HDL binding to SR-B1, which colocalizes with eNOS in endothelial caveolae, causes significant stimulation of eNOS activity in endothelial cells that results in endothelium- and NO-dependent vasodilation.[63] HDL activation of eNOS requires apolipoprotein (apo) A-I binding to SR-B1.[66]

HDL binding to SR-B1 stimulates eNOS activity by increasing intracellular ceramide levels independent of an increase in cytoplasmic Ca^{2+} or Akt kinase phosphorylation.[62,67] HDL interaction with the SR-B1 receptor also activates Akt kinase and MAPK cascades[67] via stimulation of a common upstream, nonreceptor tyrosine kinase, which leads to parallel activation of Akt kinase and MAPK. As a result, Akt and MAPK independently modulate the enzyme.[68]

eNOS Expression. HDL and apo A-I increase eNOS abundance in the human vascular endothelium. When cultured human vascular endothelial cells are exposed to HDL in vitro, expression of eNOS is enhanced with a resultant, NO-mediated platelet antiaggregatory effect.[69] eNOS protein stability is raised by a process of increased phosphorylation and activation of ERK1/ERK2 and Akt.[26]

Insulin. Insulin receptors are present in the endothelial and vascular smooth muscle cells of large and small blood vessels.[70] Because the glucose transporter GLUT4 is not expressed in endothelial cells, these cells are not responsive to the metabolic effects of insulin. Thus, **the endothelial insulin receptor appears to play a role primarily in the control of vascular tone.**[71] Insulin's effects on the vasculature involve several processes that aid glucose homeostasis:

- **insulin's vasodilatory effect may enhance glucose and insulin delivery to skeletal muscle;**
- **insulin raises endothelial NO and cGMP production, which upon diffusion into underlying muscle or adipose tissues, may act to increase glucose uptake.**[72]

Transendothelial Insulin Transport and Glucose Homeostasis. There is a need to deliver insulin across the endothelium to the underlying, metabolically active target tissues. Transendothelial transport of insulin is a rate-limiting step in insulin action on glucose disposal. **Insulin**

transport across the peripheral endothelium critically determines the kinetics of insulin action in major insulin-sensitive tissues. The transendothelial transport of insulin in vivo appears to involve the insulin receptor.[72]

Vascular Effects of Insulin. Insulin both protects and imperils normal vascular function.

Protective effects of insulin derive from its ability to

- protect against apoptosis and
- stimulate the production of NO,

which results in vasodilation and inhibits some processes that participate in atherosclerosis.

Deleterious effects of insulin derive from its mitogenic activity to

- activate vascular mediators, such as VEGF, a strong angiogenesis factor, and
- stimulate ET-1 gene transcription.[72]

Insulin Stimulation of Nitric Oxide Production. Under normal physiologic circumstances, insulin stimulates the production of NO in endothelial cells. Insulin-induced NO generation increases within minutes and is sustained for up to 2 hours.[73]

Insulin Activation of eNOS. The rapid vasodilatory effect of insulin is consistent with activation of eNOS via signal transduction. The insulin signaling pathway for eNOS sequentially entails

- activation of insulin receptor tyrosine kinase activity,
- IRS-1 complex formation with and activation of PI3K and phosphoinositide-dependent kinase-1 (PDK-1),
- phosphorylation of Ser473 PKB/Akt kinase,
- phosphorylation of Thr308 PKB/Akt kinase, and
- Ser1179 phosphorylation of a complex composed of Akt kinase and eNOS with activation of eNOS.

Correspondingly, insulin-mediated NO production is blocked by inhibitors of tyrosine kinase (genistein), PI3K (wortmannin—50% inhibition), and NOS (L-NAME).[73-75] **In effect, NO is an effector of the same proximal insulin signaling pathway that controls glucose metabolism, and the insulin-mediated metabolic and vascular pathways overlap.**[76]

Insulin Signaling Pathways and Fluid Shear Stress. In bovine aortic cells, both fluid shear stress and insulin

- stimulate IRS-1 tyrosine phosphorylation,
- increase IRS-1–associated PI3K activity,
- increase phosphorylation of Akt/PKB Ser473, and
- induce phosphorylation of eNOS Ser1179, which activates eNOS and increases NO production.74

Thus, both fluid shear stress and insulin regulate eNOS phosphorylation and NO production via overlapping mechanisms, and **the eNOS activating pathways for insulin and fluid shear stress appear to be identical. Not surprisingly, the efficacy of insulin-mediated glucose disposal correlates with preservation of endothelium-dependent vasodilation.**[76]

Insulin-Mediated Increase in eNOS Expression. Insulin increases constitutive expression of the eNOS gene through activation of PI3K in endothelial cells of the microvasculature.[70] Insulin appears to play a role in the regulation of eNOS expression in vascular tissues even in the basal state.[72]

The duration of insulin-mediated vasodilation is consistent with a gene transcription effect. Application of insulin to native endothelial cells increased eNOS mRNA, followed by a comparable increase in eNOS protein. In the process, insulin activated multiple signaling pathways in endothelial cells, including the combined activation of a PI3K- and activating protein-1 (AP-1)–dependent pathway with insulin-enhanced DNA binding activity of Sp1 and AP-1.[77]

Nitric Oxide–Mediated Anti-inflammatory Effect of Insulin. In human aortic endothelial cells, insulin, in an NO-dependent manner, inhibits the expression of

- ICAM-1,
- MCP-1, and
- NFkB,

three major proinflammatory mediators, in parallel with an increase in eNOS expression.

The inhibition of inflammatory mediators by insulin is wholly NO dependent.[78]

Antiapoptotic Effect of Insulin. By activating the PI3K-Akt pathway, insulin protects vascular smooth muscle cells from undergoing apoptosis.[79]

ENDOTHELIAL DYSFUNCTION

Given its unique anatomic location, the endothelium is a vulnerable primary target for mechanical and biochemical injuries caused by traditional and novel cardiovascular risk factors. **Injury to the endothelium alters normal endothelial physiology and is referred to as endothelial dysfunction.**[80]

Time Course of Endothelial Dysfunction. Endothelial integrity and NO activity are impaired early in the course of human vascular disease, and such impairment represents the initial lesion of the atherogenic process. Impairment of endothelial vasodilator responses, as assessed by ultrasound determination of brachial artery vasoreactivity, precedes the appearance of atherosclerotic intimal lesions[81,82] and ultimately leads to clinical events.[1,83]

Endothelial dysfunction occurs decades before the onset of symptomatic vascular disease.[84] In long-term follow-up over 10 years in women with de novo angina, angiographically normal-appearing coronary arteries, and evidence of reversible myocardial perfusion defects on single-photon emission computed tomography, the presence of endothelial dysfunction was a sign of the future development of atherosclerosis.[85]

The Impairment of Dysfunctional Endothelium. The decreased NO production by a dysfunctional endothelium is implicated in the clinical course of all known cardiovascular disease.[86]

Cardiovascular Risk Factors. The functional response of the endothelium to increased blood flow is a major independent predictor of atheromatous disease progression and clinical outcome in patients at risk for CHD.[1] Human brachial and coronary endothelial vasodilator dysfunction is predictive of cardiovascular event rates (Fig. 8-2). **Endothelial dysfunction is associated with a growing list of cardiovascular disease risk factors** (Fig. 8-3). All known CHD risk factors such as

- hyperlipidemia,
- hypertension,
- cigarette consumption,
- established CHD,

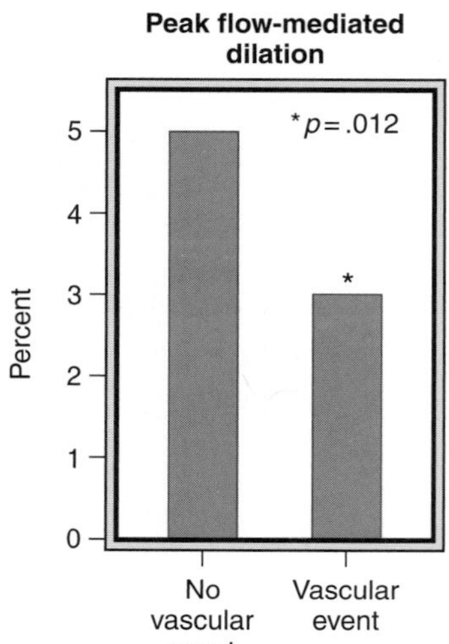

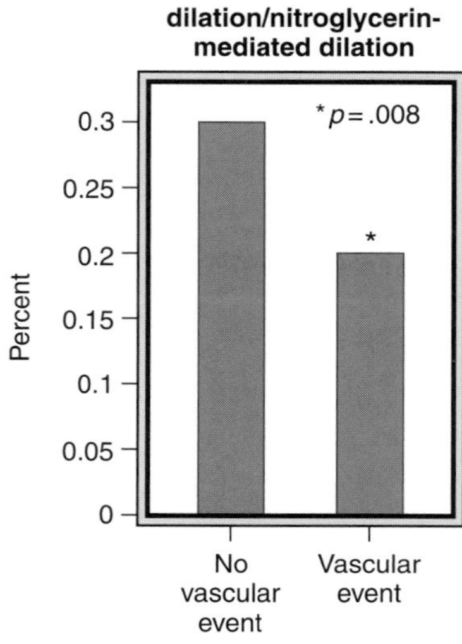

›› **Figure 8–2.**
Peak flow-mediated dilation and flow-mediated dilation/nitroglycerin-mediated dilation in 152 patients with coronary artery disease over 34-month follow-up. The incidence of vascular events was higher in patients with impaired endothelial function. *(Modified from Chan SY, Mancini GJ, Kuramoto L, et al. The prognostic importance of endothelial dysfunction and carotid atheroma burden in patients with coronary artery disease. J Am Coll Cardiol 2003;42:1037-1043.)*

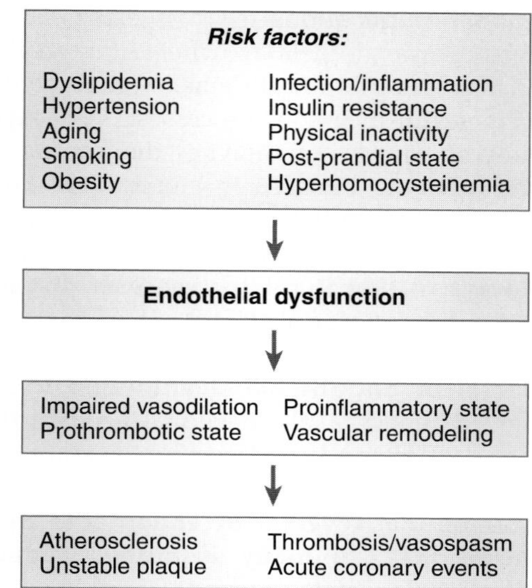

Figure 8–3.
Endothelial dysfunction and the pathogenesis of cardiovascular disease. *(Modified from Widlansky ME, Gokce N, Keaney JJ, Vita JA. The clinical implications of endothelial dysfunction. J Am Coll Cardiol 2003;42:1149-1160.)*

- peripheral/cerebrovascular disease,
- heart failure,
- increasing age,
- insulin resistance,
- hyperglycemia,
- DM,
- a family history of premature atherosclerotic disease,
- male gender,
- obesity,
- hyperhomocysteinemia,
- elevated C-reactive protein,
- chronic systemic inflammation or infection, and
- oxidative stress

reduce NO availability.[1,83,84]

Vascular Disease. NO bioavailability represents a key marker of vascular health because NO availability is inversely related to the progression of atheromatous vascular disease.[1] Endothelial dysfunction implies a permutation in endothelial phenotype to one that is atherogenic. Endothelial dysfunction engenders the loss of vasodilator and antithrombotic factors and an increase in vasoconstrictor and prothrombotic products. As a result, endothelial dysfunction increasingly gives rise to vasoconstriction, inflammation, and thrombosis, which portend ischemic symptoms and an elevated risk for cardiovascular events (Table 8-2).[1,6] Endothelial dysfunction is pathogenic and contributes to the vascular dysfunction of atherosclerosis, insulin resistance, systemic and pulmonary hypertension.[80]

A chronic deficiency or loss of NO activity contributes to medial thickening or myointimal hyperplasia, or to both. Endothelial dysfunction is associated with increased conduit vessel stiffness.[87] It accelerates the development of vascular lesions and participates in the initiation and progression of atherosclerosis.[6]

Specifically, endothelial dysfunction promotes inflammation with inflammatory cytokines, leukocyte chemotactic factors, and adhesion molecules. Inflammatory factors, in turn, promote monocyte and T-cell adhesion, foam cell formation, extracellular matrix digestion, vascular smooth muscle migration and proliferation leading to atherosclerotic plaque formation, and platelet activation. Endothelial dysfunction also participates in the later stages of the disease, ultimately culminating in plaque rupture and thrombus formation in the setting of acute coronary syndromes.[1]

Table 8-2. Consequences of Endothelial Dysfunction

Reduced nitric oxide	Reduced vasodilation Reduced anti-inflammatory impact
Increased endothelin-1	Vasoconstriction Increased thrombosis Oxidative stress
Increased adhesion/ chemotactic molecules	Monocyte recruitment Plaque rupture
Reduced protein C Increased tissue factor Increased plasminogen activator inhibitor-1	Increased thrombosis Reduced fibrinolysis

The severity of endothelial dysfunction relates to the risk for initial and recurrent cardiovascular events.[81,82] Interestingly, endothelial function is more strongly related to outcome than the actual atheroma burden is. For any degree of atherosclerosis, endothelial function modulates the prognosis (Fig. 8-4).[88]

Exercise Capacity. Endothelial dysfunction in the setting of vascular disease probably contributes to the impairment in exercise capacity.

Endothelial dysfunction limits exercise capacity through either cardiac or peripheral mechanisms. NO contributes significantly to an exercise-induced increase in limb blood flow. Conditions that reduce NO curtail exercise-induced hyperemia and impair exercise capacity.[16]

In patients with hypercholesterolemia and coronary atherosclerosis, coronary and systemic arteries may actually constrict during exercise because of the loss of vasodilatory capacity by the dysfunctional endothelium and the increased responsiveness to vasoconstrictors such as norepinephrine and ET-1.[16]

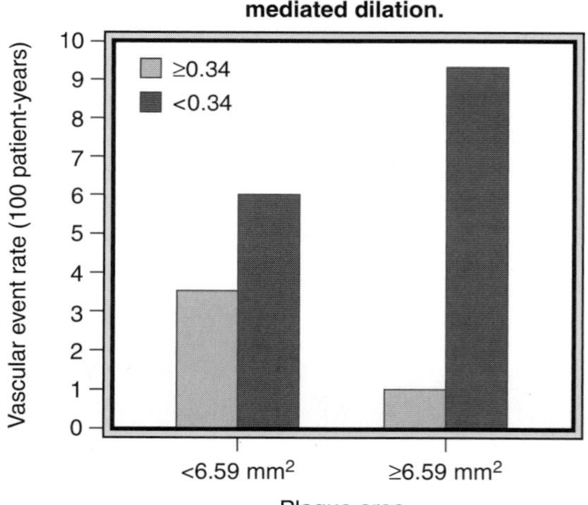

›› **Figure 8–4.**
Flow mediated dilation/nitroglycerin mediated dilation. Vascular event rate as a function of carotid plaque burden and the ratio of peak flow-mediated dilation/nitroglycerin-mediated dilation in patients with coronary artery disease over 34-month follow-up. The incidence of vascular events was higher in patients with impaired endothelial function. *(Modified from Chan SY, Mancini GJ, Kuramoto L, et al. The prognostic importance of endothelial dysfunction and carotid atheroma burden in patients with coronary artery disease. J Am Coll Cardiol 2003;42:1037-1043.)*

Metabolic Implications. NOS is expressed in the vascular endothelium, where it regulates arterial pressure, and in skeletal muscle, where it participates in metabolic processes. NOS plays an important role not only in the control of arterial pressure but also in glucose and lipid homeostasis. **Dysfunctional eNOS constitutes a link between the vascular and metabolic pathways in that it relates vascular disease and insulin resistance.**[89]

Reversal of Endothelial Dysfunction. Well-preserved endothelial function predicts the absence of CHD and good exercise tolerance.[90,91] An important corollary to this observation is the notion that **reversal of endothelial dysfunction may, in many instances, reduce cardiovascular risk.** A number of medical interventions and lifestyle changes that target an improvement in cardiovascular risk are, in fact, associated with improved vasomotor function. Thus, beneficial pharmacologic agents, such as aspirin, angiotensin-converting enzyme (ACE) inhibitors, and HMG-CoA reductase inhibitors, as well as lifestyle changes such as exercise, smoking cessation, and specific dietary interventions, all increase NO availability (Table 8-3).[1,92,93]

In several instances, enhanced endothelial function in response to an intervention does, in fact, identify a group of individuals with improved prognosis.[90,91] Unfortunately, endothelial functional improvement is not an absolute surrogate indicator for risk reduction. Antioxidants, hormone replacement therapy, phosphodiesterase-5 inhibitors, and L-arginine supplementation may

Table 8-3. Interventions with Concordant Benefit on Endothelial Function and Coronary Heart Disease Events

INTERVENTION	EFFECT ON ENDOTHELIAL FUNCTION	EFFECT ON CHD EVENTS
Lipid-lowering therapy	+	+
Smoking cessation	+	+
Exercise	+	+
Angiotensin-converting enzyme inhibitors	+	+
Angiotensin receptor blockers	+	+
n-3 fatty acids	+	+

Modified from Widlansky ME, Gokce N, Keaney JJ, Vita JA. The clinical implications of endothelial dysfunction. J Am Coll Cardiol 2003;42:1149-1160.

Table 8-4. Interventions with Discordant Effects on Endothelial Function and Coronary Heart Disease Events

INTERVENTION	EFFECT ON ENDOTHELIAL FUNCTION	EFFECT ON CHD EVENTS
Hormone replacement therapy	±	–
Cyclooxygenase-2 inhibition	+	–
Peroxisome proliferator–activated receptor-γ activation	+	?
Tumor necrosis factor-alpha inhibition	+	?
L-Arginine	+	?
Dietary flavonoids	+	?
Vitamin C	+	?
Folate	+	?
Tetrahydrobiopterin	+	?

Modified from Widlansky ME, Gokce N, Keaney JJ, Vita JA. The clinical implications of endothelial dysfunction. J Am Coll Cardiol 2003;42:1149-1160.

all improve endothelial function but are associated with controversial, neutral, or even negative cardiovascular outcomes (Table 8-4).[60,91,94,95]

MECHANISMS OF ENDOTHELIAL DYSFUNCTION

Endothelial dysfunction is characterized by reduced levels of NO. The bioavailability of NO reflects a balance between its production by eNOS and its degradation. **Diminished bioactivity of NO may arise as a result of decreased production or increased degradation of NO, or both.**

Endothelial vasodilator dysfunction is thus regulated by at least three different determinants of endothelial NO bioavailability:

1. transcriptional regulation of eNOS,
2. post-transcriptional activity of eNOS, and
3. NO half-life as determined by the balance in ROS-mediated breakdown of NO with antioxidant defense mechanisms.[6]

The pathophysiologic mechanisms of endothelial dysfunction are multifactorial and may differ with diverse causes.[80]

Decreased eNOS Expression. Impaired NO release may be due to down-regulation of eNOS expression.

Certain gene polymorphisms of the eNOS gene may be associated with functional or structural alterations in the enzyme and vascular disease. One such eNOS gene polymorphism is Glu298 → Asp. This substitution is responsible for a decrease in basal NO production.[96] Clinically, this amino acid substitution is responsible for a statistically significant higher frequency of hypertension and vasospastic angina, suggestive of endothelial dysfunction.[97] The missense mutation is also associated with an increased incidence of CHD and cardiovascular morbidity and mortality.[98,99]

In addition, in advanced CHD, the reduced expression of eNOS may be due to cytokine- or lipid-induced instability, to reduced transcription of eNOS mRNA, or to both.[6]

Decreased eNOS Activity. Diminished NO release may arise from insufficient eNOS activation. Abnormalities in

- shear stress,
- agonist-linked receptor mechanisms that activate eNOS, and
- substrate or cofactor availability

may all be playing a role.

L-Arginine Deficiency. L-Arginine substrate deficiency for eNOS is rare. Lower intracellular L-arginine bioavailability can occur with diminished L-arginine recycling or increased L-arginine metabolism.

Asymmetric Dimethylarginine. Endogenously produced competitive inhibitors of L-arginine, such as ADMA and *N*-monomethylarginine (NMA), can create a de facto relative deficiency of the natural substrate for eNOS, thus curtailing the production of NO. Endogenous inhibitors of NOS activity may be responsible for the endothelial dysfunction of many individuals with CHD risk factors or CHD.[4,6]

Asymmetric Dimethylarginine Action. ADMA is an endogenous, competitive inhibitor of NOS. It competes with L-arginine for both the active site of NOS and the Y^+ transporter.[6]

Asymmetric Dimethylarginine Formation. ADMA is formed by protein arginine *N*-methyltransferases (PRMTs), which use *S*-adenosylmethionine as a methyl group donor. Four different isoforms of human PRMTs have been identified with specificity for different proteins. A number of cells elaborate ADMA, including human endothelial cells. **Asymmetric dimethylarginine is derived from the catabolism of proteins that contain methylated arginine residues** or that have been post-translationally methylated. Such proteins are mainly found in the nucleus and are involved in RNA processing and transcriptional control. Upon hydrolysis of these proteins, their methylated arginine residues are released as ADMA and NMA. The intracellular concentration of ADMA can exceed the extracellular or circulating concentration fivefold.[6,58]

Asymmetric Dimethylarginine Metabolism and Excretion. The methylated arginine residues ADMA and NMA are excreted in urine or are metabolized.

A minor source of metabolism occurs via dimethylarginine pyruvate transferase in the kidney and possibly via acetylation in the liver.

The major metabolic pathway for NMA and ADMA occurs via DDAH. Two enzymatic isoforms of DDAH are known, I and II. Either or both isoforms are widely distributed. DDAH I is typically found in tissues expressing neuronal NOS. DDAH II predominates in tissues containing eNOS. DDAH hydrolyzes ADMA to L-citrulline and dimethylamine. Both ADMA and DDAH are widely distributed in tissues.[6,100]

Asymmetric Dimethylarginine Levels in Endothelial Dysfunction. ADMA is constantly produced as part of normal protein turnover, and increased levels are associated with endothelial dysfunction. The plasma level of ADMA is normally 1 μmol/L. Plasma ADMA levels are typically increased 2-fold in subjects with risk factors for vascular disease and up to 10-fold in subjects with clinical atherosclerosis and established cardiovascular disease. In fact, **plasma ADMA levels correlate with the severity of endothelial dysfunction.**[101]

Mechanisms of Asymmetric Dimethylarginine Elevation. ADMA levels are elevated with

- increased PRMT and
- decreased DDAH

activity.

1. PRMT. Expression of PRMTs is up-regulated in the presence of native or oxidized LDL, which may be due in part to the enhanced gene expression of PRMTs.[101] The production of ADMA by human endothelial cells is also up-regulated in the presence of methionine or homocysteine.[3,6,100]
2. DDAH. The activity of DDAH appears to be critical in regulating ADMA levels. Because ADMA is constantly produced as part of normal protein turnover, DDAH activity is essential to prevent the accumulation of ADMA.
   - DDAH is sensitive to oxidative stress. Oxidation or nitrosylation of a sulfhydryl moiety at the catalytic site impairs enzymatic activity and increases ADMA levels.[102]
   - Although oxidized LDL and TNF-α leave protein levels of DDAH unaffected, they significantly decrease the activity of DDAH.
   - Homocysteine increases ADMA levels not only by increasing ADMA production but also by decreasing DDAH activity.
   - Hyperglycemia reduces DDAH activity and increases ADMA accumulation.[3,6,100]

The resulting elevation in ADMA levels contributes to endothelial cell dysfunction.

Asymmetric Dimethylarginine Elevation in Clinical Settings. Plasma levels of ADMA are dynamically regulated by dietary factors and can be correlated with indices of endothelial dysfunction.

- A high-salt diet is associated with an increase in urinary ADMA excretion and an increase in blood pressure. A low-salt diet reverses these abnormalities.[6]
- Plasma levels of ADMA are also acutely elevated after the ingestion of a high-fat meal with a reduction in the vasodilator response of the brachial artery to reactive hyperemia, an endothelium-dependent response.[103]
- In general, cardiovascular risk factors such as hypercholesterolemia, hypertriglyceridemia, hypertension, hyperglycemia, insulin resistance, renal insufficiency, cigarette smoking,

and aging are all associated with increased plasma levels of ADMA.[102]

Decreased eNOS Cofactor Availability. BH_4 is the necessary cofactor for coupling L-arginine to the eNOS enzyme for L-arginine to be oxidized to NO and L-citrulline. It plays a crucial role not only in increasing the rate of NO production but also in limiting the formation of superoxide in endothelial cells. Additionally, BH_4 serves as an antioxidant by scavenging any ROS produced, such as superoxide and peroxynitrite.[9,4,104] **Deficiency of BH_4 or other flavonoid cofactors causes endothelial dysfunction.**

BH_4 is very susceptible to oxidation, which converts it to dihydrobiopterin (Fig. 8-5). In the absence of BH_4, electron transfer is shunted to molecular oxygen, and the eNOS reaction produces superoxide through the uncoupled NADH/NADPH oxidase reaction (Fig. 8-6). BH_4 deficiency is implicated not only in the endothelial production of ROS but also in the inadequate scavenging thereof.[9,4,104]

Decreased Nitric Oxide Half-Life. Once released, the half-life of NO is reduced under conditions of oxidative stress in the presence of free radicals.

Other Factors Underlying Endothelial Dysfunction. Oxidative stress, inflammation, mental stress, and dyslipidemia all activate pathways that impair endothelial function.

Oxidative Stress. Oxidative endothelial injury plays a major role in vascular complications.

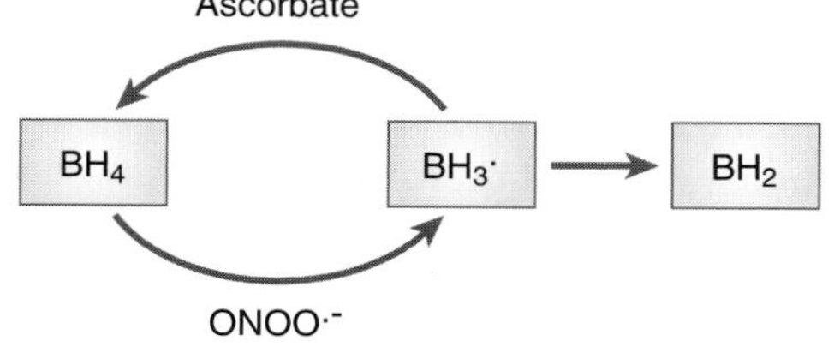

Figure 8–5.
Peroxynitrite ($ONOO^-$) oxidation of tetrahydrobiopterin (BH_4) to an intermediate radical with subsequent degradation to dihydrobiopterin (BH_2). The antioxidant action of ascorbate reverses the oxidant effect. BH_3, trihydrobiopterin.

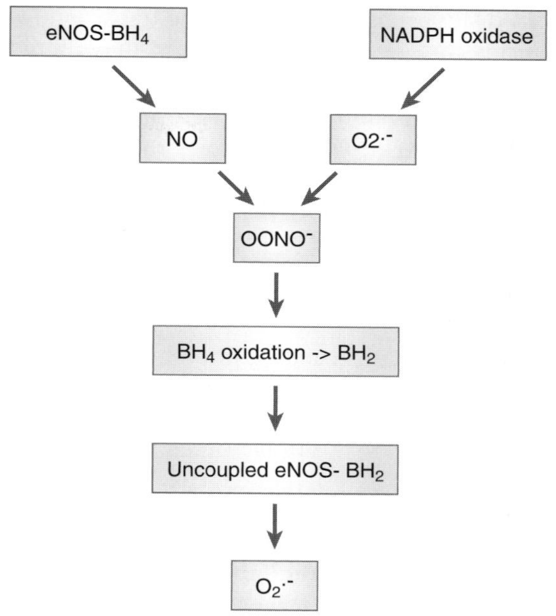

Figure 8–6.
Oxidative uncoupling of endothelial nitric oxide synthase (eNOS) with resultant eNOS-superoxide ($O_2^{\cdot-}$) production. BH_2, dihydrobiopterin; BH_4, tetrahydrobiopterin; NADPH, nicotinamide adenine dinucleotide phosphate.

Exposure to oxidative stress not only limits NO bioavailability but also inhibits NO production in endothelial cells by impairing eNOS expression and activity.[105]

NO activity is curtailed by ROS, which combines with NO to form peroxynitrite, or $ONOO^-$, a less biologically active vasodilator than NO. Formation of the peroxynitrite anion engenders lipid peroxidation and nitrosation of tyrosine moieties, thereby disrupting cell membranes, cell signaling, and cell survival. In the later stages of atherosclerosis, there is reduced sensitivity to endogenous and exogenous NO, possibly because of oxidative inactivation of NO or soluble guanylate cyclase (or both).[6,16]

Myeloperoxidase is an oxidant implicated in endothelial dysfunction. It is rapidly taken up by endothelial cells via a transcytotic process and accumulates within the subendothelial space, where it is positioned anatomically to interfere with the protective effects of NO in the vessel wall. Myeloperoxidase catalytically consumes NO. In vitro, myeloperoxidase impairs NO-dependent vasodilation in isolated arterial and tracheal rings and decreases NO bioavailability in cultured cells. It induces endothelial dysfunction in organ chamber and animal model studies. Clinically, there is a significant, strong independent relationship between the serum myeloperoxidase level and endothelial dysfunction, as reflected by brachial artery flow–mediated dilation, after adjustment for prevalent cardiovascular disease, cardiac risk factors, and C-reactive protein levels.[106]

Oxidized LDL is toxic to endothelial cells and causes decreased NO release and enhanced expression of cytokines and adhesion molecules, which leads to vascular inflammation and atherogenesis.[107]

Inflammation. Inflammatory mediators are implicated in endothelial dysfunction.[108]

Nuclear Factor KappaB. NFκB plays a central role in endothelial cell activation by proinflammatory cytokines. This pathway is rapidly activated by cytokines and peaks at 30 minutes. It has an impact on the transcription of TNF-α, preproET-1, and NOS genes.[109,110]

Tumor Necrosis Factor-α. TNF-α is elevated in diverse inflammatory conditions and impairs endothelial function.

- TNF-α down-regulates eNOS expression by shortening the half-life of eNOS mRNA.[109]
- TNF-α inhibits fluid shear stress–mediated NO production. Activation of PKC is involved with overexpression of growth factors, cytokines, and oxidative stress.[74]
- TNF-α interferes with intracellular insulin signaling in fat, skeletal muscle, endothelium, and other insulin-responsive tissues. Because of the overlap in metabolic and vascular insulin signaling pathways, TNF-α has an inhibitory effect on insulin-stimulated endothelial function in humans.[74,111]
- TNF-α also inhibits insulin-induced enhancement of eNOS expression. It lowers insulin receptor protein content and insulin receptor phosphorylation in human aortic endothelial cells.[112]
- TNF-α and interleukin-1beta (IL-1β) suppress the mRNA and protein level of cGK. In primary bovine aortic vascular smooth muscle cells, cytokines such as IL-1α and TNF-α increase iNOS expression with cross-activation of PKA, which down-regulates the expression of cGK.[113]

The Renin-Angiotensin-Aldosterone System. Although inflammation is clearly multifactorial in etiology, the renin-angiotensin-aldosterone system (RAAS) plays an important contributory role. **During inflammation, angiotensin II contributes to endothelial dysfunction.** Angiotensin II is a major factor increasing pro-oxidant stress. It decreases NO/cGMP/cGK action by stimulating the activity and expression of phosphodiesterase, which increases cGMP hydrolysis, thus decreasing cGMP levels and cGK action.[4]

Mineralocorticoid receptors are present in the vasculature. Aldosterone has been implicated in the pathogenesis of endothelial dysfunction. In normal men, acute short-term systemic administration of aldosterone results in endothelium-dependent vasodilatory dysfunction.[114] In New Zealand rabbits given a hypercholesterolemic diet, mineralocorticoid receptor antagonism reduced superoxide generation and improved endothelial function.[115]

Endothelin-1. ET-1 levels rise with inflammation and activation of the RAAS and are associated with endothelial dysfunction. NO and ET-1 have reciprocal regulation: conditions that lower NO, such as endothelial dysfunction and insulin resistance, increase ET-1, and vice versa. The balance between ET-1 and NO has great relevance for the control of vascular tone, blood pressure, and vascular remodeling. Imbalances in these factors underlie both systemic and pulmonary hypertension, as well as the atherosclerotic process.[116]

ET-1 is produced from preproET-1, cleaved by a furin protease to big ET-1, and additionally processed to bioactive ET-1 by endothelin-converting enzyme-1. Endothelin-converting enzyme-1 is up-regulated by the ERK pathway.[116]

ET-1 has a bidirectional effect on NO. Whereas the ET B receptor on endothelial cells increases NO production, the ET A receptor on smooth muscle cells lowers NO production.[116] ET-1 promotes inflammation and causes vascular smooth muscle cell contraction and growth.[117,118] ET-1 induces endothelial cell expression of NADH/NADPH oxidase. The resultant increase in oxidant stress worsens endothelial dysfunction.[119]

Rho/Rho Kinase. From a molecular perspective, inflammatory cytokines and vasoconstrictors appear to mediate endothelial dysfunction via Rho/Rho kinase, which suppresses both eNOS activity and gene expression and thereby causes a rapid and a prolonged decrease in NO production.[35]

Stress. Mental stress impairs endothelial function through activation of the sympathetic nervous system, as well as the hypothalamic-pituitary-adrenal axis.

Sympathetic activation, via an α-adrenergic mechanism, is implicated in endothelial dysfunction.[120] It also engenders RAAS activation.

Glucocorticoids have a negative impact on endothelial function, and reduced endothelium-dependent vasodilation is characteristic of glucocorticoid excess. Glucocorticoid receptors are present in endothelial cells. Via activation of glucocorticoid receptors, cortisol significantly decreases eNOS protein levels in a dose-dependent manner. In cultured bovine coronary artery endothelial cells, cortisol decreased agonist-induced, cytoplasmic Ca^{2+}-mediated NO release.[121] In rat vessels, glucocorticoids also inhibited the expression of GTP cyclohydrolase, the rate-limiting enzyme for the synthesis of BH_4, an important cofactor for eNOS.[31]

Vascular Stretch. Vascular stretch, which is increased in hypertension, is a potent stimulus for the endothelium and vascular smooth muscle cells to produce ROS, which contribute to endothelial dysfunction.[122,123]

Low-Density Lipoprotein. There is an association between dyslipidemia and endothelial dysfunction. **LDL, in particular oxidized LDL, impairs endothelial NO availability via numerous mechanisms and is implicated in atherogenesis.**

Caveolae. Oxidized LDL depletes the cholesterol content of caveolae. The depletion of caveolar cholesterol disrupts eNOS activation and causes eNOS to translocate from caveolae to an unidentified intracellular compartment.[37]

The scavenger receptor CD36 is generally thought to mediate the net uptake of cholesterol because macrophages internalize and store sterols via that receptor. However, endothelial cells are net exporters of cholesterol and do not accumulate large amounts of it. In endothelial cells, the CD36 receptor thus mediates the net efflux, not influx, of caveolar cholesterol as LDL binds to CD36. The scaffolding protein caveolin is required for the efflux of cholesterol from caveolae.[37]

Caveolin. Exposure to native LDL increases the expression of caveolin-1 in endothelial cells, thus impairing eNOS activity as a result of caveolin-eNOS inhibition.[14]

Oxidation. Oxidized LDL inactivates NO directly.[124]

Asymmetric Dimethylarginine. Another mechanism for oxidized LDL to induce endothelial dysfunction involves the inefficient utilization of L-arginine substrate by eNOS via increased concentrations of ADMA.

ENDOTHELIAL DYSFUNCTION AND INSULIN RESISTANCE

Insulin resistance is associated with endothelial dysfunction, although the cause-and-effect relationship is unclear. Endothelial dysfunction with decreased NO bioavailability has been implicated in insulin resistance, and insulin resistance, as well as hyperinsulinemia, may aggravate the vascular injury.[125] Insulin resistance is manifested at the level of the endothelium. **The degree of endothelial dysfunction is proportional to the severity of insulin resistance.**[73,126,127]

Insulin Resistance contributing to Endothelial Dysfunction. Insulin resistance plays an integral role in the development and progression of endothelial dysfunction.

A knockout mouse model for the insulin receptor and IRS-1, in addition to the expected metabolic effects, engenders impaired endothelium-dependent vascular relaxation and hypertension.[128] Insulin resistance elicits molecular mechanisms that contribute to vascular dysfunction (Fig. 8-7), including disturbances in intracellular signal transduction, increased oxidative stress, and decreased bioavailability of NO. The resulting abnormalities impair and further compromise endothelial function, thereby increasing the risk for atherosclerosis and adverse cardiovascular events.[129]

Selective Insulin Resistance. Insulin resistance is selective and applies only to the metabolic and vascular signaling pathways of insulin.
The cellular response to insulin receptor activation is mediated by at least two pathways,

1. the metabolic and vascular PI3K-Akt pathway and
2. the mitogenic Ras-MAPK pathway.[72]

In the setting of systemic insulin resistance, insulin has reduced effects only on the PI3K-Akt pathway, thereby forfeiting the insulin-mediated vasodilatory and anti-inflammatory effects of NO. Insulin signaling via the MAPK pathway remains intact.[130,131]

Vascular Effects of Hyperinsulinemia. With selective insulin resistance, the cell growth–, migration-, and thrombosis-promoting responses of the MAPK pathway are enhanced by compensatory hyperinsulinemia and other mechanisms.[131,132] In this context, with loss of insulin's vasoprotective PI3K-Akt track, high insulin levels become atherogenic and contribute to the excessive rates of cardiovascular disease in obesity, hypertension, and type 2 DM.

Because insulin signaling preferentially targets the MAPK pathway in insulin resistance, the elevated insulin level of hyperinsulinemia will

- increase the expression of PAI-1, thus impairing fibrinolysis;
- raise the expression of adhesion molecules[131]: plasma levels of E-selectin, ICAM-1, and VCAM-1 are correlated with the degree of insulin resistance[133];
- encourage monocyte adherence to the endothelium[131]: the concentration of mononuclear cells binding to cultured endothelium is significantly correlated with plasma levels of adhesion molecules[133];
- stimulate vascular and nonvascular cell growth[131]; and
- induce endothelial cell, vascular smooth muscle cell, and monocyte migration.[132]

Endothelin-1. Insulin-mediated MAPK activation induces the production of ET-1 by endothelial cells.[134] ET-1, in turn, impairs insulin signaling via the PI3K pathway in vascular smooth muscle cells. It increases oxidant stress in endothelial cells, thus worsening not only endothelial function but also insulin sensitivity.[119]

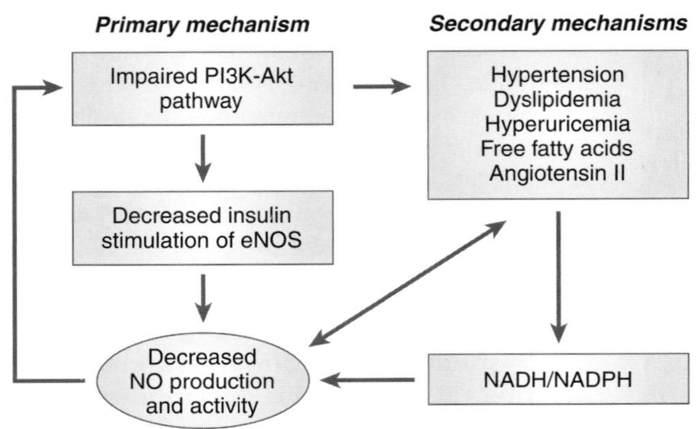

▸▸ **Figure 8–7.**
Primary and secondary mechanisms of endothelial dysfunction with insulin resistance. eNOS, endothelial nitric oxide synthase; NADH/NADPH, nicotinamide adenine dinucleotide phosphate; NO, nitric oxide; PI3K, phosphatidylinositol 3-kinase. *(Adapted from Hsueh WA, Quinones MJ. Role of endothelial dysfunction in insulin resistance. Am J Cardiol 2003;92[suppl]: 10J-17J.)*

Angiotensin II. With hyperinsulinemia, the tissue RAAS is activated.

Insulin may cross-bind to the IGF receptor, which induces the production of angiotensinogen and vascular smooth muscle growth.[135] Hyperinsulinemia induces endothelial tissue ACE and angiotensin II production as ACE enhances the conversion of angiotensin I to angiotensin II. High insulin levels induce AT_1 receptor overexpression in vascular smooth muscle cells.[119]

Angiotensin II further stimulates the mitogenic MAPK pathway. It induces cell growth and vascular remodeling. It may also increase the transcription of IGF for further angiotensinogen release.[135] Angiotensin II is implicated in the generation of ROS, thus further compromising both metabolic insulin signaling and endothelial function.[119]

Asymmetric Dimethylarginine. A significant relationship exists between insulin resistance and plasma concentrations of ADMA. Increased ADMA plasma concentrations with insulin resistance contribute to the development of endothelial dysfunction and CHD.[136]

Plasma ADMA concentrations are positively correlated with

- the degree of insulin resistance,
- impairment of insulin-mediated glucose disposal, and
- fasting triglyceride levels in nondiabetic, normotensive subjects.[137]

Tetrahydrobiopterin. Insulin resistance may induce endothelial dysfunction through a relative deficiency of BH_4 in vascular endothelial cells.

Insulin resistance is associated with abnormalities in pteridine metabolism. The resultant suboptimal levels of BH_4 allow the production of superoxide by eNOS and thus lead to endothelial dysfunction. Oral supplementation of BH_4 may help relieve oxidative tissue damage and restore endothelial function.[138]

Metabolic Syndrome. As insulin resistance worsens and progresses to the metabolic syndrome, **most components of the syndrome, such as glucose intolerance, hypertension, dyslipidemia, hyperuricemia, and elevated free fatty acid levels, further compromise endothelial function.**[125]

Hyperglycemia. With severe insulin resistance and impaired glucose uptake, hyperglycemia impairs NO bioavailability, thereby contributing to endothelial vasodilator dysfunction in insulin-resistant states, through several mechanisms:

- ADMA: glucose-induced impairment of DDAH causes ADMA accumulation[139];
- the polyol pathway: hyperglycemia can activate the polyol pathway, which leads to depletion of the NADPH essential for the regeneration of antioxidant molecules such as glutathione, tocopherol, ascorbate, and BH_4, all involved in increasing eNOS functionality or NO bioavailability[140];
- PKC activation: hyperglycemia increases the synthesis of diacylglycerol, which activates the PKC pathway and adversely affects NO production and vascular integrity[140]; and
- glycosylation modification: hyperglycemia impairs the functional properties of cytosolic and nuclear proteins via O-linked glycosylation modification. As a result, the metabolic-vascular branches of insulin signaling are further impaired, coupled with enhanced activation and expression of MMP-2 and MMP-9.[10] The production of advanced glycation end products (AGEs) also increases the oxidation of LDL and induces the release of IL-1, TNF-α, and growth factors that further stimulate vascular remodeling.[140]

Free Fatty Acids. Increased free fatty acid fluxes affect vascular reactivity and are linked to endothelial dysfunction.[141]

Insulin resistance–associated free fatty acid liberation as a result of excessive lipolysis and diminished skeletal muscle uptake mediates abnormalities in endothelial cell function by affecting the synthesis and degradation of NO.[142] Free fatty acids impair endothelial function via several mechanisms[143]:

- increased production of oxygen-derived free radicals: free fatty acid metabolites uncouple oxidative phosphorylation and generate ROS such as superoxide in mitochondria.[144] An infusion of free fatty acids reduces endothelium-dependent vasodilation in animal models and in humans. Coinfusion of the antioxidant ascorbic acid mitigates the fatty acid–induced vascular dysfunction, which suggests that oxidative stress participates in its pathogenesis[145];

- activation of PKC: free fatty acid–mediated membrane translocation and activation of PKC inhibit the PI3K-Akt pathway, thereby thwarting NO production.[146] Activation of the PKC pathway also increases the production of ET-1 and encourages the production of growth factors such as VEGF, epidermal growth factor (EGF), and TGF-α, which participate in the vascular remodeling process[140]; and
- exacerbation of dyslipidemia: the free fatty acid flux increases hepatic very-low-density lipoprotein (VLDL) production and cholesteryl ester synthesis. The resulting increased levels of triglyceride-rich lipoproteins lower HDL levels and promote the generation of atherogenic oxidized, small dense LDL, both of which processes are implicated in endothelial dysfunction.[147]

Concordance of Insulin Resistance and Endothelial Dysfunction. Insulin-resistant states exhibit

- diminished insulin-mediated glucose uptake into peripheral tissues,
- impaired insulin-mediated vasodilation, and
- deficient endothelium-dependent vasodilation in response to the muscarinic receptor agonist acetylcholine.

Because insulin signaling mechanisms in peripheral tissues and the endothelium appear to be shared, insulin action in peripheral tissues is closely linked to its action in the endothelium. Thus, sensitivity to the vasodilatory effects of insulin is positively correlated with metabolic insulin sensitivity,[148] and the molecular mechanisms causing defects in insulin signaling might be expected to be manifested in vascular and metabolically active tissues.[149]

Endothelial dysfunction occurs in the metabolic syndrome and type 2 DM.[126] Increased abdominal adiposity, as measured by the waist-hip ratio, is a strong predictor of endothelial dysfunction, independent of other risk factors. In patients without CHD, high insulin resistance and elevated remnant lipoprotein levels are correlated with coronary arterial endothelial dysfunction. Insulin resistance is associated with increased conduit vessel stiffness.[150] In a detailed study of the metabolic syndrome in 119 nondiabetic offspring of diabetic probands, hypoadiponectinemia as well as high levels of cytokines and adhesion molecules, indicative of low-grade inflammation and endothelial dysfunction, were found to be essential findings in subjects with the metabolic syndrome.[151]

Endothelial Dysfunction as a Precursor of Insulin Resistance. Endothelial dysfunction may play a major role in the pathogenesis of insulin resistance. Vascular dysfunction is associated with insensitivity to insulin. Vascular reactivity in both the microcirculation and macrocirculation is reduced

- in subjects with type 2 DM,[152]
- in those with impaired glucose tolerance, and
- in healthy, normoglycemic individuals at potential genetic risk for DM.[151,153,154]

Diminished NO availability, caused by administration of ADMA, the endogenous inhibitor of eNOS, to wild-type mice, impaired insulin sensitivity within hours.[155] In a study of both lean and obese women, microvascular dysfunction was associated with decreased insulin sensitivity and increased blood pressure.[156] In the prospective Nurses' Health Study, elevated plasma levels of biomarkers (E-selectin, ICAM-1, and VCAM-1) reflecting endothelial dysfunction were powerful predictors of type 2 DM in a large cohort of initially healthy women, independent of other known risk factors, including obesity and subclinical inflammation.[157]

These studies suggest that **endothelial dysfunction develops at an early stage, before the detection of carbohydrate intolerance,** and may constitute an early link not only to insulin resistance and hyperglycemia but also to the pathophysiologic sequelae of the metabolic syndrome.[158]

eNOS, Nitric Oxide, and Insulin Sensitivity. **eNOS and NO may play a major role in the regulation of insulin sensitivity.** NO directly improves insulin sensitivity by blocking the inhibitory interaction of Rho kinase with IRS-1.[7] **A complete loss of eNOS in an eNOS −/− knockout mouse model causes the development of insulin resistance, hypertension, and hyperlipidemia.** Thus, eNOS is implicated not only in the regulation of arterial pressure. Loss of eNOS expression at both endothelial and skeletal muscle sites also creates insulin resistance and impairs insulin-stimulated glucose uptake.[89]

Microvascular Dysfunction and Insulin Resistance. Whereas dysfunctional endothelium in large and medium-sized arteries plays a central role in atherogenesis, vascular dysfunction at the arteriolar and capillary level appears to play a primary role in the pathogenesis of both insulin resistance and the associated features of the metabolic syndrome. **Insulin resistance and the metabolic syndrome might thus be viewed as the metabolic consequence of vascular dysfunction in the peripheral, microvascular bed.**[159]

There is differential regulation of vascular tone in conduit and resistance vessels, and dysfunction of the conduit versus resistance vasculature may have different clinical implications.[1] Inflammation engenders dysfunction primarily in the microvasculature.[160] Microvascular disturbances may play a role in arousing the amplified inflammatory response of adipose tissue that is implicated in adipose tissue and systemic insulin resistance.[161]

Ultimately, eNOS and vascular dysfunction may be implicated in the pathogenesis of insulin resistance. **With defective vascular function preceding the clinical onset of metabolic disease, the metabolic syndrome may, in effect, etiologically derive from vascular disease.**

ASSESSMENT OF ENDOTHELIAL FUNCTION

Coronary and peripheral endothelial function represents a gauge of cardiovascular health independent of other cardiac risk factors. Abnormal arterial reactivity is an index of endothelial dysfunction. Assessment of endothelial function is of potential use for patient screening and the evaluation of new therapeutic strategies.[81,82] Physiologic vascular testing of the endothelium may eventually evolve into an important adjunctive tool for the assessment of cardiovascular risk and the response to treatment (Table 8-5). However, further prospective, randomized studies that focus specifically on the clinical utility of endothelial functional testing as a means of assessing cardiovascular risk and the adequacy of therapy are needed.[91]

In practice, endothelial function is measured in the coronary circulation and peripherally (Table 8-6). The assessments are indirect in that they examine the ability of an artery to dilate in response to a stimulus that induces NO release. Stimuli that increase the production of endothelium-derived NO and have proved useful in assessing endothelium-dependent vasodilation in humans include

- increased shear stress derived from increased blood flow and
- receptor-dependent agonists, such as acetylcholine, bradykinin, and substance P.

Basal NO release can be assessed through the use of specific inhibitors of NOS, such as NMA.[1]

Table 8-5. Utility of Endothelial Function Assessment

CURRENT USES

Identification of novel risk factors for atherosclerosis
Investigation of mechanisms of vascular dysfunction and atherosclerosis
Surrogate marker of cardiovascular risk for intervention studies

POTENTIAL USES

Individual screening for future cardiovascular risk
Preoperative individual screening
Evaluation of individual need for lifestyle/pharmacologic intervention
Follow-up of responses to primary and secondary prevention strategies

Modified from Widlansky ME, Gokce N, Keaney JJ, Vita JA. The clinical implications of endothelial dysfunction. J Am Coll Cardiol 2003;42:1149-1160.

Table 8-6. Techniques for Measurement of Blood Flow/Endothelial Function

TECHNIQUE	TARGET	METHOD	COMMENT
Catheterization	Vessel diameter	Angiography/intravascular ultrasonography	Costly, risks, invasive
	Microcirculation	Fick principle	
Ultrasound	Vessel diameter	Measurement	Observer dependent
	Microcirculation	Blood flow estimated	
Plethysmography	Microcirculation	Limb volume/electrical impedance change	Expertise dependent
Positron emission tomography	Microcirculation	Tracer distribution	Costly
Laser Doppler flow determination	Microcirculation	Doppler	Validation needed

Modified from Calles-Escandon J, Cipolla M. Diabetes and endothelial dysfunction: a clinical perspective. Endocr Rev 2001:22:36-52.

Assessment of Coronary Artery Endothelial Function. Coronary artery endothelial function is most commonly assessed via invasive coronary catheterization approaches that involve a comparison between the responses to endothelium-independent and endothelium-dependent vasodilators.

- Endothelium-independent dilators such as nitroglycerin and sodium nitroprusside donate NO to vascular smooth muscle cells and thus define the vasodilatory capacity of the vessel.
- Endothelium-dependent vasodilators such as acetylcholine and methacholine act via endothelial muscarinic receptors, which stimulate eNOS to generate and release NO for vasodilation. Alternatively, distal administration of direct vascular smooth muscle cell relaxing agents, such as papaverine or adenosine, which increase coronary blood flow, may elicit flow-mediated NO release and endothelium-dependent, epicardial coronary vasodilation.

Normal coronary endothelial function is defined by the occurrence of coronary epicardial vessel dilation in response to intracoronary endothelium-dependent vasodilators, as detected by angiographic techniques or intravascular ultrasonography. Endothelial dysfunction is defined by a diminished epicardial coronary vasodilatory response or by paradoxical vasoconstriction, as for example in response to muscarinic agonists, when the smooth muscle vasoconstrictor effects of these agents supersedes the endothelial NO dilator effect.[1]

Advantages. The advantages inherent in this approach are the ability to directly examine basal endothelial function via NOS antagonist infusion, direct quantification of endothelial function in the vascular bed of interest, and assessment of dose-response relationships for endothelial agonists and antagonists.[1]

Disadvantages. Widespread application of this methodology is limited primarily by the risk inherent with invasive procedures, as well as its expense.[91]

Noninvasive Alternatives. Noninvasively, Doppler echocardiography, positron emission tomography, and magnetic resonance imaging may assess microvascular vasodilatory capacity via flow measurements in response to vasodilators.[93]

Assessment of Peripheral Arterial Endothelial Function. Because atherosclerosis and its underlying endothelial dysfunction are a diffuse, systemic process, endothelial function can be assessed in either the coronary or the peripheral circulation. Thus, **brachial artery endothelial function parallels endothelial function in the coronary circulation.**[162]

Alternatives to the testing of coronary endothelial function entail the evaluation of endothelial function in peripheral arteries. Peripheral arteries that are readily studied are the

- brachial,
- carotid,
- superficial femoral, and
- radial

arteries.

High-Resolution Ultrasound Imaging. A convenient noninvasive method currently used is high-resolution ultrasound imaging of postischemic brachial artery reactivity during reactive hyperemia.

In the process, the brachial artery is imaged at the midportion of the upper part of the arm at baseline and with any intervention. Forearm and hand ischemia is induced by interrupting arterial perfusion just below the elbow via 5-minute pressure cuff occlusion at the suprasystolic pressure of 300 mm Hg. Ischemia causes dilation of the distal microvasculature. Release of the tourniquet induces reactive hyperemia because of alterations in hydrostatic pressure. The attendant hyperemic blood flow increases shear stress and results in the local endothelial release of NO.

As an alternative to forearm ischemia, an acetylcholine infusion can be administered at doses of around 3.75 to 7.5 μg/min to elicit endothelium-dependent vasodilation.[163,164]

The magnitude of the change in vessel diameter from the baseline period to the peak dilation observed during reactive hyperemia imaged over a period of 5 minutes is indicative of the degree of endothelial function.[91] The percentage of flow-mediated dilation is calculated as

$$100 \times (\text{Peak hyperemic diameter} - \text{Rest diameter}) / \text{Rest diameter.}$$

With normal endothelial function, the postischemic, reactive hyperemic flow causes dilation of the brachial artery. An abnormal response occurs with endothelial dysfunction because the vasodilatory response is dependent on shear stress and endothelial NO.[91]

A nitroglycerin infusion at doses of 1.5 and 3.0 μg/min or sublingual nitroglycerin–induced arterial dilation, monitored for 6 minutes after nitroglycerin administration, determines the vasodilatory capacity of the vessel; the ratio

$$\text{Peak flow-mediated dilation} / \text{Nitroglycerin-mediated dilation}$$

may also be of utility in risk assessment.[88]

Advantages. Because brachial reactivity correlates with endothelial dysfunction in the coronary circulation, advantages of peripheral arterial ultrasound imaging are that the technique is

- noninvasive,
- safer,
- less costly, and
- faster

than any invasive method. Furthermore, this technique generally uses flow as a physiologic stimulus for vasodilation rather than agonists such as acetylcholine.[1]

Disadvantages. To date, peripheral arterial ultrasound imaging suffers from insufficient standardization to be of clinical utility in longitudinal follow-up or in allowing comparisons between laboratories. For example, in brachial artery reactivity studies, the occluding cuff may be placed above or below the elbow. The time after cuff deflation when measurements are taken may vary between laboratories, and there is considerable operator dependence in several aspects of test performance. There is also poor image resolution relative to arterial size with significant variability in measurements.[91]

A noninvasive alternative to brachial ultrasonography is the scintigraphic assessment of hyperemic reactivity, which may be integrated into a resting myocardial perfusion scan.[165]

Digital Pulse Wave Plethysmography. Endothelial function can also be assessed by noninvasive, digital pulse wave plethysmography. This technique entails measuring volume changes in the limb by mercury strain gauges during reactive hyperemia in response to the ischemic challenge of venous occlusion.

Alternatively, more invasive studies may involve the infusion of endothelium-dependent agonists into the limb artery and measurement of the vasodilator responses of forearm resistance vessels by plethysmography. Responses to the infusion of vasoactive agents such as methacholine as an endothelium-dependent vasodilator are compared with the responses elicited by sodium nitroprusside as an exogenous NO donor and are contrasted with the responses of normal subjects.

Blood flow may be monitored in a variety of regional vascular beds. Typically, leg or forearm blood flow is examined.[91]

Advantages. Akin to studies in the coronary circulation, this approach allows the use of specific agonists and antagonists and the examination of dose-response relationships in a more accessible vascular bed.

Disadvantages. The technique requires arterial catheterization and thus has limited applicability for large-scale studies and future development as a clinical tool.[1]

Other Venues for the Assessment of Vascular Function. Numerous other measurements of vasomotor activity or biochemical markers can shed light on the health status of the vasculature.

Digital Reactive Hyperemia. Reactive hyperemia peripheral arterial tonometry (RH-PAT), an assessment of digital volume changes accompanying pulse waves, appears to provide a technically less complex, noninvasive measure of endothelial function. The process involves the use of probes placed on a finger on each hand, one side to undergo 5 minutes of pulse occlusion followed by reactive hyperemia, the other to serve as a continuous control. RH-PAT measures the changes in digital pulse volume that occur during reactive hyperemia.[166]

RH-PAT may serve as a noninvasive test to identify coronary endothelial dysfunction. The digital hyperemic response, as assessed by RH-PAT, was attenuated in patients with coronary microvascular endothelial dysfunction.[167]

Endothelium-Independent Vasodilation. Vascular smooth muscle cells are the final common pathway mediating vasorelaxation. Functional abnormalities in arterial vascular smooth muscle vasodilatory capacity may be associated with impaired vascular health. Endothelium-independent vasodilation can be evaluated in both the coronary and peripheral circulation after the administration of agents that directly relax smooth muscle cells, such as nitroglycerin or sodium nitroprusside. Typically, impaired endothelium-independent vasodilation responses also imply the presence of decreased endothelium-dependent vasodilation and endothelial dysfunction. Not surprisingly, abnormal endothelium-independent responses to nitroglycerin are also predictive of an adverse prognosis.[91]

Arterial Compliance. Measures of arterial stiffness, including pulse wave velocity and arterial distensibility, are alternative, noninvasive measures of vascular health. Although endothelial function plays a role, arterial stiffness is highly dependent on structural features of the vascular wall, such as the degree of fibrosis and calcification. Measures of arterial stiffness may predict cardiovascular events; however, the relationship between endothelial function and vascular stiffness, as well as clinical applicability, requires further definition.[1]

Nitric Oxide Metabolites. Because of the short half-life of NO, NO is rapidly oxidized to the stable end products nitrate and nitrite, which are excreted in urine. NO production, reflective of endothelial function, may thus be estimated by measuring plasma or urinary levels of the metabolic products nitrate and nitrite. Urinary excretion of NO metabolites may be reduced in individuals with atherosclerotic disease. However, this type of evaluation is complicated by the fact that many stimuli, such as exercise, perturb the release of NO and its metabolites.[168]

Urinary Albumin Excretion. The amount of the water-soluble protein albumin excreted in urine, or urinary albumin excretion, is a marker for endothelial dysfunction and the metabolic syndrome. Although numerous cellular or active transport factors and increased glomerular membrane permeability may underlie proteinuria, modest, "normal" amounts of urinary albumin excretion may reflect systemic endothelial dysfunction and preclinical vascular disease. **Microalbuminuria (30 to 300 mg/lg creatinine in spot urine or >5 μg/min in a random morning sample) is a strong risk factor of cardiovascular morbidity and mortality, independent of other risk factors** such as age, gender, renal creatinine clearance, DM, hypertension, or dyslipidemia. Sensitive testing for microalbuminuria is now available.[169,170]

Erectile Dysfunction. Erectile dysfunction correlates highly with endothelial dysfunction. Because penile erection is a vascular event that is dependent on intact endothelial function, it serves as a symptom and marker of endothelial disturbance and early vascular disease.[171] Patients with erectile dysfunction, in the absence of any evidence of obstructive vascular disease or endocrinologic, physical, or psychological impairment, have endothelial dysfunction as evidenced by abnormal brachial flow–mediated dilation.[172]

Many of the risk factors for CHD constitute risk factors for erectile dysfunction, including endothelial dysfunction, lipid disturbances, hypertension, smoking, DM, and a sedentary lifestyle.[173] In a study of erectile dysfunction in the absence of other clinical cardiovascular disease, 30 men with erectile dysfunction had reduced brachial artery flow–mediated vasodilation and nitroglycerin-mediated vasodilation when compared with men who had intact erectile function.[172]

In patients with type 2 DM, the presence of erectile dysfunction may, in fact, be associated with the presence of silent myocardial ischemia.[174]

cGMP Kinase Activity. cGMP activity may serve as an assay for endothelial function. cGK is a downstream effector of the NO/cGMP signaling chain. Its activity thus reflects the integrated activity and expression of cGK and its upstream signaling components. cGK phosphorylates a substrate VASP at Ser239. Immunoblotting techniques with antibodies to phosphorylated VASP detect cGK activity. This assay reliably reflects NO/cGMP signaling activity in platelets, in cultured endothelial and smooth muscle cells, in intact vascular tissues, and in the endothelium of intact arteries under basal NO release conditions. This assay reflects endothelial function and potentially represents a biochemical assay for the early recognition of disease states and for the evaluation of therapeutic strategies.[4]

Endothelial Progenitor Cells. Endothelial progenitor cells, derived from the bone marrow, participate in ongoing repair of the endothelium. Mobilization and differentiation of endothelial progenitor cells are also critical to the process of angiogenesis in response to myocardial ischemia. Impaired mobilization and the depletion of such progenitor cells contribute to endothelial dysfunction. Thus, the number of circulating endothelial progenitor cells correlates with flow-mediated brachial artery reactivity (Fig. 8-8), but is inversely related to an individual's combined Framingham risk score. **Levels of endothelial progenitor cells may thus be a surrogate marker for vascular function.**[175]

Inflammatory Markers. Inflammation impairs endothelial function, and **markers of systemic or vascular inflammation reflect vascular dysfunction.**

C-Reactive Protein, Myeloperoxidase. Markers of systemic inflammation, including elevated levels of C-reactive protein or myeloperoxidase, are associated with endothelial dysfunction in humans and may predict the risk for future cardiovascular events.[1,106]

Adhesion Molecules. Cellular adhesion molecules may assist in the assessment of endothelial integrity. They are expressed on the surface of injured endothelial cells and play an integral role in leukocyte adherence and transmigration. Cellular adhesion molecules and inflammatory, prothrombotic mediators are shed into the

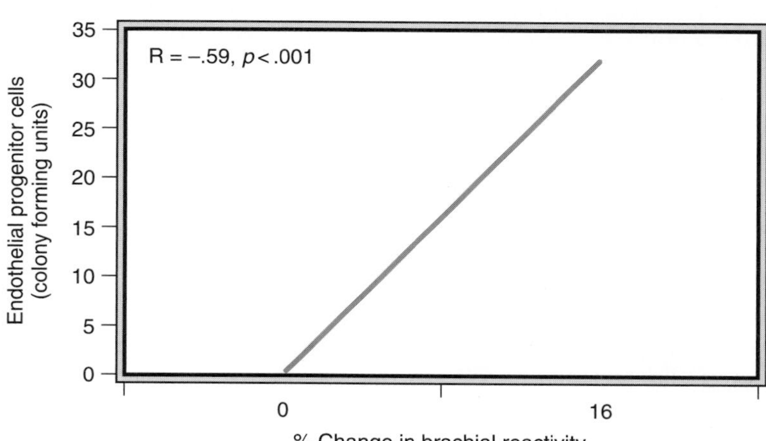

Figure 8–8. Relationship between the number of endothelial progenitor cells and endothelial function in men. *(Modified from Hill JM, Zalos G, Halcox JPJ, et al. Circulating endothelial progenitor cells, vascular function, and cardiovascular risk. N Engl J Med 2003;348:593-600.)*

circulation and are independent predictors of future cardiovascular events, even in individuals without known CHD. **In patients with known CHD, elevated levels of soluble ICAM have prognostic value.**[1]

Superoxide Dismutase. Vascular, extracellular SOD may also be of utility in the assessment of vascular function. It is an important antioxidant enzyme system and is substantially reduced in individuals with CHD.[91]

Asymmetric Dimethylarginine. Circulating levels of ADMA, an endogenous inhibitor of NOS, may provide information to assess the severity of underlying endothelial dysfunction.[84] ADMA is a potential marker of cardiovascular disease. There is significant correlation between circulating concentrations of ADMA, intima-media thickening in the carotid artery, and impaired endothelium-dependent relaxation.[58]

CONCLUSION

There is an interdependence between vascular and metabolic health, between the intact functioning of eNOS and the metabolic insulin pathway. Murine insulin receptor and IRS-1 knockout models develop endothelial dysfunction together with insulin resistance. Murine eNOS knockout models acquire insulin resistance together with endothelial dysfunction.

Anabolic metabolism requires not only the intake of nutrients and intracellular anabolic pathways. Effective macrovascular and microvascular delivery of nutrients and anabolic hormones such as insulin is also a sine qua non linking nutrient intake to cellular processes. Like the insulin receptor, NOS is expressed not only in the vascular endothelium, where it regulates arterial tone, but also in skeletal muscle, where it participates in metabolic processes. In fact, there is close anatomic linkage of the insulin receptor with eNOS. Both eNOS and the activated insulin receptor are located in caveolae. Furthermore, insulin and eNOS signaling are linked from a molecular perspective. In reciprocal fashion, insulin activates eNOS, whereas intact functioning of the NO/cGMP/cGK pathway enhances insulin sensitivity. Insulin's vasculoprotective and anti-inflammatory effects are implemented through NO as a downstream effector to insulin's PI3K-Akt signaling pathway. Furthermore, both fluid shear stress and insulin regulate eNOS phosphorylation and NO production via overlapping mechanisms. Not surprisingly, the preservation of endothelium-dependent vasodilation correlates with the integrity of anabolic, insulin-mediated glucose handling.

In contrast, stress and inflammation are catabolic processes. The inflammatory process prioritizes nutrient utilization by insulin-independent immune organs at the expense of the needs of insulin-dependent tissues such as the musculature. Thus, concomitant with its interference with insulin signaling and nutrient uptake, chronic inflammation impairs endothelial, microvascular function and nutrient delivery. Here again, the close anatomic and molecular linkage of eNOS with the insulin receptor plays a role. Both eNOS and insulin metabolic signaling are adversely affected by

- factors that disrupt caveolar membrane cholesterol content,
- disruption of caveolin scaffolding,
- caveolar crosstalk from vasoconstrictor or cytokine receptor signaling, and
- Rho kinase activation.

In short, the metabolic-vascular signaling of insulin is compromised by similar caveolar contingencies that disrupt the activity of eNOS. Not surprisingly, dysfunctional endothelium compromises insulin sensitivity, insulin resistance worsens endothelial function, and endothelial dysfunction correlates with the severity of insulin resistance and contributes to its deterioration.

The NOS-insulin interaction plays a critical role linking the control of vasomotor tone and vascular function with glucose and lipid homeostasis. In the presence of chronic stress and inflammation, dysfunctional eNOS and disturbed vascular function underlie and intensify the ensuing metabolic disturbances, thus rendering the pathogenesis of insulin resistance a vascular disease. Exercise, through its metabolic requirements, requires increased anabolic activity. The enhanced laminar shear stress associated with exercise is of particular interest in counteracting the vascular and catabolic effects of inflammation.

Laminar shear increases the number of caveolae and enhances activation of the shear-sensitive signaling molecule Akt. It antagonizes the effects of TNF-α and angiotensin II, effects that would be expected to favor not only vascular perfusion but also anabolic metabolism. It is thus not surprising that in general, numerous lifestyle, nutritional, or pharmacologic interventions that aim to enhance endothelial function and cardiovascular prognosis concomitantly improve insulin resistance and lessen the risk for the development of type 2 DM.

GLOSSARY

ACE	angiotensin-converting enzyme
ADMA	asymmetric dimethylarginine
ADP	adenosine 5′-diphosphate
AGE	advanced glycation end product
AMP	adenosine 5′-monophosphate
AMPK	5′-AMP–activated protein kinase
AP-1	activating protein-1
apo	apolipoprotein
AT_1	angiotensin II type 1 receptor
BH_4	tetrahydrobiopterin
Ca^{2+}	calcium
CAT-1	cationic amino acid-1
cGK	cGMP-dependent protein kinase
cGMP	cyclic guanosine 3′,5′-monophosphate
CHD	coronary heart disease
CoA	coenzyme A
COX	cyclooxygenase
DDAH	dimethylarginine dimethylaminohydrolase
DM	diabetes mellitus
EGF	epidermal growth factor
Egr-1	early growth response-1
eNOS	endothelial nitric oxide synthase
ERK	extracellular signal–regulated kinase
ET-1	endothelin-1
FAK	focal adhesion kinase
FGF	fibroblast growth factor
GPI	glycosylphosphatidylinositol
GTP	guanosine 5′-triphosphate
HDL	high-density lipoprotein
HMG	3-hydroxy-3-methylglutaryl
Hsp 90	heat shock protein 90
ICAM-1	intracellular adhesion molecule-1
IGF-I	insulin-like growth factor type I
IL	interleukin
iNOS	inducible nitric oxide synthase
IRS	insulin receptor substrate
JNK	c-Jun NH_2-terminal kinase
LDL	low-density lipoprotein
MAPK	mitogen-activated protein kinase
MCP-1	monocyte chemoattractant protein-1
MMP	matrix metalloproteinase
NADH/NADPH	nicotinamide adenine dinucleotide phosphate oxidase
NFκB	nuclear factor kappaB
NMA	*N*-monomethylarginine
nNOS	neuronal nitric oxide synthase
NO	nitric oxide
NOS	nitric oxide synthase
PAI-1	plasminogen activator inhibitor-1
PDGF	platelet-derived growth factor
PDK-1	phosphoinositide-dependent kinase-1
PI3K	phosphatidylinositol 3-kinase
PKA	protein kinase A
PKB	protein kinase B
PKC	protein kinase C
PPAR	peroxisome proliferator–activated receptor
PRMT	protein arginine *N*-methyltransferase
RAAS	renin-angiotensin-aldosterone system
RH-PAT	reactive hyperemia peripheral arterial tonometry
ROS	reactive oxygen species
SAPK	stress-activated protein kinase
Ser	serine
SOD	superoxide dismutase
SR-B1	scavenger receptor B1
TGF	transforming growth factor
Thr	threonine
TIMP	tissue inhibitor of matrix metalloproteinases
TNF	tumor necrosis factor
TNFR1	TNF receptor type 1
tPA	tissue plasminogen activator
TRAF	TNF receptor–associated factor
VCAM-1	vascular cell adhesion molecule-1
VEGF	vascular endothelial growth factor
VLDL	very-low-density lipoprotein

REFERENCES

1. Widlansky ME, Gokce N, Keaney JJ, Vita JA. The clinical implications of endothelial dysfunction. J Am Coll Cardiol 2003;42:1149-1160
2. Koshland DE Jr: The molecule of the year. Science 1992;258:1861
3. Hayden MR, Tyagi SC. Is type 2 diabetes mellitus a vascular disease (atheroscleropathy) with hyperglycemia a late manifestation? The role of NOS, NO, and redox stress. Cardiovasc Diabetol 2003;2:2
4. Munzel T, Feil R, Mulsch A, et al. Physiology and pathophysiology of vascular signaling controlled by guanosine 3′,5′-cyclic monophosphate–dependent protein kinase. Circulation 2003;108:2172-2183
5. Moncada S, Higgs A. The L-arginine–nitric oxide pathway. N Engl J Med 1993;329:2002-2012
6. Cooke JP. Does ADMA cause endothelial dysfunction? Arterioscler Thromb Vasc Biol 2000;20:2032-2037
7. Begum N, Sandu OA, Ito M, et al. Active Rho kinase (ROK-alpha) associates with insulin receptor substrate-1 and inhibits insulin signaling in vascular smooth muscle cells. J Biol Chem 2002;277:6214-6222
8. Wung BS, Cheng JJ, Shyue SK, Wang DL. NO modulates monocyte chemotactic protein-1 expression in endothelial cells under cyclic strain. Arterioscler Thromb Vasc Biol 2001;21:1941-1947
9. Harrison DG, Cai H. Endothelial control of vasomotion and nitric oxide production. Cardiol Clin 2003;21: 289-302
10. Federici M, Menghini R, Mauriello A, et al. Insulin-dependent activation of endothelial nitric oxide synthase is impaired by O-linked glycosylation modification of signaling proteins in human coronary endothelial cells Circulation 2002;106:466-472
11. Radomski MW, Palmer RM, Moncada S. The role of nitric oxide and cGMP in platelet adhesion to vascular endothelium. Biochem Biophys Res Commun 1987; 148:1482-1489
12. Sarkar R, Meinberg EG, Stanley JC, et al. Nitric oxide reversibly inhibits the migration of cultured vascular smooth muscle cells. Circ Res 1996;78:225-230
13. Kubes P, Suzuki M, Granger DN. Nitric oxide: an endogenous modulator of leukocyte adhesion. Proc Natl Acad Sci U S A 1991;88:4651-4655
14. Pelat M, Dessy C, Massion P, et al. Rosuvastatin decreases caveolin-1 and improves nitric oxide–dependent heart rate and blood pressure variability in apolipoprotein E–/– mice in vivo. Circulation 2003;107:2480-2486
15. Higaki Y, Hirshman MF, Fujii N, Goodyear LJ. Nitric oxide increases glucose uptake through a mechanism that is distinct from the insulin and contraction pathways in rat skeletal muscle. Diabetes 2001;50:241-247
16. Kingwell BA. Nitric oxide–mediated metabolic regulation during exercise: effects of training in health and cardiovascular disease. FASEB J 2000;14:1685-1696
17. Kone BC, Kuncewicz T, Zhang W, Yu ZY. Protein interactions with nitric oxide synthases: controlling the right time, the right place, and the right amount of nitric oxide. Am J Physiol Renal Physiol 2003;285:F178-F190
18. Sase K, Michel T. Expression of constitutive nitric oxide synthase in human blood platelets. Life Sci 1995; 57:2049-2055
19. Feron O, Zhao YY, Kelly RA. The ins and outs of caveolar signaling. m2 muscarinic cholinergic receptors and eNOS activation versus neuregulin and ErbB4 signaling in cardiac myocytes. Ann N Y Acad Sci 1999;874:11-19
20. Goligorsky MS, Li H, Brodsky S, Chen J. Relationships between caveolae and eNOS: everything in proximity and the proximity of everything. Am J Physiol Renal Physiol 2002;283:F1-F10
21. Bernier SG, Haldar S, Michel T. Bradykinin-regulated interactions of the mitogen-activated protein kinase pathway with the endothelial nitric-oxide synthase. J Biol Chem 2000;275:30707-30715
22. Shaul PW. Regulation of endothelial nitric oxide synthase: location, location, location. Annu Rev Physiol 2002;64:749-774
23. Liu P, Wang P, Michaely P, et al. Presence of oxidized cholesterol in caveolae uncouples active platelet-derived growth factor receptors from tyrosine kinase substrates. J Biol Chem 2000;275:31648-31654
24. Stulnig TM, Huber J, Leitinger N, et al. Polyunsaturated eicosapentaenoic acid displaces proteins from membrane rafts by altering raft lipid composition. J Biol Chem 2001;276:37335-37340
25. Dimmeler S, Zeiher AM. Exercise and cardiovascular health: get active to "AKTivate" your endothelial nitric oxide synthase. Circulation 2003;107:3118-3120.
26. Ramet ME, Ramet M, Lu Q, et al. High-density lipoprotein increases the abundance of eNOS protein in human vascular endothelial cells by increasing its half-life. J Am Coll Cardiol 2003;41:2288-2297
27. Hambrecht R, Adams V, Erbs S, et al. Regular physical activity improves endothelial function in patients with coronary artery disease by increasing phosphorylation of endothelial nitric oxide synthase. Circulation 2003;107:3152-3158
28. Peterson TE, Poppa V, Ueba H, et al. Opposing effects of reactive oxygen species and cholesterol on endothelial nitric oxide synthase and endothelial cell caveolae. Circ Res 1999;85:29-37
29. Feron O, Dessy C, Opel DJ, et al. Modulation of the endothelial nitric-oxide synthase–caveolin interaction in cardiac myocytes. Implications for the autonomic regulation of heart rate. J Biol Chem 1998; 273:30249-30254
30. Mann GE, Yudilevich DL, Sobrevia L. Regulation of amino acid and glucose transporters in endothelial and smooth muscle cells. Physiol Rev 2003;83:183-252
31. Johns DG, Dorrance AM, Tramontini NL, Webb RC. Glucocorticoids inhibit tetrahydrobiopterin-dependent endothelial function. Exp Biol Med 2001;226:27-31
32. Jaimes EA, Sweeney C, Raij L. Effects of the reactive oxygen species hydrogen peroxide and hypochlorite on endothelial nitric oxide production. Hypertension 2001;38:877-883
33. Nuszkowski A, Grabner R, Marsche G, et al. Hypochlorite-modified low density lipoprotein inhibits nitric oxide synthesis in endothelial cells via an intracellular dislocalization of endothelial nitric-oxide synthase. J Biol Chem 2001;276:14212-14221
34. Fleming I, Busse R. Molecular mechanisms involved in the regulation of the endothelial nitric oxide synthase. Am J Physiol Regul Integr Comp Physiol 2003;284: R1-R12
35. Barandier C, Ming XF, Rusconi S, Yang Z. PKC is required for activation of ROCK by RhoA in human endothelial cells. Biochem Biophys Res Commun 2003;304:714-719
36. Kone BC. Protein-protein interactions controlling nitric oxide synthases. Acta Physiol Scand 2000;168:27-31

37. Kincer JF, Uittenbogaard A, Dressman J, et al. Hypercholesterolemia promotes a CD36-dependent and endothelial nitric-oxide synthase–mediated vascular dysfunction. J Biol Chem 2002;277:23525-23533
38. Solomonson LP, Flam BR, Pendleton LC, et al. The caveolar nitric oxide synthase/arginine regeneration system for NO production in endothelial cells. J Exp Biol 2003;206:2083-2087
39. Sun RJ, Muller S, Zhuang FY, et al. Caveolin-1 redistribution in human endothelial cells induced by laminar flow and cytokine. Biorheology 2003;40:31-39
40. Boyd NL, Park H, Yi H, et al. Chronic shear induces caveolae formation and alters ERK and Akt responses in endothelial cells. Am J Physiol Heart Circ Physiol 2003;285:H1113-H1122
41. Park H, Go YM, St John PL, et al. Plasma membrane cholesterol is a key molecule in shear stress–dependent activation of extracellular signal–regulated kinase. J Biol Chem 1998;273:32304-32311
42. Park H, Go YM, Darji R, et al. Caveolin-1 regulates shear stress–dependent activation of extracellular signal–regulated kinase. Am J Physiol Heart Circ Physiol 2000;278:H1285-H1293
43. Davis ME, Cai H, Drummond GR, Harrison DG. Shear stress regulates endothelial nitric oxide synthase expression through c-Src by divergent signaling pathways. Circ Res 2001;89:1073-1080
44. Vita JA, Mitchell GF. Effect of shear stress and flow pulsatility on endothelial function. Insights gleaned from external counterpulsation therapy. J Am Coll Cardiol 2003;42:2095-2098
45. Rizzo V, Morton C, DePaola N, et al. Recruitment of endothelial caveolae into mechanotransduction pathways by flow conditioning in vitro. Am J Physiol Heart Circ Physiol 2003;285:H1720-H1729
46. Ceravolo R, Maio R, Pujia A, et al. Pulse pressure and endothelial dysfunction in never-treated hypertensive patients. J Am Coll Cardiol 2003;41:1753-1758
47. Yamawaki H, Lehoux S, Berk BC. Chronic physiological shear stress inhibits tumor necrosis factor–induced proinflammatory responses in rabbit aorta perfused ex vivo. Circulation 2003;108:1619-1925
48. Bonetti PO, Barsness GW, Keelan PC, et al. Enhanced external counterpulsation improves endothelial function in patients with sympathetic coronary artery disease. J Am Coll Cardiol 2003;41:1761-1768
49. Berk BC, Min W, Yan C, et al. Atheroprotective mechanisms activated by fluid shear stress in endothelial cells. Drug News Perspect 2002;15:133-139
50. Gielen S, Hambrecht R. The childhood obesity epidemic: impact on endothelial function. Circulation 2004;109:1911-1913
51. Calnek DS, Mazzella L, Roser S, et al. Peroxisome proliferator–activated receptor gamma ligands increase release of nitric oxide from endothelial cells. Arterioscler Thromb Vasc Biol 2003;23:52-57
52. Plutzky J. Peroxisome proliferator–activated receptors in endothelial cell biology. Curr Opin Lipidol 2001;12: 511-518
53. Iglarz M, Touyz RM, Amiri F, et al. Effect of peroxisome proliferator–activated receptor-alpha and -gamma activators on vascular remodeling in endothelin-dependent hypertension. Arterioscler Thromb Vasc Biol 2003;23: 45-51
54. Vita JA, Keany JF Jr. Hormone replacement therapy and endothelial function: the exception that proves the rule? Arterioscler Thromb Vasc Biol 2001;21:1867-1869
55. Brown NJ, Abbas A, Byrne D, et al. Comparative effects of estrogen and angiotensin-converting enzyme inhibition on plasminogen activator inhibitor-1 in healthy postmenopausal women. Circulation 2002;105:304-309
56. Sorensen KE, Dorup I, Hermann AP, Mosekilde L. Combined hormone replacement therapy does not protect women against the age-related decline in endothelium-dependent vasomotor function. Circulation 1998;97: 1234-1238
57. Chambliss KL, Shaul PW. Estrogen modulation of endothelial nitric oxide synthase. Endocr Rev 2002; 23:665-686
58. Holden DP, Cartwright JE, Nussey SS, Whitley GS. Estrogen stimulates dimethylarginine dimethylaminohydrolase activity and the metabolism of asymmetric dimethylarginine. Circulation 2003;108:1575-1580
59. Rossouw JE, Anderson GL, Prentice RL, et al for the Women's Health Initiative Investigators. Risks and benefits of estrogen plus progestin in healthy postmenopausal women: principal results from the Women's Health Initiative randomized controlled trial. JAMA 2002; 288:321-333
60. Hulley S, Grady D, Bush T, et al. Randomized trial of estrogen plus progestin for secondary prevention of coronary heart disease in postmenopausal women: Heart and Estrogen/progestin Replacement Study (HERS) research group. JAMA 1998;280:605-613
61. Dessy C, Kelly RA, Balligand JL, Feron O. Dynamin mediates caveolar sequestration of muscarinic cholinergic receptors and alteration in NO signaling. EMBO J 2000;19:4272-4280
62. Li XA, Titlow WB, Jackson BA, et al. High density lipoprotein binding to scavenger receptor, class B, type I activates endothelial nitric-oxide synthase in a ceramide-dependent manner. J Biol Chem 2002;277:11058-11063
63. Shaul PW. Endothelial nitric oxide synthase, caveolae and the development of atherosclerosis. J Physiol 2003;547:21-33
64. Kuvin JT, Ramet ME, Patel AR, et al. A novel mechanism for the beneficial vascular effects of high-density lipoprotein cholesterol: enhanced vasorelaxation and increased endothelial nitric oxide synthase expression. Am Heart J 2002;144:165-172
65. Uittenbogaard A, Shaul PW, Yuhanna IS, et al. High density lipoprotein prevents oxidized low density lipoprotein–induced inhibition of endothelial nitric-oxide synthase localization and activation in caveolae. J Biol Chem 2000;275:11278-11283
66. Yuhanna IS, Zhu Y, Cox BE, et al. High-density lipoprotein binding to scavenger receptor-BI activates endothelial nitric oxide synthase. Nat Med 2001;7: 853-857
67. Calabresi L, Gomaraschi M, Franceschini G. Endothelial protection by high-density lipoproteins: from bench to bedside. Arterioscler Thromb Vasc Biol 2003;23: 1724-1731
68. Mineo C, Yuhanna IS, Quon MJ, Shaul PW. High density lipoprotein–induced endothelial nitric-oxide synthase activation is mediated by Akt and MAP kinases. J Biol Chem 2003;278:9142-9149
69. Chen H, Yu Q-S, Guo Z-G. High density lipoproteins enhanced antiaggregatory activity of nitric oxide derived from bovine aortal endothelial cells. Acta Physiol Sin 2000;52:81-84
70. Kuboki K, Jiang ZY, Takahara N, et al. Regulation of endothelial constitutive nitric oxide synthase gene expression in endothelial cells and in vivo: a specific vascular action of insulin. Circulation 2000;101:676-681
71. Zeng G, Quon MJ. Insulin-stimulated production of nitric oxide is inhibited by wortmannin. J Clin Invest 1996;98:894-898

72. Vicent D, Ilany J, Kondo T, et al. The role of endothelial insulin signaling in the regulation of vascular tone and insulin resistance. J Clin Invest 2003;111:1373-1380
73. Schnyder B, Pittet M, Durand J, Schnyder-Candrian S. Rapid effects of glucose on the insulin signaling of endothelial NO generation and epithelial Na transport. Am J Physiol Endocrinol Metab 2001;282:E87-E94
74. Kim F, Gallis B, Corson MA. TNF-alpha inhibits flow and insulin signaling leading to NO production in aortic endothelial cells. Am J Physiol Cell Physiol 2001;280:C1057-C1065
75. Montagnani M, Ravichandran LV, Chen H, et al. Insulin receptor substrate-1 and phosphoinositide-dependent kinase-1 are required for insulin-stimulated production of nitric oxide in endothelial cells. Mol Endocrinol 2002;16:1931-1942
76. Mather K, Laakso M, Edelman S, et al. Evidence for physiological coupling of insulin-mediated glucose metabolism and limb blood flow. Am J Physiol Endocrinol Metab 2000;279:E1264-E1270
77. Fisslthaler B, Benzing T, Busse R, Fleming I. Insulin enhances the expression of the endothelial nitric oxide synthase in native endothelial cells: a dual role for Akt and AP-1. Nitric Oxide 2003;8:253-261
78. Dandona P, Aljada A, Mohanty P, et al. Insulin inhibits intranuclear nuclear factor kappaB and stimulates IkappaB in mononuclear cells in obese subjects: evidence for an antiinflammatory effect? J Clin Endocrinol Metab 2001;86:3257-3265
79. Goetze S, Blaschke F, Stawowy P, et al. TNFalpha inhibits insulin's antiapoptotic signaling in vascular smooth muscle cells. Biochem Biophys Res Commun 2001;287:662-670
80. Schindler TH, Nitzsche EU, Munzel T, et al. Coronary vasoregulation in patients with various risk factors in response to cold pressor testing. J Am Coll Cardiol 2003;42:814-822
81. Sorensen KE, Celermajer DS, Spiegelhalter DJ, et al. Non-invasive measurement of human endothelium dependent arterial responses: accuracy and reproducibility. Br Heart J 1995;74:247-253
82. Gokce N, Keany JF, Hunter LM, et al. Predictive value of noninvasively determined endothelial dysfunction for long-term cardiovascular events in patients with peripheral vascular disease. J Am Coll Cardiol 2003; 41:1769-1775
83. Celermajer DS, Sorensen KE, Spiegelhalter DJ, et al. Aging is associated with endothelial dysfunction in healthy men years before the age-related decline in women. J Am Coll Cardiol 1994;24:471-476
84. Engler MM, Engler MB, Malloy MJ, et al. Antioxidant vitamins C and E improve endothelial function in children with hyperlipidemia: Endothelial Assessment of Risk from Lipids in Youth (EARLY) Trial. Circulation 2003;108:1059-1063
85. Bugiardini R, Manfrini O, Pizzi C, et al. Endothelial function predicts future development of coronary artery disease: A study of women with chest pain and normal coronary angiograms. Circulation 2004; 109:2518-2523
86. Szmitko PE, Wang C-H, Weisel RD, et al. Biomarkers of vascular disease linking inflammation to endothelial activation: Part II. Circulation 2003;108:2041-2048
87. Nigam A, Mitchell GF, Lambert J Tardif J-C. Relation between conduit vessel stiffness (assessed by tonometry) and endothelial function (assessed by flow-mediated dilatation) in patients with and without coronary heart disease. Am J Cardiol 2003;92:395-399
88. Chan SY, Mancini GJ, Kuramoto L, et al. The prognostic importance of endothelial dysfunction and carotid atheroma burden in patients with coronary artery disease. J Am Coll Cardiol 2003;42:1037-1043
89. Duplain H, Burcelin R, Sartori C, et al. Insulin resistance, hyperlipidemia, and hypertension in mice lacking endothelial nitric oxide synthase. Circulation 2001; 104:342-345
90. Modena M, Bonetti L, Coppi F, et al. Prognostic role of reversible endothelial dysfunction in hypertensive postmenopausal women. J Am Coll Cardiol 2002; 40:505-510
91. Kuvin JT, Karas RH. Clinical utility of endothelial function testing: ready for prime time? Circulation 2003; 107:3243-3247
92. Perticone F, Ceravolo R, Pujia A, et al. Prognostic significance of endothelial dysfunction. Circulation 2001; 104:191-196
93. Quyyumi AA. Prognostic value of endothelial function. Am J Cardiol 2003;91(suppl):19H-24H
94. Yusuf S, Dagenais G, Pogue J, et al. Vitamin E supplementation and cardiovascular events in high-risk patients: the Heart Outcomes Prevention Evaluation Study investigators. N Engl J Med 2000; 342:154-160
95. Chauhan A, More RS, Mullins PA, et al. Aging-associated endothelial dysfunction in humans is reversed by L-arginine. J Am Coll Cardiol 1996;28:1796-1804
96. Veldman BA, Spiering W, Doevendans PA, et al. The Glu298Asp polymorphism of the NOS 3 gene as a determinant of the baseline production of nitric oxide. J Hypertens 2002;20:2023-2027
97. Miyamoto Y, Saito Y, Kajiyama N, et al.: Endothelial nitric oxide synthase gene is positively associated with essential hypertension. Hypertension 1998;32:3-8
98. Shimasaki Y, Vasue H, Yoshimura M, et al. Association of the missense Glu298Asp variant of the endothelial nitric oxide synthase gene with myocardial infarction. J Am Coll Cardiol 1998;31:1506-1510
99. Colombo MG, Andreassi MG, Paradossi U, et al. Evidence for association of a common variant of the endothelial nitric oxide synthase gene (Glu298 → Asp polymorphism) to the presence, extent, and severity of coronary artery disease. Heart 2002;87:525-528
100. Ito A, Tsao PS, Adimoolam S, et al. Novel mechanism for endothelial dysfunction: dysregulation of dimethylarginine dimethylaminohydrolase. Circulation 1999; 99:3092-3095
101. Boger RH, Sydow K, Borlak J, et al. LDL cholesterol upregulates synthesis of asymmetrical dimethylarginine in human endothelial cells: involvement of S-adenosylmethionine–dependent methyltransferases. Circ Res 2000;87:99-105
102. Stühlinger MC, Oka RK, Graf EE, et al. Endothelial dysfunction induced by hyperhomocyst(e)inemia: role of asymmetric dimethylarginine. Circulation 2003;108: 933-938
103. Fard A, Tuck CH, Donis JA, et al. Acute elevations of plasma asymmetric dimethylarginine and impaired endothelial function in response to a high-fat meal in patients with type 2 diabetes. Arterioscler Thromb Vasc Biol 2000;20:2039-2044
104. Werner-Felmayer G, Golderer G, Werner ER. Tetrahydrobiopterin biosynthesis, utilization and pharmacological effects. Curr Drug Metab 2002;3:159-173
105. Nakamura S-I, Sugiyama S, Fujioka D, et al. Polymorphism in glutamate-cysteine ligase modifier subunit gene is associated with impairment of nitric oxide–mediated

coronary vasomotor function. Circulation 2003;108: 1425-1427

106. Vita JA, Brennan M-L, Gokce N, et al. Serum myeloperoxidase levels independently predict endothelial dysfunction in humans. Circulation 2004;110:1134-1139
107. Reusch JEB. Current concepts in insulin resistance, type 2 diabetes mellitus, and the metabolic syndrome. Am J Cardiol 2002;90(suppl):19G-26G
108. Sinisalo J, Paronen J, Mattila KJ, et al. Relation of inflammation to vascular function in patients with coronary heart disease. Atherosclerosis 2000;149: 403-411
109. Paz Y, Frolkis I, Pevni D, et al. Effect of tumor necrosis factor-alpha on endothelial and inducible nitric oxide synthase messenger ribonucleic acid expression and nitric oxide synthesis in ischemic and nonischemic isolated rat hearts. J Am Coll Cardiol 2003;42:1299-1305
110. Jin W, Sun G-S, Marchadier D, et al. Endothelial cells secrete triglyceride lipase and phospholipase activities in response to cytokines as a result of endothelial lipase. Circ Res 2003;92:644-650
111. Rask-Madsen C, Domínguez H, Ihlemann N, et al. Tumor necrosis factor-alpha inhibits insulin's stimulating effect on glucose uptake and endothelium-dependent vasodilation in humans. Circulation 2003; 108:1815-1821
112. Aljada A, Ghanim H, Assian E, Dandona P. Tumor necrosis factor-alpha inhibits insulin-induced increase in endothelial nitric oxide synthase and reduces insulin receptor content and phosphorylation in human aortic endothelial cells. Metabolism 2002;51:487-491
113. Browner NC, Sellak H, Lincoln TM. Downregulation of cGMP-dependent protein kinase expression by inflammatory cytokines in vascular smooth muscle cells. Am J Physiol Cell Physiol 2004;287:C88-C96
114. Farquharson CA, Struthers AD. Aldosterone induces acute endothelial dysfunction in vivo in humans: evidence for an aldosterone-induced vasculopathy. Clin Sci (Lond) 2002;103:425-431
115. Rajagopalan S, Duquaine D, King S, et al. Mineralocorticoid receptor antagonism in experimental atherosclerosis. Circulation 2002;105:2212-2216
116. Eto M, Barandier C, Rathgeb L, et al. Thrombin suppresses endothelial nitric oxide synthase and upregulates endothelin-converting enzyme-1 expression by distinct pathways: role of Rho/ROCK and mitogen-activated protein kinase. Circ Res 2001;89:583-590
117. Piatti PM, Monti LD, Conti M, et al. Hypertriglyceridemia and hyperinsulinemia are potent inducers of endothelin-1 release in humans. Diabetes 1996;45: 316-321
118. Wolpert HA, Steen SN, Istfan NW, et al. Insulin modulates circulating endothelin-1 levels in humans. Metabolism 1993;42:1027-1030
119. Arcano G, Creti A, Balzano S, et al. Insulin causes endothelial dysfunction in humans. Sites and mechanisms. Circulation 2002;105:576-582
120. Hijmering ML, Stroes ESG, Olijhoek J, et al. Sympathetic activation markedly reduces endothelium-dependent, flow-mediated vasodilation. J Am Coll Cardiol 2002;39:683-688
121. Rogers KM, Bonar CA, Estrella JL, Yang S. Inhibitory effect of glucocorticoid on coronary artery endothelial function. Am J Physiol Heart Circ Physiol 2002;283: H1922-H1928
122. Hishikawa K, Luscher TF. Pulsatile stretch stimulates superoxide production in human aortic endothelial cells. Circulation 1997;96:3610-3616
123. Hishikawa K, Oemar BS, Yang Z, et al. Pulsatile stretch stimulates superoxide production and activates nuclear factor-kappa B in human coronary smooth muscle. Circ Res 1997;81:797-803
124. Chin JH, Azhar S, Hoffman BB. Inactivation of endothelial-derived relaxing factor by oxidized lipoproteins. J Clin Invest 1994;93:10-18
125. Hsueh WA, Quinones MJ. Role of endothelial dysfunction in insulin resistance. Am J Cardiol 2003; 92(suppl):10J-17J
126. Steinberg HO, Chaker H, Leaming R, et al. Obesity/insulin resistance is associated with endothelial dysfunction: implications for the syndrome of insulin resistance. J Clin Invest 1996;97:2601-2610
127. Williams SB, Cusco JA, Roddy MA, et al. Impaired nitric-oxide mediated vasodilation in patients with non–insulin dependent diabetes mellitus. J Am Coll Cardiol 1996;27:567-574
128. Abe H, Yamada N, Kamata K, et al. Hypertension, hypertriglyceridemia, and impaired endothelium-dependent vascular relaxation in mice lacking insulin receptor substrate-1. J Clin Invest 1998;101:1784-1788
129. Creager MA, Lüscher TF, Cosentino F, Beckman JA. Diabetes and vascular disease: pathophysiology, clinical consequences, and medical therapy: Part I. Circulation 2003;108:1527-1532
130. Cusi K, Maezono K, Osman A, et al. Insulin resistance differentially affects the PI 3-kinase– and MAP kinase–mediated-signaling in human muscle. J Clin Invest 2000;105:311-320
131. Montagnani M, Golovchenko I, Kim I, et al. Inhibition of phosphatidylinositol 3-kinase enhances mitogenic actions of insulin in endothelial cells. J Biol Chem 2002;277:1794-1799
132. Pessin JE, Saltiel AR. Signaling pathways in insulin action: molecular targets of insulin resistance. J Clin Invest 2000;106:165-169
133. Reaven G. Insulin resistance, hypertension, and coronary heart disease. J Clin Hypertens (Greenwich) 2003; 5:269-274
134. Ferri C, Pittoni V, Piccoli A, et al. Insulin stimulates endothelin-1 secretion from human endothelial cells and modulates its circulating levels in vivo. J Clin Endocrinol Metab 1995;80:829-835
135. Rakugi H, Kamide K, Ogihara T. Vascular signaling pathways in the metabolic syndrome. Curr Hypertens Rep 2002;4:105-111
136. Chan NN, Chan JC. Asymmetric dimethylarginine (ADMA): a potential link between endothelial dysfunction and cardiovascular diseases in insulin resistance syndrome? Diabetologia 2002;45:1609-1616
137. Stuhlinger MC, Abbasi F, Chu JW, et al. Relationship between insulin resistance and an endogenous nitric oxide synthase inhibitor. JAMA 2000;287:1420-1426
138. Shinozaki K, Kashiwagi A, Masada M, Okamura T. Stress and vascular responses: oxidative stress and endothelial dysfunction in the insulin-resistant state. J Pharmacol Sci 2003;91:187-191
139. Lin KY, Ito A, Asagami T, et al. Impaired nitric oxide synthase pathway in diabetes mellitus: role of asymmetric dimethylarginine and dimethylarginine dimethylaminohydrolase. Circulation 2002;106:987-992
140. Deedwania PC. Diabetes is a vascular disease: the role of endothelial dysfunction in pathophysiology of cardiovascular disease in diabetes. Cardiol Clin 2004;22:505-509
141. Sunayama S, Watanabe Y, Daida H, Yamaguchi H. Thiazolidinediones, dyslipidemia and insulin resistance syndrome. Curr Opin Lipidol 2000;11:397-402

142. King GL. The role of hyperglycaemia and hyperinsulinaemia in causing vascular dysfunction in diabetes. Ann Med 1996;28:427-432
143. Steinberg HO, Tarshoby M, Monestel R, et al. Elevated circulating free fatty acid levels impair endothelium-dependent vasodilation J Clin Invest 1997;100: 1230-1239
144. Bakker SJL, Ijzerman RG, Teerlink T, et al. Cytosolic triglycerides and oxidative stress in central obesity: the missing link between excessive atherosclerosis, endothelial dysfunction, and beta-cell failure? Atherosclerosis 2000;148:17-21
145. Pleiner J, Schaller G, Mittermayer F, et al. FFA-induced endothelial dysfunction can be corrected by vitamin C. J Clin Endocrinol Metab 2002;87:2913-2917
146. Griffin ME, Marcucci MJ, Cline GW, et al. Free fatty acid–induced insulin resistance is associated with activation of protein kinase C theta and alterations in the insulin signaling cascade. Diabetes 1999;48: 1270-1274
147. Cummings MH, Watts GF, Umpleby AM, et al. Increased hepatic secretion of very-low-density lipoprotein apolipoprotein B-100 in NIDDM. Diabetologia 1995;38:959-967
148. Laakso M, Edelman SV, Brechtel G, et al. Decreased effect of insulin to stimulate skeletal muscle blood flow in obese man. A novel mechanism for insulin resistance. J Clin Invest 1990;85:1844-1852
149. Baron AD. Insulin resistance and vascular function. J Diabetes Complications 2002;16:92-102
150. Riley WA, Freedman DS, Higgs NA, et al. Decreased arterial elasticity associated with cardiovascular risk factors in the young. Arteriosclerosis 1986;6:378-386
151. Salmenniemi U, Ruotsalainen E, Pihlajamäki J, et al. Multiple abnormalities in glucose and energy metabolism and coordinated changes in levels of adiponectin, cytokines, and adhesion molecules in subjects with metabolic syndrome. Circulation 2004;110: 3842-3848
152. Calles-Escandon J, Cipolla M. Diabetes and endothelial dysfunction: a clinical perspective. Endocr Rev 2001:22:36-52
153. Balletshofer BM, Rittig K, Enderle MD, et al. Endothelial dysfunction is detectable in young normotensive first degree relatives of subjects with type 2 diabetes in association with insulin resistance. Circulation 2000;101:1780-1784
154. Quinones MJ, Pampaloni MH, Juarez BE, et al. Insulin resistance in healthy Mexican Americans is associated with coronary artery endothelial dysfunction. Diabetes 2000;49(suppl 1):A146
155. Lin KY, Cooke JP. Acute administration of asymmetric dimethylarginine reduces insulin sensitivity in mice. J Am Coll Cardiol 2004;43(suppl A):527A
156. de Jongh RT, Serné EH, Ijzerman RG, et al. Impaired microvascular function in obesity: implications for obesity-associated microangiopathy, hypertension, and insulin resistance. Circulation 2004;109:2529-2535
157. Meigs JB, Hu FB, Rifai N, Manson JE. Biomarkers of endothelial dysfunction and risk of type 2 diabetes mellitus. JAMA 2004;291:1978-1986
158. Caballero AE, Arora S, Saouaf R et al. Microvascular and macrovascular reactivity is reduced in subjects at risk for type 2 diabetes. Diabetes 1999;48:1856-1862
159. Pinkney JH, Stehouwer CD, Coppack SW, Yudkin JS. Endothelial dysfunction: cause of the insulin resistance syndrome. Diabetes 1997;46(suppl 2):S9-S13
160. Vita JA, Keaney JF, Larson MG, et al. Brachial artery vasodilator function and systemic inflammation in the Framingham Offspring Study. Circulation 2004; 110:3604-3609
161. Wellen KE, Hotamisligil GS. Obesity-induced inflammatory changes in adipose tissue. J Clin Invest 2003;112:1785-1788
162. Anderson TJ, Uehata A, Gerhard MD, et al. Close relation of endothelial function in the human coronary and peripheral circulations. J Am Coll Cardiol 1995;26: 1235-1241
163. Celermajer DS, Sorensen KE, Gooch VM, et al. Non-invasive detection of endothelial dysfunction in children and adults at risk of atherosclerosis. Lancet 1992; 340:1111-1115
164. Corretti MC, Anderson TJ, Benjamin EJ, et al. Guidelines for the ultrasound assessment of endothelial-dependent flow-mediated vasodilation of the brachial artery: a report of the International Brachial Artery Reactivity Task Force. J Am Coll Cardiol 2002;39:257-265
165. Dupuis J, Arsenault A, Meloche B, et al. Quantitative hyperemic reactivity in opposed limbs during myocardial perfusion imaging: a marker of coronary artery disease. J Am Coll Cardiol 2004;44:1473-1477
166. Gerhard-Herman M, Creager MA, Hurley S, et al. Assessment of endothelial function (nitric oxide) at the tip of a finger. Circulation 2002;102(suppl 2):851
167. Bonetti PO, Pumper GM, Higano ST, et al. Noninvasive identification of patients with early coronary atherosclerosis by assessment of digital reactive hyperemia. J Am Coll Cardiol 2004;44:2137-2141
168. Misko TP, Schilling RJ, Salvemini D, et al. A fluorometric assay for the measurement of nitrite in biological samples. Anal Biochem 1993;214:11-16
169. Messerli AW, Seshadri N, Pearce GL, et al. Relation of albumin/creatinine ratio to C-reactive protein and to the metabolic syndrome. Am J Cardiol 2003;92:610-612
170. Klausen K, Borch-Johnson K, Feldt-Rasmussen B, et al. Very low levels of microalbuminuria are associated with increased risk of coronary heart disease and death independently of renal function, hypertension, and diabetes. Circulation 2004;110:32-35
171. Kloner RA, Mullin SH, Shook T, et al. Erectile dysfunction in the cardiac patient: how common and should we treat? J Urol 2003;170:S46-S50
172. Kaiser DR, Billups K, Mason C, et al. Impaired brachial artery endothelium-dependent and -independent vasodilation in men with erectile dysfunction and no other clinical cardiovascular disease. J Am Coll Cardiol 2004; 43:179-184
173. Feldman HA, Johannes CB, Derby CA, et al. Erectile dysfunction and coronary risk factors: prospective results from the Massachusetts Male Aging Study. Prev Med 2000;30:328-338
174. Gazzaruso C, Giordanetti S, De Amici E, et al. Relationship between erectile dysfunction and silent myocardial ischemia in apparently uncomplicated type 2 diabetic patients. Circulation 2004;110:22-26
175. Hill JM, Zalos G, Halcox JPJ, et al. Circulating endothelial progenitor cells, vascular function, and cardiovascular risk. N Engl J Med 2003;348:593-600

9 Skeletal Muscle

Animals are characterized by their ability to move. Locomotion is critical for an animal's procurement of food, self-defense, and escape from danger. Not surprisingly, **skeletal muscle is the most abundant tissue in animals.** It constitutes approximately 40% of the body mass in normal-weight humans and up to 50% in dogs and horses. **The sheer bulk of metabolically active muscle tissue renders it a critical factor in carbohydrate and lipid homeostasis. As would be expected, there is an intimate link between metabolism and vascular function, between the signaling pathways of insulin and nitric oxide (NO) in skeletal muscle.**

NORMAL SKELETAL MUSCLE METABOLISM

Free fatty acids are the predominant fuel for skeletal and cardiac muscle under normal circumstances. With exercise or cold exposure, free fatty acids essentially serve as the exclusive energy source.[1] Plasma free fatty acids, though present only in micromolar concentrations, provide the major circulating lipid fuel. With moderate-intensity exercise, free fatty acid availability may increase twofold to fourfold. Other potential sources of fatty acid fuel include circulating very-low-density lipoprotein (VLDL) triglycerides, which constitute approximately a fifth of the fuel available as free fatty acid, and intramyocellular triglycerides, or triacylglycerols, which are present at a concentration of approximately 2 mmol/kg of muscle.[2] Correspondingly, **muscle is a principal tissue responsible for lipid uptake and utilization and contributes significantly to whole-body lipid homeostasis.**[3] **Skeletal muscle can use other substrates such as glucose and lactate.**[4,5] For example, during exercise, skeletal muscle also relies on intramuscular glycogen stores as a source of energy for contractile activity.[6] **Skeletal muscle is the largest insulin-sensitive tissue in the body. It plays a primary role in glucose uptake and accounts for 60% to 80% of glucose disposal under insulin-stimulated conditions,** as opposed to 10% for adipose tissue and 30% for the liver.[7,8]

MYOCYTE STRUCTURE AND FUNCTION

The myofilament proteins actin and myosin are the major constituents of muscle cells. Tension generation in skeletal muscle, via crossbridges that the myosin heads can form with actin, occurs directly in proportion to muscle mass.

Stimulation of skeletal muscle contraction involves the integration of signal-transducing events from the plasma membrane to the cytoplasmic myofilaments. With the exception of the neuromuscular and musculotendinous junctions, the sarcolemma of mature myocytes is composed of a mosaic of transverse tubule (T tubule) domains together with sarcolemmal caveolae and β-dystroglycan domains. Caveolae and their scaffolding protein caveolin are closely associated with the underlying peripheral sarcoplasmic reticulum and play an important role in the coordination of extracellular stimuli and intracellular effectors in muscle.[9]

SKELETAL MUSCLE ADAPTATION TO EXERCISE

Although an individual's muscle tissue is determined by genetic makeup, gender, body size, and age, **skeletal muscle has a tremendous capacity to adapt structurally and functionally to specific stresses** such as exercise, temperature, or nutritional status. However, **the structural and functional modifications incurred are maintained only for the duration of the stimulus and are reversible with its cessation.**

Physical exercise is a complex physiologic stimulus that initiates multiple biophysical and biochemical aspects of myocyte function. Exercise induces changes in gene transcription that effect growth and metabolic changes in muscle. **Training alters regulatory gene expression in skeletal muscle within hours and in structural genes within weeks.**[10,11] An increase in amino acid uptake facilitates protein synthesis, and changes in glucose and glycogen metabolism take place. Each individual training session activates the initial signaling responses that lead to long-term adaptations, but ultimately, exercise-induced adaptations constitute the cumulative result of repeated bouts of exercise.[12]

The mechanisms by which exercise regulates intracellular signal transduction to modulate gene expression are not well established. Mechanical stressors and metabolic changes, such as lactate generation and depletion of oxygen, adenosine 5′-triphosphate (ATP), and fatty acids, are sensed and integrated into the transcriptional adaptations of trained muscle, possibly by modulating the rate of gene transcription and mRNA degradation. Muscle signal transduction may also be altered by increased blood flow with hormone-receptor–mediated effects, by autocrine and paracrine signaling from muscle tissue, or by mechanical tension.[12]

Mitochondria and Capillaries. Contraction is the central activity of skeletal muscle and exerts the highest metabolic demand. Capillaries deliver oxygen and nutrients to skeletal myocytes for generation of energy in the mitochondria. Both capillary density and mitochondrial volume adapt to muscle activity. **There is thus a close match between the oxidative capacity of muscle and capillary density, and maximal oxygen consumption closely tracks total mitochondrial volume.** Whereas subsarcolemmal mitochondria represent a fixed proportion of 16% to 35% of the total mitochondrial population, the number of central mitochondria, in proximity to myofilaments, correlates with the activity level. Lipid droplets, which constitute a supply of energy substrate, are strategically positioned in close contact with mitochondria.[9]

Hypertrophy. Exercise training induces muscle hypertrophy. Skeletal muscle hypertrophy is characterized, in part, by increases in protein mass per myocyte. This increased accumulation of protein results from a net increase in protein synthesis relative to breakdown. Muscle hypertrophy is also associated with higher mitochondrial and capillary mass and increased glycogen and lipid stores.[13]

Endurance and strength training induce distinct structural and functional changes in muscle fibers. Muscle hypertrophy is associated with an increased proportion of slow-twitch, oxidative myofibers.[13]

Endurance Training. Endurance training via highly repetitive, low-load exercises for 2 months increases the protein concentration of muscle. **The morphologic changes increase the respiratory capacity of muscle by engendering a metabolic shift in trained muscle to a greater reliance on fat as a fuel. There is a concomitant reduction in glycolytic flux and tighter control of the acid-base status. These adaptations cumulatively enhance performance.**[14]

In the process, the capillary supply is enhanced as capillary density expands by 30%. Concomitantly, the size and number of mitochondria increase as mitochondrial volume rises by 40%.[15] There is an associated increase in the activity of key enzymes of the mitochondrial electron transport chain, such as ATP synthase, enzymes of the citrate cycle, and fatty acid and ketone oxidation enzymes. The number of muscle glucose transporters (GLUT4) is augmented.[16]

Strength/Resistance Training. Resistance training occurs via high-load exercises with little repetition. **It increases myofibrillar volume by as much as 20%** as evidenced by hypertrophy. There is increased expression of numerous proteins, regulated in part by induction of the immediate early genes c-jun and c-fos.[17]

SIGNAL TRANSDUCTION OF THE MECHANICAL EFFECTS OF EXERCISE

Mechanical factors of physical activity have an impact both on pretranscriptional controls and on the transcription of downstream target genes.

The mitogen-activated protein kinase (MAPK) cascade links mechanical activity to nuclear signaling and cellular growth and may thus mediate exercise-induced adaptations in skeletal muscle.[18,19]

Mitogen-Activated Protein Kinase. Acute exercise elicits signal transduction via MAPK cascades in direct response to muscle contraction. MAPK is a ubiquitous series of protein kinases. Exercise can induce three limbs of the MAPK pathways:

1. p42 and p44 MAPK, or the extracellular signal–regulated protein kinases (ERK)1/2 and ERK5;
2. the c-Jun NH_2-terminal kinase (JNK), also known as stress-activated protein kinase (SAPK), SAPK1/JNK; and
3. p38 MAPK or SAPK2/p38.[12,18,20-22]

Each kinase is a member of a cascade of kinases, the structure of which is highly conserved between organisms. **The MAPK cascades relay extracellular signals from the plasma membrane to targets in the cytoplasm and the nucleus.** In response to extracellular signals such as

- growth factors,
- cytokines,
- hypoxia,
- ultraviolet light,
- stress-inducing agents,
- tension, and
- stretch,

these MAPKs regulate gene expression by phosphorylating and thus activating transcription factors and, in the process, frequently amplifying the signal.

Transcription factors that are affected include

- cyclic adenosine 3′,5′-monophosphate (cAMP) response element binding protein (CREB),
- activating transcription factor (ATF) 1 and 2,
- myocyte enhance factor 2 (MEF2) A and C, and
- c-fos and c-jun.

The activated MAPK cascades are thus associated with increased transcriptional activity linking extracellular stimuli to cellular responses.

The ensuing signal transduction pathways and biologic responses associated with these cascades are diverse and lead to a variety of cellular outcomes, including

- cellular growth,
- cell proliferation,
- cell differentiation,
- apoptosis,
- metabolic regulation, and
- adaptation to environmental stress.[23]

Distinct exercise-training protocols of different intensity and duration result in selective postexercise activation of diverse intracellular signaling pathways, which may be one of the mechanisms regulating the specific adaptations induced by disparate training programs.[24]

Mitogen-Activated Protein Kinase Activation. MAPKs are phosphorylated and activated by MAPK kinases (MAPKKs), which in turn are phosphorylated and activated by MAPKK kinases.

Mechanical tension modulates JNK and ERK1/2 directly.[25] Activation of these kinases affects the transcription factors c-fos and c-jun, as well as the ATF/CREB family, and they bind to the promoter of genes such as cytochrome *c*.[12,26]

ERK2 stimulation involves the Raf-1 and MAPKK1 signaling pathway in muscle and activates its downstream target p90 ribosomal S6 kinase (p90RSK2) and mitogen- and stress-activated protein kinases 1 and 2 (MSK1/2). ERK2 stimulation is correlated with an increase in citrate synthase activity. The exercise effect on ERK1/2 is limited to working muscle, and exercise favors ERK1/2 over p38 MAPK signaling.[12]

In contrast, the p38 pathway responds to mechanical stretch and exercise indirectly. p38 MAPK is situated downstream of MAPKK6 and MAPKK3. Phosphorylated p38 MAPK also activates p90RSK and MSK1/2. p38 MAPK activation leads to a marked down-regulation of insulin-induced glucose uptake via GLUT4.[27]

ENERGY SENSORS AND METABOLIC ADAPTATIONS IN SKELETAL MUSCLE

There is an economic need for a feedback mechanism in skeletal muscle that allows a myocyte to adjust its metabolic activity acutely and chronically to a wide range of energy requirements as it alternates between a resting state and varying workloads, between a deconditioned, active, and superbly trained status.

Adenosine Triphosphate. The high-energy phosphate bond of ATP is used as a source of energy for muscle contraction, and adenosine 5′-diphosphate (ADP) and inorganic phosphate are generated in the process. **All cells must maintain a high ratio of cellular ATP to ADP in order to survive.** For continued muscle contraction to occur, ATP needs to be reconstituted from ADP. There are several mechanisms for reestablishing ATP. Rapid nonoxidative mechanisms at the commencement of muscle contraction entail reactions of the following enzymes:

1. myokinase or adenylate kinase, which reconstitute one ATP molecule and one adenosine 5′-monophosphate (AMP) molecule from two ADP moieties:

$$2ADP \rightarrow ATP + AMP;$$

2. creatine phosphokinase, which transfers a high-energy phosphate from phosphocreatine or creatine phosphate (CP) to ADP to reconstitute ATP with creatine (Cr):

$$CP + ADP \rightarrow Cr + ATP \text{ (Fig. 9-1).}$$

ADP can also be phosphorylated to ATP via

1. glycolytic pathways in the sarcoplasm and

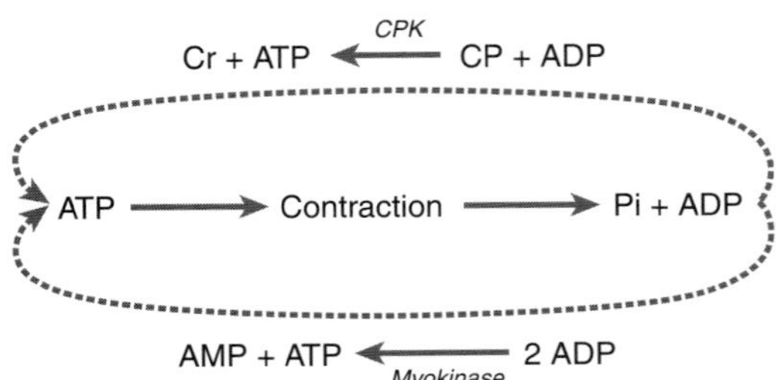

Figure 9–1.
Contraction-induced decreases in creatine phosphate (CP) and adenosine 5′-triphosphate (ATP) with generation of creatine (Cr) and adenosine 5′-monophosphate (AMP). ADP, adenosine 5′-diphosphate; CPK, creatine phosphokinase; Pi, inorganic phosphate.
(Modified from Winder WW. AMP-activated protein kinase: possible target for treatment of type 2 diabetes. Diabetes Technol Ther 2000;2:441-448.)

2. oxidative phosphorylation in the mitochondria.[28]

To replenish high-energy sources, muscle metabolism is up-regulated with exercise. The energy demands of contraction entail an increase in skeletal muscle fuel uptake. Muscle glycogen is consumed as a fuel source, and fatty acid oxidation increases with exercise. The mechanisms by which exercise signals a metabolic need and effects metabolic changes in skeletal muscle are not well established.

5′-AMP–Activated Protein Kinase. Metabolic changes in exercising muscle have an impact on 5′-AMP–activated protein kinase (5′-AMPK or AMPK). Like MAPK, AMPK and other signaling cascades are activated in response to intense exercise in skeletal muscle.[29] Via specific protein kinases and transcription factors, both mechanical and metabolic stimuli are integrated to enhance myocyte gene transcription in response to exercise training.[30]

AMPK is the downstream component of a metabolite-sensing protein kinase family that is activated in response to alterations in cellular energy levels. The AMPK pathway coordinates the energy supply and demand of the myocyte with myocyte metabolism. As such, AMPK acts as an intracellular energy sensor to maintain energy balance within the cell.[19]

AMPK is a putative regulator of multiple metabolic processes in skeletal muscle, including fatty acid and carbohydrate metabolism. It is an intermediary in the signaling cascade leading to contraction-stimulated glucose transport in skeletal muscle.[19]

AMPK Isoforms. AMPK is a heterotrimeric protein consisting of three subunits with a catalytic kinase domain (α) and two regulatory subunits (β and γ) with the ATP binding site.[31] There are two catalytic isoforms:

1. AMPK-α1 is expressed in the liver, pancreas, adipose tissue, and skeletal muscle;
2. AMPK-α2 is predominantly expressed in skeletal muscle.[31]

AMPK Activation. AMPK is activated upon depletion of fuel stores and high-energy phosphates. Two types of mechanisms activate AMPK:

1. allosteric effects and
2. phosphorylation.

Allosteric Effects. Consumption of glycogen stores, as well as an increase in the AMP/ATP and Cr/CP ratio as a result of depleted high-energy phosphates, leads to the allosteric activation of AMPK.[31]

AMP levels rise as the ATP/ADP ratio declines. Correspondingly, a high cellular ratio of AMP to ATP signals a compromise in the energy status of the cell. When inactive, AMPK is allosterically inhibited by CP. Activation occurs upon

- dissociation of CP from AMPK as CP levels drop and
- allosteric activation by AMP as AMP levels rise.[31]

AMPK Phosphorylation. AMPK is also activated via phosphorylation by AMPK kinase (AMPKK), which is itself allosterically activated by elevated levels of AMP (Fig. 9-2). Additionally,

AMPK is phosphorylated and activated by

- **leptin,**
- **adiponectin,**

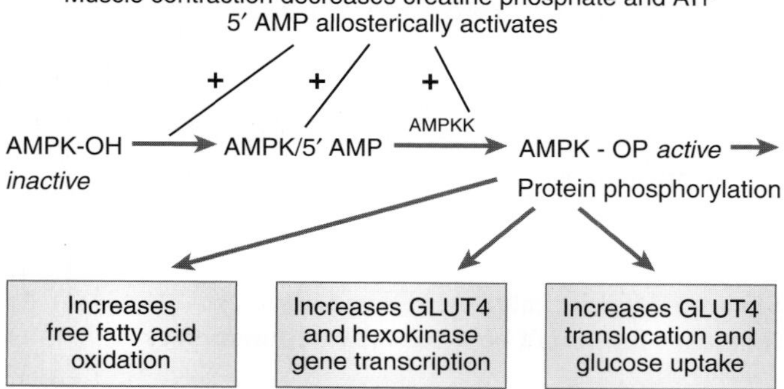

▸▸ **Figure 9–2.**
Postulated mechanism of increased skeletal muscle glucose uptake and fatty acid oxidation with contraction as 5′-AMP–activated protein kinase (AMPK) and AMPK kinase (AMPKK) are allosterically activated by elevated levels of adenosine 5′-monophosphate (5′AMP). GLUT4, glucose transporter 4. *(Modified from Winder WW, Hardie DG. AMP-activated protein kinase, a metabolic master switch: possible roles in type 2 diabetes. Am J Physiol 1999;277:E1-E10.)*

- hormones that act via G_q-coupled receptors, such as α_1-adrenoceptor–G_q agonists,
- 5′-aminoimidazole 4-carboxamide riboside (AICAR), and
- metformin.[32-34]

AMPK is deactivated by phosphatases.[35]

Coordination of Cellular Energy Supply and Demand. AMPK effectively functions as a gauge of and response element to myocyte energy status in that it is increasingly activated during muscle contractions as the ATP/ADP and CP/Cr ratios, as well as glycogen stores, decline.[32]

AMPK plays a key role in numerous metabolic processes. **Once activated, AMPK responds to the decrease in high-energy phosphate levels of myocytes by activating energy-producing processes while switching off energy-consuming processes.** AMPK effectively functions as a metabolic master switch, which by phosphorylating target proteins controls the flux through various processes.[35] Activated AMPK

- inhibits anabolic, ATP-consuming processes that are not essential for short-term cell survival, such as lipid, carbohydrate, and protein synthesis. As a result, there is a
  - reduction in adipocyte lipogenesis,
  - decrease in hepatocyte cholesterol synthesis via inactivation of 3-hydroxy-3-methylglutaryl (HMG) coenzyme A (CoA) reductase, the rate-limiting enzyme for cholesterol biosynthesis,
  - decrease in fatty acid esterification to form glycerolipids and triacylglycerols, and
  - modulation of insulin secretion from beta cells;[19]
- promotes catabolic pathways that generate ATP in response to exercise and thereby causes
  - an increase in glycolysis,
  - stimulation of adipocyte lipolysis, and
  - an increase in skeletal muscle fatty acid oxidation.[19,32]

Skeletal Muscle Fatty Acid Oxidation. AMPK increases fatty acid beta oxidation in myocytes with exercise by lowering the availability of malonyl CoA.

Malonyl CoA is an allosteric inhibitor of carnitine palmitoyltransferase I (CPT-I), the enzyme that controls the transfer of long-chain fatty acyl CoA from the cytosol to the mitochondria for oxidation. In the absence of malonyl CoA, CPT-I is disinhibited, thus allowing the transfer of long-chain fatty acids into the mitochondria for fatty acid oxidation to proceed with continued exercise.

In the process, AMPK phosphorylates and inhibits acetyl CoA carboxylase (ACC) in skeletal muscle by phosphorylating ACC at Ser79, the AMPK phosphorylation site. Inhibition of ACC impairs the synthesis of malonyl CoA. AMPK may also have an effect on enzymes that govern malonyl CoA degradation.[28]

Myocyte Triacylglycerol Accumulation. Activation of AMPK lowers the accumulation of intramyocyte lipid.

AMPK and malonyl CoA are implicated in the peripheral regulation of energy balance. Activation of AMPK increases the expression of uncoupling proteins and the transcriptional regulator peroxisome proliferator–activated receptor-gamma (PPAR-γ) coactivator-1α (PGC1α), which may raise energy expenditure. Factors that activate AMPK and lower the concentration of malonyl CoA in peripheral tissues decrease the accumulation of triacylglycerols in myocytes and in other cells by increasing energy expenditure and the oxidation of fatty acids.

Additionally, malonyl CoA and AMPK may also play a central nervous system role. They may modulate hypothalamic fuel-sensing and signaling mechanisms that regulate systemic food intake and energy expenditure.[34]

AMPK and Nitric Oxide. With increased muscle metabolic activity, AMPK activation is associated with an increase in myocyte NO production.

There is enhanced phosphorylation and activation of neuronal NO synthase (nNOS) in skeletal muscle (nNOS-μ) at Ser1451. Increased NO elaboration protects the muscle from metabolic stress and ischemia through its protective effects on muscle perfusion, substrate utilization, and contractile function.[36]

Activated AMPK may also stimulate endothelial NOS (eNOS) in the muscular microcirculation via Ser1177 phosphorylation in order to enhance the production of endothelial NO and its downstream signaling component cyclic guanosine 3′,5′-monophosphate (cGMP), an additional mechanism of local blood flow augmentation.[37,38]

AMPK Transcriptional Impact. AMPK is implicated in the transcriptional control and regulation of gene expression. Acute activation of AMPK by exercise decreases the transcription of certain genes. Chronic activation of AMPK increases the mRNA and protein content relating to other genes such as

- GLUT4,
- hexokinase II, and
- uncoupling protein-3.

Over the long term, chronic activation of AMPK increases skeletal muscle mitochondrial enzyme and glycogen content.[39] AMPK plays a role in exercise-induced alterations in protein content. **The protein targets of AMPK appear to be involved not only in the control of acute metabolic responses but also in the chronic adaptation to exercise.**[35]

Other Metabolic Sensors in Skeletal Muscle. Other myocyte signaling pathways also have an impact on skeletal muscle blood flow supply, mitochondrial biogenesis, and carbohydrate and lipid metabolism.

Peroxisome Proliferator–Activated Receptor-α. Exercise induces the activation of PPAR-α.

PPAR-α promotes the transcription of genes modulating carbohydrate metabolism and fatty acid oxidation. Although muscle has only a limited amount of PPAR-γ, PPAR-α is richly expressed in skeletal muscle, where it plays a major role in the regulation of lipid homeostasis. There is an increase in PPAR-α mRNA levels in response to training in human muscle.[40-42] **PPAR-α increases free fatty acid beta oxidation while decreasing fatty acid esterification into myocyte triacylglycerol.**[3] Unsaturated long-chain fatty acids, which are released from adipose tissue during exercise, serve as ligands for PPAR-α and stimulate PPAR-α–activated gene transcription.[43]

Hypoxia-Inducible Factor-1. Metabolic changes in exercising muscle have an impact on transcription factors such as hypoxia-inducible factor-1 (HIF-1).

Exercise increases HIF-1 levels. Whereas HIF-1 is normally unstable and is readily degraded, exercise-associated tissue hypoxia stabilizes HIF-1 by reducing the hydroxylation of particular residues.[44,45]

Upon exercise-induced activation, HIF-1 and PPAR-α bind to promoter regions in order to promote the transcription of genes. HIF-1 affects oxygen delivery by promoting the transcription of vascular endothelial growth factor (VEGF) and glycolytic genes.[40,41]

Other. Exercise-induced adaptive increases in

- PGC-1 and
- nuclear respiratory factor 1 and 2 (NRF-1/2)

coordinate the up-regulation of mitochondrial biogenesis and GLUT4 expression.[16] NRF-1, together with exercise-induced transcription of mitochondrial transcription factor A (Tfam), is involved in coordinated expression of the myocyte nuclear and mitochondrial genomes and in mitochondrial biogenesis.[46,47]

MEDIATORS OF NON–INSULIN-DEPENDENT GLUCOSE UPTAKE IN SKELETAL MUSCLE

Insulin levels fall during exercise as the organism's energy supplies are directed from anabolic storage toward utilization and consumption. Given the increased energy demands of working skeletal muscle, there is the metabolic requirement for an insulin-independent pathway to enhance fuel supply to myocytes during contraction. **Non–insulin-dependent glucose uptake is enhanced during muscle contraction by recruiting insulin-independent, separate pools of intracellular GLUT4 transporters.**[35] The mechanisms involved have not been fully delineated.

Glucose Uptake in Skeletal Muscle. The physical bulk of the skeletal musculature renders the control of myocyte glucose uptake a major factor in the maintenance of whole-body carbohydrate homeostasis. Glucose uptake into skeletal muscle involves a number of different regulatory steps, such as

- delivery of glucose to the skeletal muscle microcirculation,
- conveyance of glucose from blood into the interstitial space,
- transmembrane transport of glucose from the interstitial space into the sarcoplasm, and
- intracellular metabolism of glucose.

In most cases, transmembrane uptake of glucose into skeletal muscle is the rate-limiting step in glucose metabolism.[32]

Trans-sarcolemmal Glucose Transport and GLUT4 Pools. The skeletal muscle sarcolemma and its T-tubule extensions into the myocyte interior allow entry of glucose into the sarcoplasm via the glucose transporter GLUT4.[48] **Stimulation of glucose transport in contracting muscle entails the translocation of GLUT4-containing vesicles from exercise-sensitive, intracellular storage sites to the T tubules and the sarcolemma.** In fact, diverse stimuli for glucose uptake in skeletal muscle, such as

- contraction,
- insulin,
- hypoxia,
- NO, and
- bradykinin,

signal GLUT4 translocation by recruiting distinct intracellular GLUT pools, thereby accomplishing a rapid increase in glucose uptake capacity (Table 9-1). The maximal effects of these stimuli are all additive. **The magnitude of GLUT4 translocation to the sarcolemma determines the capacity of skeletal muscle for glucose disposal.**[5,32]

Table 9-1. Skeletal Muscle Stimuli Recruiting Distinct Intracellular Pools of the Glucose Transporter GLUT4 with Additive Maximal Effects on Glucose Uptake

Contraction
Insulin
Hypoxia
Nitric oxide
Bradykinin

Potential Stimulants for Non–Insulin-Dependent Muscle Glucose Transport. Skeletal muscle is the primary target for the stimulation of glucose transport by various stimulants. Muscle glucose transport is probably the result of the interaction of several signaling pathways that are variably activated as a function of the metabolic needs of the muscle. Specific modulators for glucose uptake are

- calcium;
- diacylglycerol;
- protein kinase C (PKC);
- AMPK activation, reflecting stimuli that increase energy demand, such as exercise, hypoxia, or any challenge to the oxidative chain;
- NO; and
- glycogen (Table 9-2).

Additional factors that may be involved in contraction-induced glucose transport are

- adenosine,
- endorphin, and
- bradykinin, which directly stimulates GLUT4 translocation.

However, the mechanisms involved are poorly understood.[49]

Calcium, Diacylglycerol, and Protein Kinase C Isoforms. Calcium (Ca^{2+}), diacylglycerol, and PKC isoforms may be early participants in the signaling pathway for contraction-induced glucose transport:

Calcium. It is likely that Ca^{2+} may play a role in the activation of glucose transport via insulin-independent mechanisms.

Table 9-2. Stimuli for GLUT4 Translocation in Exercising Muscle

Sarcoplasmic reticular release of cytoplasmic Ca^{2+}
Metabolic stress activation of AMPK
PKC isoforms
Diacylglycerol
NOS activation
Myocyte glycogen stores

AMPK, adenosine 5′-monophosphate–activated protein kinase; GLUT4, glucose transporter 4; NOS, nitric oxide synthase; PKC, protein kinase C.

The neural stimulation that initiates the development of force in skeletal muscle triggers sarcolemmal depolarization with an increase in cytoplasmic Ca^{2+} levels. Together with other mediators, the rise in intracellular Ca^{2+} may contribute to the increment in glucose uptake during muscle contractions. The Ca^{2+}-sensitive modulation of glucose transport occurs early in excitation-contraction coupling.[32]

Diacylglycerol. The intracellular concentration of diacylglycerol is also increased during contraction and plays a role in myocyte glucose transport.[32]

Protein Kinase C Isoforms. Muscle contraction is associated with the translocation of PKC from the cytosol to the particulate fraction. PKC isoforms play an essential role in contraction-stimulated glucose transport. Several conventional and atypical protein kinases, such as the PKC isoforms for glucose transport, are Ca^{2+} sensitive and require diacylglycerol for optimal activation.[5,32]

AMPK-Mediated Glucose Uptake. With continued muscle contraction, the level of glucose transport needs to respond to the balance of energy supply and demand in the myocyte, as reflected by high-energy phosphate reserves and tension development.[5] Exercise may increase glucose transport into skeletal muscle by activating AMPK as a fuel sensor. Although other factors may be involved in the metabolic control of glucose transport and questions remain regarding a true causal link between AMPK activation and glucose transport, **AMPK involvement appears to occur with relatively intense contractions and exercises that are associated with some degree of hypoxia and depletion of high-energy phosphates.**[32]

Principally, **the AMPK-α2 isoform is increased by physical exercise, with the increase being a function of exercise intensity. AMPK enhances GLUT4 translocation,** but specific mechanisms are not well defined.[35]

AMPK-dependent effects of exercise on glucose transport may in part be mediated by

- proline-rich tyrosine kinase 2 (PYK2),
- the ERK pathway,
- phospholipase D (PLD), and
- atypical PKCs.[50]

Additionally, there appears to be crosstalk between the AMPK and MAPK signaling pathways inasmuch as AMPK activates p38 MAPK, which may be required for AMPK-mediated glucose transport.[19] AMPK activation in muscle may also stimulate glucose transport via activation of eNOS coupled to downstream signaling components.[35]

Nitric Oxide. NO modulates carbohydrate metabolism to preserve intracellular energy stores by promoting glucose uptake (Fig. 9-3).[51] However, the role of NO in exercise-induced muscle glucose uptake is currently controversial. It is also not clear whether there is, in fact, an

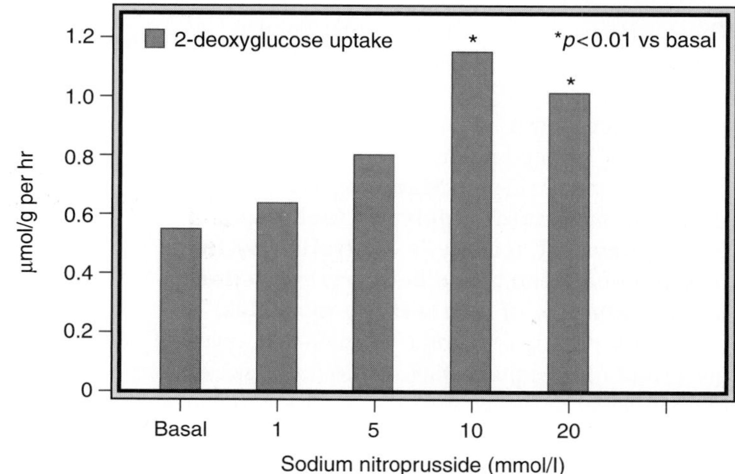

Figure 9–3. Sodium nitroprusside–stimulated glucose uptake in isolated rat skeletal muscle. *(Modified from Higaki Y, Hirshman MF, Fujii N, Goodyear LJ. Nitric oxide increases glucose uptake through a mechanism that is distinct from the insulin and contraction pathways in rat skeletal muscle. Diabetes 2001;50:241-247.)*

interaction between NO and AMPK signaling to stimulate glucose transport in skeletal muscle.[32,35]

Glycogen Stores. Not surprisingly, the magnitude of glycogen stores in skeletal muscle modulates glucose transport. **High glycogen levels in muscle, appropriately, inhibit both contraction- and insulin-stimulated GLUT4 translocation.**

It has been hypothesized that glycogen particles are structurally attached to GLUT4 vesicles, although no biochemical evidence for a physical link has been found. Physical linkage of glycogen with GLUT4 might render GLUT4 unable to translocate to the sarcolemma for glucose uptake as long as glycogen stores are ample in muscle. Conversely, in this construct, as soon as glycogen stores are depleted, GLUT4 would be unbound and available for translocation and glucose uptake at the sarcolemma. Alternatively, glycogen may regulate glucose transport by modulating signal transduction pathways.[32]

Not only is glucose transport dependent on glycogen, but muscle glycogen content is also an important regulator of contraction- and insulin-induced glycogen synthase activity. The ability of factors such as insulin and contraction to regulate glycogen synthase activity is diminished in glycogen-replete muscle and increased in glycogen-depleted tissue. **The lower the glycogen content in muscle, the stronger the response to insulin and other factors.**[32]

ENDOTHELIAL FUNCTION, NITRIC OXIDE, AND SKELETAL MUSCLE METABOLISM

The vascular system controls the delivery of nutrients and hormones to skeletal muscle. Modulation of blood flow within the skeletal muscle interstitium has an impact on substrate delivery to myocytes, muscle metabolism, and contractile performance. **Matching tissue oxygen and substrate supply to fuel demand during physical activity is controlled by the interplay between blood delivery, extraction, and metabolism of nutrients by myocytes.**

Multiple neuronal, endothelial, metabolic, myogenic, and muscle pump factors modulate skeletal muscle blood flow via effects on perfusion pressure and arteriolar resistance. NOS in skeletal muscle plays a major role in this respect. **With neuronal NOS, nNOS-μ, in skeletal muscle governing metabolic processes and eNOS in the vascular endothelium regulating perfusion pressure, the NOS system plays a pivotal role not only in the control of arterial pressure but also in the regulation of glucose and lipid homeostasis. Vascular NO effects enhance nutrient supply to skeletal muscle, whereas within skeletal muscle, the net effect of NO appears to be one of lowering oxygen demand.**[51,52]

Nitric Oxide Synthase in Muscle. Of the three isoforms of the NOS family that have been identified, termed

1. neuronal NOS-1 (nNOS),
2. inducible NOS-2 (iNOS), and
3. endothelial NOS-3 (eNOS),

nNOS and eNOS are constitutively expressed in skeletal muscle. They are low-output isoforms that produce NO as a signaling mechanism. nNOS is found not only in skeletal muscle but also in

- neuronal tissue (brain, spinal cord, sympathetic ganglia, peripheral nerves),
- the pancreas,
- epithelial cells of the stomach,
- the lung, and
- the uterus.[53]

In skeletal muscle, nNOS, or nNOS-μ, is homogeneously distributed between type I and type II muscle fibers, near the sarcolemma, and localized to motor end plates. The dystrophin-glycoprotein complex mediates the association of nNOS with the sarcolemma.[51]

Myocyte Effects of Nitric Oxide. NO enhances the blood perfusion of skeletal muscle. **In addition to its vascular, anti-inflammatory, and antiplatelet effects, NO is implicated in the control of multiple aspects of skeletal muscle metabolism and function.** NO modulates

- metabolic regulation through its impact on glucose homeostasis and oxidative phosphorylation. NO enhances glucose uptake but decreases glycolysis, mitochondrial respiration, and the breakdown of CP;
- excitation-contraction coupling and contractility;

- immune function;
- cell growth; and
- neurotransmission.[51,52]

Modulation of Muscle Perfusion. NO may play a role in matching tissue substrate supply with fuel demand. It is constitutively released from muscles at rest. **Exercise and contractile activity in skeletal muscle increase the release of NO. In effect, as muscle physical activity and metabolic demand rise, so does the production of NO.** NO diffuses into the vasculature, where it promotes vasodilation and increases the nutritive blood perfusion of skeletal muscle.[35]

NO in skeletal muscle is derived from eNOS and nNOS through a number of stimuli. Specifically,

- acetylcholine from the neuromuscular junctions may diffuse to the vascular endothelium and activate muscarinic receptors, thereby promoting endothelial NO release and smooth muscle cell relaxation;
- metabolite accumulation in contracting muscle engenders resistance vessel dilation, which promotes the resultant increase in flow-related shear stress and further release of endothelially derived NO;
- exercise-mediated central and peripheral elevations in sympathetic tone to conductance vessels promote NO release via stimulation of endothelial β-adrenergic type 2 receptors. NO also inhibits the prejunctional release of norepinephrine;
- NO of skeletal muscle origin can be produced in response to the elevation in cytoplasmic Ca^{2+} induced by Ca^{2+} release from the sarcoplasmic reticulum during excitation-contraction coupling[51]; and
- AMPK activation during exercise can phosphorylate and activate eNOS, which increases NO production in muscle.[37,38]

Nitric Oxide Impact on Glucose Uptake. NO and cGMP promote glucose uptake by myocytes.[51]

NOS may play a direct role in GLUT4 translocation. The mechanism by which NO stimulates glucose transport appears to be distinct from and additive to the exercise/contraction mechanism and may entail the NO-stimulated activation of AMPK-α1 rather than AMPK-α2 (Fig. 9-4).[32,35]

Nitric Oxide–Mediated Reduction in Oxygen Consumption. NO reduces skeletal muscle oxygen extraction by decreasing both energy demand and the consumption of oxygen. This dual effect occurs as a result of its negative effects on contractility and on enzymes involved in oxidative phosphorylation and the transfer of high-energy phosphates.[51]

Directly, **NO dampens contractile activity and its associated metabolism** through modulation of excitation-contraction coupling by causing nitrosation or metal nitrosylation of

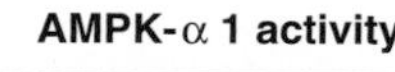

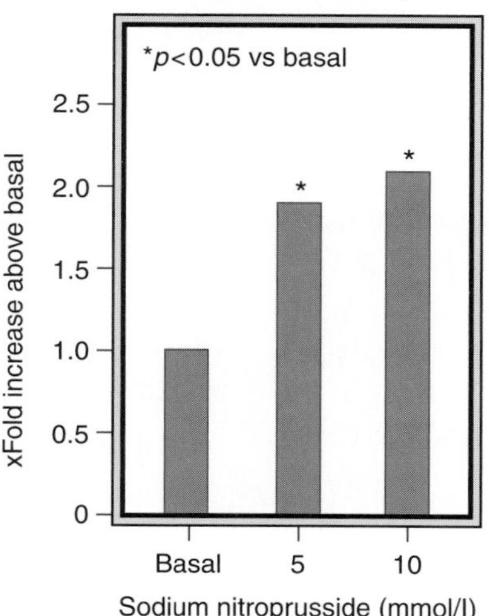

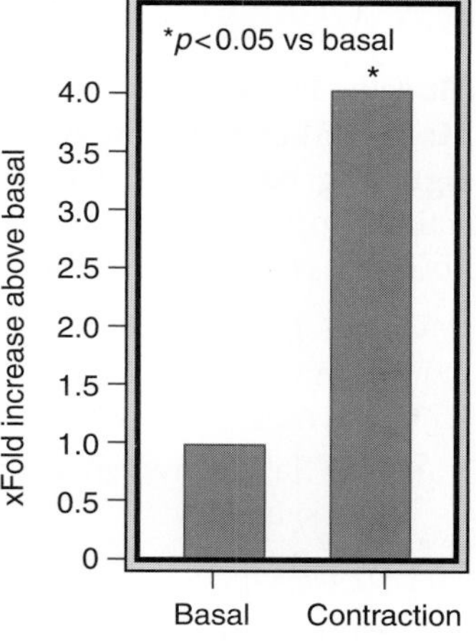

Figure 9–4. Effect of sodium nitroprusside and contraction on rat skeletal muscle adenosine 5′-monophosphate–activated protein kinase alpha 1 (AMPK-alpha 1) and AMPK-alpha 2 activity, respectively. *(Modified from Higaki Y, Hirshman MF, Fujii N, Goodyear LJ. Nitric oxide increases glucose uptake through a mechanism that is distinct from the insulin and contraction pathways in rat skeletal muscle. Diabetes 2001;50:241-247.)*

target proteins and thereby resulting in a depression in

- isometric force,
- shortening velocity of contractions,
- glycolysis, and
- mitochondrial respiration.

There is a reduction in myofilament Ca^{2+} sensitivity. The effect on L-type calcium currents varies, being inhibitory at low and stimulatory at high NO concentrations.[53,54]

In contrast, cGMP actually improves aspects of mechanical and metabolic muscle performance. cGMP increases

- the shortening velocity of contractions,
- the maximal mechanical power,
- the initial rate of force development,
- glucose uptake,
- glycolysis, and
- mitochondrial respiration

and decreases twitch time to peak force. However, despite the opposing effects attributable to cGMP, the net result of exposure of skeletal muscle to NO is a reduction in contractility and submaximal skeletal muscle force.[53,54]

INSULIN-STIMULATED GLUCOSE UPTAKE IN SKELETAL MUSCLE

In the postabsorptive, resting state, skeletal muscle is the predominant site for insulin-stimulated glucose disposal; it is critical for systemic glucose homeostasis in that it encompasses greater than 60% to 80% of insulin-stimulated glucose uptake.[6-8]

Muscle Fiber Type and Insulin Signaling. Muscle fiber types have an effect on insulin signaling pathways. Based on myosin ATPase staining or enzymatic analysis, skeletal muscle fibers are classified into three distinct categories:

- type I, slow-twitch, oxidative fibers, high in mitochondrial density, rich in oxidative enzymes;
- type IIa, fast-twitch, oxidative and glycolytic fibers; and
- type IIb, fast-twitch, glycolytic fibers.

Insulin-mediated glucose uptake is proportional to the oxidative capacity of the muscle fiber: it is highest for type I, intermediate for type IIa, and lowest for type IIb fibers. Correspondingly, type I fibers have greater levels of GLUT4 expression, increased insulin action at the level of insulin receptor binding and tyrosine phosphorylation, increased insulin receptor substrate (IRS)-1/2 and class IA phosphatidylinositol 3-O kinase (PI3K) activity, and higher Akt phosphorylation. Whole-body glucose uptake is positively correlated with an individual's proportion of type I muscle fibers and negatively correlated with the proportion of type IIb fibers.[55] **Exercise increases, whereas obesity and inactivity decrease the number of type I fibers.**[56]

Insulin-Stimulated Glucose Uptake. Although glucose uptake in skeletal muscle during contractions has to occur via insulin-independent mechanisms, insulin-stimulated glucose uptake in striated muscle occurs in the postprandial state and after exercise.

Postprandial Glucose Disposal. Insulin-stimulated glucose uptake in muscle is pivotal for the disposal of postprandial glycemia.

Disposal of postprandial glucose entails a rise in insulin levels leading to an increase in glucose transport in fast- and slow-twitch muscles. Insulin activates the PI3K pathway and downstream effectors such as atypical PKCs and protein kinase B (PKB)/Akt kinase. The latter are implicated in translocating the insulin-responsive glucose transporter GLUT4 from intracellular storage sites to the sarcolemma to effect transmembrane glucose transport (Fig. 9-5).[32]

Postexercise Glucose Uptake and Disposal. Insulin also plays an important role in the period after prolonged and heavy physical activity, when glycogen stores have been depleted. **For previously exercised muscles, glycogen resynthesis is a high priority. Restoration of glycogen reserves is thought to be partly responsible for the prolonged enhancement of sensitivity to insulin's metabolic action,** which results in increased

- muscle glucose transport and
- glycogen synthase activity and glycogen synthesis.

Insulin sensitization is restricted to the muscle actually performing the work and is positively

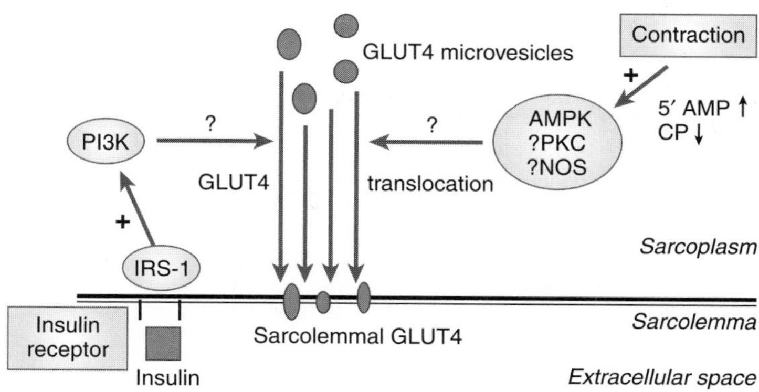

Figure 9–5.
Skeletal muscle glucose uptake mediated by insulin and by contraction. AMP, adenosine 5′-monophosphate; AMPK, 5′-AMP–activated protein kinase; CP, creatine phosphate; GLUT4, glucose transporter 4; IRS-1, insulin receptor substrate-1; NOS, nitric oxide synthase; PI3K, phosphatidylinositol 3′-OK-kinase; PKC, protein kinase C. *(Adapted from Winder WW, Hardie DG. AMP-activated protein kinase, a metabolic master switch: possible roles in type 2 diabetes. Am J Physiol 1999;277:E1-E10.)*

correlated with the amount of glycogen used during the previous exercise bout. It may last up to 48 hours and thus contribute to the restoration or even super-compensation of glycogen stores. However, in the absence of insulin, exercise or contractions activate these same metabolic processes.[32]

Vasodilation and Glucose Uptake. Insulin is a potent stimulator of glucose transport in skeletal muscle. Clearly, for its greatest efficacy, two components of the process must be facilitated:

1. delivery of glucose and insulin from blood to the myocyte and
2. transmembrane transport of glucose into the myocyte.

In addition to its metabolic actions in skeletal muscle, part of the mechanism whereby insulin increases glucose transport in vivo involves an increase in muscle perfusion in order to enhance the delivery of insulin and glucose to the target organ.[57] Insulin directly affects the endothelium and smooth muscle tone of the vasculature by causing the release of NO and engendering vasodilation and increased blood flow to the affected muscle.[58]

Insulin's metabolic and vascular actions are not only linked molecularly but also complement each other physiologically. Physiologic levels of insulin have a significant impact on muscle metabolism, as well as on NO-dependent vasodilation and capillary recruitment, switching from non-nutritive to nutritive perfusion. Capillary recruitment may be an important aspect of insulin's role in increasing the uptake of glucose in muscle both at rest and in the postexercise period.[57]

Distinct Metabolic Pathways for Glucose Transport in Skeletal Muscle. Of the diverse mechanisms that mediate glucose uptake in skeletal muscle, at least three, specifically,

1. insulin,
2. contraction-hypoxia, and
3. NO,

appear to utilize not only diverse GLUT pools but also biochemically distinct signaling pathways. **This redundancy of glucose uptake mechanisms reflects the importance of glucose metabolism in skeletal muscle; such redundancy allows for the additive effect of diverse stimuli and affords the use of alternative mechanisms of glucose uptake in the event that one pathway should be impaired.**[5,32]

Although activation of PI3K is essential for insulin-mediated glucose transport, this step is not required for the non–insulin-dependent stimuli that induce GLUT4 translocation. Muscle contraction, as well as hypoxia-mediated glucose transport, is distinct from insulin signaling and is mediated via activation of AMPK-α2 (Fig. 9-6). NO stimulates glucose uptake through a mechanism that differs from both the insulin and contraction signaling pathways; it is associated with activation of the AMPK-α1 catalytic subunit of AMPK.[35,37]

SKELETAL MUSCLE METABOLISM IN INFLAMMATION AND INSULIN RESISTANCE

A systemic inflammatory state and insulin resistance have a negative impact on skeletal muscle performance. **Inflammation is a catabolic state**

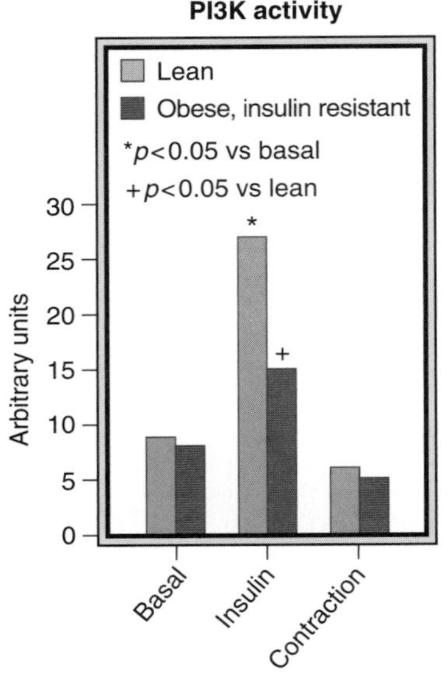

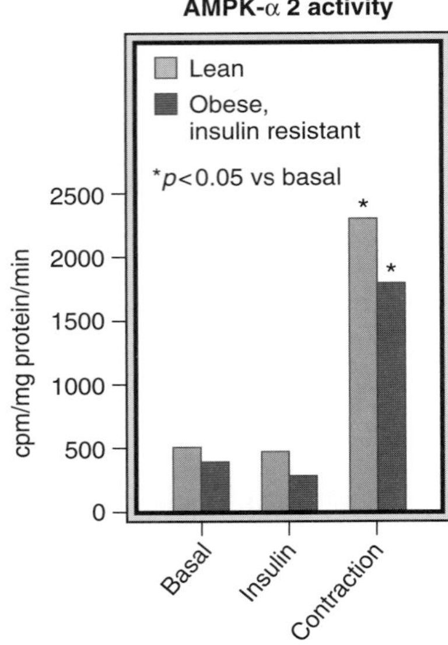

▸▸ **Figure 9–6.** Muscle phosphatidylinositol 3-O kinase (PI3K) and adenosine 5′-monophosphate–activated protein kinase alpha 2 (AMPK-α 2) activity in response to insulin and contraction, respectively, in lean and in obese, insulin-resistant Zucker rats. *(Modified from Barnes BR, Ryder JW, Steiler TL, et al. Isoform-specific regulation of 5′ AMP–activated protein kinase in skeletal muscle from obese Zucker [fa/fa] rats in response to contraction. Diabetes 2002;51:2703-2708.)*

that prioritizes nutrient delivery to inflammatory tissues via insulin resistance mechanisms at the expense of anabolic pathways in insulin-sensitive tissues.

Skeletal Muscle and Inflammation. Inflammation compromises blood perfusion to skeletal muscle and interferes with muscle metabolism, contractile function, and structural integrity. Inflammatory cytokines mediate these effects on skeletal muscle function by affecting gene expression and adaptive responses.

Blood Perfusion. Inflammation diminishes microvascular nutritive muscle perfusion.

Endotoxin-activated, proinflammatory cytokines in sepsis impair nutritive blood flow to skeletal muscle.[59] Because type I oxidative fibers are more sensitive to the vasoconstrictive effects of norepinephrine, the high sympathetic tone in chronic inflammation and insulin resistance diverts blood flow from efficient, oxidative type I to the inefficient, glycolytic type II fibers.[60-62]

Insulin Resistance. Proinflammatory cytokines induce insulin resistance.

During inflammatory processes in skeletal muscle, principally four proinflammatory cytokines, interleukin (IL)-1, IL-6, tumor necrosis factor-alpha (TNF-α), and interferon-γ, induce metabolic alterations that include enhanced protein breakdown, decreased protein synthesis, decreased fatty acid uptake and oxidation, increased expression of iNOS, and insulin resistance.[63] TNF-α is the cytokine most prominently linked to muscle pathophysiology.

Tumor Necrosis Factor-α. **Skeletal muscle myocytes synthesize TNF-α, and angiotensin II may be one of the factors that induce the expression of TNF-α in skeletal muscle.**[64] TNF-α functions as an endogenous modulator of muscle adaptation via autocrine/paracrine effects. TNF-α exerts several significant biologic actions on skeletal muscle myocytes:

- insulin resistance,
- contractile dysfunction,
- inhibition of myocyte differentiation,
- disruption of myogenesis,
- accelerated catabolism, and
- muscle protein loss.[65,66]

TNF-α causes insulin resistance in myocytes. In primary neonatal rat myotubes, TNF-α, through activation of p38 MAPK and inhibitor kappaB kinase (IKK), induces serine phosphorylation of the insulin receptor and IRS-1, thereby impairing its tyrosine phosphorylation by insulin and the corresponding activation of PI3K and Akt. As a result, insulin-mediated GLUT4 translocation and glucose uptake are inhibited.[67] The degree of intramyocyte expression of TNF-α mRNA is inversely related to the sarcolemmal expression of GLUT4.[59]

TNF-α induces selective insulin resistance. In skeletal muscle, TNF-α selectively impairs the metabolic-vascular pathway, with no effect on insulin's mitogenic activity.[68]

Other Inflammatory Mediators. Other inflammatory cytokines alter insulin action in skeletal muscle as well, and some of the mechanisms may entail cytokine-induced alterations in intramyocyte fatty acid content.

In awake mice, acute treatment with IL-6 reduced insulin-stimulated glucose uptake in skeletal muscle, and this was associated with defects in insulin-stimulated IRS-1–associated PI3K activity and increases in fatty acyl CoA levels in skeletal muscle. In contrast, cotreatment with IL-10, a predominantly anti-inflammatory cytokine, protected skeletal muscle from IL-6–induced defects in insulin signaling while lowering intramuscular fatty acyl CoA levels.[69]

Other cytokines released from activated adipose tissue may impair insulin activity in skeletal muscle. The release of fat cell factors from an adipocyte-conditioned culture medium or from human fat and muscle cell coculture may rapidly induce insulin resistance in human skeletal muscle cells by a process implicating the IKK/nuclear factor kappaB (NFκB)-dependent pathway.[70]

iNOS activation during inflammatory processes impairs myocyte insulin resistance via oxidative stress pathways.[63]

Contractile Dysfunction. Proinflammatory cytokines and TNF-α in inflammation induce contractile dysfunction.

Contractile dysfunction is an acute response to inflammation that develops over a period of hours and results in diminished force production. Inflammatory cytokines affect the expression of sarcoplasmic reticular Ca^{2+}-ATPase and phospholamban. They activate iNOS via NFκB. Excessive cytoplasmic levels of NO will cause Ca^{2+} desensitization of the myofilaments and also inhibit aerobic enzymes such as cytochrome-*c* oxidase. High levels of cytosolic pro-oxidant species, derived from mitochondrial electron transport, contribute to the contractile dysfunction.[59,71-73]

Muscle Atrophy. Chronic exposure to inflammatory cytokines engenders the loss of muscle mass.

TNF-α is associated with muscle catabolism and loss of muscle function in human diseases ranging from heart failure to arthritis, acquired immunodeficiency syndrome, and cancer. The protein loss induced by TNF-α is a chronic response that occurs over a period of days to weeks. Changes in gene expression required for TNF-α–induced catabolism are regulated by the transcription factor NFκB, which is essential for the net loss of muscle protein. TNF-α–induced atrophy as a result of postreceptor TNF-α signal transduction is mediated by

- an NFκB-dependent increase in a ubiquitin-proteasome degradation pathway,
- opposition to the trophic effects of insulin, and
- a rapid rise in endogenous oxidants.[72,73]

Metabolic Derangements of Skeletal Muscle with Insulin Resistance. Insulin resistance is the metabolic manifestation of a chronic, proinflammatory state.

Insulin resistance in skeletal muscle is the earliest detectable defect in individuals at risk for the development of type 2 diabetes mellitus (DM) at a later date.[74] With skeletal muscle being a principal determinant of insulin sensitivity, insulin resistance in skeletal muscle is a major defect.

Glucose Transport. Insulin-mediated glu-cose transport in skeletal muscle is the rate-limiting step for insulin-mediated glucose metabolism. Its dysregulation is a hallmark of insulin resistance.[75] Given the importance of glucose delivery to working muscle, however, non–insulin-sensitive, contraction-mediated mechanisms for glucose uptake are preserved.

Insulin resistance not only decreases the efficacy of PI3K-mediated glucose uptake but also impairs the response of AMPK-α1 to contractile activity. Because NO-stimulated glucose uptake is associated with increased activity of the AMPK-α1 subunit, **NO-mediated glucose uptake, albeit distinct from insulin- or contraction-stimulated glucose uptake, is also impaired with insulin resistance.**

Insulin resistance, however, has no effect on AMPK-α2. Skeletal muscle glucose transport elicited by metabolic stimuli such as

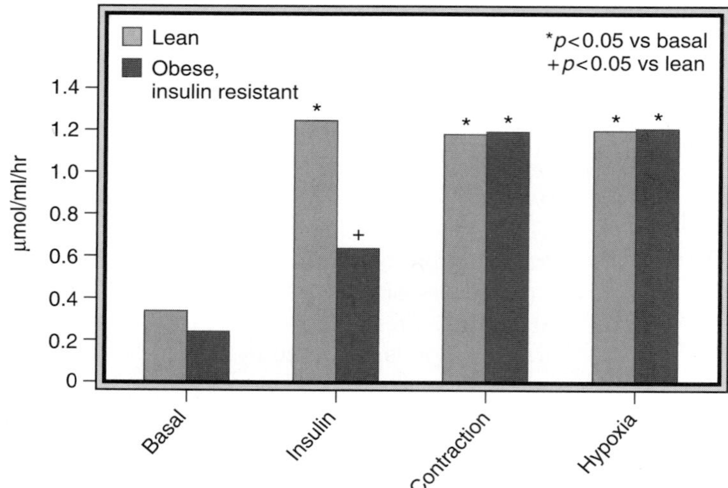

▸▸ **Figure 9–7.** Muscle deoxyglucose uptake in lean and obese, insulin-resistant Zucker rats. Despite insulin resistance, contraction- and hypoxia-mediated deoxyglucose uptake is preserved. *(Modified from Barnes BR, Ryder JW, Steiler TL, et al. Isoform-specific regulation of 5′ AMP–activated protein kinase in skeletal muscle from obese Zucker [fa/fa] rats in response to contraction. Diabetes 2002;51:2703-2708.)*

contraction and hypoxia remains intact (Fig. 9-7).[76]

Glycogen Synthesis. The dysregulation of insulin-mediated glucose transport in skeletal muscle is the rate-limiting step for insulin-mediated glycogen synthesis. Glycogen synthesis in muscle is the primary pathway for nonoxidative glucose disposal and a major aspect of overall glucose metabolism. **Impaired glycogen synthesis is a major intracellular metabolic defect associated with insulin resistance.**[77]

Metabolic and Vascular Insulin Resistance. The metabolic action of insulin in peripheral tissues is closely linked to its vascular action in the endothelium. Because insulin signaling mechanisms in peripheral, metabolically active tissues and the vascular endothelium appear to be shared, the molecular mechanisms causing resistance to insulin signaling are manifested in skeletal muscle as well as in the vasculature. Insulin-resistant states thus exhibit diminished

- insulin-mediated glucose uptake into muscle tissue,
- insulin-mediated vasodilation, and
- endothelium-dependent vasodilation.[78]

Activity and Expression of Constitutive Nitric Oxide Synthase. In insulin resistance, both endothelial and skeletal muscle NOS activity is lessened. There is reduced skeletal muscle nNOS expression in insulin-resistant states.[51]

Impact on Metabolic Insulin Sensitivity. Diminished NO- and insulin-mediated capillary recruitment leads to impaired nutritive, microcirculatory perfusion of skeletal muscle. The vascular dysfunction compounds the cellular derangement of glucose uptake, further aggravating the overall resistance to insulin action and contributing to secondary hyperinsulinemia.[57]

Impact on Exercise Capacity. The dysfunctional NOS signaling may contribute to the impairment in exercise capacity in insulin resistance. Whereas dysfunctional NOS reduces nutritive skeletal blood flow and glucose uptake during exercise, insulin resistance diminishes muscle perfusion, glucose uptake, and glycogen restoration during recovery. As a result, insulin resistance lowers functional exercise capacity by decreasing the anaerobic threshold and peak oxygen consumption.[51,79,80]

In a detailed study of the metabolic syndrome in 119 nondiabetic offspring of diabetic probands, the metabolic syndrome was associated with low maximum oxygen uptake. These subjects also had lower energy expenditure during the hyperinsulinemic clamp, findings suggestive of a lower increase in meal-induced thermogenesis and a consequent tendency to gain weight when compared with individuals with normal metabolism.[81]

Structural Changes in Skeletal Muscle with Insulin Resistance. Insulin resistance is associated with a number of changes in skeletal muscle phenotype.

Skeletal Muscle Fiber Type. Insulin resistance is linked to a reduction in the highly efficient, oxidative type I skeletal muscle fibers. Instead, there is an increase in the metabolically inefficient, type IIb glycolytic fibers, as seen on muscle biopsy of overweight, insulin-resistant, first-degree relatives of patients with type 2 DM.[82,83]

Fatty Acid Membrane Composition of Skeletal Muscle. The fatty acid composition of sarcolemmal phospholipids in skeletal muscle is closely related to insulin sensitivity. Specifically, increased saturation of sarcolemmal fatty acids with decreased activity of delta 5 desaturase is associated with resistance to insulin.[84]

Intramyocyte Fatty Acid Accumulation. Insulin-resistant offspring of individuals with type 2 DM have increases in plasma fatty acid concentrations and intramyocellular lipid content.

Muscle biopsy measurement of triacylglycerol content, or proton (^{1}H) magnetic resonance spectroscopic assessment of intramyocyte triacylglycerol, indicates a strong relationship between intramuscular lipid content and insulin resistance in skeletal muscle.[82] Increased intramyocyte triacylglycerol concentrations are inversely proportional to the expression of GLUT4 mRNA[59,85] and predate the clinical onset of type 2 DM by many years.[74]

Dysregulation of Fatty Acid Metabolism with Insulin Resistance. The insulin-resistant state impairs free fatty acid utilization, as well as glucose metabolism, in skeletal muscle.[85] **As a result, fatty acids, rather than being oxidized, accumulate as storage triacylglycerols in skeletal muscle,** as they do in the liver.

Specifically, mitochondrial rates of ATP production are reduced by approximately 30% in the muscle of insulin-resistant subjects as compared with insulin-sensitive controls. Consistent with decreased mitochondrial oxidative phosphorylation, reflecting in part a lower mitochondrial content in muscle, there is a reduced ratio of inorganic phosphate to CP, as may occur with a lower ratio of oxidative type I fibers to glycolytic type II fibers in insulin-resistant subjects.[82]

Causes of Decreased Oxidative Metabolism. The reason for the reduction in fatty acid beta-oxidative capacity is unclear, but a number of factors appear to play a role, as discussed in greater detail earlier in this chapter (AMPK section) and in the chapter on insulin resistance. For purposes of this discussion, although a genetic predisposition is important,[82] external factors such as physical inactivity and obesity modulate an individual's propensity toward decreased oxidative metabolism. Chronic inflammation is similarly an underlying factor inasmuch as intramyocyte triacylglycerol concentrations are proportional to skeletal muscle TNF-α mRNA.[59,85]

CONCLUSION

Barring morbid obesity and excessive adipose tissue expansion, skeletal muscle is the most abundant tissue in our bodies. The musculature is structurally, functionally, and biochemically malleable and adaptive to training. A well-trained muscle hypertrophies. With muscle work and conditioning, there is a switch from glycolytic type II to oxidative type I muscle fibers together with mitochondrial biogenesis. Capillary density increases to enhance perfusion.

Contractile performance and adaptation are critically dependent on the supporting metabolic activity. When appropriately used, working skeletal muscle is a metabolically very active and responsive organ. Activation of PPAR-α and AMPK up-regulates oxidative metabolism and the metabolic rate to match energy demand. Insulin sensitivity is enhanced for postexercise, com-pensatory, anabolic action.

Muscle metabolic activity, in turn, is intricately linked with vasodilatory capacity. In working, metabolically active muscle, AMPK signaling increases the constitutive production of NO by myocyte nNOS and endothelial eNOS. After exercise, insulin similarly enhances eNOS activity. Both insulin and AMPK activate vascular eNOS to control vascular perfusion and activate muscle nNOS to govern metabolic processes, thus linking metabolic with vascular function. As a result, there is concurrent facilitation of

- delivery of fuel from blood to the working and recovering myocytes,

- transmembrane transport of fuel into myocytes,
- increased oxidative consumption of fuel to meet working energy demands, and
- enhanced glycogen synthesis for restoration of fuel supplies during recovery

in order to effect the greatest availability and utilization of nutrients. Insulin, AMPK, and NOS signaling thus plays a critical and complementary role not only in controlling muscle perfusion but also in governing glucose and lipid homeostasis.

Inflammatory pathways aim to secure and maximize nutritional support for the immune system cells at the expense of other, "less critical" tissues such as adipose tissue and muscle. Thus, inflammation in adipose tissue storage depots causes insulin resistance with antiadipogenesis and lipolysis; in working muscle, inflammation similarly induces insulin resistance, contractile dysfunction, and decreased oxidative phosphorylation with impaired myogenesis and myocyte differentiation and actual loss of muscle mass. In this construct as well, there is a concordance of the metabolic and vascular changes as AMPK, adiponectin, insulin, and constitutive NOS signaling are all down-regulated. The changes evoked by these altered metabolic parameters, in positive feedback, further aggravate inflammatory activation and insulin resistance through alterations in myocyte phenotype, endothelial function, and intramyocellular lipid accumulation.

In this respect, the greatest promise for interrupting the vicious circle of insulin resistance lies in the very plasticity and bulk of skeletal muscle. In contrast to adipose tissue, muscle is not a passive, reactive, cytokine-producing mass. Muscle is exquisitely responsive to the multiplicity of benefits arising from moderate exercise training and conditioning, as reflected in the high number of exercise studies performed in chronic inflammatory conditions such as coronary heart disease, heart failure, and type 2 DM. Exercise conditioning and fitness have the greatest potential for exchanging a catabolic, insulin-resistant milieu for an anabolic, insulin-sensitive one with systemic benefit. Aside from exercise, there is also promise for angiotensin II antagonism to interrupt the stimulus for TNF-α generation in skeletal muscle, with a potential role for appropriate antioxidants.

GLOSSARY

ACC	acetyl CoA carboxylase
ADP	adenosine 5′-diphosphate
AICAR	5′-aminoimidazole 4-carboxamide riboside
AMP	adenosine 5′-monophosphate
AMPK	5′-AMP–activated protein kinase
AMPKK	AMPK kinase
ATF	activating transcription factor
ATP	adenosine 5′-triphosphate
Ca^{2+}	calcium
cAMP	cyclic 3′,5′-adenosine monophosphate
cGMP	cyclic guanosine 3′,5′-monophosphate
CoA	coenzyme A
CP	creatine phosphate
CPT-I	carnitine palmitoyltransferase I
Cr	creatine
CREB	cyclic AMP response element binding protein
DM	diabetes mellitus
eNOS	endothelial NOS
ERK	extracellular signal–regulated kinase
GLUT	glucose transporter
HIF-1	hypoxia-inducible factor-1
HMG	3-hydroxy-3-methylglutaryl
IKK	inhibitor kappaB kinase
IL	interleukin
iNOS	inducible NOS
IRS	insulin receptor substrate
JNK	c-Jun NH_2-terminal kinase
MAPK	mitogen-activated protein kinase
MAPKK	MAPK kinase
MEF2	myocyte enhance factor 2
MSK	mitogen- and stress-activated protein kinase
NFκB	nuclear factor kappaB
NO	nitric oxide
NOS	nitric oxide synthase
nNOS	neuronal NOS
NRF	nuclear respiratory factor
p90RSK2	p90 ribosomal S6 kinase
PGC1α	PPAR-gamma coactivator-1alpha

PI3K	phosphatidylinositol 3-O kinase
PKB	protein kinase B
PKC	protein kinase C
PLD	phospholipase D
PPAR	peroxisome proliferator–activated receptor
PYK2	proline-rich tyrosine kinase 2
SAPK	stress-activated protein kinase
Tfam	mitochondrial transcription factor A
TNF	tumor necrosis factor
T tubule	transverse tubule
VEGF	vascular endothelial growth factor
VLDL	very-low-density lipoprotein

REFERENCES

1. Boden G, Hoeldtke RD. Nerves, fat, and insulin resistance. N Engl J Med 2003;349:1966-1967
2. Jensen MD. Fate of fatty acids at rest and during exercise: regulatory mechanisms. Acta Physiol Scand 2003; 178:385-390
3. Muoio DM, Way JM, Tanner CJ, et al. Peroxisome proliferator–activated receptor-alpha regulates fatty acid utilization in primary human skeletal muscle cells. Diabetes 2002;51:901-909
4. Gunn HM. Heart weight and running ability. J Anat 1989;167:225-233
5. Henriksen EJ. Exercise effects of muscle insulin signaling and action. Invited review: Effects of acute exercise and exercise training on insulin resistance. J Appl Physiol 2002;93:788-796
6. Wojtaszewski JFP, Nielsen JN, Richter EA. Exercise effect on muscle insulin signaling and action. Invited review: Effect of acute exercise on insulin signaling and action in humans. J Appl Physiol 2002;93:384-392
7. Katz L, Glickman M, Rapoport S, et al. Splanchnic and peripheral disposal of oral glucose in man. Diabetes 1983;32:675-679
8. Smith U. Impaired ("diabetic") insulin signaling and action occur in fat cells long before glucose intolerance—is insulin resistance initiated in the adipose tissue? Int J Obes 2002;26:897-904
9. Rahkila P, Takala TE, Parton RG, Metsikko K. Protein targeting to the plasma membrane of adult skeletal muscle fiber: an organized mosaic of functional domains. Exp Cell Res 2001;267:61-72
10. Kadi F, Thornell LE. Concomitant increases in myonuclear and satellite cell content in female trapezius muscle following strength training. Histochem Cell Biol 2000; 113:99-103
11. Booth FW, Tseng BS, Fluck M, Carson JA. Molecular and cellular adaptation of muscle in response to physical training. Acta Physiol Scand 1998;162:343-350
12. Widegren U, Ryder JW, Zierath JR. Mitogen-activated protein kinase signal transduction in skeletal muscle: effects of exercise and muscle contraction. Acta Physiol Scand 2001;172:227-235
13. Booth FW, Thomason RB. Molecular and cellular adaptation in response to exercise: perspectives of various models. Physiol Rev 1991;71:541-585
14. Hawley JA. Adaptations of skeletal muscle to prolonged, intense endurance training. Clin Exp Pharmacol Physiol 2002;29:218-222
15. Hoppeler H, Howald H, Conley K, et al. Endurance training in humans: aerobic capacity and structure of skeletal muscle. J Appl Physiol 1985;59:320-327
16. Baar K, Wende AR, Jones TE, et al. Adaptations of skeletal muscle to exercise: rapid increase in the transcriptional coactivator PGC-1. FASEB J 2002;16:1879-1886
17. Luthi JM, Howald H, Claassen H, et al. Structural changes in skeletal muscle tissue with heavy-resistance exercise. Int J Sports Med 1986;7:123-127
18. Aronson D, Violan MA, Dufresne SD, et al. Exercise stimulates the mitogen-activated protein kinase pathway in human skeletal muscle. J Clin Invest 1997;99: 1251-1257
19. Zierath JR. Invited review: Exercise training–induced changes in insulin signaling in skeletal muscle. J Appl Physiol 2002;93:773-781
20. Aronson D, Wojtaszewski JF, Thorell A, et al. Extracellular-regulated protein kinase cascades are activated in response to injury in human skeletal muscle. Am J Physiol 1998;275:C555-C561.
21. Henriksen EJ. Effects of acute exercise and exercise training on insulin resistance. J Appl Physiol 2002;93: 788-796
22. Boppart MD, Aronson D, Gibson L, et al. Eccentric exercise markedly increases c-Jun NH(2)-terminal kinase activity in human skeletal muscle. J Appl Physiol 1999; 87:1668-1673
23. Park H, Go YM, St John PL, et al. Plasma membrane cholesterol is a key molecule in shear stress–dependent activation of extracellular signal–regulated kinase. J Biol Chem 1998;273:32304-32311
24. Lee JS, Bruce CR, Spurrell BE, Hawley JA. Effect of training on activation of extracellular signal–regulated kinase 1/2 and p38 mitogen-activated protein kinase pathways in rat soleus muscle. Clin Exp Pharmacol Physiol 2002;29:655-660
25. Martineau LC, Gardiner PF. Insight into skeletal muscle mechanotransduction: MAPK activation is quantitatively related to tension. J Appl Physiol 2001;91: 693-702
26. Hunter T, Karin M. The regulation of transcription by phosphorylation. Cell 1992;70:375-387
27. Fujishiro M, Gotoh Y, Katagiri H, et al. MKK6/3 and p38 MAPK pathway activation is not necessary for insulin-induced glucose uptake but regulates glucose transporter expression. J Biol Chem 2001;276:19800-19806
28. Winder WW. AMP-activated protein kinase: possible target for treatment of type 2 diabetes. Diabetes Technol Ther 2000;2:441-448
29. Yu M, Stepto NK, Chibalin AV, et al. Metabolic and mitogenic signal transduction in human skeletal muscle after intense cycling exercise. J Physiol 2003;546:327-335
30. Hoppeler H, Fluck M. Normal mammalian skeletal muscle and its phenotypic plasticity. J Exp Biol 2002; 205:2143-2152
31. Hayashi T, Hirshman MF, Fujii N, et al. Metabolic stress and altered glucose transport: activation of AMP-activated protein kinase as a unifying coupling mechanism. Diabetes 1999;49:527-531

32. Richter EA, Derave W, Wojtaszewski JF. Glucose, exercise and insulin: emerging concepts. J Physiol 2001;535: 313-322
33. Hardie DG. Minireview: the AMP-activated protein kinase cascade: the key sensor of cellular energy status. Endocrinology 2003;144:5179-5183
34. Ruderman NB, Saha AK, Kraegen EW. Minireview: malonyl CoA, AMP-activated protein kinase, and adiposity. Endocrinology 2003;144:5166-5171
35. Higaki Y, Hirshman MF, Fujii N, Goodyear LJ. Nitric oxide increases glucose uptake through a mechanism that is distinct from the insulin and contraction pathways in rat skeletal muscle. Diabetes 2001;50: 241-247
36. Chen ZP, McConell GK, Michell BJ, et al. AMPK signaling in contracting human skeletal muscle: acetyl-CoA carboxylase and NO synthase phosphorylation. Am J Physiol Endocrinol Metab 2000;279:E1202-E1206
37. Fryer LG, Hajduch E, Rencurel F, et al. Activation of glucose transport by AMP-activated protein kinase via stimulation of nitric oxide synthase. Diabetes 2000;49: 1978-1985
38. Morrow VA, Foufelle F, Connell JM, et al. Direct activation of AMP-activated protein kinase stimulates nitric-oxide synthesis in human aortic endothelial cells. J Biol Chem 2003;278:31629-31639
39. Fryer LG, Foufelle F, Barnes K, et al. Characterization of the role of the AMP-activated protein kinase in the stimulation of glucose transport in skeletal muscle cells. Biochem J 2002;363:167-174
40. Wojtaszewski JF, Jorgensen SB, Frosig C, et al. Insulin signalling: effects of prior exercise. Acta Physiol Scand 2003;178:321-328
41. Semenza GL. Regulation of hypoxia-induced angiogenesis: a chaperone escorts VEGF to the dance. J Clin Invest 2001;108:39-40
42. Escher P, Wahli W. Peroxisome proliferator–activated receptors: insight into multiple cellular functions. Mutat Res 2000;448:121-138
43. Kliewer SA, Sundseth SS, Jones SA, et al. Fatty acids and eicosanoids regulate gene expression through direct interactions with peroxisome proliferator–activated receptors alpha and gamma. Proc Natl Acad Sci U S A 1997;94:4318-4323
44. Jewell UR, Kvietikova I, Scheid A, et al. Induction of HIF-1alpha in response to hypoxia is instantaneous. FASEB J 2001;15:1312-1314
45. Wenger RH, Bauer C. Oxygen sensing: "hydroxy" translates "oxy." News Physiol Sci 2001;16:195-196
46. Hood DA. Invited review: contractile activity-induced mitochondrial biogenesis in skeletal muscle. J Appl Physiol 2001;90:1137-1157
47. Bengtsson J, Gustafsson T, Widegren U, et al. Mitochondrial transcription factor A and respiratory complex IV increase in response to exercise training in humans. Pflugers Arch 2001;443:61-66
48. Goodyear LJ, Kahn BB. Exercise, glucose transport, and insulin sensitivity. Annu Rev Med 1998;49:235-261
49. Shiuchi T, Cui T-X, Wu L, et al. ACE inhibitor improves insulin resistance in diabetic mouse via bradykinin and NO. Hypertension 2002;40:329-334
50. Chen HC, Bandyopadhyay G, Sajan MP, et al. Activation of the ERK pathway and atypical protein kinase C isoforms in exercise- and aminoimidazole-4-carboxamide-1-beta-D-riboside (AICAR)-stimulated glucose transport. J Biol Chem 2002;277:23554-23562
51. Kingwell BA. Nitric oxide–mediated metabolic regulation during exercise: effects of training in health and cardiovascular disease. FASEB J 2000;14:1685-1696
52. Duplain H, Burcelin R, Sartori C, et al. Insulin resistance, hyperlipidemia, and hypertension in mice lacking endothelial nitric oxide synthase. Circulation 2001;104: 342-345
53. Marechal G, Gailly P. Effects of nitric oxide on the contraction of skeletal muscle. Cell Mol Life Sci 1999; 55:1088-1102
54. Feron O, Dessy C, Opel DJ, et al. Modulation of the endothelial nitric-oxide synthase–caveolin interaction in cardiac myocytes. Implications for the autonomic regulation of heart rate. J Biol Chem 1998;273:30249-30254
55. Megeney LA, Neufer PD, Dohm GL, et al. Effects of muscle activity and fiber composition on glucose transport and GLUT-4. Am J Physiol 1993;264:E583-E593
56. Ryder JW, Gilbert M, Zierath JR. Skeletal muscle and insulin sensitivity: pathophysiological alterations. Front Biosci 2001;6:154-163
57. Clark MG, Wallis MG, Barrett EJ, et al. Blood flow and muscle metabolism: a focus on insulin action. Am J Physiol Endocrinol Metab 2003;284:E241-E258
58. Steinberg HO, Baron AD. Vascular function, insulin resistance and fatty acids. Diabetologia 2002;45:623-634
59. Hotamisligil GS. Mechanisms of TNF-alpha–induced insulin resistance. Exp Clin Endocrinol Diabetes 1999;107:119-125
60. Soop M, Duxbury H, Agwunobi AO, et al. Euglycemic hyperinsulinemia augments the cytokine and endocrine responses to endotoxin in humans. Am J Physiol Endocrinol Metab 2002;282:E1276-E1285
61. Gray SD. Responsiveness of the terminal vascular bed in fast and slow skeletal muscles to alpha-adrenergic stimulation. Angiologica 1971;8:285-296
62. Youd JM, Rattigan S, Clark MG. Acute impairment of insulin-mediated capillary recruitment and glucose uptake in rat skeletal muscle in vivo by TNF-alpha. Diabetes 2000;49:1904-1909
63. Zhang Y, Pilon G, Marette A, Baracos VE. Cytokines and endotoxin induce cytokine receptors in skeletal muscle. Am J Physiol Endocrinol Metab 2000;279:E196-E205
64. Togashi N, Ura N, Higashiura K, et al. The contribution of skeletal muscle tumor necrosis factor-alpha to insulin resistance and hypertension in fructose-fed rats. J Hypertens 2000;18:1605-1610
65. Li YP, Reid MB. Effect of tumor necrosis factor-alpha on skeletal muscle metabolism. Curr Opin Rheumatol 2001;13:483-487
66. Halse R, Pearson SL, McCormack JG, et al. Effects of tumor necrosis factor-alpha on insulin action in cultured human muscle cells. Diabetes 2001;50:1102-1109
67. de Alvaro C, Teruel T, Hernandez R, Lorenzo M. Tumor necrosis factor alpha produces insulin resistance in skeletal muscle by activation of inhibitor kappaB kinase in a p38 MAPK-dependent manner. J Biol Chem 2004; 279:17070-17078
68. Yamaguchi K, Higashiura K, Ura N, et al. The effect of tumor necrosis factor-alpha on tissue specificity and selectivity to insulin signaling. Hypertens Res 2003; 26:389-396
69. Kim HJ, Higashimori T, Park SY, et al. Differential effects of interleukin-6 and -10 on skeletal muscle and liver insulin action in vivo. Diabetes 2004;53:1060-1067
70. Dietze D, Ramrath S, Ritzeler O, et al. Inhibitor kappaB kinase is involved in the paracrine crosstalk between human fat and muscle cells. Int J Obes Relat Metab Disord 2004;28:985-992
71. Gielen S, Adams V, Moebius-Winkler S, et al. Anti-inflammatory effects of exercise training in the skeletal muscle of patients with chronic heart failure. J Am Coll Cardiol 2003;42:861-868

72. Mann DL, Reid MB. Exercise training and skeletal muscle inflammation. In chronic heart failure: feeling better about fatigue. J Am Coll Cardiol 2003;42:869-872
73. Reid MB, Li YP. Cytokines and oxidative signalling in skeletal muscle. Acta Physiol Scand 2001;171:225-232
74. Taylor R. Causation of type 2 diabetes—the Gordian knot unravels. N Engl J Med 2004;350:639-641
75. Cline GW, Petersen KF, Krssak M, et al. Impaired glucose transport as a cause of decreased insulin-stimulated muscle glycogen synthesis in type 2 diabetes. N Engl J Med 1999;341:240-246
76. Barnes BR, Ryder JW, Steiler TL, et al. Isoform-specific regulation of 5′ AMP–activated protein kinase in skeletal muscle from obese Zucker (fa/fa) rats in response to contraction. Diabetes 2002;51:2703-2708
77. Shulman GI, Rothman DL, Jue T, et al. Quantitation of muscle glycogen synthesis in normal subjects and subjects with non–insulin-dependent diabetes by ^{13}C nuclear magnetic resonance spectroscopy. N Engl J Med 1990;322:223-228
78. Baron AD. Insulin resistance and vascular function. J Diabetes Complications 2002;16:92-102
79. Borghouts LB, Wagenmakers AJ, Goyens PL, Keizer HA. Substrate utlilization in non-obese type II diabetic patients at rest and during exercise. Clin Sci (Lond) 2002;103:559-566
80. Regensteiner JG, Sippel J, McFarling ET, et al. Effects of non–insulin-dependent diabetes on oxygen consumption during treadmill exercise. Med Sci Sports Exerc 1995;27:875-881
81. Salmenniemi U, Ruotsalainen E, Pihlajamäki J, et al. Multiple abnormalities in glucose and energy metabolism and coordinated changes in levels of adiponectin, cytokines, and adhesion molecules in subjects with metabolic syndrome. Circulation 2004;110:3842-3848
82. Petersen KF, Dufour S, Befroy D, et al. Impaired mitochondrial activity in the insulin-resistant offspring of patients with type 2 diabetes. N Engl J Med 2004;350: 664-671
83. Hickey MS, Carey JO, Azevedo JL, et al. Skeletal muscle fiber composition is related to adiposity and in vitro glucose transport rate in humans. Am J Physiol 1995;268: E453-E457
84. Vessby B. Dietary fat and insulin action in humans. Br J Nutr 2000;83(suppl 1):S91-S96
85. Kelley DE, Simoneau JA. Impaired free fatty acid utilization by skeletal muscle in non–insulin-dependent diabetes mellitus. J Clin Invest 1994;94:2349-2356

Section IV

Manifestations of Insulin Resistance

Lipids and Atherogenic Dyslipidemia 10

Dyslipidemia is a manifestation of insulin resistance in the metabolic syndrome. Disturbances in lipid homeostasis play an important role in the cardiovascular complications of the metabolic syndrome and type 2 diabetes mellitus (DM).

APOLIPOPROTEINS

There are at least 12 apolipoproteins (apo), named alphabetically starting with A. They are synthesized and secreted by both the intestine and the liver. **Apolipoproteins are amphipathic molecules, which implies that they have both polar hydrophilic and nonpolar hydrophobic aspects. This characteristic allows apolipoproteins to solubilize nonpolar lipids, thus providing a mechanism for the transport of lipids in blood.**

Apolipoproteins serve a number of functions:

- they contribute to the structural integrity of lipoproteins;
- they are active in lipoprotein metabolism and secretion; and
- they serve as ligands for lipoprotein receptors, as cofactors for lipolytic enzymes, and as lipid transferases.[1]

LIPOPROTEINS

Lipoproteins are large, multimolecular particles that package hydrophobic lipid molecules, such as triglycerides and cholesteryl esters, for transport in blood. En route from the intestines and the liver, they deliver lipids to specific target tissues in the organism. Targeting occurs via apolipoproteins, which serve as ligands for cell surface receptors or as cofactors for cell surface lipases such as lipoprotein lipase (LPL).[2]

Lipoproteins are typically spherical particles composed of one or more amphipathic carrier apolipoproteins that present their polar, hydrophilic aspect to the plasma. The hydrophilic, outer coat of the lipoprotein complex is also composed of phospholipids and free cholesterol. Cholesteryl esters and triglycerides bind to the internal, nonpolar, hydrophobic moiety of the complex (Fig. 10-1).[3]

The size and density of lipoproteins are of clinical relevance. In that respect, the relative amounts of core lipids and proteins are determining factors. The larger lipoproteins contain an abundance of core lipids. Small lipoproteins have less core lipid and are correspondingly denser.[3]

The apolipoprotein content of lipoproteins has an impact on cardiovascular risk. Elevated levels of apolipoprotein B (apo B)- and low levels of apo A-I–containing lipoproteins constitute adverse cardiovascular risk factors. Conversely, low levels of apo B– and high levels of apo A-I–containing lipoproteins are protective of vascular health.[3]

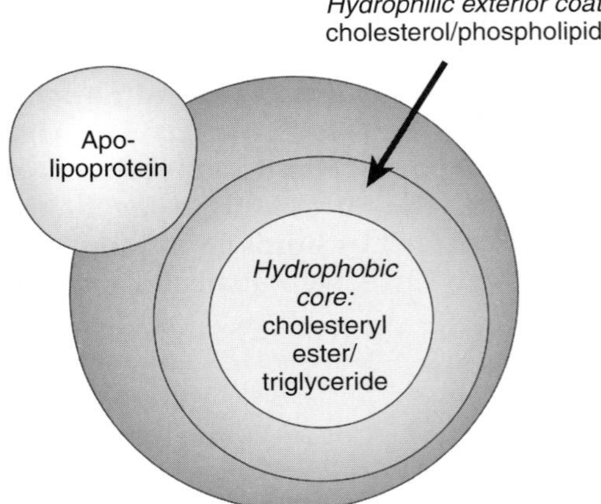

›› **Figure 10–1.**
Schematic lipoprotein structure.

APOLIPOPROTEIN A-I–CONTAINING LIPOPROTEINS: STRUCTURE AND FUNCTION

High-Density Lipoprotein. High-density lipoprotein (HDL) is the major apo A-I–containing lipoprotein, although the complex is also composed of other apolipoproteins. Apo A-I is expressed in the liver and the small intestine. Its secretion into plasma results in de novo HDL production. There are a variety of HDL subfractions based on differential molecular densities: HDL2b, HDL2c, and HDL3.[4]

HDL Composition. Human HDLs are a heterogeneous class of lipoproteins. As their name implies, HDL particles are dense, with a density of 1.063 to 1.21 g/mL. They are correspondingly small and measure only about 5 to 17 nm in diameter.[5] Fifty percent of the HDL particle mass is composed of protein. Upon secretion from the liver and the intestine, the pre-β_1 HDL complex is disk shaped and composed of

- protein: apo A-I (70% of the protein mass) and other apolipoproteins (A-II, A-IV, C, E, and minor apolipoproteins),
- phospholipids, and
- minimal cholesterol.[1]

Lecithin-cholesterol acyltransferase (LCAT), paraoxonase (PON), and platelet-activating factor acetylhydrolase (PAF-AH) are also associated with HDL and participate in significant physiologic functions.[4]

Reverse Cholesterol Transport. Approximately 9 mg of cholesterol per kilogram of body weight is synthesized on a daily basis by nonhepatic, peripheral tissues. This quantity of cholesterol has to be transferred to the liver for catabolism to maintain global lipid homeostasis.[5] **One of the functions of HDL is to lower the cholesterol content in the periphery via a net flux of cholesterol to the liver and steroidogenic organs. This process is termed reverse cholesterol transport.**[3]

Reverse cholesterol transport occurs as HDL extracts excess cholesterol from peripheral cells, such as foam cell macrophages in the vessel wall, for transport back to the liver and for removal from the body. Cholesterol is derived for reverse transport via three mechanisms:

1. diffusion,
2. scavenger receptor class B, type 1 (SR-B1)-mediated efflux, and
3. apolipoprotein-mediated efflux via the adenosine triphosphate–binding cassette transporter A-1 (ABCA-1), which moves free, unesterified cholesterol out of a cell onto the cell surface–bound HDL moiety.[6,7]

Adenosine Triphosphate–Binding Cassette Transporters. Normally, the cellular cholesterol concentration is tightly controlled. To prevent excessive accumulation, cholesterol is translocated to the cell membrane. ABCA-1 transports cholesterol and phospholipids from the cytosol to the plasmalemma.[1]

The ABCA-1 transporter is highly expressed in hepatocytes, macrophages, and other peripheral cells. One regulatory element in the promoter region for the ABCA-1 gene is the liver X receptor. Elevated cytosolic levels of cholesterol, as well as its oxidized derivative oxysterols, stimulate the liver X receptor pathway to enhance the expression of ABCA-1.[8]

Cholesterol Extraction from Cells. The ABCA-1 transporter cycles between the endocytic compartment and the plasmalemma to facilitate the movement of cytoplasmic cholesterol to the plasmalemma. Cholesterol enrichment of the plasmalemma, in turn, facilitates the lipidation of apo A-I, which is the major apolipoprotein acceptor for ABCA-1–mediated cholesterol efflux. As pre-β or nascent HDL is formed, it facilitates the further removal of excess cellular cholesterol and initiates the reverse transport of cholesterol out of peripheral, nonhepatic tissues.[8]

Maturation of High-Density Lipoprotein. Within the HDL particle, free cholesterol is esterified by LCAT, with apo A-I acting as its cofactor. In the process, a fatty acid from phosphatidylcholine is transferred to free cholesterol to create a cholesteryl ester, which is stored in the lipophilic core of the HDL particle.[7]

With the accumulation of cholesterol, HDL grows in size and becomes spherical. It first turns into the smaller HDL3 complex and then matures into the larger HDL2-type particle after further accretion of cholesteryl esters.[7] The nascent HDL and HDL3 particles accomplish reverse cholesterol transport more efficaciously than mature HDL2 does.[1]

High-Density Lipoprotein Cholesterol Delivery. The HDL complex delivers cholesteryl esters via a different plasmalemmal HDL receptor, the scavenger receptor SR-B1. SR-B1 is found on hepatocytes and at other sites such as the adrenals, the ovaries, and endothelial cells.[9] Upon binding to that receptor, cholesteryl esters are released into the recipient cell.[1]

Alternatively, cholesteryl ester transfer protein (CETP) can mediate an exchange of cholesteryl esters from HDL for triglycerides from apo B–containing lipoproteins such as very-low-density lipoproteins (VLDLs) and low-density lipoproteins (LDLs). Similarly, the phospholipid transfer protein mediates the transfer of phospholipids from apo B–containing lipoproteins to the HDL particle. Some of the cholesteryl esters transferred to apo B lipoproteins may then return to the liver via the LDL receptor. Approximately 50% of the reverse cholesterol transport occurs through this route.[10]

As cholesteryl ester is exchanged for triglyceride, HDL, now enriched in triglyceride, is rendered subject to the action of triglyceride lipases. Hepatic lipase (HL) hydrolyzes the triglyceride and phospholipid component of HDL, which allows the HDL cholesteryl esters to then be cleared by the SR-B1 receptor.[10]

Lipase Action on High-Density Lipoprotein. Other triglyceride lipases affect the metabolism of triglyceride-enriched HDL in additional ways. LPL contributes to HDL formation by hydrolyzing triglyceride in triglyceride-rich apo B–containing lipoproteins, which results in the transfer of redundant phospholipid and apolipoprotein surface materials from VLDL to HDL3, a necessary step in the formation of cholesterol-rich HDL2.[11] Endothelial lipase (EL) hydrolyzes HDL phospholipids, thereby generating a lipid-depleted HDL and ultimately promoting HDL catabolism. EL is more effective at hydrolyzing lipids pertaining to HDL than LPL and HL are.[10]

Cholesterol Excretion and High-Density Lipoprotein Catabolism. In the liver cells, the transferred cholesteryl esters are hydrolyzed into free cholesterol to be converted to bile acids or to be secreted directly into bile for further elimination into the gastrointestinal tract.[10]

The lipid-depleted HDL can then be recycled for further reverse cholesterol transport. However, the resultant small, senescent apo A-I particles are susceptible to glomerular filtration in the proximal renal tubule, as well as to catabolism by other tissues.[10]

Factors That Modulate High-Density Lipoprotein Levels and Reverse Cholesterol Transport. Numerous genetic, lifestyle, habitus, hormonal, and pharmacologic factors have an impact on HDL levels and function (Table 10-1).

Non–High-Density Lipoprotein Factors. Factors that will enhance net reverse cholesterol transport are

- activation of LCAT,
- inhibition of CETP,
- balanced activity of HL,
- adequate adipose tissue and muscle LPL activity,
- suppression of EL, and
- enhanced hepatic cholesteryl ester uptake from HDL via SR-B1–dependent pathways.[10,12]

Table 10-1. Factors Influencing High-Density Lipoprotein Levels

DECREASE HDL	INCREASE HDL
Male gender	Female gender
Genetic disorders	Hyperalphalipoproteinemia
Sedentary lifestyle	Aerobic exercise
Overweight	Lean body mass index/ weight loss
Inflammation	Smoking cessation
Insulin resistance	Estrogen
Hypertriglyceridemia	Low-carbohydrate diet
Increased apolipoprotein B	Moderate alcohol use
Diabetes mellitus	Niacin
Anabolic steroids	Peroxisome proliferator–activated receptor-α agonists
Diet very low in fat	+/– Thiazolidinediones
Tobacco use	Statins (moderate effect)
β-Blockers	Cholesterol ester transfer protein inhibitors
Androgens	? Fish oils
Progestins	Biochemically reconstituted high-density lipoprotein
Benzodiazepines	

High-Density Lipoprotein Factors. The functional effect of HDL is variable. It may act via

- specific protein-receptor interactions,
- charged phospholipid-phospholipid contact,
- activation of cellular signaling pathways resulting in the regulation of genes, or
- modification of proteins for various functions.

The activity of HDL is a function of the lipoprotein's

- cholesterol content,
- lipid and phospholipid composition,
- apolipoprotein composition,
- apo A-I genotype,
- enzymes, and
- size.

Although in general, elevated levels of HDL are of benefit, the appropriate functionality of HDL is of greater importance than the actual levels of HDL.[10]

The apo A-I genotype, in particular, affects HDL function. Certain apo A-I mutations have deleterious effects on endothelial function.[13] In contrast, apo A-I_{Milano} (apo A-I_M) is a naturally occurring molecular variant of apo A-I characterized by a cysteine-for-arginine substitution and the tendency to form apo A-I_M/apo A-I_M dimers. These dimers have a prolonged circulation time in plasma and offer greater capacity for reverse cholesterol transport. These variants improve endothelial function and have antiatherogenic, antiproliferative, antirestenotic, antiplatelet, and antithrombotic properties that confer protection from cardiovascular disease despite markedly reduced HDL levels in human carriers of the mutation.[14]

Clinical Impact of Reverse Cholesterol Transport. The association of high levels of HDL with a decreased incidence of cardiovascular events implies a central involvement of HDL in the retardation of the atherosclerotic process. HDL lowers cardiovascular risk in part by promoting the efflux of excessive

cholesterol from arterial wall macrophages via reverse cholesterol transport. It may thereby inhibit plaque expansion and enhance the stability of existing atheromata.[15]

Beyond Reverse Cholesterol Transport. In addition to its effects on reverse cholesterol transport, **HDL has a variety of other properties that may contribute to its antiatherogenic actions, such as its**

- **antioxidant,**
- **anti-inflammatory,**
- **anticoagulant, and**
- **vascular protective**

effects (Table 10-2).[10]

Antioxidant Effects. HDL has antioxidant properties and interferes with the proatherogenic oxidation of LDL. Through its association with antioxidant enzymes such as

- PON and
- PAF-AH,

HDL may inhibit LDL oxidation and decrease the expression of adhesion molecules. PON-1 is a serum esterase bound to HDL, first recognized for its ability to hydrolyze a metabolite of the insecticide parathion. **Oxidized LDL may actually be reduced by the transfer of oxidized lipids to HDL,** where such lipids are cleaved by the enzymes associated with HDL.[16]

Table 10-2. High-Density Lipoprotein and Atherosclerosis: Beyond Reverse Cholesterol Transport

HDL INHIBITS	HDL STIMULATES
Endothelial dysfunction	Nitric oxide availability
Endothelial cell apoptosis	Synthesis of prostacyclin
Adhesion of leukocytes	Synthesis of natriuretic peptide C
Chemotaxis of monocytes	Activation of proteins C, S
Low-density lipoprotein oxidation	Proliferation of endothelial cells
Complement activation	
Platelet activation	
Platelet aggregation	
Factor X activation	
Proliferation of smooth muscle cells	

Caveolae. **HDL antagonizes the adverse endothelial effects of oxidized LDL.** As HDL binds to the scavenger receptor SR-B1, which colocalizes with endothelial nitric oxide synthase (eNOS) in endothelial caveolae, it donates cholesteryl esters to caveolae, thereby preserving their structure and function.[17] **Some of the atheroprotective features of HDL may, in fact, be due to direct effects of HDL on the signal transduction mechanisms of endothelial cells that are localized in plasmalemmal caveolae.**[18]

Anti-inflammatory Effects. HDL has anti-inflammatory properties. It reduces complement activation and cytokine-induced up-regulation of adhesion molecules, such as vascular cell adhesion molecule-1 (VCAM-1) and E-selectin, by endothelial cells. HDL inhibits the chemotaxis of monocytes and the adhesion of leukocytes to the endothelium.[8] In cultured human umbilical vein endothelial cells, preincubation with physiologic concentrations of HDL suppresses the C-reactive protein (CRP)-induced expression of inflammatory adhesion molecules via oxidized phospholipid components of HDL.[19]

Anticoagulant Effects. HDL has antiplatelet and anticoagulant effects. It may promote the release and stability of prostacyclin. HDL directly enhances the activation of proteins C and S, as well as nitric oxide (NO) platelet antiaggregatory activity.[5]

Vascular Protective Effects. HDL is protective of vascular health (Fig. 10-2).

Endothelial Function. **Clinically, HDL exerts direct, beneficial effects on endothelial function.** It normalizes abnormal endothelial function by increasing NO bioavailability. As a result, **in general the HDL plasma concentration is proportional to the sum of all plasma nitrite/nitrate metabolites of NO.** Thus, in type 2 diabetic patients without clinical vascular disease, low HDL is associated with low, and high HDL with high plasma NO end products. HDL directly modulates vascular cell proliferation, apoptosis, vasomotion, and the synthesis of natriuretic peptide C.[5]

Endothelial Nitric Oxide Synthase. **HDL induces significant stimulation of eNOS**

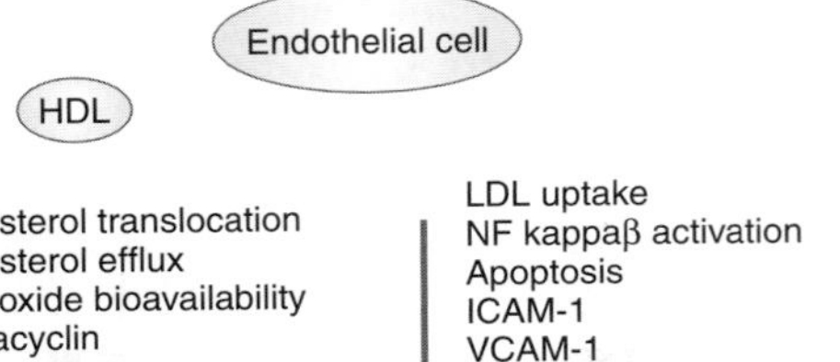

Figure 10–2.
Protective anti-inflammatory and antithrombotic high-density lipoprotein (HDL) effects on vascular endothelial cells. ICAM, intercellular adhesion molecule; LDL, low-density lipoprotein; NF, nuclear factor; PAI, plasminogen activator inhibitor; tPA, tissue plasminogen activator; VCAM, vascular cell adhesion molecule. *(Modified from Genest J. Genetics and prevention: A new look at high-density lipoprotein cholesterol. Cardiol Rev 2002;10:61-71.)*

activity in endothelial cells that results in endothelium- and NO-dependent vasodilation.[17]

HDL activation of eNOS requires apo A-I binding to the scavenger receptor SR-B1, which may stimulate eNOS activity by increasing intracellular ceramide levels.[18,20] HDL stimulation of eNOS also entails activation of a common upstream, nonreceptor tyrosine kinase, which leads to parallel activation of Akt kinase and mitogen-activated protein kinase (MAPK) and their resultant, independent modulation of the enzyme (Fig. 10-3).[21]

Clinical Impact of High-Density Lipoprotein Plasma Levels. Elevated levels of apo A-I–containing HDL, in particular, of the larger HDL2, lower cardiovascular risk and are directly protective against atherosclerosis via lipid-lowering and pleiotropic mechanisms. Plasma levels of HDL are proportional to longevity and inversely proportional to the incidence of coronary heart disease (CHD), independent of other known CHD risk factors (Fig. 10-4).[22]

The effects of apo A-II on atherogenesis are controversial, but apo A-II does not appear to be a strong determinant but rather a modulator of effects.[15] Apo A-II may have a role in visceral fat accumulation.[22]

Low High-Density Lipoprotein Levels. **Low levels of HDL cholesterol serve as a metabolic marker for increased cardiovascular risk and the metabolic syndrome** (Table 10-3). **A low plasma HDL concentration is an independent predictor of endothelial dysfunction in healthy individuals, as well as in hyperlipidemic diabetic persons and CHD patients.**[4]

Endothelial dysfunction has been reported in individuals with primary hypoalphalipoproteinemia, a genetic lipoprotein disorder characterized by low plasma HDL and apo A-I levels. Loss-of-function mutations in the ABCA-1 gene locus cause familial hypoalphalipoproteinemia and constitute a human isolated, low-HDL model. As expected, in ABCA-1 heterozygotes, isolated, low HDL is associated with endothelial dysfunction.[23]

The inverse association of HDL concentration and CHD incidence is robust. **Even with low LDL levels, a low HDL level remains an important predictor of CHD risk.**[1,24] Low HDL and low apo A-I levels are frequently observed with cardiovascular risk factors such as

- cigarette consumption,
- physical inactivity,

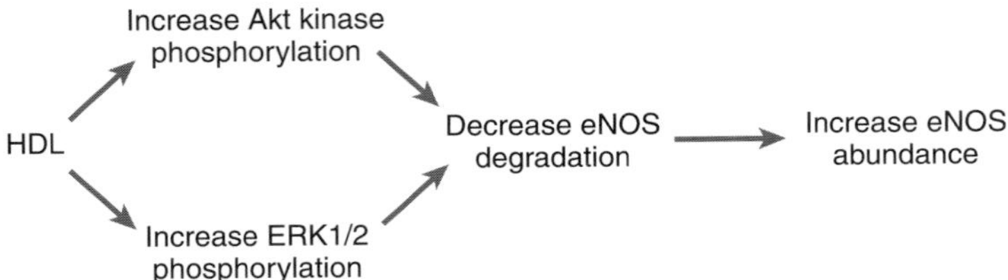

Figure 10–3.
High-density lipoprotein (HDL) increases endothelial nitric oxide synthase (eNOS) expression via kinase-dependent pathways. ERK, extracellular signal–regulated protein kinase. *(Modified from Ramet ME, Aamet M, Lu Q, et al. High-density lipoprotein increases the abundance of eNOS protein in human vascular endothelial cells by increasing its half-life. J Am Coll Cardiol 2003;41:2288-2297.)*

Figure 10-4.
Framingham Heart Study: relative coronary heart disease (CHD) risk adjustment as a function of high-density lipoprotein (HDL) and low-density lipoprotein (LDL) levels in men aged 50 to 70 years. *(Modified from Castelli WP. Cholesterol and lipids in the risk of coronary artery disease—the Framingham Heart Study. Can J Cardiol 1988;4(suppl A):5A-10A.)*

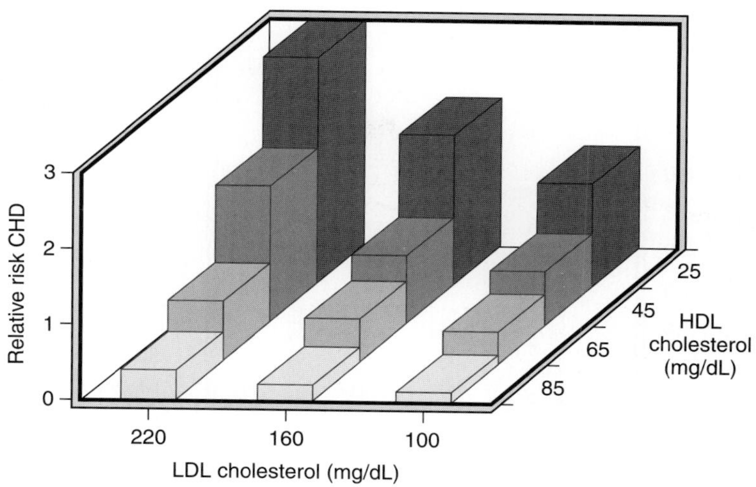

- hypertriglyceridemia, and
- the metabolic syndrome.

Low HDL,

- <40 mg/dL in men and
- <50 mg/dL in women,

is now one of the Adult Treatment Panel III criteria for diagnosis of the metabolic syndrome.[25] As triglyceride levels progressively increase, a lower HDL level promotes increasing risk for CHD.[26]

Table 10-3. Adult Treatment Panel III Classification of Total, High-Density Lipoprotein, and Low-Density Lipoprotein Cholesterol

Total Cholesterol (mg/dL)	
<200	Desirable
200-239	Borderline high
≥240	High
High-Density Lipoprotein (mg/dL)	
<40	Low
≥60	High
Low-Density Lipoprotein (mg/dL)	
<100	Optimal
100-129	Near optimal/above optimal
130-159	Borderline high
160-189	High
≥190	Very high

Adapted from http://www.guidelines.gov/VIEWS/summary.asp?guidelines=00219.

Therapeutic Improvement of High-Density Lipoprotein Levels. Elevation of plasma HDL levels by drug treatment or infusion of synthetic HDL significantly improves cardiovascular risk.[4] An increase in HDL by 1 mg/dL (0.026 mmol/L) is associated with a 2% to 4% reduction in the risk for cardiovascular events.[27,28] Over 12 years' follow-up, a 10-mg/dL increase in HDL cholesterol causes a 50% lowering of CHD risk.[26]

Even in the short term, however, infusion of HDL improves endothelial function. In hypoalphalipoproteinemic individuals, endothelial function was completely restored after a single, rapid infusion of apo A-I/phosphatidylcholine.[23] In a similar study, infusion of reconstituted HDL containing apo A-I and phosphatidylcholine in a molar ratio of 1:150 in healthy, hypercholesterolemic men restored and normalized endothelium-dependent vasodilation in an NO-dependent manner (Fig. 10-5).[29]

Modulation of HDL may in fact exert antiatherogenic effects and cause lesion regression. In apo E–null mice with native aortic and vein graft atherosclerosis, 4 weeks of daily oral and intraperitoneal administration of the apo A-I mimetic, amphipathic, helical peptide D4F significantly reduced evolving atherosclerotic vein graft lesions but not established aortic sinus disease.[30] In a trial of 46 patients with acute coronary syndrome, five weekly infusions of a recombinant apo A-I_M/phospholipid complex produced a modest but rapid and

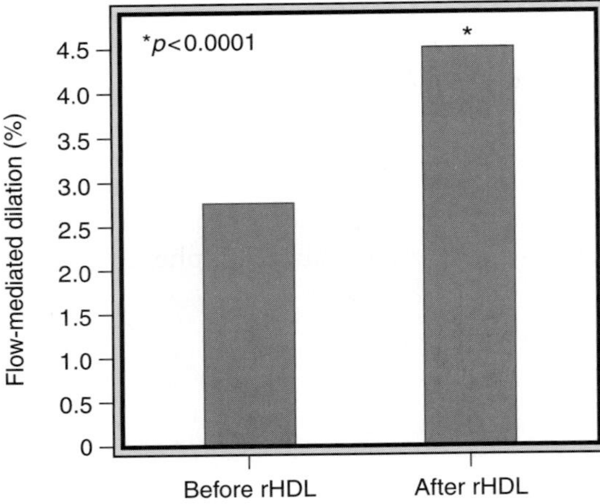

⏩ **Figure 10–5.**
Enhanced brachial artery flow–mediated dilation in hypercholesterolemic men after the administration of intravenous reconstituted HDL (rHDL). *(Modified from Spieker LE, Sudano I, Huerlimann D, et al. High-density lipoprotein restores endothelial function in hypercholesterolemic men. Circulation 2002;105:1399-1402.)*

statistically significant regression of coronary atherosclerosis when measured by intravascular ultrasonography.[31] Other HDL mimetic compounds that may induce lesion regression, such as phospholipid liposomes in unilamellar vesicles and other apo A-I mimetic peptides, are now being tested in animal models and patients.[13]

APOLIPOPROTEIN B–CONTAINING LIPOPROTEINS: STRUCTURE AND FUNCTION

There are numerous lipoproteins that incorporate apo B. Apo B–containing lipoproteins are

- chylomicrons,
- VLDL,
- the metabolic remnants of VLDL and chylomicrons,
- intermediate-density lipoprotein (IDL),
- LDL, and
- lipoprotein (a) (Lp[a]).

These lipoproteins all have one molecule of apo B-100.

Chylomicrons. Chylomicrons are very large. Because of their size they contain several apolipoproteins,

- apo B-100,
- apo C-I,
- apo C-II,
- apo C-III, and
- apo E.

Apo E is a truncated version of apo B-100 and is required for lipid secretion from intestinal cells. Chylomicrons are, in fact, synthesized in the intestine. Their purpose is to transport exogenous dietary fat in the form of triglycerides and cholesteryl esters via the portal circulation to the liver. Triglycerides constitute more than 90% of the weight of chylomicrons.

Very-Low-Density Lipoproteins. VLDL is also a large lipoprotein. Like chylomicrons, VLDL contains several types of apolipoproteins, but apo B-100 is essential for its secretion by the liver. The liver releases VLDL in order to transport lipids from the liver to the periphery. Triglycerides constitute 50% to 60% of VLDL weight; cholesteryl esters make up the rest.

Intermediate-Density Lipoproteins. In the peripheral circulation, as LPL interacts with VLDL, triglycerides are hydrolyzed. This reaction reduces the size and weight of the complex and generates IDL in the process, which carries an equivalent amount of triglycerides and cholesteryl esters.

Remnant Lipoproteins. Chylomicron remnants and VLDL remnants are derived from lipoprotein hydrolysis of their respective core triglycerides.

Lipoprotein(a). Lp(a) is a complex of LDL linked by an interchain disulfide bridge of two free cysteine residues to a glycoprotein, apoprotein(a), which is structurally homologous to plasminogen. Lp(a) is rich in cholesteryl ester and is assembled extracellularly. **Lp(a) appears to play a vital role in atherothrombogenesis**[22] and is associated with endothelial dysfunction. Lp(a) may induce inflammation by activating monocytes, colocalizing with plaque macrophages, and stimulating smooth muscle cells. It has been implicated in the initiation, progression, and destabilization of atheromata. Because of the structural homology of apoprotein(a) with plasminogen, **Lp(a) may compete with plasminogen and inhibit its thrombolytic effect.**[32]

Low-Density Lipoproteins. Further hydrolysis of triglyceride in IDL by both LPL and HL removes most of the triglyceride, with only cholesteryl esters and nonesterified cholesterol remaining in the complex. Upon the loss of apo E, the particle is now called LDL. The LDL particle consists of a cholesteryl ester core surrounded by apo B-100.

The lipoprotein's apo B-100 binds to LDL(B,E) receptors in tissues. Upon binding of the LDL complex, the cholesteryl esters of LDL are hydrolyzed in lysosomes to produce free intracellular cholesterol.[2,33]

The sterol regulatory element binding protein (SREBP) increases the transcription of two genes:

1. the LDL receptor gene and
2. the gene for 3-hydroxy-3-methylglutaryl–coenzyme A (HMG-CoA) reductase, which is the rate-limiting enzyme of cholesterol synthesis.

As free cholesterol accumulates intracellularly upon LDL binding to the LDL(B,E) receptor, it inhibits the release of SREBP and thereby causes down-regulation of the synthesis of cholesterol and the LDL receptor in a negative feedback loop.[34]

LDL is the major supply vector of cholesterol to the periphery. It supplies the cholesterol used in the composition of cell membranes and for the synthesis of steroid hormones and bile acids.[2]

Elevated levels of LDL play a central role in mediating vascular pathology (see Table 10-3) (Fig. 10-6).

Small, Dense Low-Density Lipoproteins. With excessive VLDL production, CETP exchanges the triglycerides of VLDL for cholesteryl esters in normal LDL. The resulting triglyceride-enriched LDL is subject to hydrolysis by HL, which leaves a cholesteryl ester–depleted, small and dense LDL complex.

The three predominant LDL phenotypes are

1. pattern A, with an LDL diameter larger than 255 Å;
2. pattern B, with an LDL diameter smaller than or equal to 255 Å; and
3. an intermediate pattern with characteristics of both A and B.

Small, dense LDL of pattern B is more atherogenic than regular LDL. Small, dense LDL

- can penetrate the endothelium and bind to intimal proteoglycans more effectively than large, buoyant LDL can, thereby resulting in prolonged retention in the arterial wall matrix;
- has poor binding affinity to the LDL(B,E) receptor, which causes decreased clearance and elevated plasma levels of small, dense LDL;
- is preferentially taken up by the scavenger receptor pathway of macrophages and thus contributes to atherogenesis; and
- is particularly susceptible to oxidation and glycation, which may induce antibody production against the modified apo B-100, as well as the formation of immune complexes.[3,22,35]

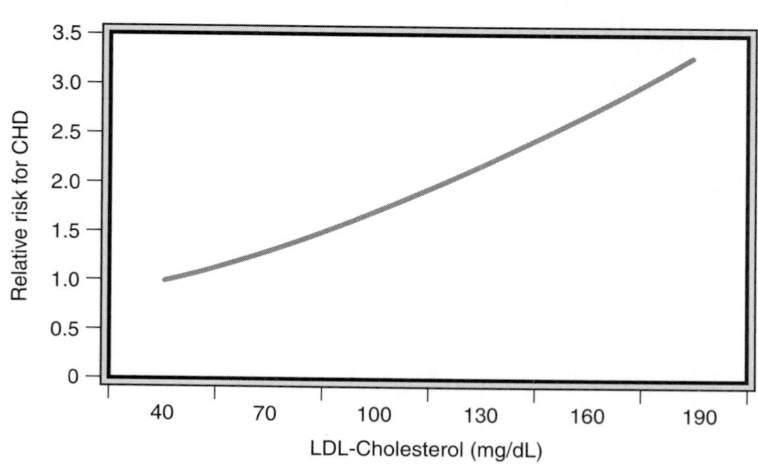

Figure 10–6. Low-density lipoprotein (LDL) level and the relative risk for coronary heart disease (CHD) from clinical trials and epidemiologic data: every 30-mg/dL increase in LDL level raises CHD risk by approximately 30%. *(Modified from Grundy SM, Cleeman JI, Merz CN, et al. Implications of recent clinical trials for the National Cholesterol Education Program Adult Treatment Panel III guidelines. Circulation 2004;110:227-239.)*

Small, dense LDL particles are less effectively cleared by the liver than normal LDL is.

Oxidized Low-Density Lipoprotein. Elevated levels of small, dense LDL complexes are more susceptible to oxidation. Oxidative modification of lipoproteins plays a central role in the pathogenesis of atherosclerosis.

Oxidized LDL promotes inflammation, in part through its uptake by macrophage scavenger receptors and subsequent nuclear factor kappaB (NFκB) activation.[36] It exerts several proatherogenic effects, including

- cytotoxicity to endothelial cells,
- impairment of vascular NO release,
- increased synthesis and secretion of cytokines and adhesion molecules,
- monocyte chemotaxis and adhesion,
- greater smooth muscle cell proliferation, and
- enhanced foam cell formation,[37]

all resulting in vascular inflammation, atherogenesis, and a worsened cardiovascular outcome.[35]

The Lectin-like Oxidized Low-Density Lipoprotein Receptor-1. Oxidized LDL participates in the pathogenesis of atherosclerosis also by activation of the lectin-like oxidized low-density lipoprotein receptor-1 (LOX-1). LOX-1 is the major receptor for oxidized LDL in

- endothelial cells,
- smooth muscle cells, and
- macrophages,

in which it mediates endothelial injury and dysfunction.

Vascular LOX-1 expression is stimulated by

- angiotensin II,
- endothelin-1,
- tumor necrosis factor-alpha (TNF-α),
- other cytokines, and
- oxidized LDL.

LOX-1 has the ability to bind

- pathogenic organisms,
- damaged or apoptotic cells,
- activated platelets,
- advanced glycation end products, and
- proatherogenic materials such as oxidized LDL

for endocytosis or phagocytosis into the cell. With LOX-1 highly expressed in blood vessels, increased amounts of oxidized LDL can undergo endocytosis, which further enhances LOX-1 expression in a positive feedback loop, with adverse outcomes.[38]

Endothelial Dysfunction. Oxidized LDL prevents agonist stimulation of eNOS and impairs endothelial function. Plasma levels of oxidized LDL may, in fact, serve as a surrogate for the assessment of coronary endothelium–dependent vasomotor function. In a clinical study of 94 individuals with normal coronary arteriograms, the level of oxidized LDL was an independent determinant of the coronary macrovasomotive and microvasomotive response to intracoronary bradykinin.[39]

Caveolae. eNOS normally functions in a signaling module within cholesterol-enriched caveolae. **Oxidized LDL binds to the CD36 receptor of endothelial cells and depletes the caveolae of cholesterol. Cholesterol depletion of the caveolar plasmalemma disrupts the structural integrity of caveolae, which ultimately interferes with the eNOS activation process** and precipitates the translocation of eNOS from caveolae to an inactive, intracellular membrane compartment.[17]

Asymmetric Dimethylarginine. **Oxidized LDL increases the production and interferes with the degradation of asymmetric dimethylarginine (ADMA), thus further impairing endothelial function.** Plasma levels of ADMA, an endogenous eNOS inhibitor, correlate with the severity of endothelial dysfunction.[40]

Endothelin-1 and Oxidant Stress. Activated platelets interact with the endothelium via LOX-1; they promote the release of endothelin-1 from endothelial cells and stimulate the generation of reactive oxygen species that inactivate NO and reduce its intracellular availability.[38]

Endothelial Cell Apoptosis. Oxidized LDL uptake by LOX-1 mediates endothelial cell apoptosis, potentially via NFκB activation.[38]

The Renin-Angiotensin-Aldosterone System. There is a positive feedback interaction

between oxidized LDL and the vascular renin-angiotensin-aldosterone system (RAAS):

- lipid accumulation in the blood vessel walls enhances expression of the local RAAS,
- angiotensin II stimulates expression of the vascular LOX-1 receptor, and
- activation of the RAAS further stimulates the accumulation of oxidized LDL in blood vessels.[41]

Oxidized LDL, through the LOX-1 receptor, increases the expression of angiotensin-converting enzyme for further angiotensin II generation, thereby aggravating vascular wall inflammation in a vicious circle.[38]

Atherogenesis. **Oxidized LDL with LOX-1 activation contributes to atherogenesis.** Up-regulation of LOX-1 induces the enhanced expression of

- P-selectin,
- VCAM-1,
- intercellular adhesion molecule-1 (ICAM-1), and
- monocyte chemoattractant protein-1 (MCP-1),

thereby engendering monocyte adhesion to and migration into the endothelium. Oxidized LDL, through LOX-1, triggers the CD40/CD40L signaling pathway and perpetuates the inflammatory response.[38]

Oxidized LDL can be taken up by macrophages to facilitate their transformation into the foam cells of atherosclerotic plaque. In contrast to the LDL(B,E) receptor pathway, the macrophage receptor pathway for the scavenger receptors SR-A and CD36 is not subject to negative feedback regulation, thus allowing unabated binding of oxidized LDL complexes. As a result, there is continuing uptake and storage of cholesteryl esters in macrophages, which prompts their subsequent conversion into foam cells. The LOX-1 receptor may also mediate the uptake of oxidized LDL by macrophages.[37]

LOX-1 activation contributes to the instability of atheromata. Oxidized LDL, binding to LOX-1, induces smooth muscle cell apoptosis and stimulates matrix metalloproteinase activity, thus compromising the physicochemical integrity of the fibrous cap.[38]

APOLIPOPROTEINS C AND E: STRUCTURE AND FUNCTION

Apolipoprotein C. Apo C-II is a component of HDL and VLDL. It is an essential cofactor and activator for the action of LPL.[2]

Apo C-III is a small protein on the surface of the apo B lipoproteins VLDL, IDL, and LDL. It delays the catabolism of these triglyceride-rich particles. Specifically, in contrast to apo C-II, apo C-III

- inhibits LPL from hydrolyzing triglycerides in apo B lipoproteins, which would facilitate their plasma clearance[42];
- prevents triglyceride-rich lipoproteins from binding to the endothelial surface and to hepatic lipoprotein receptors, which would aid in their removal from plasma; and
- interferes with apo E–mediated receptor clearance of remnant particles from plasma.[43]

Apolipoprotein E. Apo E structurally resembles a truncated version of apo B-100. Apo E is a critical participant in plasma lipid metabolism. It is required for the secretion of lipids from enteric cells into the circulation. Apo E functions as a ligand for the surface receptors of cells that take up triglyceride-rich lipoproteins from the plasma, thus mediating the uptake of chylomicron and VLDL remnants by the LDL(B,E) receptor and its cousin, LDL receptor–related protein. As such, it plays a crucial role in the metabolism of triglyceride-rich lipoproteins and in the hepatic clearance of their remnants. Because apo E appears to coexist with apo C-III in apo B lipoproteins, the beneficial effect of the former may be thwarted by the latter.[16,44]

There are common polymorphisms of apo E associated with hypercholesterolemia, type III hyperlipidemia, and Alzheimer's disease. As compared with the E3 allele (population frequency, 60%), the apo E4 allele (frequency of 30%) increases plasma cholesterol levels, whereas the apo E2 allele (frequency of 10%) decreases plasma cholesterol levels. These common variations of apo E explain 5% of the genetic variation in cholesterol levels in the U.S. population.[16]

NORMAL METABOLISM OF FREE FATTY ACIDS

Triacylglycerols, commonly termed triglycerides in clinical usage, are extremely energy dense. They serve as important fuel for oxidative phosphorylation in many metabolically active tissues, such as

- cardiac muscle,
- skeletal muscle, and
- the liver.

Triacylglycerols play a particularly important role as an energy source during starvation or exercise. Being lipophilic, they are insoluble in water and thus require transport in the circulation via lipoprotein complexes.[1]

Dietary Fatty Acids. Fatty acids, derived from dietary sources and packaged as triglycerides, are incorporated into chylomicrons by the intestinal epithelium to be delivered to the liver. As such, they also enter the systemic circulation via lymphatic flow.[1]

The Liver and Normal Very-Low-Density Lipoprotein Secretion. Hepatic assembly plus secretion of VLDL is a complex process involving the interaction of apo B with both core and surface lipids to form a lipoprotein particle. It depends mainly on the availability of

- free fatty acids,
- triglycerides,
- cholesteryl esters,
- apo B, and
- microsomal triglyceride transfer protein,

as modulated by the sensitivity to insulin signaling.[45] Insulin regulates the production of triglyceride-rich VLDL particles.

The Role of Free Fatty Acids. Partitioning of free fatty acids toward esterification rather than oxidation in the liver is critical in regulating the synthesis of VLDL. Enhanced fatty acid esterification leads to increased VLDL secretion. Four sources of fatty acids are used for lipoprotein synthesis:

- de novo lipogenesis, which quantitatively plays a minor role in regulating VLDL synthesis, but is elevated under conditions of high-carbohydrate feeding;
- cytoplasmic triglyceride stores, which importantly contribute to VLDL triglycerides;
- fatty acids derived from lipoproteins taken up directly by the liver, which are either oxidized or esterified; and
- plasma free fatty acids, which enter hepatocytes and play an important role in stimulating hepatic VLDL production.

Normally, with intact insulin signaling, plasma levels of free fatty acids are typically low and play little role in VLDL secretion. Fatty acid levels are physiologically elevated postprandially, as well as during starvation. In the absence of starvation or a need to metabolize free fatty acids for increased energy demands, postprandial acute elevations of plasma free fatty acids up-regulate hepatic de novo lipogenesis. Surplus fat is then stored as hepatocyte triacylglycerol and is secreted as VLDL.[46]

Insulin Impact on Apo B-100 Availability. Insulin normally profoundly influences a number of processes in VLDL secretion via a phosphatidylinositol 3-kinase–dependent pathway:

- Insulin physiologically suppresses apo B synthesis by attenuating the rate of apo B mRNA translation.
- An important determinant of apo B lipoprotein secretion is the intracellular stability of apo B. With sensitivity to insulin signaling, a substantial amount of newly synthesized apo B is normally subjected to intracellular degradation via the ubiquitin-proteasome system, although other proteases have been implicated in apo B degradation.
- Insulin also suppresses the secretion of VLDL by negatively regulating the expression of microsomal triglyceride transfer protein.[45]

Fatty Acid Distribution and Uptake. From the liver, triglycerides, incorporated primarily into triglyceride-enriched VLDL, are transported to the periphery as a fuel source. Triglycerides cannot cross cell membranes, but require hydrolysis by LPL or HL in tissue capillary beds. Hydrolysis generates

$$\text{Triglyceride} \rightarrow \text{Free fatty acids} + \text{Free glycerol or monoacylglycerol.}$$

About 40 LPL molecules may act on a triglyceride-rich lipoprotein simultaneously. Hydrolysis end products can then be transported into adipocytes and myocytes.[47]

Although free fatty acid uptake into adipocytes may occur by diffusion, it is primarily a transporter-mediated process. Induction of fatty acid transport proteins (FATPs) 1 and 4 occurs during adipocyte differentiation. Insulin induces the translocation of fatty acid translocase/CD36 from the intracellular, perinuclear compartment to the plasma membrane. As a result, the uptake of long-chain fatty acids increases within a matter of minutes.[47]

After triglyceride hydrolysis, the smaller, residual remnants of chylomicrons and VLDL are transported back to the liver, where the specific LDL(B,E) receptor, recognizing the apo E component, enables their uptake into hepatocytes.[2,33]

Fatty Acid Storage versus Oxidation. Further disposition of fatty acids depends on the tissue and the nutritional state.

In adipocytes, the presence or absence of insulin directs fatty acids toward storage versus lipolysis, respectively. In the sated state, fatty acids within adipocytes are re-esterified and stored as triglyceride.[2,33] In the postabsorptive state, fatty acids, released from adipocytes via lipolysis, are transported back to the liver from the periphery.

In skeletal or myocardial muscle in the sated state, free fatty acids may be esterified to enter a triacylglycerol pool for temporary storage. Postabsorptively, fatty acids are beta-oxidized as fuel for energy.[2,33]

INFLAMMATION AND HEPATIC INSULIN RESISTANCE

There is a critical linkage between the development of a proinflammatory state, insulin resistance, intrahepatocellular lipid accumulation, derangement of hepatic lipoprotein metabolism, overproduction of apo B–containing lipoproteins, and the dyslipidemia of metabolic syndrome.

Ectopic Fat Deposition in the Liver with Inflammation. One of the consequences of the metabolic changes initiated by inflammatory pathways is the ectopic deposition of fat in the liver, which engenders hepatic steatosis and the entire spectrum of nonalcoholic fatty liver disease.

Inflammatory cytokine–induced fat accumulation in hepatocytes results from an imbalance in the input, output, and oxidation of fatty acids. **The impairment in hepatocyte oxidative capacity by inflammatory pathways facilitates the accumulation of ectopic fat in the liver.**

There are underlying mitochondrial morphologic and functional alterations with fatty liver disease.[48,49] Specifically, the mitochondrial dysfunction of hepatic steatosis entails the impairment of mitochondrial fatty acid beta oxidation, inhibition of mitochondrial respiration, and damage to mitochondrial DNA.[50]

Proinflammatory cytokines, free fatty acids, and inflammation-related down-regulation of adiponectin and peroxisome proliferator–activated receptor-alpha (PPAR-α) action may contribute to hepatic steatosis.

Proinflammatory Cytokines. Proinflammatory cytokines inhibit hepatic fatty acid oxidative capacity and thus cause free fatty acids in the liver to be re-esterified with reconstitution of triacylglycerols.[22,51]

The proinflammatory cytokines interleukin-12 (IL-12) and IL-18 may mediate hepatosteatosis through impairment of the microcirculation, thereby leading to mitochondrial dysfunction in hepatocytes.[52]

In an in vitro rat hepatocyte model, TNF-α blocked fatty acid oxidation and shunted fatty acids from oxidation to synthesis. The inhibitory effects of TNF-α on fatty acid oxidation were enhanced by either IL-1 or IL-6 and were associated with increased production of malonyl CoA.[53]

Suppressors of Cytokine Signaling. Suppressors of cytokine signaling (SOCS) proteins play an important role in the cytokine-mediated pathogenesis of hepatosteatosis. TNF-α, IL-1, IL-6, and interferon-γ cause sustained induction of SOCS-3, which directly impairs both early and late steps in the metabolic insulin signaling cascade.[54] In mice, overexpression of SOCS-1 and SOCS-3 in the liver causes insulin resistance and an increase in SREBP-1c, the key regulator of fatty acid synthesis in the liver, and thus engenders hepatic steatosis and hypertriglyceridemia. In the process, increased levels of SOCS proteins disinhibit and enhance the expression of SREBP-1c by antagonizing the signal transducer and activator of transcription (STAT-3)-mediated inhibition of SREBP-1c promoter activity.[55]

Free Fatty Acids. The release of free fatty acids from adipose tissue as a result of proinflammatory cytokine-induced lipolysis may contribute to the development of fatty liver as a result of lipotoxicity and lysosomal destabilization. Hepatocyte exposure to free fatty acids engenders the destabilization of lysosomes with the release of cathepsin B, a lysosomal cysteine protease, into the cytosol. Release of cathepsin B into the cytoplasm in humans with fatty liver disease correlates with disease severity. Lysosomal destabilization results in NFκB-dependent TNF-α expression. In a murine model of fatty liver disease, inactivation of cathepsin B protected against the development of hepatic steatosis, liver injury, insulin resistance, and dyslipidemia.[56]

Adiponectin. Inflammation and TNF-α suppress adiponectin production and also antagonize adiponectin action in target tissues, including the liver.

Subjects with fatty liver disease have increased levels of TNF-α and soluble TNF receptor 2, but reduced adiponectin. **Adiponectin deficiency is closely correlated with hepatic lipid accumulation in patients with insulin resistance,** and hypoadiponectinemia is at least partly responsible for the hepatic steatosis and liver injury in insulin resistance.[57,58]

Adiponectin is anti-inflammatory and plays a hepatoprotective role against liver injury, in part because of its antagonism against TNF-α and suppression of TNF-α production in the liver. It also opposes hepatic steatosis directly through

- induction of hepatic fatty acid oxidation and
- inhibition of fatty acid synthesis.

Accordingly, inflammation-related loss of adiponectin forfeits its hepatoprotective effects and facilitates fatty liver disease.[57,58]

The administration of recombinant adiponectin to nonalcoholic, obese ob/ob mice with nonalcoholic fatty liver disease dramatically alleviated hepatomegaly, steatosis, and alanine aminotransferase abnormalities. Specifically, adiponectin increased carnitine palmitoyltransferase I activity and enhanced hepatic fatty acid oxidation, and it decreased the activity of two key enzymes involved in fatty acid synthesis, acetyl CoA carboxylase and fatty acid synthase. Furthermore, adiponectin suppressed the hepatic production and plasma levels of TNF-α.[57,58]

Peroxisome Proliferator–Activated Receptor-α. Inflammatory pathways antagonize the expression of PPAR-α,[59] thus favoring intrahepatocellular lipid accumulation and hepatic steatosis. PPAR-α and the classic peroxisomal fatty acyl CoA oxidase are critically important in energy metabolism. Down-regulation of PPAR-α expression impairs hepatic fatty acid oxidation and contributes to the development of hepatic steatosis.

Fatty Acid Beta Oxidation. Beta oxidation of fatty acids in the liver occurs in both mitochondria and peroxisomes.

- Mitochondria are involved in fatty acid beta oxidation, the tricarboxylic acid cycle, and oxidative phosphorylation. They catalyze beta oxidation of the bulk of nutritionally derived short-, medium-, and long-chain fatty acids. This pathway constitutes the major process by which fatty acids are oxidized to generate energy.[48,49] PPAR-α is the predominant PPAR subtype in the liver, where it controls the transcription of genes of mitochondrial fatty acid metabolizing proteins. PPAR-α activation increases the fatty acid beta oxidation rate in liver mitochondria.[60]
- Peroxisomes are involved in the beta oxidation chain shortening of long-chain and very-long-chain fatty acyl CoAs, long-chain dicarboxylyl CoAs, eicosanoid CoAs, 2-methyl–branched fatty acyl CoAs, and the CoA esters of the bile acid intermediates dihydroxycoprostanoic and trihydroxycoprostanoic acids, with H_2O_2 generated in the process. There are two complete sets of beta oxidation enzymes present in peroxisomes, and each set consists of three distinct enzymes. The peroxisomal beta oxidation system consists of

1. the classic PPAR-α–regulated and inducible set, which participates in the beta

oxidation of straight-chain fatty acyl CoAs via
- fatty acyl CoA oxidase, which initiates the beta oxidation spiral,
- L-bifunctional protein, and
- thiolase.

The genes encoding the classic beta oxidation pathway in the liver are transcriptionally regulated by PPAR-α;

2. the noninducible pathway, which catalyzes the oxidation of 2-methyl–branched fatty acyl CoAs via
   - branched-chain acyl CoA oxidase (pristanoyl CoA oxidase/trihydroxycoprostanoyl CoA oxidase),
   - D-bifunctional protein, and
   - sterol carrier protein (SCP) x.

The cytochrome P-450 CYP4A system also metabolizes long-chain and very-long-chain fatty acids through omega oxidation to dicarboxylic acids, which serve as substrates for peroxisomal beta oxidation.[61,62]

In Otsuka Long-Evans Tokushima fatty rats with hepatic steatosis, reduced expression of PPAR-α and acyl CoA oxidase preceded the definitive development of hepatic steatosis.[63]

Metabolic Manifestations with Fatty Liver Disease. Ectopic accumulation of triacylglycerols, or triglycerides, in hepatocytes is associated with insulin resistance and dyslipidemia.

Insulin Resistance. Inflammation causes insulin resistance. Nonalcoholic fatty liver disease is reproducibly associated with insulin resistance and the metabolic syndrome.[63] Hepatic steatosis is intimately related to markers of insulin resistance, and **insulin resistance plays a major role in the initial accumulation of fat in the liver.** Both the prevalence and the severity of fatty liver disease are related to hyperinsulinemia and hypertriglyceridemia.[48,49] Nonalcoholic fatty liver disease is an early predictor of insulin resistance and metabolic disorders, particularly in the normal-weight population.[64]

Dyslipidemia. Nonalcoholic fatty liver disease is implicated in the dyslipidemia of insulin resistance. With steatosis, after a fat load there is a greater triglyceride-rich lipoprotein response, a larger area under the postprandial curve, and a longer duration of the hypertriglyceridemic peak, coupled with lower plasma HDL2 levels and a higher ratio of triglyceride to apo B in VLDL.[65] Nonalcoholic fatty liver disease is a significant predictor of hypertriglyceridemia and lower levels of HDL in normal-weight and overweight nondiabetic individuals.[64]

Dyslipidemia with Infection and Inflammation. Infection and inflammation induce the acute phase response and insulin-resistant metabolism. Insulin resistance in the liver causes fatty liver changes and multiple alterations in lipid and lipoprotein metabolism supportive of the host response. These acute phase alterations include

- mobilization of lipid from adipose stores in order to fuel the immune response to infection, and
- activation of an innate, nonadaptive host immune response to infection. Triglyceride-rich lipoproteins, such as VLDL and chylomicrons, bind and neutralize lipopolysaccharide and protect the host from the harmful effects of bacteria, viruses, and parasites.

The molecular mechanisms underlying the acute phase changes involve a coordinated decrease in the expression of several nuclear hormone receptors with inflammation, including the PPARs, the liver X receptor, the farnesoid X receptor, and the retinoid X receptor.[66,67]

As a result of infection or inflammation, hypercholesterolemia may at times occur as a result of

- increased hepatic cholesterol synthesis,
- decreased LDL clearance,
- impaired reverse cholesterol transport,
- lower conversion of cholesterol to bile acids, and
- diminished secretion of cholesterol into bile.

During an inflammatory state, plasma triglyceride levels rise as a result of

- adipose tissue lipolysis,
- decreased LPL activity,
- suppression of hepatic and myocellular fatty acid oxidation,
- increased de novo hepatic fatty acid synthesis,

- increased hepatic secretion of triglyceride-rich lipoproteins,
- lower apo E content in VLDL, and
- decreased VLDL clearance.[67]

Additionally, with inflammation, marked alterations in proteins important for HDL metabolism render HDL a proinflammatory entity that causes impaired reverse cholesterol transport and increased cholesterol delivery to immune cells. Oxidation of LDL and VLDL increases. Lipoproteins become enriched in ceramide, glucosylceramide, and sphingomyelin, which enhances their uptake by macrophages.[67]

As a result, **a lipid disturbance characterized by**

- **hypertriglyceridemia,**
- **high levels of VLDL,**
- **low plasma HDL, and**
- **small, dense LDL particles**

accompanies the insulin-resistant conditions occurring during infections and inflammatory processes.[67]

ATHEROGENIC DYSLIPIDEMIA IN INSULIN RESISTANCE

If protracted, the cytokine-induced dyslipidemia, implemented via changes in the structure and function of lipoproteins, becomes proatherogenic and constitutes a major risk factor for cardiovascular disease.[67]

The metabolic syndrome is a proinflammatory state. Atherogenic dyslipidemia is thus a hallmark of the metabolic syndrome. It derives from a resistance to insulin signaling in the liver that engenders dysregulation of free fatty acid and lipoprotein metabolism. Akin to the dyslipidemia of inflammation, it is characterized by a lipid disturbance, also termed the "lipid triad":

1. elevated triglyceride levels with increased VLDL secretion from the liver,
2. low HDL and apo A-I levels, and
3. frequently normal levels of plasma LDL with particles that are smaller, denser, and more atherogenic than normal (Table 10-4).

Table 10-4. Dyslipidemia of the Metabolic Syndrome

LIPID	METABOLIC SYNDROME
Triglyceride	Increased
High-density lipoprotein	Decreased
Apolipoprotein A-I	Decreased
Low-density lipoprotein	Neutral
Small, dense LDL	Increased
Apolipoprotein B	Increased

The lipid disturbance is very highly atherogenic and constitutes a major risk for premature cardiovascular disease.[68] Each component is a powerful, independent CHD risk factor in its own right. The insulin resistance dyslipidemia accounts for a significant part of the increased CHD risk in individuals with the metabolic syndrome.[2,22]

Hypertriglyceridemia with Insulin Resistance. Insulin-resistant states induce elevated levels of triglyceride-rich lipoproteins and remnant particles with exaggerated and prolonged postprandial hypertriglyceridemia.[2,22] Although there are other causes, **80% to 85% of individuals with hypertriglyceridemia have the metabolic syndrome** (Table 10-5).[1]

Impaired insulin signaling in the liver is the pathophysiologic basis for hypertriglyceridemia in atherogenic dyslipidemia (Table 10-6). Additionally, insulin resistance in adipose tissue and impaired oxidative capacity in metabolically active organs such as skeletal and cardiac muscle and the liver are factors.

Insulin-resistant states induce elevated levels of VLDL because of inadequate clearance and overproduction of the lipoprotein. With insulin resistance, the insulin-induced LPL activity in adipose tissue and skeletal muscle is reduced, thereby decreasing peripheral VLDL degradation.[2,22] Underlying the insulin-resistant overproduction of triglyceride-rich lipoproteins are complex interactions between

- the enhanced flux of free fatty acids from peripheral tissues to the liver arising from impaired insulin suppression of adipose lipolysis and from compromised fatty acid oxidative capacity in metabolically active tissues,
- attenuated insulin signaling in the liver and the intestine, and
- chronic up-regulation of de novo lipogenesis by hyperinsulinemia.[69]

Table 10-5. Secondary Causes of Hypertriglyceridemia with Underlying Insulin Resistance

Lifestyle and Habitus
Obesity
Diet with a high glycemic index
Alcohol consumption
Diseases
Metabolic syndrome
Type 2 diabetes mellitus
Cushing's syndrome
Renal failure
Chronic systemic inflammation
Chronic infections
Sepsis
Pharmacologic Agents
β-Blockers
Thiazides
Oral contraceptives
Hormone replacement therapy
Human immunodeficiency virus protease inhibitors
Immunosuppressants

Adapted from Rosas S, Szapary P, Pader DJ. Management of selected lipid abnormalities: hypertriglyceridemia, isolated low HDL-cholesterol, lipoprotein(a), and lipid abnormalities in renal diseases and following solid organ transplantation. Cardiol Clin 2003;21:377-392.

Adipose Tissue. The dyslipidemia is partly caused by resistance to insulin signaling in the adipose lipid depots. With loss of adipose sensitivity to insulin action, insulin-resistant adipocytes are unable to store lipid, which allows lipolysis of triglycerides to proceed. Defective storage and enhanced mobilization of triglycerides from adipose tissue release elevated levels of fatty acids into the bloodstream.[70]

The increased flux of free fatty acids into nonadipose tissues such as the liver contributes to the ectopic storage of fat in the liver, which as in the case of intramyocellular lipid accumulation, further compromises hepatocellular sensitivity to insulin signaling.[70]

Table 10-6. Adult Treatment Panel III Classification of Serum Triglycerides

Normal triglycerides	<150 mg/dL
Borderline high	150-199 mg/dL
High	200-499 mg/dL
Very high	>500 mg/dL

Adapted from http://www.guidelines.gov/VIEWS/summary.asp?guidelines=00219.

Visceral/Omental Adipose Tissue. In particular, visceral/omental fat is the metabolically most active adipose depot with the highest turnover of free fatty acids. In contrast to subcutaneous fat, **visceral fat is less sensitive to insulin suppression of lipolysis and is, in general, metabolically very susceptible to lipid mobilization.**[71] Furthermore, visceral adipose tissue is a prolific producer of proinflammatory cytokines and is exquisitely sensitive to their autocrine/paracrine/endocrine antiadipogenic and prolipolytic effects, thus contributing to the increased flux of fatty acids toward the liver.

Portal Vein Free Fatty Acid Fluxes. The venous effluent from visceral/omental fat drains into the portal vein, with visceral free fatty acids and other substances delivered directly and exclusively to the liver. **The anatomic proximity of visceral fat to the liver as part of the portal circulation renders the liver particularly vulnerable to proinflammatory and metabolic mediators released from the visceral fat depot.**

Very-Low-Density Lipoprotein Secretion with Insulin Resistance. Hypertriglyceridemia occurs largely as a result of the overproduction of triglyceride-rich, apo B–containing lipoproteins with insulin resistance. Specifically, **hepatic overproduction of VLDL is a crucial, underlying factor in the development of hypertriglyceridemia and metabolic dyslipidemia.** In the fructose-fed hamster model of insulin resistance, there is oversecretion of both hepatically derived apo B-100–containing VLDL and intestinal apo B-48–containing triglyceride-rich lipoproteins.[69]

Fatty Liver and Increased Very-Low-Density Lipoprotein Secretion. With insulin resistance, the mechanisms that suppress the release of VLDL particles fail. Because proinflammatory insulin resistance chronically curtails fatty acid oxidation, fatty acids taken up by the liver are shunted to esterification. Upon increased hepatic triacylglycerol production, the lipid is stored in cytosolic triacylglycerol pools, and a smaller portion is secreted in the form of VLDL. **Increasing cytosolic lipid pool size, or hepatic steatosis, correlates with higher VLDL secretion.**[22,51] As a result, in insulin-resistant individuals with fatty liver conditions, basal VLDL secretion is persistently increased when compared with insulin-sensitive subjects. Under these conditions, approximately 30% of the total VLDL triglycerides coming out of the liver are derived from cytoplasmic triglyceride stores.[46]

Up-regulated Apo B Secretion. With up-regulated de novo lipogenesis in insulin resistance, **hepatic synthesis and secretion of apo B-100 are increased and its degradation reduced.**[22,45,51] Insensitivity to insulin contributes to the enhanced VLDL particle assembly and causes overexpression of the microsomal triglyceride transfer protein to promote the secretion of triglyceride-rich VLDL particles.[45]

In hepatocytes of the fructose-fed hamster model of insulin resistance, hepatic insulin resistance was manifested by significantly reduced tyrosine phosphorylation of the insulin receptor and the insulin receptor substrates 1 and 2. Phosphatidylinositol 3-kinase activity, as well as insulin-stimulated Akt-Ser473 and Akt-Thr308 phosphorylation, was consequently reduced. Interestingly, there was a corresponding significant increase in the expression and activity of protein tyrosine phosphatase 1B, which coincided with marked suppression of ER-60, a cysteine protease that plays a role in the intracellular degradation of apo B. There was an ensuing increase in the synthesis and secretion of apo B.[45]

Hepatic Glucocorticoid Effects. Glucocorticoid effects on the liver play a role in hepatic insulin resistance during the activation of stress pathways, as well as in the setting of visceral-omental adiposity with increased expression of the glucocorticoid regenerating enzyme 11β-hydroxysteroid dehydrogenase type 1 (11β-HSD-1). Enhanced hepatic glucocorticoid effects engender fatty liver changes, dyslipidemia with increased hepatic lipid synthesis/flux, and impaired hepatic lipid clearance.[72]

Low High-Density Lipoprotein with Insulin Resistance. HDL levels are inversely correlated with plasma triglyceride in a curvilinear relationship.[1] Low levels of HDL are secondary manifestations emanating from the triglyceride excess (see Table 10-3).[2,22] The hypertriglyceridemia of insulin resistance, together with the decreased LPL and increased CETP and HL activities in insulin-resistant states,

- reduces HDL cholesterol via a triglyceride-cholesterol exchange transfer of lipids,
- impairs HDL function, and
- lowers HDL levels as a result of greater apo A-I plasma clearance.[22]

Bimolecular Transfer between Very-Low-Density Lipoprotein and High-Density Lipoprotein via CETP. There is an inverse relationship between VLDL triglyceride and HDL cholesterol. With diminished peripheral lipolysis of triglyceride-rich lipoproteins by LPL, there is less transfer of their apolipoproteins and phospholipids to HDL, which impairs its function. Additionally, in the circulation, CETP is associated with the HDL lipoprotein. As increased numbers of VLDL interact with HDL lipoproteins, CETP exchanges HDL cholesteryl esters for VLDL triglycerides. This process lowers HDL cholesterol with the transfer of cholesterol to VLDL and raises HDL triglyceride (Fig. 10-7).

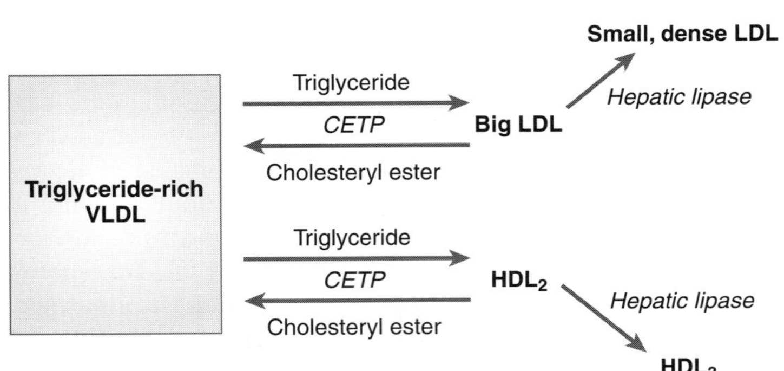

Figure 10–7. Impact of cholesteryl ester transfer protein (CETP) and hepatic lipase on lipoproteins. HDL, high-density lipoprotein; LDL, low-density lipoprotein; VLDL, very-low-density lipoprotein. *(Adapted from Brunzell JD, Hokanson JE. Dyslipidemia of central obesity and insulin resistance. Diabetes Care 1999 (Suppl 3): c10-c13.)*

Triglyceride-enriched HDL is less effective in removing cholesterol from peripheral cells.[22]

Hepatic Lipase and High-Density Lipoprotein Dissolution. The triglyceride-enriched HDL lipoproteins are subject to further lipolysis, particularly by the increased activity of HL in insulin resistance. Lipolysis causes further compositional and structural alterations of the HDL complex as HDL diminishes in size with progressive loss of triglyceride. As a result, the association of apo A-I with the complex is compromised, which eventually causes the dissociation of apo A-I and dissolution of the erstwhile HDL complex.

The dissociated apo A-I is readily cleared from the circulation.[10] Because apo A-I is the essential lipid-carrying entity for HDL, its loss impinges on the number of available HDL complexes. **With insulin-resistant states, there is, in particular, a decrease in the larger HDL2 as compared with HDL3** (see Fig. 10-7).[22]

Low-Density Lipoprotein Changes with Insulin Resistance. Individuals with the highest resistance to insulin have the pattern B LDL phenotype, characterized by small, dense LDL, whereas pattern A individuals are most insulin sensitive.[73] **Elevated fasting triglyceride and small, dense LDL concentrations are positively correlated.**[74] Increased small, dense LDL is a secondary manifestation of triglyceride excess. In insulin-resistant states, hypertriglyceridemia, as well as the decreased LPL and increased CETP and HL actions,

- reduces LDL cholesterol via a triglyceride-cholesterol exchange and
- renders the LDL complex small and dense (see Fig. 10-7).[22]

Bimolecular Transfer between Very-Low-Density Lipoprotein and Low-Density Lipoprotein via CETP. Although LDL should constitute the final product of VLDL metabolism, the increased plasma levels of VLDL in insulin resistance lead to the exchange of LDL cholesteryl ester for VLDL triglyceride via the same CETP-mediated bimolecular transfer that occurs between VLDL and HDL. This transfer renders LDL cholesterol poor and triglyceride rich.

Like HDL, the triglyceride-enriched LDL is subject to lipolysis by LPL or HL. As lipolysis breaks down the triglycerides, the LDL core is compromised and LDL diminishes in size. The resultant LDL particle is small and dense.[22]

Very-Low-Density Lipoprotein Changes with Insulin Resistance and Remnant Lipoproteins. The transfer of cholesteryl esters from both HDL and LDL onto VLDL renders VLDL enriched in cholesteryl ester and significantly more atherogenic. These altered VLDL complexes and their remnant derivatives readily permeate the vessel wall to deposit cholesterol and enhance atherogenesis.[22] **Increased levels of remnant lipoproteins are a significant and independent risk factor for CHD and predict future coronary events.**[75]

Lipid Deposition in the Arterial Wall. Remnant lipoproteins have been found within the arterial wall, and lipoprotein core lipids such as cholesteryl and retinyl esters are deposited in heart, muscle, and adipose tissue.[2]

Lipoprotein penetration into the vascular wall is facilitated through the increased permeability of the endothelial vascular barrier. Although lipoproteins are normally too large to cross the capillary endothelium, several factors, including proinflammatory molecules such as P-selectin and fatty acids, enhance endothelial permeability. The pool of LPL located on the macrophage surface may also be playing a role.[2]

Additionally, VLDL, via protein kinase C (PKC)-mediated activation of MAPK, may increase plasminogen activator inhibitor-1 (PAI-1) biosynthesis in endothelial cells by inducing transcription of the PAI-1 gene promoter and stabilizing the mRNA transcript for PAI-1.[2,22]

THE TRIGLYCERIDE LIPASE FAMILY

Lipases hydrolyze lipids. They play an important role in lipid homeostasis by modulating lipoprotein metabolism, as well as tissue uptake and disposal of lipids. Insulin resistance and other pathologic states have an effect on lipase action thus contributing to the dysregulation of lipid metabolism.

Lipoprotein Lipase. LPL plays a central role in energy homeostasis and triglyceride-rich lipoprotein catabolism. LPL is the primary enzyme that hydrolyzes triglycerides in chylomicrons and VLDLs in adipose tissue and muscle.[11]

Synthesis of Lipoprotein Lipase. LPL has an unusual intercellular itinerary. It is synthesized by parenchymal cells in

- myocardium,
- skeletal muscle,
- adipose tissue,
- lactating mammary glands,
- macrophages,
- adrenals,
- ovaries,
- testes,
- spleen,
- lungs,
- kidneys,
- thoracic aorta, and
- certain neuronal cells.[2]

To attain physiologic activity, after intraparenchymal synthesis LPL is thought to transfer to the vascular endothelial cells near its tissue of origin, such as muscle or adipose tissue. It then transcytoses to the luminal surface. LPL is bound to the luminal aspect of the endothelial cell plasmalemma by highly charged interactions with membrane-bound chains of heparan sulfate proteoglycans. Configured as a homodimer, LPL is enzymatically active on the surface of capillary endothelial cells[76] and mediates lipolysis mainly within the vascular lumen.[77] LPL requires apo C-II as its specific cofactor.[2]

Function of Lipoprotein Lipase. LPL has a central role in overall lipid metabolism and lipid transport. It is a key enzyme in regulating the disposal of lipid fuel in the body. It catalyzes the key step in the removal of lipids from the circulation in order to generate free fatty acids for conversion to storage triacylglycerol in adipocytes or for oxidative energy generation in skeletal and cardiac myocytes.[11]

Tissue Partitioning of Free Fatty Acids. LPL has an important role in the disposition of dietary fatty acids. Acting as a metabolic gatekeeper, LPL catalyzes triglyceride hydrolysis, preferentially on chylomicrons but also on other circulating, triglyceride-rich lipoproteins such as VLDL. Luminal triglyceride hydrolysis generates

- free fatty acids,
- monoglycerides, and
- remnant lipoproteins.

Nonesterified fatty acids and 2-monoacylglycerols are then available for transport into the subjacent tissue for oxidation or storage.[78]

The level of LPL expression in any tissue is a rate-limiting process for the uptake of triglyceride-derived fatty acids. LPL activity is regulated in a tissue-specific manner according to the tissue needs for fatty acids.[33]

Feeding and Fasting. Because LPL plays a role in the partitioning of dietary free fatty acids and because fatty acid uptake correlates with tissue LPL activity, feeding and fasting affect LPL function:

- In white fat, LPL is active in the sated state in order to facilitate fatty acid uptake into adipose tissue for fatty acid re-esterification and deposition as triacylglycerol. During a fast, white adipose tissue LPL is suppressed.[33] In adipose tissue, LPL constitutes only one of a series of metabolic steps involving insulin, acylation-stimulating protein, leptin, and other factors in the disposition of fatty acids.[11]
- In myocardial and skeletal muscle, LPL is suppressed in the sated state. It is enhanced in a fast to allow free fatty acid uptake for use as oxidative fuel during starvation.[33]

Lipoprotein Modulation. LPL synthesized by adipose tissue and skeletal muscle is antiatherogenic.[2]

- LDL: Because non–macrophage-expressed LPL catabolizes circulating, triglyceride-rich lipoproteins, it directly enhances the formation of less atherogenic, cholesterol-rich LDL.
- HDL: Adipose tissue and muscle LPL increases HDL indirectly via catabolism of triglyceride-rich lipoproteins, which also causes the transfer of redundant phospholipids and apolipoproteins from VLDL to HDL and lowers the occurrence of bimolecular triglyceride–cholesteryl ester exchange.[11,78]

Thus, postheparin plasma levels of LPL are

- correlated with HDL levels and
- inversely correlated with the triglyceride level, body mass index, and intra-abdominal visceral fat.

There is no correlation of LPL levels with subcutaneous fat.[78]

Macrophage Lipoprotein Lipase. In contrast to LPL present on endothelial cells, the LPL enzyme expressed by macrophages is proatherogenic. In that location, LPL can assume a noncatalytic, bridging function that contributes to atherogenesis:

- LPL can act as a monocyte adhesion protein and bridge heparan sulfate proteoglycans on the monocyte surface to endothelial cells.
- By binding simultaneously to lipoproteins and cell surface receptors or proteoglycans, this LPL can lead to the accumulation and cellular uptake of lipoproteins into macrophages.
- When attached to the surface of vascular smooth muscle cells, enzymatically activated LPL, with activated PKC, can induce smooth muscle cell proliferation.[2]

Macrophage LPL is also proinflammatory and contributes to vascular inflammation and atherogenesis:

- It induces expression of the TNF-α gene.
- In conjunction with interferon-γ, LPL stimulates macrophage inducible NOS expression and activates endothelial nicotinamide adenine dinucleotide phosphate (NADH/NADPH) oxidase.[2]

Hormonal and Cytokine Impact on Lipoprotein Lipase Activity. LPL expression and activity are modulated not only by nutritional status but also by hormonal activity and inflammation.

Because LPL participates in directing triglyceride deposition within adipocytes, it has an impact on the regional accumulation of adipose tissue. For example, during lactation there is increased LPL activity in the mammary glands that causes enlargement of mammary tissues (Table 10-7). Regional variations in LPL density account for some of the gender-related differences in fat distribution.[11] Testosterone, via the androgenic receptor and human growth hormone, inhibits LPL and stimulates lipolysis. Estrogen's net effect matches that of testosterone.[2]

Table 10-7. Lipoprotein Lipase Activities in Different Tissues According to Nutritional and Physiologic State

TISSUE	LPL UNITS
Mammary gland	
Before pregnancy	1
End of pregnancy	7
Lactation	50
Adipose tissue	
Fed	3.6
Starved	0.6
Heart	
Fed	3.5
Starved	7.2
Skeletal muscle	
Untrained	0.9
Trained	1.4

Modified from Fielding B, Frayn KN. Lipoprotein lipase and the disposition of dietary fatty acids. Br J Nutr 1998;80:495-502.

Other hormones and cytokines modulate LPL activity and fatty acid uptake for lipid deposition or oxidative metabolism as follows:

- Cortisol, via the glucocorticoid receptor, increases LPL expression and facilitates lipid accumulation in adipose tissue.
- LPL is insulin sensitive. Expression of LPL in myocytes and adipocytes and its translocation to the luminal surface of endothelial cells are both insulin-related processes.
- Human growth hormone abolishes LPL activity by turning metabolism into a lipid-mobilizing state.
- Inflammatory cytokines, such as TNF-α, IL-1, IL-6, and interferon-γ, all decrease the expression of LPL mRNA and reduce LPL activity.
- Macrophage LPL is induced by elevated levels of glucose, free fatty acids, and homocysteine.[2,12]

Lipoprotein Lipase Dysfunction. Abnormalities in LPL function occur in numerous clinical situations.

Overexpression of Lipoprotein Lipase. In obesity, adipose tissue LPL is elevated. It may be further increased after efforts to induce weight loss in an attempt to replenish lipid stores during refeeding.[76]

Underexpression of Lipoprotein Lipase. Expression of LPL is an insulin-sensitive process that is suppressed with insulin resistance.[22] Low LPL activity is thus found in

- central visceral-omental obesity, the degree of visceral adiposity correlating inversely with postheparin plasma LPL levels,
- inflammation,
- insulin resistance,
- chylomicronemia,
- dyslipidemia,
- atherosclerosis,
- DM,
- aging,
- cachexia, and
- Alzheimer's disease.

In all these conditions, low LPL contributes to postprandial hypertriglyceridemia as a result of the delayed clearance of triglyceride-rich lipoproteins by LPL. Because hypertriglyceridemia engenders low HDL levels, defective LPL function is thus partly implicated in the central lipoprotein abnormalities of inflammation and insulin resistance.[2,79,80]

Other Variations in Regional Lipoprotein Lipase Expression. Selected differences in LPL expression have the following implications:

- absent LPL in macrophages yields a very low propensity to atherogenesis;
- low LPL in adipose tissue and high LPL in muscle imparts resistance to obesity; and
- extremely high LPL in muscle will produce increased ectopic, intramyocellular triglyceride, thereby engendering insulin resistance.[47]

Hepatic Lipase. HL is a lipolytic enzyme synthesized by hepatocytes. It plays a role in lipoprotein metabolism by hydrolyzing the triglycerides and phospholipids of remnant lipoproteins and HDL in the liver. HL is located on the surface of

- hepatocytes,
- sinusoid endothelial cells of hepatic sinusoid capillaries,
- macrophages, and
- the endothelium within the adrenals, the thyroid gland, and the gonads.[12]

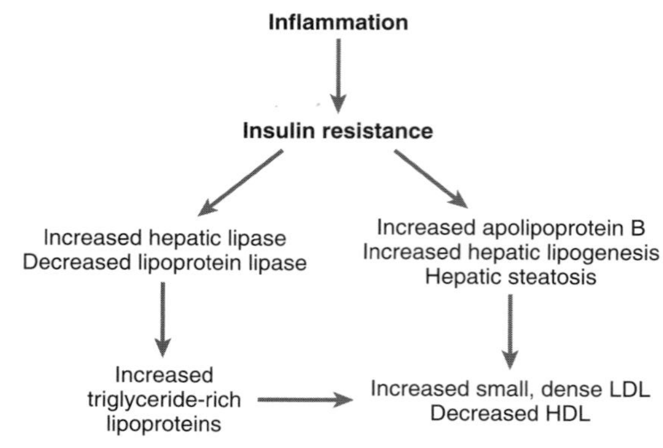

Figure 10–8.
Selected factors contributing to the dyslipidemia of the metabolic syndrome. HDL, high-density lipoprotein; LDL, low-density lipoprotein. *(Adapted from Ayyobi AF, Brunzell JD. Lipoprotein distribution in the metabolic syndrome, type 2 diabetes mellitus, and familial combined hyperlipidemia. Am J Cardiol 2003;92(4A):27J-33J.)*

HL shares a number of functional domains with LPL. Expression of HL is increased in the presence of increased visceral fat and insulin resistance (Fig. 10-8).[12,81]

Hepatic Lipase Impact on High-Density Lipoprotein and Other Lipoproteins. HL has a role in HDL metabolism. The level of HDL and its function in reverse cholesterol transport are at least partly regulated by the expression of HL. HL not only hydrolyzes triglycerides and phospholipids in the larger, less dense HDL2 but also stimulates the uptake of HDL cholesteryl esters by hepatocytes. HL can thus decrease HDL2 levels by remodeling the lipoprotein to the smaller HDL3. High plasma HL activity appears to correlate with reduced levels of HDL.[82]

HL also plays a key role in remnant lipoprotein catabolism, as well as in the remodeling of LDL particles (see Fig. 10-7). The antiatherogenic or proatherogenic role of HL is modulated by the presence of other lipid disturbances, as well as by genetic regulation of other enzymes involved in lipoprotein metabolism.[81]

Endothelial Lipase. EL is synthesized in endothelial cells and has 41% to 44% homology with LPL and HL. EL plays a role in the lipid metabolism of the vessel wall, and EL expression appears to be an important modulator of HDL metabolism. Relative to LPL and HL, EL has greater phospholipase than triglyceride lipase activity.[12,78,83]

In nonatherosclerotic coronary arteries, EL is located on vascular endothelial cells and medial smooth muscle cells and functions at these sites. In addition, with atheromatous disease, EL is expressed on infiltrating macrophage cells within atherosclerotic plaque and in the neovasculature within the atheromata of atherosclerotic coronary arteries.[78,83]

EL is not secreted by endothelial cells under basal conditions. The activity of EL is highly regulated by physical forces and is up-regulated by inflammatory cytokines such as IL-1β and TNF-α, which seem to increase the rate of transcription of the EL gene.[12]

Overexpression of EL leads to lowering of HDL, whereas a deficiency in EL causes a marked increase in HDL. Akin to the effects of macrophage LPL, the presence of EL in the vascular wall has been implicated in the progression of atherosclerosis through facilitation of lipoprotein uptake into the vascular wall by its noncatalytic bridging function between lipoprotein particles and matrix proteoglycans.[78,83]

Hormone-Sensitive Lipase. Hormone-sensitive lipase (HSL) is the enzyme responsible for intracellular triacylglycerol hydrolysis within adipocytes.

- Postprandially, whereas insulin activates LPL to facilitate fatty acid uptake, HSL, and thus lipolysis, are suppressed by insulin, with the free fatty acids taken up by adipocytes targeted toward re-esterification and storage as triacylglycerol.
- In the fasting state, with low insulin levels, HSL is most active, and free fatty acids are released into the plasma.[84]

Insulin suppression of HSL is lost with insulin-resistant states, thus facilitating adipose tissue lipolysis and an increased efflux of free fatty acids.

CONCLUSION

Acute inflammatory states, such as sepsis, are associated with hypertriglyceridemia and profoundly reduced HDL levels. Chronic inflammatory states, such as rheumatoid arthritis and systemic lupus erythematosus, exhibit similar disturbances in the lipid profile. During inflammatory processes, energy demands are increased. Inflammatory pathways consequently alter lipid homeostasis by engendering insulin resistance, switching from anabolic to catabolic metabolism, as a means for generating fatty acids as fuel sources for participating inflammatory cells.

The catabolic state of insulin resistance, spawned by a systemically aroused inflammatory response, enhances free fatty acid flux via a coordinated, multifaceted response:

- Antilipogenic pathways prevent fatty acid uptake in adipose tissue.
- Lipolysis in adipose tissue further increases plasma free fatty acid efflux.
- Uptake and oxidative metabolism of fatty acids in the musculature are thwarted.
- Oxidative metabolism in the liver is down-regulated, and the liver produces triglyceride for export into the systemic circulation.
- Down-regulation of LPL delays VLDL processing and also directs lipoprotein-derived fatty acids away from the musculature and adipose tissue.

In the presence of large free fatty acid fluxes, hepatic insulin resistance generates hepatic steatosis and dyslipidemia. The latter appears to participate in the innate, nonadaptive immune response and delivers a generous fatty acid fuel supply for immune organs.

In this context, the vasculature becomes an innocent bystander and default recipient of the undifferentiated immune assault. Inflammation and inflammatory cytokines impair endothelial function concurrent with insulin resistance. Suppression of eNOS signaling and endothelial dysfunction promote vascular inflammation and the up-regulation of EL. EL and macrophage LPL and expression of the vascular RAAS and the LOX-1 receptor all allow the vascular wall to evolve into a recipient of lipoprotein lipids, a process further facilitated by increased endothelial permeability and inflammatory cell chemotaxis.

Inflammatory pathways, unless curtailed, amplify. The atherosclerotic process may eventually evolve into a chronic inflammatory condition in its own right. As such, it will perpetuate and further magnify inflammatory, insulin-resistant pathways and the maladaptive, highly atherogenic dyslipidemia, ultimately engendering atherothrombosis and acute ischemic syndromes. In this respect, the severity of the dyslipidemia, though participating in the vascular disease process, is reflective and essentially a symptom of the underlying inflammatory activation.

Lifestyle modifications, such as exercise, stress relaxation, weight control, and nutritional choices that ameliorate or eliminate stress and inflammatory pathways, may be of benefit in curtailing the inflammatory stimulus for insulin-resistant dyslipidemia. Beyond therapeutic lifestyle changes, lipid-modulatory therapy is nearly always required. Although the dyslipidemia is not always characterized by high levels of LDL, statin therapy is highly desirable in view of the beneficial anti-inflammatory, pleiotropic effects of HMG-CoA reductase inhibitors. Measures that enhance the level or the functionality of HDL (or both) may be of significant benefit. Additionally, PPAR-α and PPAR-γ ligands would be expected to have a very favorable impact on the underlying causes of this lipid disturbance.

GLOSSARY

ABCA-1	adenosine triphosphate–binding cassette transporter A-1
ADMA	asymmetric dimethylarginine
apo	apolipoprotein
CETP	cholesterol ester transfer protein
CHD	coronary heart disease
CoA	coenzyme A
CRP	C-reactive protein
DM	diabetes mellitus
EL	endothelial lipase
eNOS	endothelial nitric oxide synthase
ERK	extracellular signal–regulated protein kinase
FATP	fatty acid transport protein
HDL	high-density lipoprotein
HL	hepatic lipase
HMG-CoA	3-hydroxy-3-methylglutaryl–CoA
11β-HSD-1	11β-hydroxysteroid dehydrogenase type 1
HSL	hormone-sensitive lipase
ICAM	intercellular adhesion molecule
IDL	intermediate-density lipoprotein
IL	interleukin
LCAT	lecithin-cholesterol acyltransferase
LDL	low-density lipoprotein
LOX-1	lectin-like oxidized low-density lipoprotein receptor-1
LPL	lipoprotein lipase
Lp(a)	lipoprotein(a)
MAPK	mitogen-activated protein kinase
MCP	monocyte chemoattractant protein
NADH/NADPH	nicotinamide adenine dinucleotide phosphate oxidase
NFκB	nuclear factor kappaB
NO	nitric oxide
PAF-AH	platelet-activating factor acetylhydrolase
PAI-1	plasminogen activator inhibitor-1
PKC	protein kinase C
PON	paraoxonase
PPAR	peroxisome proliferator–activated receptor
RAAS	renin-angiotensin-aldosterone system
SCP	sterol carrier protein
SOCS	suppressor of cytokine signaling
SR-B1	scavenger receptor class B type 1
SREBP	sterol regulatory element binding protein
STAT	signal transducer and activator of transcription
TNF	tumor necrosis factor
tPA	tissue plasminogen activator
VCAM	vascular cell adhesion molecule
VLDL	very-low-density lipoprotein

REFERENCES

1. Genest J. Genetics and prevention: A new look at high-density lipoprotein cholesterol. Cardiol Rev 2002;10:61-71
2. Mead JR, Irvine SA, Ramji DP. Lipoprotein lipase: structure, function, regulation, and role in disease. J Mol Med 2002;80:753-769
3. Kwiterovich PO Jr. Lipoprotein heterogeneity: diagnostic and therapeutic implications. Am J Cardiol 2002;90(8A): 1i-10i
4. Calabresi L, Gomaraschi M, Franceschini G. Endothelial protection by high-density lipoproteins: from bench to bedside. Arterioscler Thromb Vasc Biol 2003;23:1724-1731
5. Nofer J-R, Kehrel B, Fobker M, et al. HDL and arteriosclerosis: beyond reverse cholesterol transport. Atherosclerosis 2002;161:1-16
6. Bortnick AE, Rothblat GH, Stoudt G, et al. The correlation of ATP-binding cassette I mRNA levels with cholesterol

efflux from various cell lines. J Biol Chem 2000;275: 28634-28640
7. Asztalos BF, Schaefer EJ. High-density lipoprotein subpopulations in pathologic conditions. Am J Cardiol 2003;91(suppl):12E-17E
8. Brewer HB, Santamarina-Fojo S. Clinical significance of high-density lipoproteins and the development of atherosclerosis: focus on the role of the adenosine triphosphate-binding cassette protein A1 transporter. Am J Cardiol 2003;92(4B):10K-16K
9. Trigatti B, Rigotti A, Krieger M. The role of the high-density lipoprotein receptor SR-BI in cholesterol metabolism. Curr Opin Lipidol 2000;11:123-131
10. Rader DJ. Regulation of reverse cholesterol transport and clinical implications. Am J Cardiol 2003;92(4A): 42J-49J
11. Ukkola O, Garenc C, Perusse L, et al. Genetic variation at the lipoprotein lipase locus and plasma lipoprotein and insulin levels in the Quebec family study. Atherosclerosis 2002;158:199-206
12. Jin W, Sun G-S, Marchadier D, et al. Endothelial cells secrete triglyceride lipase and phospholipase activities in response to cytokines as a result of endothelial lipase. Circ Res 2003;92:644-650
13. Hovingh GK, Brownlie A, Bisoendial RJ, et al. HDL and coronary artery disease. A novel apoA-I mutation (L178P) leads to endothelial dysfunction, increased arterial wall thickness, and premature coronary artery disease. J Am Coll Cardiol 2004;44:1429-1435
14. Kaul S, Coin B, Hedayiti A, et al. Rapid reversal of endothelial dysfunction in hypercholesterolemic apolipoprotein E–null mice by recombinant apolipoprotein A-I_{Milano}–phospholipid complex. Circulation 2004; 44:1311-1319
15. Libby P. Managing the risk of atherosclerosis: the role of high-density lipoprotein. Am J Cardiol 2001;88(12A): 3N-8N
16. Lusis AJ, Fogelman AM, Fonarow GC. Genetic basis of atherosclerosis: Part I. New genes and pathways. Circulation 2004;110:1868-1873
17. Shaul PW. Endothelial nitric oxide synthase, caveolae and the development of atherosclerosis. J Physiol 2003; 547:21-33
18. Li XA, Titlow WB, Jackson BA, et al. High density lipoprotein binding to scavenger receptor, class B, type I activates endothelial nitric-oxide synthase in a ceramide-dependent manner. J Biol Chem 2002;277: 11058-11063
19. Wadham C, Albanese N, Roberts J, et al. High-density lipoproteins neutralize C-reactive protein proinflammatory activity. Circulation 2004;109:2116-2122
20. Yuhanna IS, Zhu Y, Cox BE, et al. High-density lipoprotein binding to scavenger receptor-BI activates endothelial nitric oxide synthase. Nat Med 2001;7: 853-857
21. Mineo C, Yuhanna IS, Quon MJ, Shaul PW. High density lipoprotein–induced endothelial nitric-oxide synthase activation is mediated by Akt and MAP kinases. J Biol Chem 2003;278:9142-9149
22. Ruotolo G, Howard BV. Dyslipidemia of the metabolic syndrome. Curr Cardiol Rep 2002;4:494-500
23. Bisoendial RJ, Hovingh GK, Levels JHM, et al. Restoration of endothelial function by increasing high-density lipoprotein in subjects with isolated low high-density lipoprotein. Circulation 2003;107:2944-2948
24. Gordon DJ, Rifkind BM. High-density lipoprotein: the clinical implications of recent studies. N Engl J Med 1989;321:1311-1316
25. Expert Panel on Detection, Evaluation, and Treatment of High Blood Cholesterol in Adults. Executive Summary of the Third Report of the National Cholesterol Education Program (NCEP) Expert Panel on Detection, and Treatment of High Blood Cholesterol in Adults (Adult Treatment Panel III). JAMA 2001;285:2486-2497
26. Sprecher DL, Watkins TR, Behar S, et al. Importance of high-density lipoprotein cholesterol and triglyceride levels in coronary heart disease. Am J Cardiol 2003;91: 575-580
27. Gordon DJ, Probstfield JL, Garrison RJ, et al. High-density lipoprotein cholesterol and cardiovascular disease: four prospective American studies. Circulation 1989;79:8-15
28. Rubens HB, Robins SJ, Collins D, et al. The Veterans Affairs High-Density Lipoprotein Cholesterol Intervention Trial Study Group. Gemfibrozil for the secondary prevention of coronary heart disease in men with low levels of high-density lipoprotein cholesterol. N Engl J Med 1999;341:410-418
29. Spieker LE, Sudano I, Huerlimann D, et al. High-density lipoprotein restores endothelial function in hypercholesterolemic men. Circulation 2002;105: 1399-1402
30. Li X, Chyu K-Y, Faria Neto JR, et al. Differential effects of apolipoprotein A-I–mimetic peptide on evolving and established atherosclerosis in apolipoprotein E–null mice. Circulation 2004;110:1701-1705
31. Nissen SE, Tsunoda T, Tuzcu EM, et al. Effect of recombinant Apo A-I Milano on coronary atherosclerosis in patients with acute coronary syndromes: a randomized controlled trial. JAMA 2003;290:2292-2300
32. Ariyo AA, Thach C, Tracy R. Lp(a) lipoprotein, vascular disease, and mortality in the elderly. N Engl J Med 2003;349:2109-2115
33. Fielding B, Frayn KN. Lipoprotein lipase and the disposition of dietary fatty acids. Br J Nutr 1998;80: 495-502
34. Sowers J. Effects of statins on the vasculature: implication for aggressive lipid management in the cardiovascular metabolic syndrome. Am J Cardiol 2003; 91(4A):14B-22B
35. Reusch JEB. Current concepts in insulin resistance, type 2 diabetes mellitus, and the metabolic syndrome. Am J Cardiol 2002;90(5A):19G-26G
36. Boullier A, Bird DA, Chang MK, et al. Scavenger receptors, oxidized LDL, and atherosclerosis. Ann N Y Acad Sci 2001;947:214-222
37. Memon RA, Staprans I, Noor M, et al. Infection and inflammation induce LDL oxidation in vivo. Arterioscler Thromb Vasc Biol 2000;20:1536-1542
38. Szmitko PE, Wang C-H, Weisel RD, et al. Biomarkers of vascular disease linking inflammation to endothelial activation: Part II. Circulation 2003;108:2041-2048
39. Matsumoto T, Takashima H, Ohira N, et al. Plasma level of oxidized low-density lipoprotein is an independent determinant of coronary macrovasomotor and microvasomotor responses induced by bradykinin. J Am Coll Cardiol 2004;44:451-457
40. Boger RH, Sydow K, Borlak J, et al. LDL cholesterol upregulates synthesis of asymmetrical dimethylarginine in human endothelial cells: involvement of *S*-adenosylmethionine–dependent methyltransferases. Circ Res 2000;87:99-105
41. Singh BM, Mehta JL. Interactions between the renin-angiotensin system and dyslipidemia: relevance in the therapy of hypertension and coronary heart disease. Arch Intern Med 2003;163:1296-1304

42. McConathy WJ, Gesquiere JC, Bass H, et al. Inhibition of lipoprotein lipase activity by synthetic peptides of apolipoprotein CIII. J Lipid Res 1992;33:995-1003
43. Fruchart J-C, Staels B, Duriez P. PPARs, metabolic disease and atherosclerosis. Pharmacol Res 2001;44:345-352
44. Lee S-J, Sacks FM. Effect of pravastatin on intermediate-density and low-density lipoproteins containing apolipoprotein CIII in patients with diabetes mellitus. Am J Cardiol 2003;92:121-124
45. Taghibiglou C, Rashid-Kolvear F, Van Iderstine SC, et al. Hepatic very low density lipoprotein–ApoB overproduction is associated with attenuated hepatic insulin signaling and overexpression of protein-tyrosine phosphatase 1B in a fructose-fed hamster model of insulin resistance. J Biol Chem 2002;277:793-803
46. Julius U. Influence of plasma free fatty acids on lipoprotein synthesis and diabetic dyslipidemia. Exp Clin Endocrinol Diabetes 2003;111:246-250
47. Pulawa LK, Eckel RH. Overexpression of muscle lipoprotein lipase and insulin sensitivity. Curr Opin Clin Nutr Metab Care 2002;5:569-574
48. Mendez-Sanchez N, Chavez-Tapia NC, Uribe M. An update on non-alcoholic fatty liver disease. Rev Invest Clin 2004;56:72-82
49. Zafrani ES. Non-alcoholic fatty liver disease: an emerging pathological spectrum. Virchows Arch 2004;444:3-12
50. Jaeschke H, Gores GJ, Cederbaum AI, et al. Mechanisms of hepatotoxicity. Toxicol Sci 2002;65:166-176
51. Adeli K, Taghibiglou C, Van Iderstine SC, Lewis GF. Mechanisms of hepatic very low-density lipoprotein overproduction in insulin resistance. Trends Cardiovasc Med 2001;11:170-176
52. Kaneda M, Kashiwamura S, Ueda H, et al. Inflammatory liver steatosis caused by IL-12 and IL-18. J Interferon Cytokine Res 2003;23:155-162
53. Nachiappan V, Curtiss D, Corkey BE, Kilpatrick L. Cytokines inhibit fatty acid oxidation in isolated rat hepatocytes: synergy among TNF, IL-6, and IL-1. Shock 1994;1:123-129
54. Marette A. Mediators of cytokine-induced insulin resistance in obesity and other inflammatory settings. Curr Opin Clin Nutr Metab Care 2000;5:377-383
55. Ueki K, Kondo T, Tseng YH, Kahn CR. Central role of suppressors of cytokine signaling proteins in hepatic steatosis, insulin resistance, and the metabolic syndrome in the mouse. Proc Natl Acad Sci U S A 2004;101: 10422-10427
56. Feldstein AE, Werneburg NW, Canbay A, et al. Free fatty acids promote hepatic lipotoxicity by stimulating TNF-alpha expression via a lysosomal pathway. Hepatology 2004;40:185-194
57. Xu A, Wang Y, Keshaw H, et al. The fat-derived hormone adiponectin alleviates alcoholic and nonalcoholic fatty liver diseases in mice. J Clin Invest 2003;112:91-100
58. Hui JM, Hodge A, Farrell GC, et al. Beyond insulin resistance in NASH: TNF-alpha or adiponectin? Hepatology 2004;40:46-54
59. Tham DM, Martin-McNulty B, Wang YX, et al. Angiotensin II is associated with activation of NF-kappaB–mediated genes and downregulation of PPARs. Physiol Genomics 2002;11:21-30
60. Grav HJ, Tronstad KJ, Gudbrandsen OA, et al. Changed energy state and increased mitochondrial-oxidation rate in liver of rats associated with lowered proton electrochemical potential and stimulated uncoupling protein 2 (UCP-2) expression. Evidence for peroxisome proliferator–activated receptor–independent induction of UCP-2 expression. J Biol Chem 2003;278: 30525-30533
61. Reddy JK, Hashimoto T. Peroxisomal beta-oxidation and peroxisome proliferator–activated receptor alpha: an adaptive metabolic system. Annu Rev Nutr 2001;21: 193-230
62. Reddy JK. Nonalcoholic steatosis and steatohepatitis. III. Peroxisomal beta-oxidation, PPAR alpha, and steatohepatitis. Am J Physiol Gastrointest Liver Physiol 2001; 281:G1333-G1339
63. Yeon JE, Choi KM, Baik SH, et al. Reduced expression of peroxisome proliferator–activated receptor-alpha may have an important role in the development of non-alcoholic fatty liver disease. J Gastroenterol Hepatol 2004;19:799-804
64. Kim HJ, Kim HJ, Lee KE, et al. Metabolic significance of nonalcoholic fatty liver disease in nonobese, nondiabetic adults. Arch Intern Med 2004;164:2169-2175
65. Cassader M, Gambino R, Musso G, et al. Postprandial triglyceride-rich lipoprotein metabolism and insulin sensitivity in nonalcoholic steatohepatitis patients. Lipids 2001;36:1117-1124
66. Harris HW, Gosnell JE, Kumwenda ZL. The lipemia of sepsis: triglyceride-rich lipoproteins as agents of innate immunity. J Endotoxin Res 2000;6:421-430
67. Khovidhunkit W, Kim MS, Memon RA, et al. Effects of infection and inflammation on lipid and lipoprotein metabolism: mechanisms and consequences to the host. J Lipid Res 2004;45:1169-1196
68. Austin MA, McKnight B, Edwards KL. Cardiovascular disease mortality in familial forms of hypertriglyceridemia: a 20-year prospective study. Circulation 2000; 101:2777-2782
69. Avramoglu RK, Qiu W, Adeli K Mechanisms of metabolic dyslipidemia in insulin resistant states: deregulation of hepatic and intestinal lipoprotein secretion. Front Biosci 2003;8:d464-d476
70. Ginsberg HN. Insulin resistance and cardiovascular disease. J Clin Invest 2000;106:453-458
71. Zierath JR, Livingston JN, Thoerne A, et al. Regional difference in insulin inhibition of non-esterified fatty acid release from human adipocytes: relation to insulin receptor phosphorylation and intracellular signalling through the insulin receptor substrate-1 pathway. Diabetologia 1998;41:1343-1354
72. Paterson JM, Morton NM, Fievet C, et al. Metabolic syndrome without obesity: Hepatic overexpression of 11beta-hydroxysteroid dehydrogenase type 1 in transgenic mice. Proc Natl Acad Sci U S A 2004; 101:7088-7093
73. Reaven GM, Chen YDI, Jeppesen J, et al. Insulin resistance and hyperinsulinemia in individuals with small, dense, low-density lipoprotein particles. J Clin Invest 1993;92:141-146
74. Lamarche B, Tchernof A, Moorjani S, et al. Small, dense, low-density lipoprotein particles as a predictor of the risk of ischemic heart disease in men: prospective results from the Quebec Cardiovascular Study. Circulation 1997;95:69-75
75. Fukushima H, Sugiyama S, Honda O, et al. Prognostic value of remnant-like lipoprotein particle levels in patients with coronary artery disease and type II diabetes mellitus. Am J Coll Cardiol 2004;43:2219-2224
76. Nicklas BJ, Rogus EM, Berman DM, et al. Responses of adipose tissue lipoprotein lipase to weight loss affect lipid levels and weight regain in women. Am J Physiol Endocrinol Metab 2000;279:E1012-E1019
77. Yagyu H, Chen G, Yokoyama M, et al. Lipoprotein lipase (LpL) on the surface of cardiomyocytes increases lipid uptake and produces a cardiomyopathy. J Clin Invest 2003;111:419-426

78. Jin W, Marchadier D, Rader DJ. Lipases and HDL metabolism. Trends Endocrinol Metab 2002;13:174-176
79. Smith SR. The endocrinology of obesity. Endocrinol Metab Clin North Am 1996;25:921-941
80. Kobayashi J, Saito K, Fukamachi I, et al. Pre-heparin plasma lipoprotein lipase mass: correlation with intra-abdominal visceral fat accumulation. Horm Metab Res 2001;33:412-416
81. Zambon A, Deeb SS, Pauletto P, et al. Hepatic lipase: a marker for cardiovascular disease risk and response to therapy. Curr Opin Lipidol 2003;14:179-189
82. Thuren T. Hepatic lipase and HDL metabolism. Curr Opin Lipidol 2000;11:277-283
83. Azumi H, Hirata K-I, Ishida T, et al. Immunohistochemical localization of endothelial cell–derived lipase in atherosclerotic human coronary arteries. Cardiovasc Res 2003;58:647-654
84. Imbeault P, Couillard C, Tremblay A, et al. Reduced alpha2-adrenergic sensitivity of subcutaneous abdominal adipocytes as a modulator of fasting and postprandial triglyceride levels in men. J Lipid Res 2000;41:1367-1375

Comorbidities of the Metabolic Syndrome 11

Systemic insulin resistance affects a number of organ systems. It is an inflammatory state that engenders a panoply of metabolic, vascular, hemostatic, and hormonal disturbances that devolve into discrete pathophysiologic entities associated with the metabolic syndrome (Table 11-1).

HYPERTENSION

A correlation has been established between insulin resistance and hypertension. Although an increase in blood pressure does not occur in all subjects who are insulin resistant, hypertension is more likely to develop in hyperinsulinemic, insulin-resistant individuals than in insulin-sensitive ones. **Hypertension is, in fact, present in a significant percentage of persons with evidence of insulin resistance, and it is estimated to occur in a third of people with the metabolic syndrome.** Conceivably, hypertension emerges when undefined corrective responses no longer compensate for the metabolic and vascular changes associated with insulin resistance that predispose to an increase in blood pressure.[1]

Normal blood pressure is defined as systolic pressure lower than 120 mm Hg and diastolic pressure lower than 80 mm Hg, although even lower systolic pressure down to 100 mm Hg may be preferable. Prehypertension (120 to 139 mm Hg and 80 to 89 mm Hg, respectively) should be treated in higher-risk individuals with diabetes mellitus (DM) or vascular or renal disease. Blood pressure targets are generally set at 130/80 mm Hg for such higher-risk individuals.[2,3]

Insulin Signaling Pathways. The cellular response to insulin is mediated by at least two pathways:

1. the phosphatidylinositol 3-kinase (PI3K)-Akt kinase pathway, associated with the glucose and lipid metabolic and endothelial nitric

Table 11-1. Comorbid Conditions Associated with the Metabolic Syndrome

Hypertension
Cardiomyopathy
Atherogenic dyslipidemia
Coronary, peripheral, and cerebrovascular disease
Calcific aortic valvular disease
Fatty liver diseases
Type 2 diabetes mellitus
Cancer of the cervix/endometrium, ovaries, prostate, breast, esophagus, liver, gallbladder, pancreas, kidney, colon/rectum
Lymphoma, multiple myeloma
Gallbladder disease
Polycystic ovary syndrome
Depression
Frailty
Dementia and Alzheimer's disease

oxide synthase (eNOS) regulatory effects of insulin, and

2. the mitogen-activated protein kinase (MAPK) pathway, associated with mitogenic effects such as cell growth and proliferation.[4]

Vascular Implications of Selective Insulin Resistance. In the setting of insulin resistance, insulin has reduced effects only on the PI3K pathway while maintaining MAPK activity.[4] **Adverse effects on vascular function derive from**

- **endothelial dysfunction,**
- **increased mitogenic effects, and**
- **secondary changes,**

which cumulatively increase vascular resistance, plasma volume, cardiac output, smooth muscle cell proliferation, and arterial rigidity.[2,3]

Endothelial Dysfunction. Insulin resistance in vascular endothelial and smooth muscle cells is manifested primarily through vascular endothelial dysfunction. Disturbances in the generation of endothelial nitric oxide (NO), abnormal endothelial signaling via NO-dependent pathways, and loss of insulin-mediated vasodilation all constitute contributing factors to hypertension in the metabolic syndrome.

Mitogenic Effects. Insulin resistance is associated with compensatory hyperinsulinemia. Hyperinsulinemia is mitogenic, and the effect appears to be mediated via the sustained activation of MAPK.

MAPK activation is, in fact, accentuated with insulin resistance because of decreased mRNA expression of insulin-mediated MAPK phosphatase, which would act as an inhibitory feedback loop to attenuate MAPK signaling.[5] Growth factor production is accentuated. As a result, **there is stimulation of vascular and nonvascular cell growth and increased arterial stiffness.**[6]

Sympathetic Nervous System. Insulin resistance and hyperinsulinemia stimulate activation of the sympathetic nervous system,[7] which raises systemic blood pressure by increasing cardiac output, vasomotor tone, and vascular resistance and by stimulating activation of the renin-angiotensin-aldosterone system (RAAS).

Renin-Angiotensin-Aldosterone System. The RAAS contributes to the development of hypertension in patients with insulin resistance. Insulin activates the RAAS by increasing the expression of angiotensinogen, angiotensin II, and the angiotensin II type 1 (AT_1) receptor. As a result, there is increased activation of the RAAS and enhanced responsiveness to angiotensin II.[7,8]

The hypertensive actions of angiotensin II are multifactorial. Its actions on the vasculature, the kidneys, and the nervous system engender direct vasoconstriction, an increase in sympathetic outflow, and retention of sodium and water:

- **Angiotensin II induces hypertension as a result of its direct vasoconstrictive effects.** It engenders endothelial dysfunction. Under normal conditions, endothelium-derived NO continuously and significantly lowers vascular resistance. Angiotensin II enhances the generation of superoxide within the vasculature. Superoxide rapidly depletes NO, thereby limiting the bioavailability of this endogenous vasodilator. In the process, peroxynitrite is generated, a highly aggressive compound that oxidizes proteins, lipids, and enzyme cofactors.[9]
- **Angiotensin-induced oxidative stress in the kidney plays a role in hypertension, as does oxidative stress in the vasculature** by

mediating vascular smooth muscle hypertrophy and remodeling.[9,10]

- **Angiotensin II has potent effects on blood pressure and cardiovascular function by inducing oxidative stress in neurons located in a specialized brain region called the subfornical organ.** The subfornical organ belongs to the circumventricular organs of the brain, which are unprotected by the blood-brain barrier. It is one of the regions of the brain most densely populated with angiotensin II receptors. The subfornical organ is considered to be a neuronal sensor for angiotensin II and is thought to couple the circulating angiotensin II signal with the neural networks of the paraventricular nucleus, the ventrolateral medulla, the nucleus tractus solitarius, and the nucleus ambiguus. These neural networks are involved in the control of various effector systems such as sympathetic outflow, vasopressin release, thirst, and salt appetite, all involved in maintaining blood pressure and body fluid homeostasis. In a "slow-pressor" model of experimental hypertension in mice, 2-week exposure to angiotensin II stimulated a gradually developing hypertension that was correlated with marked elevations in intracellular superoxide production in the subfornical organ.[9,10]

Endothelin-1. The expression of vasoconstrictors such as endothelin-1 is increased in insulin resistance. Endothelin-1 is a very potent vasoconstrictor. Elaboration of endothelin-1 is increased, in part via a conventional protein kinase C (PKC)-dependent pathway in which PKC-β_2 is translocated to the plasma membrane and induces increased expression of endothelin-1.[11]

Sodium Retention. Blood pressure in obese patients is sensitive to sodium intake. Adipocytes express natriuretic clearance receptors, and these receptors engender a state of reduced natriuretic peptide concentration in obesity associated with sodium retention and volume expansion.[12]

Sodium retention is higher with insulin resistance. A high-salt diet worsens insulin resistance–associated hypertension. Insulin has antinatriuretic effects, which are exacerbated by hyperinsulinemia because renal epithelial cells remain sensitive to insulin. As a result, hyperinsulinemia stimulates enhanced renal tubular sodium reabsorption.[2,3,8,13]

Increased renal tubular reabsorption of sodium is also engendered by heightened renal sympathetic nerve activity, by the direct effect of aldosterone, and possibly by an alteration in intrarenal physical forces.[14,15]

These cellular cation transport abnormalities induce volume overload. High salt intake also increases vascular activation of p70s6k and other factors that affect cell growth and protein synthesis.[2,3]

Other Factors. Leptin and free fatty acids may act synergistically with insulin to raise blood pressure.

Enhanced sympathetic, RAAS, and leptin activity additionally stimulates small guanosine 5′-triphosphatase (GTPase) RhoA and Rho kinase activity, which increases vascular smooth muscle calcium sensitivity and vasomotor tone. RhoA activation is common in hypertension.[16]

CARDIOMYOPATHY

Insulin resistance can lead to a cardiomyopathic process that may range from subclinical disease to full-blown congestive heart failure (CHF) with type 2 DM. Insulin resistance may predate the development of heart failure by 20 years or more.[17] Treatment of impaired glucose metabolism may reverse systolic dysfunction in animal models.[18]

Cardiac Remodeling. The cardiomyopathy of insulin resistance is characterized by diastolic dysfunction with interstitial collagen deposition and myocardial fibrosis. Abnormal cardiac structure and function may precede the onset of overt DM.[19,20]

Biventricular cardiac function is impaired with obesity. In a study of 51 obese individuals with a body mass index (BMI) greater than 35 kg/m^2 versus normal-weight controls, severe obesity was associated with elevated left ventricular filling pressure and left atrial enlargement, biventricular diastolic dysfunction, eccentric left ventricular hypertrophy, and early left ventricular systolic dysfunction.[21] Although obesity is associated with left ventricular remodeling,[22] **an**

expansion of visceral adiposity as expressed by the amount of metabolically active epicardial fat, more than BMI alone, is related to an increase in left ventricular mass.[23]

In the Framingham offspring study, a large community-based sample, **diastolic dysfunction was associated with impaired insulin resistance even in the presence of normal ventricular mass.** Left atrial size, reflecting the diastolic dysfunction, was related to the severity of insulin resistance. Left ventricular mass and wall thickness increased with worsening glucose tolerance. Particularly in women, insulin resistance was related to increased ventricular mass.[24]

Diastolic dysfunction is, in fact, the hallmark of diabetic cardiomyopathy. There is prolonged relaxation and decreased chamber compliance, with elevation of ventricular filling pressure. Diastolic dysfunction precedes systolic dysfunction.[25]

Insulin Resistance as a Cause of Cardiomyopathy. As a result of insulin resistance–related neurohormonal and cytokine activation, there is a panoply of vascular and cardiomyocellular disturbances. Altered signaling pathways caused by sympathetic and RAAS hyperactivity contribute to the pathogenesis of myocyte dysfunction. There are defects in sarcolemmal and sarcoplasmic reticular calcium transport and in myocardial contractile protein and collagen formation. These abnormalities induce myocyte hypertrophy and interstitial collagen accumulation and cause disturbances in diastolic and, ultimately, systolic function.[25]

Endothelial, Metabolic, and Inflammatory Disturbances. The causes of a myopathic process with insulin resistance are manifold. Inflammatory, vascular, and metabolic disturbances are implicated.

- With insulin resistance, there is increased expression of proinflammatory cytokines, adhesion molecules, growth factors, procoagulant activity, and endothelin-1.[26] Activation of tumor necrosis factor-alpha (TNF-α) and inducible NOS (iNOS), in particular, has a negative impact on contractility. Interstitial fibrosis compromises diastolic function.
- Endothelial dysfunction impairs small vessel nutritive blood flow, thereby compromising nutrient delivery to the myocardium and resulting in microvascular tissue injury.
- Deficient leptin signaling with concurrent leptin resistance leads to the myocardial hypertrophy seen with obesity, type 2 DM, or hypertension.[27,28]
- Deranged fatty acid and glucose metabolism as a result of insulin resistance contributes to energy deprivation and myocardial dysfunction.[29]

Sympathetic Hyperactivity. Hyperinsulinemia engenders sympathetic hyperactivity. **Excessive, chronic sympathetic nervous system activation causes myocyte toxicity and apoptosis.** Hyperinsulinemia and sympathetic activation alter β-adrenergic receptor densities, with downregulation of β_1- and β_2-receptors, which mediate positive inotropy and chronotropy, and upregulation of the cardiosuppressant β_3-receptor. Additionally, there may be impairment of baroreceptor reflex sensitivity and decreased heart rate variability.[30]

Renin-Angiotensin-Aldosterone System. Myocardial RAAS activation with insulin resistance has multiple detrimental consequences on myocardial function:

- Angiotensin II plays an important role in myocyte apoptosis.
- Local tissue angiotensin II and aldosterone induce collagen synthesis and impede collagen degradation. The resulting fibrosis impairs the electrical and mechanical behavior of the hypertrophied myocardium.
- PKC activation by angiotensin II has negative inotropic and lusitropic effects. PKC phosphorylation of troponins inhibits myofibrillar adenosine triphosphatase (ATPase) activity and contractility. Sarcoplasmic reticular calcium uptake is slowed and inhibited by PKC.[30]

Protein Kinase C Activation. In general, overexpression or activation of conventional PKC-β_2 may play a role in the cardiomyopathic process associated with insulin resistance. Targeted overexpression of PKC-β_2 causes pathologic changes in myocardial function in mice that result in reduced cardiac contractility, cell death, and severe fibrosis. These pathologies are induced through the phosphorylation of troponin I and increased expression of transforming growth factor-beta 1 (TGF-β_1), connective tissue growth factor, and basement membrane proteins, similar to diabetic cardiomyopathy.[11]

Heart Failure as a Cause of Insulin Resistance. Insulin resistance causes myocardial dysfunction. Conversely, **many patients with CHF are insulin resistant.** Glucose intolerance is a common characteristic of patients with idiopathic dilated cardiomyopathy. In a study of 230 patients from a heart failure clinic, half the individuals with idiopathic dilated cardiomyopathy had either impaired fasting glucose, impaired glucose tolerance, or DM, a significantly greater prevalence than in the control population.[31] Heart failure is associated with an increased risk for the development of type 2 DM. Worsening New York Heart Association (NYHA) functional status of patients correlates with worsening glucose homeostasis.[32] In a cohort of ischemic cardiomyopathy patients, the development of new-onset DM over a 7-year period correlated with NYHA class.[26,33]

Insulin resistance in CHF is an indicator of a poor prognosis independent of NYHA class, left ventricular ejection fraction, norepinephrine or free fatty acid levels, peak oxygen consumption,[34] or anaerobic threshold during cardiopulmonary exercise testing.[35] In a longitudinal study of patients with valvular cardiomyopathy, increasing severity of heart failure and decreased survival time were related to worsening insulin resistance independent of other measured variables, including peak oxygen consumption.[36]

Insulin resistance in CHF is independent of the cause of heart disease[37] and is probably multifactorial.

- Sympathetic and RAAS overactivity with increased levels of endothelin-1,
- increased circulating proinflammatory cytokines such as TNF-α,
- secondary elevations in plasma free fatty acids,
- impaired endothelial function, and
- loss of skeletal muscle mass

associated with CHF may all contribute to the development of insulin resistance in that condition.

Implications of Insulin Resistance in Heart Failure. Normal myocardium predominantly uses free fatty acid beta oxidation as a source for the generation of adenosine triphosphate (ATP). **Fatty acids account for approximately 70% of the energy source for the myocardium. During myocardial ischemia or injury, glucose becomes the preferred metabolic substrate. A similar metabolic shift takes place with advanced cardiomyopathy.**[26]

The main reason for such a metabolic shift is the relative economy of oxygen consumption with glucose use. Although the use of free fatty acids yields a higher absolute number of ATP molecules with oxidative phosphorylation,

$$1 \text{ mol free fatty acid} \rightarrow 130 \text{ ATP},$$

$$1 \text{ mol glucose} \rightarrow 38 \text{ ATP},$$

glucose utilization is associated with greater energetic efficiency:

$$\text{Free fatty acids yield } 2.83 \text{ ATP}/O_2,$$

$$\text{Glucose yields } 3.17 \text{ ATP}/O_2.$$[26]

The metabolic change is regulated at the genetic level. With CHF in adult life, myocardial gene expression shifts to favor the metabolic enzyme profile prevalent in fetal life, when glucose oxidation prevails as the predominant source of myocardial energy. Additionally, free fatty acid oxidation in CHF is impaired as a result of decreased levels of carnitine, which is necessary for the mitochondrial transport of fatty acids to undergo beta oxidation.[26]

Because the shift to myocardial glucose consumption constitutes the metabolic adaptation to the heart failure state, insulin resistance, with the attendant impairment in insulin-mediated glucose uptake, undermines this adaptive mechanism. Insulin resistance thus forces the dysfunctional myocardium to resort to higher consumption of oxygen for diminished ATP availability, thereby engendering energy deprivation.[26]

In a vicious circle, as heart failure worsens insulin resistance, insulin resistance further compromises cardiac function by jeopardizing carbohydrate and free fatty acid metabolism of the failing heart. Insulin resistance may play an integral role in the skeletal muscle derangements and exercise intolerance of heart failure.[20]

CORONARY HEART DISEASE

Individuals with the metabolic syndrome have a significantly higher incidence of coronary heart disease (CHD) and peripheral and cerebrovascular disease than do individuals without the metabolic syndrome (Table 11-2). **Subjects with the metabolic syndrome also suffer from disproportionately more acute ischemic events for the same amount of atherosclerosis than do individuals without the metabolic syndrome.**[38]

The prothrombotic risk, when combined with vascular inflammation and atherogenic dyslipidemia, largely accounts for the increased incidence of acute ischemic events with the metabolic syndrome. The presence of the metabolic syndrome is associated with odds ratios of 3 for CHD and 1.8 for cardiovascular mortality when compared with age-matched controls.[38]

Causes of Atherosclerosis in Insulin Resistance. The underlying reasons for active vascular disease with insulin resistance and the metabolic syndrome are multifactorial and complex. Among other factors, **endothelial dysfunction and insulin resistance induce an inflammatory response in the vessel wall that is evident in patients as an elevation in circulating levels of C-reactive protein (CRP) and other inflammatory mediators that serve as markers of poor prognosis in patients with the metabolic syndrome** (Table 11-3).

Table 11-2. Prevalence of Coronary Heart Disease with the Metabolic Syndrome or Diabetes Mellitus from NHANES III Data for Persons 50 Years or Older

HEALTH STATUS	PERCENT AGE-ADJUSTED CHD PREVALENCE
– Metabolic syndrome / – DM	8.7
– Metabolic syndrome / + DM	7.5
+ Metabolic syndrome / – DM	13.9
+ Metabolic syndrome / + DM	19.2

NHANES, National Health and Nutrition Examination Survey.
Modified from Alexander CM, Landsman PB, Teutsch SM, et al. Diabetes NCEP-defined metabolic syndrome, diabetes, and prevalence of coronary heart disease among NHANES III participants age 50 years and older. 2003;52:1210-1214.

Table 11-3. Risk Factors for Patients with the Metabolic Syndrome

TRADITIONAL RISK FACTORS
Hypertension
Atherogenic dyslipidemia
Obesity
Sedentary lifestyle
Type 2 diabetes mellitus
Cigarette smoking
Family history of coronary heart disease in a first-degree relative (men <55 years, women <65 years)
Age ≥45 years for men, ≥55 years for women
Male sex
NONTRADITIONAL RISK FACTORS
Remnant lipoproteins
Lipoprotein(a)
Lipoprotein-associated phospholipase A
Abnormal fibrinolysis (plasminogen activator inhibitor-1)
Hypercoagulability (fibrinogen)
Endothelial dysfunction
Microalbuminuria
Inflammatory markers (C-reactive protein, tumor necrosis factor-alpha, interleukin-6, serum amyloid A, myeloperoxidase)
Hyperhomocysteinemia

Endothelial Dysfunction. Endothelial dysfunction is the initial lesion of atherosclerosis. It evolves concurrently with insulin resistance and is associated with the metabolic syndrome and type 2 DM. Increased abdominal adiposity, as measured by the waist-hip ratio, is a strong predictor of endothelial dysfunction, independent of other risk factors.[39]

In insulin resistance, the defect in metabolic signaling parallels defective endothelial function. **Inhibition of vascular eNOS activity impairs endothelium-dependent vasodilation, coupled with activation of inflammatory pathways and the expression of matrix metalloproteinases 2 and 9.**[40]

Vascular Smooth Muscle Dysfunction. Patients with insulin resistance manifest abnormal vascular smooth muscle function independent of endothelial dysfunction. The mitogenic effects of insulin, through direct trophic effects and via generation of reactive oxygen species (ROS), PKC, and activation of nuclear factor kappaB (NFκB), promote smooth muscle cell growth, migration, and proliferation.

With insulin resistance there is increased smooth muscle cell tone mediated by endogenous endothelin-1, a resultant decreased vasoconstrictor response to exogenous endothelin-1, and diminished NO-mediated vasodilation.[41]

Inflammation and Oxidative Stress. Insulin resistance intensifies inflammatory pathways. With preserved insulin sensitivity, insulin, in parallel with increased elaboration of NO, inhibits the expression of major proinflammatory mediators such as

- intracellular adhesion molecule-1 (ICAM-1),
- monocyte chemoattractant protein-1 (MCP-1), and
- NFκB.

Resistance to insulin signaling entails a loss of these moderating, anti-inflammatory effects of insulin and NO.[40]

Though instigated by an inflammatory process, insulin resistance and the metabolic syndrome perpetuate the proinflammatory state with elevated levels of proinflammatory cytokines such as

- TNF-α,
- interleukin-6 (IL-6), and
- CRP.

The ensuing heightened expression of proinflammatory mediators and cytokines generates an overexpression of growth factors and oxidant stress. ROS play a pivotal role in vascular disease and complications.[40]

Additionally, adipokine factors in the metabolic syndrome aggravate the inflammatory state. Directly, such adipokines may have an atherothrombotic impact via activation of monocytes/macrophages. Indirectly, the development of leptin resistance and hypoadiponectinemia promotes the development of atherosclerotic cardiovascular events.[40]

Angiotensin II. The activated RAAS and angiotensin II contribute to plaque formation by promoting macrophage and T-lymphocyte recruitment through the generation of adhesion molecules and cytokines. Angiotensin II is a powerful stimulus for the generation of ROS in blood vessels from nicotinamide adenine dinucleotide phosphate (NADH/NADPH) oxidases. Angiotensin II induces arterial wall remodeling through smooth muscle cell growth, migration, and proliferation and by altering the composition of the extracellular matrix of atheromata.[8]

The RAAS is implicated in the pathogenesis of plaque rupture and thrombosis, with increased angiotensin-converting enzyme (ACE) and angiotensin II activity observed primarily on macrophages within atherosclerotic lesions.[8]

Dyslipidemia. The dyslipidemia of the metabolic syndrome further jeopardizes vascular health. Insulin resistance in adipose tissue, the musculature, and the liver increases free fatty acid fluxes, triglyceride synthesis, and very-low-density lipoprotein (VLDL) secretion. Elevated triglyceride-rich lipoproteins set the stage for a highly atherogenic, proinflammatory, and oxidant milieu encompassing higher levels of remnant lipoproteins, the formation of small, dense, oxidized low-density lipoprotein (LDL), and low levels of dysfunctional high-density lipoprotein (HDL).[38] Especially in women, there is a very strong association of CHD events with high triglyceride levels.[42]

Hypercoagulability. The increased coagulopathy that is seen with insulin resistance and the metabolic syndrome is engendered by impairment of the fibrinolytic system complemented by activation of the coagulation cascade and platelets. The presence of the metabolic syndrome thus identifies a population that is at substantial risk for acute ischemic events.

Impaired Fibrinolysis. The fibrinolytic dysfunction of the metabolic syndrome plays a major role in the pathogenesis of cardiovascular atherothrombotic events.

Plasminogen Activator Inhibitor-1. Fibrinolysis in the metabolic syndrome is impaired. **Insulin resistance is associated with elevated levels of plasminogen activator inhibitor-1 (PAI-1), and PAI-1 levels correlate with plasma insulin. Elevated levels of PAI-1 predict myocardial infarction, stroke, and mortality.**[38,42]

PAI-1 is a natural inhibitor of tissue plasminogen activator (tPA) in atherosclerotic vessels. As a result, the actions of plasmin are inhibited, thus preventing the plasmin-mediated breakdown of fibrin clots. PAI-1 also has profibrotic properties.[8,38]

Factors That Increase PAI-1 Expression. Several factors increase PAI-1 elaboration from adipose tissue, endothelial cells, the liver, and platelets:

- Insulin stimulates the production of PAI-1 from adipose tissue. Accumulation of visceral fat seems to be an important determinant of prevailing concentrations of PAI-1 in blood. Release of PAI-1 from adipose tissue is stimulated by cytokines such as tumor growth factor-β and TNF-α. Activation of the adipose RAAS promotes the synthesis of PAI-1. Oxygen-centered free radicals and NFκB augment PAI-1 synthesis by diverse cells.[43]
- Endothelial dysfunction increases PAI-1. There is increased elaboration of PAI-1 from endothelial cells in response to IL-1 and CRP. t-PA augments the elaboration of PAI-1 from venous human umbilical cord endothelial cells, and proinsulin augments it in aortic endothelial cells.[43]
- Insulin, proinsulin, proinsulin split products, and insulin-like growth factor type I (IGF-I) stimulate PAI-1 synthesis in a human hepatoma cell line via stabilization of PAI-1 mRNA through the MAPK pathway. Liver steatosis is a determinant of elevated concentrations of PAI-1, and hyperinsulinemia increases the expression of PAI-1. Free fatty acids, as well as enhancement of hepatic VLDL synthesis, also augment PAI-1 expression.[43]
- There is increased PAI-1 activity in platelets, and platelets may be contributing to the elevated PAI-1 concentrations in blood.[43]

Although endogenous tPA levels are elevated in response to endogenous fibrinolytic inhibitors such as PAI-1, a prothrombotic dysequilibrium favoring inhibitors over activators of plasminogen persists.[8,38]

Prothrombotic State. In the metabolic syndrome, impaired fibrinolysis is further aggravated by a prothrombotic state. Visceral obesity and insulin resistance increase the risk for venous thrombosis and arterial thrombo-occlusive disease.[38] Insulin resistance is associated with hypercoagulability as reflected by increased concentrations of prothrombin fragment 1, thrombin-antithrombin complexes, and fibrinopeptide A in blood.[43] Many circulating coagulation factors are present in increased concentrations. **Activation of the PKC pathway seems to be one of the most likely elements responsible for the increased production of a variety of prothrombotic factors,** and the resulting higher levels of

- serum fibrinogen,
- von Willebrand factor,
- factor VII, VIII, XI, and XII, and
- thrombin

create a prothrombotic milieu. Mediators of inflammation, such as kallikrein, are also increased, and stimulate activation of coagulation factor XII. Concentrations of natural inhibitors of coagulation, such as protein C, are decreased.[43,44]

Platelet Hyperreactivity. Alterations in platelet function contribute to the activated coagulation cascade and heighten the risk for atherothrombosis. There is enhanced

- platelet activation and
- platelet aggregability.

Increased platelet reactivity is reflected by higher levels of platelet products such as β-thromboglobulin, thromboxane B_2, and platelet factor 4, an inhibitor of heparin.[43]

Incidence of Insulin Resistance and Impaired Glucose Metabolism with Coronary Heart Disease. There is a high incidence of mostly unrecognized insulin resistance in patients with CHD. Impaired carbohydrate metabolism is associated with a higher cardiovascular event rate in CHD patients.

Insulin Resistance. Insulin resistance is a common finding even with newly diagnosed CHD.

In 40 patients with newly diagnosed CHD, no previous history of metabolic disorders, and no treatment with medications that might disturb insulin sensitivity, relative to 15 healthy controls, insulin suppression testing demonstrated the presence of insulin resistance in 82.5% of patients. Changes in the lipid profile and in uric acid levels paralleled the changes in insulin sensitivity such that serum triglycerides and uric acid were higher and HDL levels lower in patients than they were in healthy controls. Additionally, 68% of new CHD patients had abnormal glucose tolerance test results.[45]

Impaired Glucose Tolerance. There is also a high frequency of disturbed glucose metabolism in CHD patients, detected primarily via glucose tolerance testing. Glucose tolerance testing, albeit more sensitive than a fasting glucose level, still underestimates the actual prevalence of insulin resistance.

In the Nateglinide and Valsartan in Impaired Glucose Tolerance Outcomes Research (NAVIGATOR) trial, oral glucose tolerance screening was performed on 43,509 potential study participants with risk factors for or diagnosed CHD. Approximately two thirds of subjects had abnormal glucose testing.[46] An oral glucose tolerance test was performed in 160 consecutive subjects undergoing elective coronary angiography for suspected CHD; normal glucose tolerance was observed in only 15% of patients, and 55% had DM.[47] In the Euro Heart survey, 30% of 4961 CHD patients with stable and unstable ischemic syndromes had known DM. Of the 1920 patients without known DM who underwent glucose tolerance testing, more than two thirds had abnormal test results.[48] In the Glucose Abnormalities in Patients with Myocardial Infarction (GAMI) study, of 168 Swedish patients with acute myocardial infarction who were free of known DM, 67% had either new-onset DM or abnormal glucose tolerance, again leaving only a third of patients with normal test results. During 2.8 years of follow-up, the event-free survival rate was 75% in patients with abnormal glucose handling versus 90% in patients with normal test results. Abnormal glucose regulation conferred a 4.18-fold increased risk for future cardiovascular events.[46]

The European Society of Cardiology may recommend that all patients with acute myocardial infarction and, in fact, all patients with acute and stable ischemic heart disease undergo glucose tolerance testing.[46]

NONALCOHOLIC FATTY LIVER DISEASE

Hepatic steatosis occurs with hepatic insulin resistance. Nonalcoholic fatty liver disease comprises a spectrum of liver injury that ranges from benign hepatic steatosis to potentially fatal cirrhosis. According to the third National Health and Nutrition Examination Survey, 6.4 million adults in the United States have nonalcoholic fatty liver disease. It is the most common cause of elevated liver enzyme levels, and elevated alanine transaminase (ALT) levels predict type 2 DM independently of obesity.[49]

Nonalcoholic steatohepatitis (NASH) represents an advanced stage within the spectrum of nonalcoholic fatty liver disease and is defined histologically by the presence of steatosis along with areas of necrosis and inflammation. By definition, NASH describes hepatic histologic changes consistent with alcoholic hepatitis in the absence of excessive alcohol intake. The liver shows fatty changes and hepatocyte injury, with or without fibrosis. There may be cirrhotic changes. Known risk factors are

- obesity with a BMI greater than 30 kg/m^2,
- age older than 45 years,
- dyslipidemia, and
- type 2 DM.

The condition is usually asymptomatic. Modest elevation of aminotransferases and hepatomegaly are common. The aspartate transaminase (AST)/ALT ratio is greater than 1. Although the course is generally indolent, cirrhosis may occur in a small number of patients.[49-51]

GLUCOSE INTOLERANCE AND TYPE 2 DIABETES MELLITUS

Insulin resistance is a precursor to impaired glucose tolerance and type 2 DM. In the initial stages of insulin resistance, the majority of individuals have a compensatory increase in insulin secretion that causes hyperinsulinemia. Because pancreatic incompetence supervenes in some individuals, insulin secretion is no longer commensurate to match the high levels of insulin required to overcome the resistance to insulin signaling. The ensuing result is glucose intolerance and ultimately type 2 DM.[52]

Macrovascular Atherothrombotic Disease. Insulin resistance–related mechanisms underlie the macrovascular complications of metabolic syndrome. Thus, the risk for macrovascular atherothrombotic complications, such as myocardial infarction or stroke, is

inherent in the metabolic syndrome regardless of the presence or absence of type 2 DM.[42]

However, hyperglycemia may further augment the risk for CHD. The cardiovascular risk associated with insulin resistance and the metabolic syndrome increases continuously as fasting glucose values rise from 90 to 125 mg/dL. Similarly, cardiovascular morbidity with glycosylated hemoglobin (HbA1c) values between 5.0% and 5.4% exceeds CHD morbidity at lower values (<5.0%).[52]

Microvascular Diabetic Complications. Although insulin resistance–related pathways are implicated in the genesis of the macrovascular complications of the metabolic syndrome, **hyperglycemia-related injury is a major cause of diabetic microvascular disease.** In both type 1 and type 2 DM, the late neuronal, retinal, and renal diabetic complications arise from chronic elevations in glucose and possibly other metabolites, including free fatty acids. Activation of the common stress-activated signaling pathways relating to

- NFκB,
- p38 MAPK,
- c-Jun NH_2-terminal kinase (JNK)/stress-activated protein kinase (SAPK),
- advanced glycosylation end products (AGEs),
- receptor for AGEs (RAGE),
- PKC, and
- sorbitol stress pathways

is implicated in the genesis of the microvascular diabetic end-organ complications.[53,54]

POLYCYSTIC OVARY SYNDROME

The polycystic ovary syndrome is characterized by anovulation with irregular or absent menstrual periods. Affected women have hyperandrogenism with elevated serum testosterone and androstenedione. This syndrome is associated with

- infertility,
- obesity,
- excess male pattern hair growth,
- male pattern hair loss, and
- acne.

Polycystic ovary syndrome affects approximately 6% to 10% of women of reproductive age. The disorder appears to have a genetic component. Affected individuals may have both male and female relatives with aspects of the metabolic syndrome and type 2 DM and have female relatives with features of the polycystic ovary syndrome.[55,56]

One of the major biochemical features of the polycystic ovary syndrome is profound insulin resistance with compensatory hyperinsulinemia. Hyperinsulinemia induces the hyperandrogenism of the polycystic ovary syndrome by increasing the ovarian production of androgens, specifically, testosterone and androstenedione, and by decreasing the serum concentration of sex hormone–binding globulin. The elevated levels of unbound androgenic hormones interfere with the pituitary-ovarian axis and lead to increased luteinizing hormone (LH) levels, anovulation, amenorrhea, and infertility. Interventions that reduce insulin levels, such as weight loss and medications, reduce insulin resistance and decrease the hyperandrogenism.[49,55,56]

MALIGNANCY

Insulin resistance is the metabolic manifestation of a systemic inflammatory state with oxidative stress. **Insulin resistance constitutes a risk factor for numerous malignancies. The causes are probably multifactorial and encompass diverse factors such as impairment of the immune response, the impact of adipose tissue on hormone levels, and the systemic trophic effects of hyperinsulinemia.**

Insulin resistance leads to elevated levels of IGF-I and decreased levels of IGF binding protein-3, its main binding protein. IGF-I is mitogenic and antiapoptotic, modulates cell growth and survival, and is thought to be important in tumor development. Elevated circulating concentrations of IGF-I are associated with an increased risk for cancer.[57]

Chronically elevated levels of proinflammatory cytokines may cause persistent activity of Rac1 GTPases in insulin-resistant states, which may induce malignant transformation. Leptin may also be implicated in increasing the risk for malignancy. Leptin signaling entails activation of the Rho and Rac family of small GTPases.[58,59] Rac1 activates NFκB, which leads to transcriptional induction of the IL-6 gene. IL-6, in autocrine fashion via the IL-6 receptor, stimulates the Janus kinase/signal transducer and activator of transcription 3 (STAT-3) signal pathway, which is a potential oncogene.[60]

Breast Cancer. Obesity and insulin resistance are risk factors for breast cancer. Elevated levels of adipokines may provide one of the mechanisms whereby obesity and insulin resistance are causally associated with a risk for breast cancer and a poor prognosis.[61] Adiponectin, which is closely and inversely associated with insulin resistance, may also underlie the association between breast cancer and obesity/insulin resistance. Adiponectin is inversely related not only to endometrial cancer but also to the development of breast cancer, with an odds ratio of 0.84.[62] Additionally, in concert with insulin resistance, elevated levels of IGF may synergistically increase the risk for breast carcinoma.[63] In a meta–regression analysis of 26 case-control studies of 3609 prostate, colorectal, and premenopausal and postmenopausal breast and lung cancer cases versus 7137 controls, high concentrations of IGF-I were associated with an increased risk for premenopausal breast and prostate cancer.[57]

Benign Prostatic Hypertrophy and Prostate Cancer. Benign prostatic hypertrophy may be associated with the metabolic syndrome, and the metabolic syndrome may confer an increased risk for incident prostate cancer. Obesity, dyslipidemia, hyperuricemia, hypertension, high ALT levels, hyperinsulinemia, vascular disease, and type 2 DM are all risk factors for the development of prostatic hypertrophy and clinical prostate cancer.[64] In a prospective population-based study of 1880 middle-aged Finnish men, prostate cancer was more likely to develop in those with the metabolic syndrome. After adjustment for other risk factors and dietary intake, the metabolic syndrome was related to a 1.9-fold risk for prostate cancer. The association between metabolic syndrome and risk for prostate cancer was even stronger in overweight and obese men (BMI >27 kg/m^2), with an adjusted relative risk of 3.0.[65]

Colorectal Cancer. Insulin resistance may be associated with the development of colorectal cancer. Mechanistically, increased levels of growth factors, including IGF-I, activation of NFκB, and altered peroxisome proliferator–activated receptor (PPAR) signaling may promote colon cancer through their effects on colonocyte kinetics.[66] Leptin may also be directly involved in colon tumorigenesis, or it may serve as a marker of an adverse endocrine environment. In a case-control study nested in the Janus Biobank, Norway, of cryopreserved, prediagnostic sera from 235 men with a median age of 45 years in whom cancer of the colon was diagnosed a median of 17 years after blood collection, there was an approximately threefold increase in colon cancer risk, relative to 378 controls, with increasing concentrations of leptin.[67]

FRAILTY

In individuals 65 years and older, 6% to 25% suffer from frailty. Frailty is a complex syndrome that is not fully defined. Individuals afflicted with frailty are typically physically inactive. They have poor appetite and experience unintentional weight loss. They are physically weak, fatigue easily, and ambulate unsteadily with an increased risk of falling. Relative to nonfrail persons, frail individuals are more likely to suffer from impaired cognition and depression and to have higher mortality.[68]

Frailty is characterized by osteopenia, sarcopenia, inflammation with a rise in inflammatory cytokines, and coagulopathy with a rise in several markers of coagulation.[68] Sarcopenia is a major cause of frailty and morbidity. With frailty, there is a loss of many anabolic signals and an increase in catabolic signals to skeletal muscle. Apoptosis contributes to the loss of skeletal myocytes.[69]

Inflammatory signals may trigger the loss of muscle cells, and insulin resistance may be playing a role. There is activation of NFκB. High levels of proinflammatory cytokines such as IL-6 are associated with frailty and carry a poor prognosis. These cytokines suppress the expression and function of local anabolic factors such as growth hormone and IGF-I. They exert direct catabolic effects and lead to anorexia and the induction of insulin resistance. Cytokines induce the atrophy-related expression of a number of E3 ligases, highly specific regulators of the ubiquitin-proteasome pathway that target proteins for proteolytic breakdown in proteasomes.[69,70]

DEMENTIA

The metabolic syndrome contributes to cognitive impairment in the elderly, particularly those with high levels of inflammatory markers. Inflammation is associated with an accelerated decline in cognitive function and Alzheimer's disease.[71-74]

Cognitive Impairment. In a 5-year prospective, observational study conducted from 1997 to 2002 at community clinics involving 2632 highly functioning African American and white participants without dementia who had a mean age of 74 years, individuals with the metabolic syndrome were significantly more likely to have cognitive impairment relative to subjects without the metabolic syndrome. There was a statistically significant interaction of inflammation and the metabolic syndrome with cognitive impairment (P = .03). After stratifying for inflammation, only individuals with the metabolic syndrome and high levels of inflammatory markers (IL-6 and CRP), not those with low levels, had an increased likelihood of cognitive impairment with a multivariate adjusted relative risk of 1.66.[75]

Alzheimer's Disease. Affective disorders and Alzheimer's disease are associated, and their linkage is based on insulin resistance. Impairment of glucose metabolism with insulin resistance may promote neurodegeneration and facilitate affective disorders. Persistent regional hypometabolism and vascular changes resulting from long-standing insulin resistance may contribute to irreversible structural changes and the onset of Alzheimer's disease.[76]

Insulin resistance is associated with Alzheimer's disease. Patients with Alzheimer's disease, randomly selected from the Bristol Memory Disorders Clinic, had a higher incidence of hyperinsulinemia and insulin resistance than controls did.[77]

Insulin resistance is associated with Alzheimer's disease independently of the apolipoprotein E4 phenotype. Among 980 people 69 to 78 years of age from Kuopio, Finland, 46 (4.7%) were classified as having probable or possible Alzheimer's disease. Although hyperinsulinemia had no effect on the risk for disease in the presence of the apolipoprotein E4 allele, in 532 nondiabetic subjects without the apolipoprotein E4 allele, hyperinsulinemia was associated with an increased risk for Alzheimer's disease (prevalence of disease, 7.5% versus 1.4% in normoinsulinemic subjects; P =.0004).[78]

Insulin resistance in the brain may directly contribute to Alzheimer's disease pathology by increasing β-amyloid peptide production in the brain. In Tg2576 mice, a model for Alzheimer's disease–like neuropathology, diet-induced insulin resistance promoted amyloidogenic β-amyloid 1-40 and 1-42 peptide generation in the brain that corresponded with increased γ-secretase activity and decreased insulin degrading enzyme activity. Increased amyloidogenic β-amyloid production also coincided with increased Alzheimer's disease–type amyloid plaque burden in the brain and impaired performance in a spatial water maze task. In the affected brain regions, there was a functional decrease in insulin receptor–mediated signal transduction, decreased phosphorylation of the insulin receptor β-subunit, and reduced activation of PI3K and Akt/protein kinase B. Akt/protein kinase B plays an inhibitory role on glycogen synthase kinase-3α activity, which promotes amyloidogenic β-amyloid peptide generation. Correspondingly, in this murine model, insulin resistance in the brain increased glycogen synthase kinase activation, as reflected by decreased glycogen synthase kinase-3α and -3β phosphorylation, which positively correlated with γ-secretase activity and the generation of amyloid precursor protein.[79]

LIPODYSTROPHIES

In contrast to other comorbid conditions devolving from insulin resistance and the metabolic syndrome, **lipodystrophies and sleep apnea, albeit associated with insulin resistance, appear to be causes rather than consequences of insulin resistance.**

Lipodystrophy is characterized by an almost complete lack of subcutaneous fat and is associated with insulin resistance. **The absence of an appropriate adipose storage site for free fatty acids engenders ectopic lipid deposits in skeletal muscle and the liver and thereby results in severe resistance to insulin signaling and DM.**

By far the most common form of lipodystrophy is that associated with the use of highly active antiretroviral therapy in patients with human immunodeficiency virus (HIV) disease.

Affected patients characteristically have wasting of the face and limbs along with accumulation of adipose tissue in the abdomen and at the back of the neck ("buffalo hump"). Lipodystrophy, especially facial lipoatrophy, can be quite disfiguring and stigmatizing. In approximately half the patients treated with antiretroviral therapy, at least one lipodystrophy-related symptom develops after 1 to 1½ years of treatment. There are, to date, no pharmacologic therapies for lipoatrophy.[49]

SLEEP APNEA

Sleep apnea is defined as the occurrence of repeated episodes of decreased or total cessation of respiratory airflow during sleep that lead to a fall of greater than 4% in oxygen saturation and to sleep fragmentation. Sleep apnea is associated with numerous afflictions, such as

- hypertension,
- CHD,
- cerebrovascular disease,
- heart failure,
- stroke,
- cardiac arrhythmias,
- pulmonary hypertension, and
- cognitive decline.

The diagnosis of sleep apnea is made by overnight polysomnography.

Sleep apnea can be obstructive or central:

1. Obstructive sleep apnea (OSA) occurs when collapse of the upper airway encumbers inspiration and precipitates strenuous, stentorian breathing efforts.
2. Central sleep apnea occurs when dysfunction of the central respiratory control mechanisms leads to diminution or cessation of thoracoabdominal respiratory muscle contraction.

When defined as more than five episodes of apnea or hypopnea per hour of sleep, sleep apnea is relatively common and affects 24% and 9% of middle-aged men and women, respectively.[80]

Sleep apnea occurs frequently in individuals with central adiposity and features of the metabolic syndrome and engenders disturbances in the autonomic nervous system:

1. Sleep apnea can induce a reflex increase in vagal tone triggered by a diving reflex caused by apnea and hypoxemia. The increased vagotonus is manifested as sinus arrest, atrioventricular nodal block, and secondary arrhythmias.
2. Sleep apnea increases sympathetic nervous system activity. Nocturnal chemoreflex activation by hypoxia and hypercapnia induces nighttime sympathetic activation and increased blood pressure. Eventually, ensuing chemoreceptor resetting and tonic chemoreceptor activation extend the sympathetic hyperactivity and hypertension even into daytime periods of normoxia.

Sleep apnea is also associated with

- endothelial dysfunction,
- lower NO availability,
- increased endothelin-1 levels,
- elevated CRP,
- elevated plasma levels and cell expression of adhesion molecules, and
- heightened oxidant stress.[80]

The sympathetic and inflammatory activation associated with the hypoxemic stress of sleep-disordered breathing promotes insulin resistance and hyperinsulinemia. OSA thus evolves into an independent, comorbid risk factor for insulin resistance and the metabolic syndrome, as it is for CHD and cerebrovascular disease.[80,81]

CONCLUSION

Insulin resistance targets many tissues, including adipose tissue, the vasculature, the musculature, the myocardium, the pancreas, the liver, and the brain. The metabolic, vascular, proinflammatory, and oxidant pathways of insulin resistance, unless curtailed, generate positive feedback systems that result in incremental and cumulative perturbations in multiple organ systems. After years of resistance to insulin signaling, the associated comorbidities of the metabolic syndrome become fully manifested as serious and, in many instances, life-threatening conditions such as hypertension; cardiomyopathy; diffuse coronary, cerebral, and peripheral vascular disease; type 2 DM; and nonalcoholic fatty liver disease (Fig. 11-1). In a number of instances, malignancies, calcific aortic valvular disease, renal impairment, the frailty of old age, depression, and dementia may ultimately also

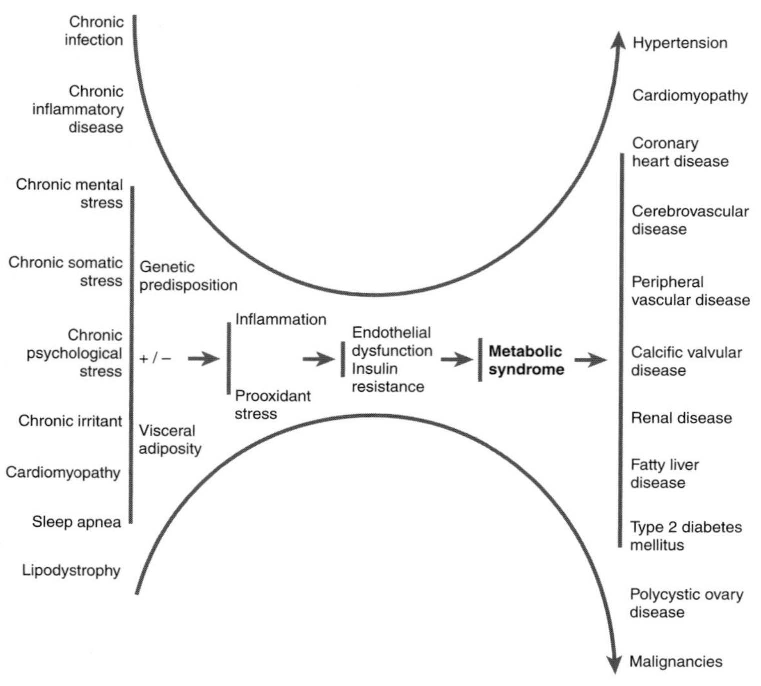

Figure 11–1. Factors leading to the metabolic syndrome and its ramifications.

evolve from a proinflammatory, insulin-resistant pathophysiology. It is the serious nature of these metabolic syndrome comorbidities that render the obesity epidemic a very significant public health concern.

Although the inflammatory pathways of insulin resistance are implicated in the etiology of its comorbid conditions, many of the disease entities discussed, such as cardiomyopathy, CHD, vascular disease in general, and type 2 DM, develop a proinflammatory milieu in their own right. Cardiomyopathy, like sleep apnea, constitutes a risk factor for insulin resistance and, as such, further amplifies the vicious circle of insulin-resistant systemic disease.

The evolution of metabolic syndrome comorbidities is protracted. That aspect renders the current obesity epidemic a truly daunting medical concern for the future. Therefore, it is a mandate for health care professionals to motivate individuals at risk to implement preventive lifestyle, dietary, and pharmacologic measures that will prevent systemic progression of the metabolic syndrome. To do less would be a public health disaster.

GLOSSARY

ACE	angiotensin-converting enzyme
AGE	advanced glycosylation end product
ALT	alanine transaminase
AST	aspartate transaminase
AT_1	angiotensin II type 1
ATP	adenosine 5′-triphosphate
BMI	body mass index
CHD	coronary heart disease
CHF	congestive heart failure
CRP	C-reactive protein
DM	diabetes mellitus
eNOS	endothelial nitric oxide synthase
GTP	guanosine triphosphate
HbA1c	glycosylated hemoglobin
HDL	high-density lipoprotein
HIV	human immunodeficiency virus
ICAM-1	intercellular adhesion molecule-1
IGF-I	insulin-like growth factor type I
IL	interleukin
iNOS	inducible nitric oxide synthase
JNK	c-Jun NH_2-terminal kinase
LDL	low-density lipoprotein
LH	luteinizing hormone
MAPK	mitogen-activated protein kinase

MCP-1	monocyte chemoattractant protein-1
NADH/NADPH	nicotinamide adenine dinucleotide phosphate oxidase
NASH	nonalcoholic steatohepatitis
NFκB	nuclear factor kappaB
NO	nitric oxide
NYHA	New York Heart Association
OSA	obstructive sleep apnea
PAI-1	plasminogen activator inhibitor-1
PI3K	phosphatidylinositol 3-kinase
PKC	protein kinase C
PPAR	peroxisome proliferator–activated receptor
RAAS	renin-angiotensin-aldosterone system
RAGE	receptor for AGEs
ROS	reactive oxygen species
SAPK	stress-activated protein kinase
STAT	signal transducer and activator of transcription
TGF	transforming growth factor
TNF	tumor necrosis factor
tPA	tissue plasminogen activator
VCAM	vascular cell adhesion molecule
VLDL	very-low-density lipoprotein

REFERENCES

1. Reaven G. Insulin resistance, hypertension, and coronary heart disease. J Clin Hypertens 2003;5:269-274
2. Rakugi H, Kamide K, Ogihara T. Vascular signaling pathways in the metabolic syndrome. Curr Hypertens Rep 2002;4:105-111
3. Chobanian AV, Bakris GL, Black HR, et al. The Seventh Report of the Joint National Committee on Prevention, Detection, Evaluation, and Treatment of High Blood Pressure: the JNC 7 report. JAMA 2003;289:2560-2571
4. Cusi K, Maezono K, Osman A, et al. Insulin resistance differentially affects the PI 3-kinase– and MAP kinase–mediated-signaling in human muscle. J Clin Invest 2000; 105:311-320
5. Begum N, Song Y, Rienzie J, Ragolia L. Vascular smooth muscle cell growth and insulin regulation of mitogen-activated protein kinase in hypertension. Am J Physiol 1998;275:C42-C49
6. Salomaa V, Riley W, Kark JD, et al. Arterial disease/hypertension/angiotensin system: non–insulin-dependent diabetes mellitus and fasting glucose and insulin concentrations are associated with arterial stiffness indexes: the ARIC study. Circulation 1995;91:1432-1433
7. Landsberg L. Insulin-mediated sympathetic stimulation: role in the pathogenesis of obesity-related hypertension (or, how insulin affects blood pressure and why). J Hypertens 2001;19:523-528
8. Deedwania PC. Metabolic syndrome and vascular disease. Is nature or nurture leading the new epidemic of cardiovascular disease? Circulation 2004;109:2-4
9. Brandes RP. And what about the endothelium? On the predominance of cerebral superoxide formation for angiotensin II–induced systemic hypertension. Circ Res 2004;95:122-124
10. Zimmerman MC, Lazartigues E, Sharma RV, Davisson RL. Hypertension caused by angiotensin II infusion involves increased superoxide production in the central nervous system. Circ Res 2004;95:210-216
11. He Z, King GL. Protein kinase Cβ isoform inhibitors. A new treatment for diabetic cardiovascular diseases. Circulation 2004;110:7-9
12. Mehra MR, Uber PA, Park MH, et al. Obesity and suppressed B-type natriuretic peptide levels in heart failure. J Am Coll Cardiol 2004;43:1590-1595
13. Schnyder B, Pittet M, Durand J, Schnyder-Candrian S. Rapid effects of glucose on the insulin signaling of endothelial NO generation and epithelial Na transport. Am J Physiol Endocrinol Metab 2001;282:E87-E94
14. Reaven GM, Lithell H, Landsberg L. Mechanisms of disease: hypertension and associated metabolic abnormalities. The role of insulin resistance and the sympathoadrenal system. N Engl J Med 1996;334:374-381
15. Ginsberg HN. Insulin resistance and cardiovascular disease. J Clin Invest 2000;106:453-458
16. Seko T, Ito M, Kureishi Y, et al. Activation of RhoA and inhibition of myosin phosphatase as important components in hypertension in vascular smooth muscle. Circ Res 2003;92:411-418
17. Arnlov J, Lind L, Zethelius B, et al. Several factors associated with the insulin resistance syndrome are predictors of left ventricular systolic dysfunction in a male population after 20 years of follow-up. Am Heart J 2001;142:720-724
18. Stroedter D, Schmidt T, Bretzel RG, Federlin K. Glucose metabolism and left ventricular dysfunction are normalized by insulin and islet transplantation in mild diabetes in the rat. Acta Diabetol 1995;32:235-243
19. Kenchaiah S, Evans JC, Levy D, et al. Obesity and the risk of heart failure. N Engl J Med 2002;347:305-313
20. Taegtmeyer H, McNulty P, Young ME. Adaptation and maladaptation of the heart in diabetes, part I: general concepts. Circulation 2002;105:1727-1733
21. Willens HJ, Chakko SC, Lowery MH, et al. Tissue Doppler imaging of the right and left ventricle in severe obesity (body mass index >35 kg/m^2). Am J Cardiol 2004;94:1087-1090
22. Gates PE, Gentile CL, Seals DR, Christou DD. Adiposity contributes to differences in left ventricular structure and diastolic function with age in healthy men. J Clin Endocrinol Metab 2003;88:4884-4890
23. Iacobellis G, Ribaudo MC, Zappaterreno A, et al. Relation between epicardial adipose tissue and left ventricular mass. Am J Cardiol 2004;94:1084-1087
24. Rutter MK, Parise H, Benjamin EJ, et al. Impact of glucose intolerance and insulin resistance on cardiac structure and function. Sex related differences in the Framingham Heart Study. Circulation 2003;107:448-454

25. Fang ZY, Najos-Valencia O, Leano R, Marwick TH. Patients with early diabetic heart disease demonstrate a normal myocardial response to dobutamine. J Am Coll Cardiol 2003;42:446-453
26. Nikolaidis LA, Levine TB. Peroxisome proliferator activator receptors (PPAR), insulin resistance, and cardiomyopathy. Friends or foe for the diabetic patient with heart failure. Cardiol Rev 2004;12:158-170
27. Paolisso G, Tagliamonte MR, Galderisi M, et al. Plasma leptin level is associated with myocardial wall thickness in hypertensive insulin-resistant men. Hypertension 1999;34:1047-1052
28. Sader S, Nian M, Liu P. Leptin: a novel link between obesity, diabetes, cardiovascular risk, and ventricular hypertrophy. Circulation 2003;108:644-646
29. Van der Vusse GJ, van Bilsen M, Glatz JF. Cardiac fatty acid uptake and transport in health and disease. Cardiovasc Res 2000;45:279-293
30. Kirpichnikov D, McFarlane SI, Sowers JR. Heart failure in diabetic patients: utility of beta-blockade. J Card Failure 2003;9:333-344
31. Witteles RM, Tang WHW, Jamali AH, et al. Insulin resistance in idiopathic dilated cardiomyopathy: a possible etiologic link. J Am Coll Cardiol 2004;44:78-81
32. Suskin N, McKelvie RS, Burns RJ, et al. Glucose and insulin abnormalities relate to functional capacity in patients with congestive heart failure. Eur Heart J 2000; 21:1368-1375
33. Tenenbaum A, Motro M, Fisman EZ, et al. Risk of developing diabetes increases with heart failure progression. Am J Cardiol 2003;114:271-275
34. Amato L, Paolisso G, Cacciatore F, et al. Congestive heart failure predicts the development of non–insulin dependent diabetes mellitus in the elderly. Diabetes Metab 1997;23:213-218
35. Levya F, Chua TP, Goldsland IF, et al. Loss of the normal coupling between the anaerobic threshold and insulin sensitivity in chronic heart failure. Heart 1999;82: 348-351
36. Paolisso G, Tagliamonte MR, Rizzo MR. Prognostic importance of insulin-mediated glucose uptake in aged patients with congestive heart failure secondary to mitral and/or aortic valve disease. Am J Cardiol 1999;83: 1338-1344
37. Swan JW, Walton C, Godsland IF, et al. Insulin resistance in chronic heart failure. Eur Heart J 1994;15:1528-1532
38. Anand SS, Yi Q, Gerstein H, et al for the Study of Health Assessment and Risk in Ethnic Groups (SHARE) and Study of Health Assessment and Risk Evaluation in Aboriginal Peoples (SHARE-AP) Investigators. Relationship of metabolic syndrome and fibrinolytic dysfunction to cardiovascular disease. Circulation 2003;108:420-425
39. Brook RD, Bard RL, Rubenfire M, et al. Usefulness of visceral obesity (waist/hip ratio) in predicting vascular endothelial function in healthy overweight adults. Am J Cardiol 2001;88:1264-1269
40. Reilley MP, Rader DJ. The metabolic syndrome: more than the sum of its parts? Circulation 2003;108:1546-1551
41. Prasad A, Quyyumi AA. Renin-angiotensin system and angiotensin receptor blockers in the metabolic syndrome. Circulation 2004;110:1507-1512
42. Deedwania PC. Metabolic syndrome and vascular disease. Is nature or nurture leading the new epidemic of cardiovascular disease? Circulation 2004;109:2-4
43. Sobel BE, Schneider DJ. Platelet function, coagulopathy, and impaired fibrinolysis in diabetes. Cardiol Clin 2004; 22:511-526
44. Deedwania PC. Diabetes is a vascular disease: the role of endothelial dysfunction in pathophysiology of cardiovascular disease in diabetes. Cardiol Clin 2004;22: 505-509
45. Piedrola G, Novo E, Serrano-Gotarredona J, et al. Insulin resistance in patients with a recent diagnosis of coronary artery disease. J Hypertens 1996;14: 1477-1482
46. Jancin B. Glucose tolerance test advocated for all CAD patients. Int Med News 2004;37:1,50
47. Wascher TC, Sourij H, Roth M, Dittrich P. Prevalence of pathological glucose metabolism in patients undergoing elective coronary angiography. Atherosclerosis 2004; 176:419-421
48. Bartnik M, Ryden L, Ferrari R, et al. The prevalence of abnormal glucose regulation in patients with coronary artery disease across Europe. The Euro Heart Survey on diabetes and the heart. Eur Heart J 2004;25:1880-1890
49. Yki-Järvinen H. Thiazolidinediones. N Engl J Med 2004; 351:1106-1118
50. Kumar KS, Malet PF. Nonalcoholic steatohepatitis. Mayo Clin Proc 2000;75:733-739
51. Angulo P. Nonalcoholic fatty liver disease. N Engl J Med 2002;346:1221-1231
52. Felber JP, Golay A. Pathways from obesity to diabetes. Int J Obes Relat Metab Disord 2002;26(suppl 2):S39-S45
53. Evans JL, Goldfine ID, Maddux BA, Grodsky GM. Oxidative stress and stress-activated signaling pathways: a unifying hypothesis of type 2 diabetes. Endocr Rev 2002;23:599-622
54. Chen J, Muntner P, Hamm LL, et al. Insulin resistance and risk of chronic kidney disease in nondiabetic US adults. J Am Soc Nephrol 2003;14:469-477
55. Utiger RD. Insulin and the polycystic ovary syndrome. N Engl J Med 1996;335:657–658
56. Renehan AG, Zwahlen M, Minder C, et al. Insulin-like growth factor (IGF)-I, IGF binding protein-3, and cancer risk: systematic review and meta-regression analysis. Lancet 2004;363:1346-1353
57. Dunaif A, Thomas A. Current concepts in the polycystic ovary syndrome. Annu Rev Med 2001;52:401-419
58. Attoub S, Noe V, Pirola L, et al. Leptin promotes invasiveness of kidney and colonic epithelial cells via phosphoinositide 3-kinase–, rho-, and rac-dependent signaling pathways. FASEB J 2000;14:2329-2338
59. Mareel M, Leroy A. Clinical, cellular, and molecular aspects of cancer invasion. Physiol Rev 2003;83:337-376
60. Faruqi TR, Gomez D, Bustelo XR, et al. Rac1 mediates STAT3 activation by autocrine IL-6. Proc Natl Acad Sci U S A 2001;98:9014-9019
61. Rose DP, Komninou D, Stephenson GD. Obesity, adipocytokines, and insulin resistance in breast cancer. Obes Rev 2004;5:153-165
62. Mantzoros C, Petridou E, Dessypris N, et al. Adiponectin and breast cancer risk. J Clin Endocrinol Metab 2004; 89:1102-1107
63. Malin A, Dai Q, Yu H, et al. Evaluation of the synergistic effect of insulin resistance and insulin-like growth factors on the risk of breast carcinoma. Cancer 2004;100: 694-700
64. Hammarsten J, Hogstedt B. Clinical, haemodynamic, anthropometric, metabolic and insulin profile of men with high-stage and high-grade clinical prostate cancer. Blood Press 2004;13:47-55
65. Laukkanen JA, Laaksonen DE, Niskanen L, et al. Metabolic syndrome and the risk of prostate cancer in Finnish men: a population-based study. Cancer Epidemiol Biomarkers Prev 2004;13:1646-1650
66. Komninou D, Ayonote A, Richie JP Jr, Rigas B. Insulin resistance and its contribution to colon carcinogenesis. Exp Biol Med (Maywood) 2003;228:396-405

67. Stattin P, Lukanova A, Biessy C, et al. Obesity and colon cancer: does leptin provide a link? Int J Cancer 2004; 109:149-152
68. Vanitallie TB. Frailty in the elderly: contributions of sarcopenia and visceral protein depletion. Metabolism 2003;52(suppl 2):22-26
69. Roubenoff R. Catabolism of aging: is it an inflammatory process? Curr Opin Clin Nutr Metab Care 2003;6: 295-299
70. Spate U, Schulze PC. Proinflammatory cytokines and skeletal muscle. Curr Opin Clin Nutr Metab Care 2004; 7:265-269
71. Yaffe K, Lindquist K, Penninx BW, et al. Inflammatory markers and cognition in well-functioning African-American and white elders. Neurology 2003;61:76-80
72. McGeer EG, McGeer PL. Brain inflammation in Alzheimer disease and the therapeutic implications. Curr Pharm Des 1999;5:821-836
73. Jones RW. Inflammation and Alzheimer's disease. Lancet 2001;358:436-437
74. Engelhardt MJ, Geerlings MI, Meijer J, et al. Inflammatory proteins in plasma and the risk of dementia: the Rotterdam Study. Arch Neurol 2004;61:668-672
75. Yaffe K, Kanaya A, Lindquist K, et al. The metabolic syndrome, inflammation, and risk of cognitive decline. JAMA 2004;292:2237-2242
76. Rasgon N, Jarvik L. Insulin resistance, affective disorders, and Alzheimer's disease: review and hypothesis. J Gerontol A Biol Sci Med Sci 2004;59:178-183
77. Razay G, Wilcock GK. Hyperinsulinemia and Alzheimer's disease. Age Ageing 1994;23:396-399
78. Kuusisto J, Koivisto K, Mykkanen L, et al. Association between features of the insulin resistance syndrome and Alzheimer's disease independently of apolipoprotein E4 phenotype: cross sectional population based study. BMJ 1997;315:1045-1049
79. Ho L, Qin W, Pomp PN, et al. Diet-induced insulin resistance promotes amyloidosis in a transgenic mouse model of Alzheimer's disease. FASEB J 2004;18: 902-904
80. Wolk R, Kara T, Somers VK. Sleep-disordered breathing and cardiovascular disease. Circulation 2003;108: 9-12
81. Ip MSM, Lam B, Ng MMT, et al. Obstructive sleep apnea is independently associated with insulin resistance. Am J Respir Crit Care Med 2002;165:670-676

Section V

Interventions

Peroxisome Proliferator–Activated Receptors 12

Peroxisome proliferator–activated receptors (PPARs) play an important role in modulating pathways of glucose and lipid metabolism and inflammation.

DEFINITION

Peroxisomes are subcellular organelles. Their functions encompass

- the catabolism of hydrogen peroxide and glyoxylic acids,
- beta oxidation of very-long-chain fatty acids, and
- biosynthesis of plasmalogens.

Peroxisome proliferators are agents that increase the number of peroxisomes and activate peroxisomal beta oxidation enzymes. Peroxisome proliferators activate the expression of genes involved in fatty acid oxidation via a receptor-mediated mechanism. That receptor, functioning as a transcription factor, is termed the peroxisome proliferator–activated receptor, or PPAR.[1]

PPARs are a subfamily of the 48-member steroid/thyroid hormone nuclear receptor superfamily of transcription factors that regulate the expression of genes in response to the binding of ligands to receptors.[2] The PPARs comprise a group of three nuclear receptor isoforms, termed

1. PPAR-α (NR1C1),
2. PPAR-γ (NR1C3), and
3. PPAR-β/δ (NR1C2 or nuc1),

that are encoded by different genes. PPARs have a heterogeneous distribution in tissue (Table 12-1). They were originally identified as critical controllers for key enzymes that catalyze the oxidation of free fatty acids.[3,4]

PPAR STRUCTURE

The PPAR isoforms are proteins with similar molecular structures. The PPAR structure has at least three different functional domains:

1. the DNA binding domain,
2. the ligand binding domain, and

Table 12–1. Tissue Distribution of Peroxisome Proliferator–Activated Receptor Types

PPAR-α	PPAR-β	PPAR-γ
Liver	Ubiquitous	Adipose tissue
Heart		Large intestine
Muscle		Pancreas
Kidney		Immune cells
Intestines		Muscle
Vascular cells		Heart
Atheroma		Vascular cells
Immune cells		Liver
Testicular cells		Atheroma

Adapted from Girard J. [PPARgamma and insulin resistance.] Ann Endocrinol (Paris) 2002;63:1S19-1S22.

3. the ligand-dependent activation domain (Fig. 12-1).

The DNA binding domains of the PPAR subtypes are comparable, with 80% homology between the different isoforms.[5]

OVERVIEW OF PPAR ROLE IN METABOLISM AND INFLAMMATION

PPARs are lipid-activated nuclear receptors that mediate pleiotropic effects encompassing the control of

- growth,
- metabolism, and
- inflammation

by controlling the expression of target genes.

Tissue Growth. PPARs affect aspects of tissue growth. They play a role in

- fertility,
- cell differentiation,
- cell proliferation,
- angiogenesis,
- apoptosis,
- central nervous system (CNS) myelogenesis, and
- CNS glial cell maturation.[5]

Excessive PPAR Activation. In mice, excessive PPAR activation leads to a net loss of cholesterol and lipids from the plasma membrane caveolae that results in perturbed cellular signaling and atrophy of adipose tissue, the thymus, and the spleen. Furthermore, as the cholesterol content of hepatocyte plasma membranes is correspondingly increased, hepatocyte signaling is enhanced, which may lead to hepatic hypertrophy and actual hepatic carcinogenesis. The systemic effects of excessive PPAR activation thus bear watching.[5]

Carbohydrates. PPARs are involved in the control of glucose and in glucose homeostasis during metabolic stress. With glucose intolerance in the metabolic syndrome, dual activation of PPAR-α and PPAR-γ lowers glucose in a dose-dependent manner, thereby correcting the metabolic derangement and improving insulin sensitivity.[5]

Lipids. PPARs have a critical role as lipid sensors and are metabolic regulators affecting lipid and lipoprotein metabolism, energy balance, and lipoprotein lipase (LPL) activity. PPARs are hypolipidemic. PPAR-α and PPAR-γ use different mechanisms of lipid lowering (Table 12-2). Their dual activation lowers low-density lipoprotein (LDL) and triglyceride levels while increasing high-density lipoprotein (HDL). Dual activation lowers the respiratory quotient and decreases fat accumulation (Table 12-3).[5]

Inflammation and Atherosclerosis. PPARs are implicated in inflammatory disorders. They play a role in

- inflammatory pathways,
- insulin resistance,

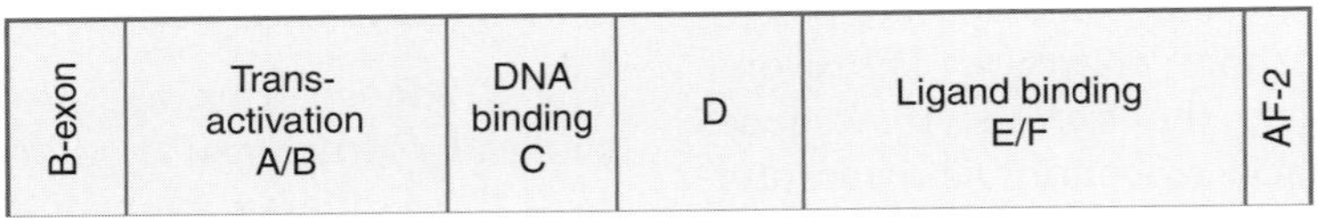

B-exon	Trans-activation A/B	DNA binding C	D	Ligand binding E/F	AF-2

▸▸ **Figure 12–1.**
Human peroxisome proliferator–activated receptor-gamma with DNA and ligand binding domains. *(Modified from Zhang X, Young HA. PPAR and the immune system—what do we know? Int Immunopharm 2002;2:1029-1044.)*

Table 12-2. Role of Peroxisome Proliferator–Activated Receptors in Regulating the Expression of Genes Involved in Lipoprotein Metabolism

PPAR-α	PPAR-γ	EFFECT
Increase		
ABCA-1	ABCA-1	Increased HDL level with enhanced reverse cholesterol transport
apo A-I apo A-II SR-B1	SR-B1	
LPL	LPL	Clearance of fasting and postprandial triglyceride
Decrease		
apo C-III		Decreased small, dense LDL with higher clearance of LDL and greater reverse cholesterol transport

ABCA-1, adenosine triphosphate–binding cassette transporter-1; apo, apolipoprotein; HDL, high-density lipoprotein; LDL, low-density lipoprotein; LPL, lipoprotein lipase; SR-B1, scavenger receptor class B type 1. Adapted from Ruotolo G, Howard BV. Dyslipidemia of the metabolic syndrome. Curr Cardiol Rep 2002;4: 494-500.

- CNS demyelination,
- infertility,
- cancer, and
- vascular inflammation and atherosclerosis.

Table 12-3. Role of Peroxisome Proliferator–Activated Receptors in Regulating the Expression of Genes Involved in Fatty Acid Metabolism

PPAR-α	PPAR-γ	EFFECT
Increase		
FATP-1 uptake	FATP-1	Increased fatty acid and storage
FAT CD36	ACS LPL	
	Adipocyte differentiation	Increased adipogenesis
CPT-1,2	Adiponectin	Increased fatty acid oxidation
Decrease		
	11β-HSD-1	Reduced visceral fat

ACS, acyl CoA synthase; CPT-1, carnitine palmitoyltransferase-1; FAT, fatty acid translocase; FATP-1, fatty acid transport protein-1; 11β-HSD-1, 11β-hydroxysteroid dehydrogenase type 1; LPL, lipoprotein lipase. Adapted from Yki-Jarvinen H. Thiazolidinediones. N Engl J Med 1004;351:1106-1118.

PPARs modulate the recruitment of leukocytes to the endothelium, regulate inflammatory cytokine production by vascular smooth muscle cells, and control the inflammatory response. Dual PPAR-α and PPAR-γ activation has an anti-inflammatory and antiatherogenic effect.[5]

PPAR MODULATION OF GENE EXPRESSION

PPARs are nuclear receptors that are activated upon the binding of ligands. PPARs affect the transcription of genes via DNA-independent and DNA-dependent pathways.

Transrepression is a DNA-independent mechanism whereby PPARs interfere with the signaling of other transcription factors. Specifically, PPARs can repress inflammatory gene transcription by negatively interfering with other signal transduction pathways, such as nuclear factor kappaB (NFκB). This approach may explain some of the anti-inflammatory actions of PPARs.[2]

Transactivation is DNA dependent, and PPARs undergo a series of steps to become transcriptionally active.[2]

Ligand Binding and Corepressor Release. PPARs are ligand-regulated transcription factors. When inactive, PPARs complex with nuclear corepressors. PPAR activation occurs upon ligand binding to the ligand binding site, which changes the conformation of PPAR and releases the corepressor. Through this conformational change, the ligand-dependent activation domain creates another PPAR binding cleft, the binding pocket for the PPAR coactivator. PPAR coactivator recruitment to the receptor is a requisite event in ligand-mediated gene activation.[1,5]

The PPAR–Retinoid X Receptor Heterodimer. The PPAR activation sequence mimics that of other nuclear receptors, such as the triiodothyronine receptor (TR) and the all-*trans* retinoic acid receptor (RAR). Upon ligand activation, these receptors, as well as the PPARs, become transcriptionally active only as heterodimers complexed with a common partner, another transcription factor, the retinoid X receptor (RXR-α, -β, or -γ). Like PPAR, the RXRs require activation by a ligand, specifically by the endogenous agonist 9-*cis* retinoic acid.[5]

PPAR Response Elements. The PPAR heterodimers control the expression of genes by binding, via the DNA binding site, to specific PPAR response elements (PPREs) within the promoter domains of target genes. Because of the similarity of the DNA binding domains, the different PPAR isoforms bind to similar PPREs.[1]

The PPREs belong to the direct-repeat (DR) category of nuclear response elements. They are composed of two hexanucleotides of the consensus nucleotide sequence AGGTCA, separated by one or two nucleotide spacers (DR1, DR2). Similar sequences are found on numerous PPAR-inducible genes.[1]

Heterodimer Coactivator. The ligand-activated, PPAR-RXR heterodimer, bound to PPRE, recruits a transcriptional coactivator to its coactivator binding pocket. The coactivator, containing histone acetylase activity, disrupts nucleosomes by opening up the chromatin structure in the vicinity of the regulatory region of the target gene. Other complexes are then recruited to provide a direct link to the basal transcription machinery, which results in the induction or increased expression of genes. The transcription of PPAR-targeted genes is thus induced or further enhanced, and new or augmented protein synthesis takes place (Fig. 12-2).[1,5]

PPAR Gene Targets. PPARs effect most of their diverse range of activities via transcription control of target genes.

PPREs have been found in the genes that encode proteins implicated in aspects of fatty acid metabolism, such as oxidation, transport, and synthesis:

- LPL,
- adipocyte fatty acid binding protein (aP2),
- fatty acid synthase,
- phosphoenolpyruvate carboxykinase (PEPCK), and
- acyl coenzyme A (CoA) oxidase.[6]

PPREs have also been found on genes encoding proteins involved in glucose homeostasis, such as

- the insulin receptor,
- components of the insulin signaling cascade,
- the p85α subunit of phosphatidylinositol 3-kinase (PI3K),
- c-Cbl–associated protein (CAP),
- glucose transporter 4 (GLUT4),
- glucokinase, and
- malic enzyme,[6]

as well as the mitochondrial uncoupling proteins (UCPs), leptin, and tumor necrosis factor-alpha (TNF-α).[7]

PPAR LIGANDS

Lipids are the principal endogenous ligands for the PPAR nuclear receptors.

The PPAR Ligand Binding Domain. The ligand binding domain in the C-terminal half of the receptor has only 65% homology between the different PPAR isoforms, thus allowing differentiation between PPAR-specific ligands. However, the PPAR ligand binding pocket is quite large, which results in low ligand specificity.[8]

PPAR Ligands. Endogenous PPAR ligands are derived from fatty acids. LPL is an endogenous pathway for generating fatty acid ligands for the

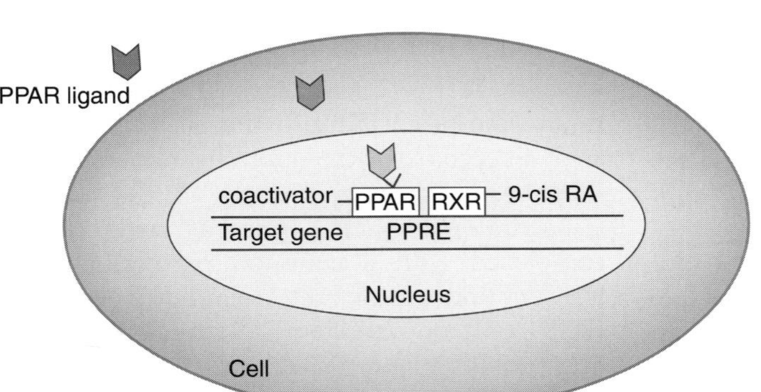

▸▸ **Figure 12–2.**
Mechanism by which peroxisome proliferator–activated receptor (PPAR) ligands alter the transcription of target genes via binding of the activated PPAR–retinoid X receptor (RXR) heterodimer plus coactivators to the PPAR response element (PPRE). *(Modified from Fruchart J-C. Peroxisome proliferator–activated receptor-alpha activation and high-density lipoprotein metabolism. Am J Cardiol 2001;88(suppl): 24N-29N.)*

PPARs via lipolysis. **The PPARs are implicated in the modification of gene expression via nutrients and may mediate some of the cardiovascular benefits accruing to high fish consumption.**[2,9] **Pharmacologic ligands have much higher binding affinity.**

Lipid-Derived Ligands. Free fatty acids and prostaglandins derived from free fatty acids have long been thought to have a regulatory role in immune functions. They participate in the complement-dependent inflammatory pathway. **Free fatty acids and their derivatives also have an impact on inflammation and metabolism by modulating DNA transcription via PPAR.** These naturally occurring PPAR ligands are active at micromolar concentrations and are composed of

- >6-carbon, long-chain, saturated and unsaturated free fatty acids,
- the esters derived from free fatty acids with CoA,
- further derivatives of free fatty acids via the cyclooxygenase (COX) or the lipoxygenase pathway, before fatty acid beta oxidation, and
- derivatives of arachidonic acid via the lipoxygenase and COX pathways, leukotriene, and prostaglandin eicosanoids.[10]

PPAR-γ has polyunsaturated fatty acids—linoleic acid, linolenic acid, arachidonic acid, eicosapentaenoic acid, and prostaglandins—as preferred ligands. PPAR-α is readily activated by a variety of saturated and unsaturated fatty acids, including palmitic, oleic, linoleic, and arachidonic acids. PPAR-δ interacts with saturated and unsaturated fatty acids, with a ligand specificity intermediate to that of PPAR-γ and PPAR-α.[10]

Pharmacologic Agents. The natural, fatty acid–derivative ligands are less potent than the pharmacologic, synthetic ligands, which may be active at nanomolar concentrations.[6] Pharmacologic ligands have not yet been optimized. **Fibric acids are activators for PPAR-α, whereas thiazolidinediones are ligands for PPAR-γ.** Nonsteroidal anti-inflammatory agents are also low-affinity ligands for PPAR-α and PPAR-γ. Dual PPAR-α and PPAR-γ activators are under development and may be of interest because they combine the insulin-sensitizing effects of PPAR-γ and the lipid-modulating activities of PPAR-α agonists. Dual PPAR activators may diminish the undesirable PPAR-γ side effect of enhanced adipogenesis via PPAR-α–stimulated lipid catabolism.[10]

PPAR-α

PPAR-α is a specific transcription factor. Upon ligand activation, it is responsible for pleiotropic effects encompassing metabolic, antioxidant, anti-inflammatory, vascular-protective, and insulin-sensitizing actions.

Tissue Expression. PPAR-α is highly expressed in tissues with high rates of fatty acid beta oxidation, such as

- hepatocytes,
- cardiac myocytes,
- skeletal myocytes,
- renal cells, and
- brown adipocytes.

PPAR-α is moderately expressed in

- enterocytes,
- vascular endothelial cells,
- vascular smooth muscle cells,
- monocytic cells,
- the thymus, and
- testicular cells.[11]

PPAR-α Activators. Fatty acids are known to activate PPAR-α. Structurally diverse ligands such as

- saturated and unsaturated fatty acids,
- unsaturated fatty acid derivatives,
- leukotriene eicosanoids (8*S*-hydroxyeicosatetraenoic acid [8*S*-HETE], leukotriene B_4), and
- fibric acid derivatives such as fenofibrate, bezafibrate, ciprofibrate, and gemfibrozil

activate PPAR-α (Table 12-4). Fasting also increases hepatic PPAR–α mRNA levels.[10,12]

PPAR-α Effects. Activation of PPAR-α influences lipoprotein metabolism, enhances free fatty acid uptake and oxidation, and controls the expression of multiple genes regulating

Table 12-4. Peroxisome Proliferator–Activated Receptor-α Activators

Saturated, unsaturated, and polyunsaturated fatty acids
Eicosanoids
Fibric acid derivatives

lipoprotein concentrations. **PPAR-α agonists have anti-inflammatory effects. They prevent or retard atherosclerosis in mice and humans and have insulin-sensitizing effects** (Table 12-5).[2]

Free Fatty Acid Metabolism. PPAR-α plays a critical role in maintaining the constitutive beta oxidation of fatty acids, as well as in mediating the metabolic responses to starvation. PPAR-α mechanisms provide energy primarily to cardiac and skeletal myocytes and are implicated in thermogenesis via UCPs 1, 2, and 3.[13-15]

Specifically, PPAR-α actions control fatty acid metabolic pathways such as

- fatty acid uptake into mitochondria,
- fatty acid activation into acyl CoA esters,
- fatty acid degradation via peroxisomal and mitochondrial beta oxidation,
- ketone body synthesis, and
- thermogenesis.[16]

To that effect, PPAR-α ligands regulate mRNA levels for enzymes and proteins that play an important role in global fatty acid homeostasis, such as

- fatty acid transport protein (FATP and FAT),
- fatty acid binding protein,
- 3-hydroxyacyl CoA dehydrogenase (HAD),
- long-chain fatty acyl CoA synthase (ACS),
- enoyl CoA hydratase,
- keto-acyl CoA thiolase,
- carnitine palmitoyltransferase I (CPT-I),
- pyruvate dehydrogenase kinase 4 (PDHK4),
- malonyl CoA decarboxylase (MCD),
- acyl CoA dehydrogenase,
- 3-hydroxy-3-methylglutaryl CoA (HMG-CoA) synthase, and
- UCPs 1, 2, and 3.

Table 12-5. Peroxisome Proliferator–Activated Receptor-α Biologic Functions

Fatty acid metabolism
Lipoprotein metabolism
Anti-inflammatory activities
Insulin sensitization

Adapted from Duval C, Chinetti G, Trottein F, et al. The role of PPARs in atherosclerosis. Trends Mol Med 2002;8:422-430.

The metabolic effects of pharmacologic PPAR-α activation may prevent high-fat diet–induced gains in body weight and adipose tissue mass in the absence of reducing caloric intake.[13]

PPAR-α ligands stimulate diverse aspects of fatty oxidative metabolism in different organs.

Skeletal Muscle. In humans, PPAR-α protein expression occurs during muscle cell differentiation, and skeletal muscle is a major site of PPAR-α expression. Skeletal muscle is the principal tissue responsible for fatty acid uptake and utilization. **PPAR-α activation increases the beta oxidation of fatty acids while decreasing the esterification of fatty acids for ectopic triacylglycerol storage in myocytes.**[15]

Hepatic–Plasma Lipid Effects. Promotion of muscle lipid catabolism suggests one mechanism for the hypolipidemic effects of PPAR-α activation. Perhaps more importantly, PPAR-α agonists stimulate reverse cholesterol transport.

PPAR-α activation in the liver regulates hepatic lipid metabolism and up-regulates the expression of genes encoding proteins involved in HDL structure, function, and metabolism. Five of these genes code for

1. apolipoprotein (apo) A-I,
2. apo A-II,
3. LPL,
4. scavenger receptor class B type 1 (SR-B1) or its human analogue CLA-I, and
5. adenosine triphosphate–binding cassette transporter-1 (ABCA-1) (Fig. 12-3).[17]

With activation of PPAR-α, peripheral cholesterol efflux is enhanced. By inducing the expression of apo A-I and A-II, PPAR-α ligands

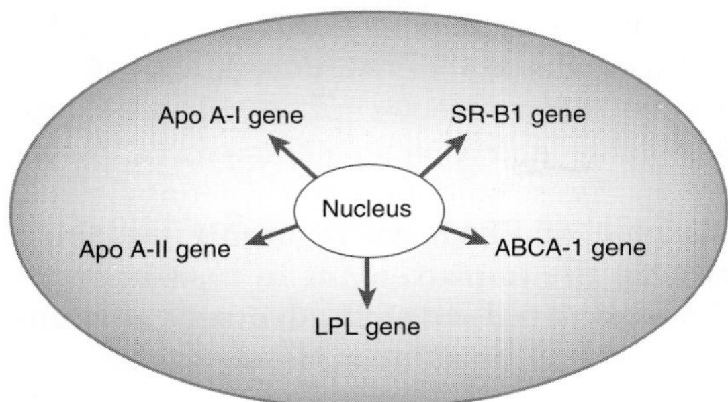

Figure 12–3.
Five key genes in high-density lipoprotein metabolism that are up-regulated by peroxisome proliferator–activated receptor-alpha ligands. ABCA-1, adenosine triphosphate–binding cassette transporter-1; Apo, apolipoprotein; LPL, lipoprotein lipase, SR-B1, scavenger receptor class B type 1. *(Modified from Fruchart J-C. Peroxisome proliferator–activated receptor-alpha activation and high-density lipoprotein metabolism. Am J Cardiol 2001;88(suppl):24N-29N.)*

increase HDL production.[18] The increased expression of ABCA-1 enhances the early steps of unesterified cholesterol and phospholipid efflux from cells such as macrophages and foam cells for uptake by HDL and reverse cholesterol transport. PPAR-α induces expression of the scavenger receptor SR-B1 or its human analogue CLA-I, thereby allowing these cell surface receptors to more effectively bind HDL and mediate the uptake of cholesteryl esters from HDL into steroidogenic tissues and the liver.[4,17] The higher expression of LPL, together with suppression of hepatic apo C-III genes, lowers the level of circulating triglycerides, which benefits HDL levels.[5]

Antioxidant Effects. PPAR-α agonists decrease oxidant stress. Activation of PPAR-α decreases expression of the superoxide-generating enzyme nicotinamide adenine dinucleotide phosphate (NADH/NADPH) oxidase and increases expression of the superoxide scavenger enzyme Cu^{2+}, Zn^{2+}-superoxide dismutase (CuZn-SOD), thereby reducing endothelial oxidative stress.[4,19]

Anti-inflammatory Effects. Activated PPAR-α has multiple anti-inflammatory effects in endothelial and smooth muscle cells and macrophages:

- Leukotriene B_4, actually a proinflammatory molecule, is a ligand agonist for PPAR-α and appears to inhibit the inflammatory response by augmenting the expression of enzymes involved in leukotriene catabolism, effectively stimulating its own degradation via negative feedback.[5]
- PPAR-α activation induces inhibitory protein IkappaB (IκB) levels, thereby suppressing NFκB signaling and inhibiting both macrophage and vascular smooth muscle cell inflammatory responses.[5]
- PPAR-α activation lowers basal and elevated C-reactive protein (CRP) levels in humans via suppression of interleukin-1 (IL-1)-, but not IL-6–induced expression of CRP in primary human hepatocytes at the transcriptional level. IL-1 induces CRP expression through two overlapping response elements, the binding sites for CCAAT-box/enhancer-binding protein-beta (C/EBP-β) and p50-NFκB. PPAR-α suppresses CRP by enhancing IκB-α expression and by preventing p50-NFκB translocation to the nucleus.[19-21]
- In human aortic smooth muscle cells, PPAR-α ligands inhibit IL-1–induced IL-6 and COX-2 gene transcription, thereby decreasing IL-6 and 6-keto-prostaglandin $F_{1\alpha}$ ($PGF_{1\alpha}$) secretion.[19]
- PPAR-α agonists thwart cytokine-induced expression of vascular cell adhesion molecule-1 (VCAM-1)[22] and inhibit the expression of monocyte chemotactic protein-1 (MCP-1) by endothelial cells stimulated by CRP. Via suppression of NFκB, PPAR-α inhibits the TNF-α–induced endothelial production of intercellular adhesion molecule-1 (ICAM-1).[23]
- PPAR-α activators inhibit expression of macrophage-inducible nitric oxide synthase (iNOS).[4,19]
- PPAR-α ligands down-regulate platelet-activating factor (PAF) receptor gene expression by human monocytes and macrophages.[4,19]

Patients receiving fenofibrate as a PPAR-α activator have lower plasma CRP, fibrinogen, and IL-6 concentrations. TNF-α levels are also lowered in hyperlipidemics.[23]

Stress Impact on PPAR-α. Angiotensin II is a negative modulator of PPAR-α. It down-regulates PPAR-α mRNA and protein, thus

diminishing the anti-inflammatory potential of PPAR-α and enhancing vascular inflammation.[24]

Antithrombotic Effects. PPAR-α has an effect on thrombogenesis.

PPAR-α mechanisms negatively regulate the surface elaboration of tissue factor by human monocytes and macrophages. Levels of plasma fibrinogen, a procoagulant factor, are decreased in a PPAR-α–dependent manner.[4] Effects on plasminogen activator inhibitor-1 (PAI-1) are inconsistent.[13]

Vascular Effects. PPAR-α affects vasomotion. It negatively interferes with the DNA binding activities of the heterodimer transcription factor AP-1, thus repressing thrombin-induced expression of the vasoconstrictor endothelin-1.[4,25]

The anti-inflammatory and antithrombotic effects of PPAR-α activation suggest its potential impact on lowering the risk for coronary heart disease (CHD) (Table 12-6). Beneficial effects have been seen in a mouse model of atherosclerosis and in several clinical and angiographic end point trials.[4]

Insulin Sensitization. The metabolic, anti-inflammatory, and antioxidant impact of PPAR-α activation would also be expected to have a favorable impact on insulin sensitivity.

Table 12-6. Peroxisome Proliferator–Activated Receptor-α Antiatherogenic Effects

SITE	ANTIATHEROGENIC SUPPRESSION
Endothelial cells	VCAM-1
	ICAM-1
	Endothelin-1
	MCP-1
Smooth muscle cells	IL-6
	COX-2
	Prostaglandin F1-alpha
Monocytes/ macrophages	Tissue factor
	NFκB
	TNF-α
	PAF
	iNOS
Hepatocytes	CRP

COX-2, cyclooxygenase-2; CRP, C-reactive protein; ICAM-1, intercellular adhesion molecule-1; IL-6, interleukin-6; iNOS, inducible nitric oxide synthase; MCP-1, monocyte chemotactic protein-1; NFκB, nuclear factor kappaB; PAF, platelet-activating factor; TNF, tumor necrosis factor; VCAM-1, vascular cell adhesion molecule-1.

Glucose Metabolism. PPAR-α activation reduces insulin resistance. In genetic and dietary rodent models of insulin resistance, fenofibrate and ciprofibrate improved insulin action, glucose utilization, and hyperinsulinemia. **Because of PPAR-α's favorable metabolic effects, the improvement in insulin sensitivity occurred without adversely affecting body weight or adipose tissue mass.**[13]

Hepatic Insulin Sensitivity. PPAR-α agonists beneficially affect hepatic glucocorticoid metabolism, which may also benefit glucose homeostasis. 11β-Hydroxysteroid dehydrogenase type 1 (11β-HSD-1) is an enzyme that converts cortisone to the active glucocorticoid cortisol. 11β-HSD-1 is highly expressed in the visceral adipose depot and is also present in the liver. Cortisol-cortisone interconversion is instrumental in the hepatic regulation of glucose metabolism inasmuch as higher cortisol levels may be formed directly in the liver or be presented to the liver via the portal vein in the presence of visceral adiposity. **PPAR-α ligands down-regulate hepatic 11β-HSD-1 expression and activity after chronic treatment, thus decreasing the hepatic glucocorticoid effects favoring glycogenolysis and gluconeogenesis.**[26]

Ectopic Intracellular Lipid. Intrahepatocellular and intramyocellular lipid concentrations correlate with insulin resistance in humans. Cytosolic lipids may accumulate via increased fluxes of fatty acids into nonadipose tissues as engendered by antiadipogenic forces, or via reduced beta oxidation of fatty acid in the affected recipient organs (or via both mechanisms).

Important determinants of the partitioning of fatty acids toward oxidation and consumption versus esterification and storage are

- CPT-I, the enzyme that catalyzes the rate-limiting step in the translocation of long-chain fatty acyl CoAs into the inner membrane of mitochondria to be oxidized;
- malonyl CoA, a potent, allosteric inhibitor of CPT-I and thus a key regulator favoring fatty acid biosynthesis over oxidation; and
- acetyl CoA carboxylase (ACC), the rate-limiting enzyme for malonyl CoA formation.[15,27]

PPAR-α activation increases fatty acid oxidation and decreases ectopic intracellular triacylglycerol content by

- decreasing malonyl CoA formation via ACC,
- increasing malonyl CoA degradation, and
- increasing CPT-I expression,

thus enhancing sensitivity to insulin signaling.

Acetyl CoA Carboxylase. ACC, the rate-limiting enzyme for malonyl CoA formation, exists as two major isoforms:

1. ACC1 (ACC-α), implicated in fatty acid synthesis, and
2. ACC2 (ACC-β), implicated in the control of mitochondrial beta oxidation.

The ACC isoforms can be regulated at the level of

- gene expression,
- allosteric regulation of the enzyme, and
- reversible phosphorylation by adenosine 5′-monophosphate–activated protein kinase (AMPK), which inactivates ACC in cardiac and skeletal myocytes.

ACC is an important target for PPAR-α agonists, which repress expression of the ACC gene. As a result,

1. **PPAR-α inhibition of ACC-α decreases synthesis of the lipid component of very-low-density lipoprotein (VLDL), and**
2. **PPAR-α inhibition of ACC-β leads to a decrease in malonyl CoA levels and disinhibition of fatty acid oxidation,**

thus partitioning fatty acids toward oxidation and consumption and away from esterification and storage.[28]

Malonyl CoA Decarboxylase. Activated PPAR-α enhances fatty acid oxidation by lowering the concentration of malonyl CoA. MCD catalyzes the decarboxylation of malonyl CoA. As such, it plays an important role in the regulation of intracellular malonyl CoA concentration and fatty acid metabolism. Increased expression of MCD corresponds with lower levels of malonyl CoA and a higher rate of fatty acid oxidation.[29]

1. Liver. PPAR-α ligands activate the transcription of rat hepatic MCD by binding to PPREs in the promoter region, thus lowering malonyl CoA and enhancing fatty acid oxidation.[30]
2. Muscle. Mature skeletal muscle in humans is a major site for PPAR-α expression. A highly selective PPAR-α agonist, GW7647, induces mRNA expression of mitochondrial enzymes that promote fatty acid catabolism, such that CPT-I and MCD increase approximately twofold.[15] Similar effects of specific PPAR-α stimulation are seen in cardiac muscle.[29,31]

Carnitine Palmitoyltransferase I. CPT-I catalyzes the translocation of activated fatty acids into mitochondria for oxidation. PPAR-α activation increases expression of the CPT-I gene.[32] In a spontaneous type 2 diabetic animal model, the Otsuka Long-Evans Tokushima Fatty rat, 7-week chow supplementation with fenofibrate significantly increased hepatic mRNA levels of FAT/CD36 and mitochondrial CPT-I.[33]

Safety Considerations. There are residual concerns about the long-term impact of PPAR-α activation. PPAR-α ligands affect gene transcription, secretion, and the gelatinolytic activity of matrix metalloproteinase-9 (MMP-9) in response to cytokines, which might destabilize atheromatous plaque.[4]

PPAR-α activation induces peroxisome proliferation and DNA synthesis in hepatocytes. It may contribute to hepatic hypertrophy and tumorigenesis, as observed in rodent models.[3]

PPAR-γ

By activating the transcription of genes involved in lipogenesis, fatty acid esterification, adipocyte differentiation, and inflammation, PPAR-γ plays a key role in adipogenesis, control of insulin sensitivity, and inflammation (Table 12-7).

Tissue Expression. PPAR-γ is primarily expressed in

- brown and white adipocytes,
- enterocytes,
- pancreatic beta cells,

Table 12-7. Changes in Gene Expression in Adipose Tissue by Peroxisome Proliferator–Activated Receptor-γ Agonists and Their Function

INCREASED EXPRESSION	FUNCTION
Adipocyte fatty acid binding protein	Intracellular fatty acid binding
Acyl CoA synthase	Lipogenesis or catabolism
Lipoprotein lipase	Hydrolysis of triglyceride-bound particles
CD36	Cell surface fatty acid transporter
Fatty acid transport protein-1	Cell surface fatty acid transporter
Uncoupling proteins 1/3	Uncouple mitochondrial respiration
Carnitine palmitoyltransferase-1	Fatty acid translocation into mitochondria
c-Cbl–associated protein	Insulin signaling for glucose transport
Adiponectin	Beneficial metabolic effects
Insulin receptor substrate-2	Insulin receptor signaling
DECREASED EXPRESSION	**FUNCTION**
Tumor necrosis factor-alpha	Proinflammatory cytokine, potential mediator of insulin resistance
Leptin	Proinflammatory cytokine, inhibits food intake
11β-Hydroxysteroid dehydrogenase type 1	Intracellular conversion to active cortisol

Adapted from Berger J, Moller DE. The mechanisms of action of PPARs. Annu Rev Med 2002;53:409-435.

- activated lymphocytes, and
- monocytes/macrophages.

PPAR-γ is also expressed in

- skeletal muscle,
- cardiac myocytes,
- vascular endothelial cells,
- vascular smooth muscle cells,
- the liver, and
- human atherosclerotic lesions.[2,24,34]

PPAR-γ mRNA levels are up to 50-fold higher in adipose tissue than in skeletal muscle. In general, PPAR-γ expression is low in tissues that express predominantly PPAR-α, such as the liver, heart, and skeletal muscle.[2]

PPAR-γ is expressed as two major isoforms that are structurally very similar and have no clear functional differences:

1. PPAR-γ_1 is expressed in a variety of tissues, including adipose tissue, liver, skeletal and cardiac muscle, and macrophages;
2. PPAR-γ_2 is highly and specifically expressed in adipocytes.

Ectopic expression of PPAR-γ_2 has been shown to promote adipogenesis. The ratio of PPAR-γ_2 to PPAR-γ_1 is positively correlated with body mass index (BMI), with PPAR-γ_1 decreasing and PPAR-γ_2 increasing as a function of BMI.[6,35,36]

PPAR-γ Activators. Fatty acids and their derivatives are known to activate PPAR-γ. Natural ligands for PPAR-γ are

- the leukotriene 15-HETE,
- the prostanoid 15δ-PGJ_2,
- pristanic acid,
- phytanic acid,
- oxidized linoleic acid, and
- some components of oxidized LDL, such as hydroxyoctadecadienoic acid (9-HODE), 13-HODE, and 15-HODE, and
- polyunsaturated fatty acids,

all with relatively low binding affinity in the micromolar range. 15δ-PGJ_2 also signals through other means, such as by stabilizing Iκ kinase.[37] Thiazolidinediones are pharmacologic ligands with PPAR-γ binding affinity in the nanomolar range (Table 12-8).[6]

PPAR-γ Effects. Activation of PPAR-γ regulates genes involved in adipocyte differentiation, intravascular lipolysis, fatty acid uptake and storage, and glucose uptake. It also modulates inflammatory pathways, vascular health, and insulin sensitivity (Table 12-9).[2]

Plasma Lipids. PPAR-γ agonists may have a favorable impact on plasma lipids by lowering plasma triglyceride levels while increasing HDL. They enhance the expression of

Table 12-8. Peroxisome Proliferator–Activated Receptor-γ Activators

Polyunsaturated fatty acids
The prostaglandin 15δ -PGJ_2
15-Hydroxyeicosatetraenoic acid
Oxidized linolenic acid: 9*S*, 13*S*-hydroxyoctadecadienoic acid
Thiazolidinediones

Table 12-9. Peroxisome Proliferator–Activated Receptor-γ Biologic Functions

Lipid metabolism
Cellular differentiation
Adipogenesis
Lipid storage
Anti-inflammatory activities
Vascular effects
Macrophage lipid homeostasis
Modulation of insulin action
Carbohydrate metabolism

genes for proteins involved in lipid metabolism, such as

- LPL,
- ACS,
- FATP-1, and
- CD36,[38]

thereby increasing intravascular lipolysis and clearance of triglyceride-rich lipoproteins while enhancing fatty acid uptake and lipid storage in adipocytes.[5,6,18]

PPAR-γ ligands may also contribute to reverse cholesterol transport. The apo E gene in macrophages, which encodes a protein promoting cholesterol efflux to HDL, is increased by PPAR-γ ligands. PPAR-γ is also implicated in up-regulating the macrophage scavenger receptor SR-B1/CLA-I and ABCA-1, which are involved in the early steps of cholesterol efflux from foam cells.[4]

Antioxidant Effects. PPAR-γ agonists reduce vascular oxidative stress. Activation of PPAR-γ decreases expression of the superoxide-generating enzyme NADH/NADPH and increases expression of the superoxide scavenger enzyme CuZn-SOD. A reduction in endothelial oxidative stress may lower LDL oxidation and ultimately lessen foam cell formation in atheromata.[4]

Anti-inflammatory Effects. PPAR-γ activation has anti-inflammatory effects. In the vascular wall, in immune cells, and in lymphoid organs, in concert with RXR, PPAR-γ can inhibit the activation of NFκB by negatively interfering with the NFκB, signal transducer and activator of transcription (STAT), and AP-1 signaling pathways.[5,39-41] PPAR-γ activators thus inhibit the induction of genes for biologically active, proinflammatory compounds derived from vascular and immune cells, such as

- IL-1β,
- IL-2,
- IL-6,
- IL-8,
- TNF-α, and
- MMPs.

With lower levels of IL-6, plasma levels of CRP are also decreased.[4]

Immune Cell Modulation. Endogenous PPAR-γ ligands modulate immune and inflammatory cells:

- Suppression of the activated transcription factors NFκB and AP-1 by PPAR-γ activators blocks T-lymphocyte proliferation and inflammatory cytokine expression.
- In T lymphocytes, PPAR-γ ligands inhibit IL-2 production by negatively interacting with the T-cell–specific transcription factor NFAT.
- PPAR-γ ligands decrease T-lymphocyte viability via apoptosis, thus further impairing T-lymphocyte proliferation.[23]
- PPAR-γ ligands inhibit the interferon-γ–mediated endothelial elaboration of major chemoattractants for T lymphocytes, the cysteine X–amino acid–cysteine (CXC) chemokines.[38] CXC chemokines participate in the differentiation and development of type 1 and type 2 T lymphocytes and natural killer cells.
- In antigen-presenting dendritic cells, PPAR-γ agonists down-modulate the secretion of IL-12, thereby interfering with the polarization of acquired immune responses.
- Surface expression of the costimulatory surface molecules CD80 and CD86 is negatively affected by PPAR-γ ligands, as is the synthesis of interferon-γ–inducible protein-10 and RANTES, all chemokines involved in the recruitment of type 1 T cells. This alters the balance of type 1/type 2 vascular T cells to favor a type 2 response.[23]

Vascular Inflammation. PPAR-γ has an impact on vascular inflammatory processes. The effects are most pronounced with the least selective PPAR–γ agonist, 15δ-PGJ$_2$.[4] All the major cell types in the vasculature express PPAR-γ, including endothelial cells, vascular smooth muscle cells, and monocytes/macrophages. Activation of PPAR–γ in these vascular cells modulates the production of chemokines and adhesion molecules. **These PPAR-γ effects may contribute to a reduction in arterial inflammation, atherosclerotic plaque remodeling, extracellular matrix degradation, and plaque rupture[23]:**

- PPAR-γ activators inhibit the cytokine-induced expression of VCAM-1 at the transcriptional level.
- PPAR-γ attenuates the endothelial cell production of CXC chemokines and IL-8, thereby interfering with the recruitment of activated T cells.
- In endothelial cells, PPAR-γ activators inhibit the TNF-α–induced expression of lectin-like, oxidized, LDL receptor-1 (LOX-1).
- PPAR-γ ligands decrease the promoter activity for genes such as iNOS by macrophages.
- PPAR-γ activation inhibits monocyte expression of chemokine receptors such as the CCR2 receptor for MCP-1, thus impeding MCP-1–instigated chemotaxis and trans-endothelial migration of monocytes.
- PPAR-γ activators reduce the uptake of lipids by macrophages from LPL hydrolysis of chylomicron and VLDL triglycerides.
- PPAR-γ effects on the macrophage scavenger receptor SR–A may decrease foam cell formation.[4]
- PPAR-γ activity limits inflammation by inducing apoptosis in monocytes/macrophages.[38]
- PPAR-γ ligands repress the gene transcription and activity of MMP-9 in monocytes/macrophages in response to cytokines.[4]

Inflammation/Stress Impact on PPAR-γ. Modulators of stress and inflammation decrease the expression of PPAR-γ, thus diminishing the anti-inflammatory potential of PPAR-γ and contributing to enhanced vascular inflammation and insulin resistance:

- Angiotensin II is a negative modulator of PPAR-γ. It down-regulates PPAR-γ mRNA and protein.[24]
- TNF-α significantly decreases the expression of both isoforms of PPAR-γ. In human adipocytes, the attenuated expression of PPAR-γ mRNA mediated by TNF-α limits the expansion of adipose tissue (Fig. 12-4).[35]

Vascular Smooth Muscle Antiproliferative and Antimigratory Effects. Activation of PPAR-γ interferes with smooth muscle cell contraction, proliferation, and migration.

Proliferation. PPAR-γ ligands inhibit vascular smooth muscle cell proliferation. The antiproliferative effects of PPAR-γ ligands are mediated by targeting critical cell cycle regulators, including Rb and p27(Kip1), that regulate the progression of cells from the G_1 phase to the S phase for DNA synthesis.[42] Crucial factors for this transition are blocked, such as the induction

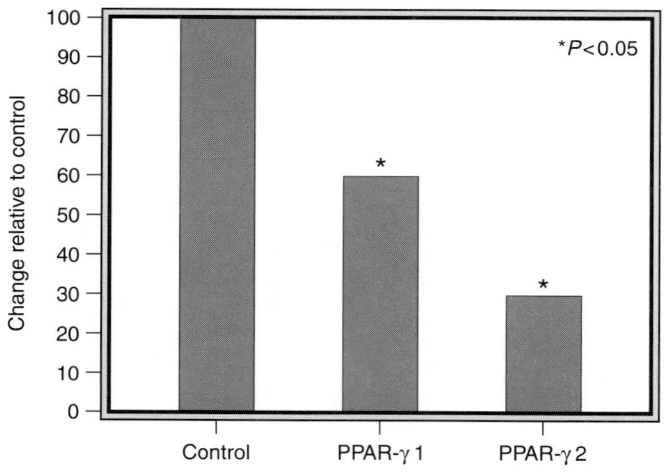

▸▸ **Figure 12–4.** Impaired expression of peroxisome proliferator–activated receptor (PPAR)-gamma isoforms in human adipocytes consequent to tumor necrosis factor-alpha exposure. *(Modified from Sewter C, Blows F, Considine R, et al. Differential effects of adiposity on peroxisomal proliferator–activated receptor gamma1 and gamma2 messenger ribonucleic acid expression in human adipocytes. J Clin Endocrinol Metab 2002;87:4203-4207.)*

of cyclin D1 and the degradation of cyclin-dependent kinase inhibitors, which leads to inhibition of retinoblastoma protein phosphorylation.[4]

Furthermore, PPAR-γ ligands thwart the expression of receptors implicated in vascular smooth muscle contraction, hypertrophy, proliferation, and migration. Specifically, the IL-1β–induced expression of the receptor for the potent smooth muscle mitogen platelet-derived growth factor-alpha (PDGF-α) is inhibited, as is expression of the angiotensin II type 1 (AT_1) receptor.[4]

Migration. PPAR-γ activation inhibits vascular smooth muscle cell migration. In addition to effects on the AT_1 receptor, vascular smooth muscle migration is inhibited by blocking expression of the transcription factor Ets-1, which is required for the induction of MMPs.[4]

Antithrombotic Effects. PPAR-γ mechanisms have an effect on thrombotic processes. In macrophages, transcription of thromboxane synthase mRNA is suppressed, and in vascular smooth muscle cells, expression of the thromboxane receptor is decreased, thus resulting in diminished thromboxane-mediated platelet aggregation and vasoconstriction. PPAR-γ effects on PAI-1 are conflicting.[4]

Endothelial Function. PPAR-γ agonists have a favorable impact on endothelial function. They suppress the secretion of endothelin-1 and stimulate the release of endothelial-derived nitric oxide (NO) from multiple vascular sites.[25] PPAR-γ ligands appear to increase the release of NO through a transcriptional mechanism that is unrelated to the expression of endothelial nitric oxide synthase (eNOS).[43] PPAR-γ activators also enhance secretion of the endothelially derived vasodilator C-type natriuretic peptide (CNP), and they promote endothelial cell growth.[4]

Vasculoprotective Effects. PPAR-γ ligands have vasculoprotective, antiatherogenic effects (Table 12-10). The expression and activation of PPAR-γ in vascular cells may protect the vasculature against injury by

- lowering oxidative stress,
- suppressing vascular inflammation,
- improving endothelial function, and
- inhibiting cell growth and migration.

In experimental models of atherosclerosis, PPAR-γ ligands prevent the progression of lesions. In humans, treatment with PPAR-γ agonists decreases the intimal and medial thickness of carotid arteries and improves coronary endothelial function.[4] A reduction in insulin resistance may play a contributory role.

Insulin Sensitization. Activation of PPAR-γ potentiates adipogenesis with adipocyte differentiation and anabolic lipid metabolism. Enhanced adipogenesis, with a concomitant reduction in visceral adiposity, contributes to the adipocyte-centered, insulin-sensitizing effects of PPAR-γ agonists.

Table 12-10. Peroxisome Proliferator–Activated Receptor-γ: Potential Antiatherogenic Effects

SITE	ANTIATHEROGENIC EFFECTS	
	Decreased	*Increased*
Endothelial cells	CXC chemokine Endothelin-1 PAI-1 IL-8 LOX-1 VCAM-1 NADH/NADPH	NO production CNP Growth
Smooth muscle cells	Migration Growth AT_1 receptor	
Monocyte/macrophage	CCR2 receptor iNOS SR-A MMP-9 Thromboxane	Apoptosis
Lymphocytes	NFκB IL-2 IL-12 CD80, CD86	Apoptosis
Circulation	IL-6 TNF-α CRP Triglycerides Free fatty acids Small, dense LDL	Adiponectin HDL

AT_1, angiotensin II type 1; CNP, C-type natriuretic peptide; CRP, C-reactive protein; CXC, cysteine X–amino acid–cysteine; HDL, high-density lipoprotein; IL, interleukin; iNOS, inducible nitric oxide synthase; LDL, low-density lipoprotein; LOX-1, lectin-like, oxidized, LDL receptor-1; MMP-9, matrix metalloproteinase-9; NFκB, nuclear factor kappaB; NO, nitric oxide; PAI-1, plasminogen activator inhibitor-1; SR-A, scavenger receptor A; TNF, tumor necrosis factor; VCAM-1, vascular cell adhesion molecule-1.

Adipogenesis. PPAR-γ engenders the expansion of adipose tissue, thereby enhancing the disposal of surplus calories within an appropriate lipid storage depot. In effect, **PPAR-γ ligands counteract factors conducive to the genesis of insulin resistance, such as elevated levels of free fatty acids and ectopic lipid storage.**

There is ectopic expression of PPAR-γ in adipocyte precursors, fibroblasts, and myoblasts in order to facilitate adipogenesis. Transient overexpression of PPAR-γ in fibroblasts induces an adipocyte-like phenotype.[44] PPAR-γ activation triggers the differentiation of fibroblasts or other undifferentiated cells into mature adipocytes.[5,6,18]

Decreased Visceral Adiposity. Although PPAR-γ agonists increase subcutaneous adiposity, they decrease visceral/omental fat by lowering glucocorticoid metabolism within adipose tissue. In contrast to subcutaneous fat, visceral/omental fat is metabolically labile and endocrinologically very active. Visceral, not subcutaneous, fat is primarily associated with the development of insulin resistance. **The reduction in the visceral adipose depot and fat redistribution to a subcutaneous locale may contribute to the insulin-sensitizing effects of PPAR-γ agonists by favorably diminishing the visceral release of humoral mediators of insulin resistance.**

In adipocytes, PPAR-γ ligands markedly inhibit gene expression for the enzyme 11β-HSD-1, which converts cortisone to the active glucocorticoid agonist cortisol. As a result of PPAR-γ activation, the level of active glucocorticoid within adipose tissue is lower, thereby diminishing the induction of adipogenesis by glucocorticoids. Because 11β-HSD-1 is predominantly expressed in visceral/omental adipose tissue, this effect of PPAR-γ activation principally decreases visceral adiposity. In contrast, the effects of enhanced adipogenicity associated with PPAR-γ activation are manifested primarily in the subcutaneous adipose tissue depot.[36]

Impact on Adipokine Signaling. PPAR-γ activation modulates endocrine signaling from adipocytes and in the process enhances adipose sensitivity to insulin.

PPAR-γ activation enhances insulin sensitivity in adipose tissue by suppressing the elaboration of mediators that induce insulin resistance and by enhancing the production of factors that improve insulin signaling[5]:

- Activation of PPAR-γ inhibits the expression of TNF-α, which interferes with insulin signaling.
- PPAR-γ agonists inhibit expression of the leptin (*ob*) gene via a receptor-mediated mechanism whereby leptin is down-regulated, which may lower leptin resistance.
- PPAR-γ activation increases the expression of insulin receptor substrate-2 (IRS-2), which is involved in insulin signal transduction in adipose tissue.
- In cultured adipocytes, PPAR-γ increases the expression of CAP, which plays a positive role in insulin signaling pathways.
- PPAR-γ activation increases the mRNA expression and plasma level of adipocyte complement-related protein of 30 kDa (ACRP30), or adiponectin. The PPAR-γ–induced reduction in TNF-α activity probably plays a contributory role.[5]

Skeletal Muscle and Liver Insulin Sensitivity. Insulin sensitization of skeletal muscle and hepatic tissue via PPAR-γ activation probably devolves from the humoral effects engendered by the improved metabolic milieu of visceral/omental adipose tissue. Because adiponectin, in particular, is a circulating adipokine with systemic, hormonal effects, up-regulation of the adiponectin pathway by PPAR-γ probably has a favorable impact on mediators of systemic insulin sensitivity, in part by activating AMPK and lowering plasma glucose, triglycerides, and free fatty acids, as well as ectopic lipid deposition, in the process (Fig. 12-5).

Skeletal Muscle. In skeletal muscle, PPAR-γ pathways and adiponectin-activated AMPK increase the beta oxidation of lipids, which lowers the ectopic intramyocellular triglyceride content and consequently ameliorates the insulin resistance of skeletal muscle.[45]

Liver. In the liver, PPAR-γ–induced adiponectin also activates AMPK, thereby down-regulating PEPCK and glucose-6-phosphatase and engendering lower glucose output from the liver.[45]

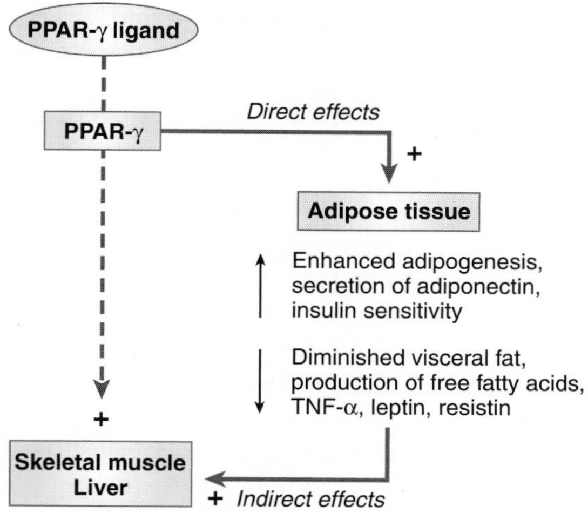

Figure 12–5.
Potential mechanism for improvement of insulin resistance via peroxisome proliferator–activated receptor (PPAR)-gamma ligands. TNF, tumor necrosis factor. *(Adapted from Girard J. [PPARgamma and insulin resistance.] Ann Endocrinol (Paris) 2002;63:1S19-1S22.)*

Energy Homeostasis. PPAR-γ regulates cellular energy homeostasis, which contributes to insulin sensitivity. Such regulation is essential for modulating thermogenesis. It increases the expression of mitochondrial UCPs 1, 2, and 3.[5]

Potential Adverse Effects. Some effects deriving from PPAR-γ activation may be potentially proatherogenic.

Although certain PPAR-γ ligands may manifest antiatherogenic effects by blocking the early process of monocyte adhesion and entry into the arterial wall, these same agents may also aggravate preexisting disease. Specifically,

- PPAR-γ ligands may not affect pathways involving E-selectin and neutrophil binding in vascular atheromata.[23,38]
- PPAR-γ agonists may promote foam cell formation in atherosclerotic plaque because PPAR-γ–related mechanisms appear to be involved in the differentiation of monocytes into macrophages.[23,38] Natural, high-affinity ligands for PPAR-γ in monocytes/macrophages, such as hexadecyl azelaoyl phosphatidylcholine, an oxidized phospholipid derived from oxidized LDL, as well as 9-HODE and 13-HODE, induce expression of the scavenger receptor CD36. CD36 promotes the uptake of oxidized LDL by macrophages, thereby promoting foam cell differentiation and rendering activation of PPAR-γ by these ligands proatherogenic.[38]
- These same PPAR-γ ligands induce COX-2.[1,24]
- PPAR-γ activators reduce the gene expression of osteopontin by macrophages in atherosclerotic plaque. A reduction in osteopontin, a component of the extracellular matrix of atherosclerotic plaque, destabilizes atheromata.
- PPAR-γ pathways increase the apoptosis of neointimal vascular smooth muscle cells, possibly by inhibiting the degradation of iNOS mRNA.
- PPAR-γ mechanisms stimulated by oxidized LDL increase the elaboration of vascular endothelial growth factor (VEGF) from macrophages. Although VEGF is potentially protective against endothelial injury, it leads to microangiogenesis in atheromatous lesions, which undermines plaque stability.[4]

PPAR-β/δ

PPAR-β/δ is found in most cell types. Its highest expression is in the skin, the brain, and adipose tissue. Although its actions remain an enigma, PPAR-β/δ appears to play a key role in basic cell functions such as cell proliferation, differentiation, and survival (Table 12-11). PPAR-δ participates in embryonic development.[46] PPAR-δ–null mice display alterations such as delayed wound closure and diminished neuronal myelination.[2] PPAR-β/δ may control brain lipid metabolism,[18] as well as lipid metabolism in peripheral tissues. It may modulate fatty acid–induced adipogenesis

Table 12-11. Peroxisome Proliferator–Activated Receptor-β/δ Biologic Functions

Brain lipid metabolism
Preadipocyte proliferation
Fatty acid–induced adipogenesis
Embryo implantation
Macrophage cholesterol homeostasis

Adapted from Duval C, Chinetti G, Trottein F, et al. The role of PPARs in atherosclerosis. Trends Mol Med 2002;8:422-430.

and preadipocyte proliferation.[46] PPAR-β/δ may increase the expression of ABCA-1 in macrophages, thus enhancing apo A-I–specific cholesterol efflux and reverse cholesterol transport.[18]

However, PPAR-β/δ may promote cholesterol accumulation by macrophages via up-regulation of genes for the scavenger receptors CD36 and SR-A and down-regulation of genes involved in lipid metabolism and cholesterol efflux, such as cholesterol 27-hydroxylase (CYP27) and apo E. The net effect of PPAR-β/δ on lipid and cholesterol homeostasis and atherogenesis thus remains unclear.[4]

CONCLUSION

Two major elements contribute to the development of insulin resistance: hormonal effects and ectopic lipid storage. Hormonal, proinflammatory mediators promote systemic endothelial dysfunction and insulin resistance. The associated reduction of adiponectin secretion contributes to insulin resistance and constitutes an important basis for the establishment of ectopic fat stores. The reduction in fatty acid beta-oxidative capacity through the loss of adiponectin action complements cytokine antiadipogenic forces and thereby engenders the ectopic storage of excess fat in muscle and liver and launches the additional insulin resistance mechanisms derived from that pathophysiology.

PPAR-α and PPAR-γ indirectly and directly enhance sensitivity to insulin signaling. Both PPARs have anti-inflammatory effects and lower plasma levels of culpable, proinflammatory cytokines. In addition, PPAR-γ activity countermands the antiadipogenic forces of proinflammatory mediators by effecting the appropriate storage of lipid in adipose tissue via adipogenesis. PPAR-α activation entails the oxidative consumption of lipids in metabolically active tissues and thus supersedes the inflammation-related reduction in beta-oxidative capacity that triggered the ectopic storage. Increased adiponectin secretion and AMPK activation support this PPAR-α effect.

Joint activation of PPAR-γ and PPAR-α would appear to be ideally suited to comprehensively target the hormonal and ectopic fat storage derangements of insulin resistance, with complementary effects: whereas PPAR-γ mechanisms alone entail adipose tissue expansion and greater nonvisceral ponderosity, the addition of PPAR-α effects may partially obviate excessive adipose weight gain as a result of the higher oxidative consumption of fatty acids.

The anti-inflammatory and insulin-sensitizing PPAR-α and PPAR-γ are, however, themselves vulnerable to down-regulation by inflammatory stress mediators, thus diminishing their anti-inflammatory potential. The tenuous balance between proinflammatory and anti-inflammatory forces determines whether insulin resistance or insulin sensitivity will ultimately prevail.

Lifestyle choices weigh in on the outcome of this tug of war and constitute a natural venue for joint PPAR-γ and PPAR-α activation without the potentially harmful hepatic and vascular effects seen with excessive pharmacologic stimulation. Aside from their role as energy-rich fuel sources, dietary fatty acids effectively function as natural ligands for the PPARs and thereby regulate gene expression. Prudent choices of appropriate dietary fats will have a favorable impact on PPAR modulation, for example, by mediating some of the cardiovascular and metabolic benefits accruing to high fish oil consumption. Additionally, exercise enhances PPAR-α expression.

Pharmacologic stimulation of PPAR-γ and PPAR-α holds significant promise. The results of trials of selective PPAR-γ and PPAR-α agonists—and more especially agents combining PPAR-α/PPAR-γ action—in treating the metabolic syndrome and cardiovascular disease are eagerly anticipated.

GLOSSARY

ABCA-1	adenosine triphosphate–binding cassette transporter-1
ACC	acetyl-CoA carboxylase
ACRP30	adipocyte complement-related protein of 30kDa, or adiponectin
ACS	acyl CoA synthase
AMPK	adenosine 5′-monophosphate–activated protein kinase
Apo	apolipoprotein
AT_1	angiotensin II type 1
BMI	body mass index

CAP	c-Cbl–associated protein
C/EBP-β	CCAAT-box/enhancer-binding protein-beta
CHD	coronary heart disease
CNP	C-type natriuretic peptide
CNS	central nervous system
CoA	coenzyme A
COX	cyclooxygenase
CPT-I	carnitine palmitoyltransferase I
CRP	C-reactive protein
CXC	cysteine X–amino acid–cysteine
CYP27	cholesterol 27-hydroxylase
DR	direct repeat
eNOS	endothelial NOS
FAT	fatty acid translocase
FATP-1	fatty acid transport protein-1
GLUT	glucose transporter
HAD	3-hydroxyacyl CoA dehydrogenase
HDL	high-density lipoprotein
HETE	hydroxyeicosatetraenoic acid
HMG CoA	3-hydroxy-3-methylglutaryl CoA
HODE	hydroxyoctadecadienoic acid
11β-HSD-1	11β-hydroxysteroid dehydrogenase type 1
ICAM-1	intercellular adhesion molecule-1
IκB	inhibitory protein IkappaB
IL	interleukin
INOS	inducible NOS
IRS	insulin receptor substrate
LDL	low-density lipoprotein
LOX-1	lectin-like, oxidized, LDL receptor-1
LPL	lipoprotein lipase
MCD	malonyl CoA decarboxylase
MCP-1	monocyte chemotactic protein-1
MMP	matrix metalloproteinase
NADH/ NADPH	nicotinamide adenine dinucleotide phosphate oxidase
NFκB	nuclear factor kappaB
NO	nitric oxide
NOS	nitric oxide synthase
PAF	platelet-activating factor
PAI-1	plasminogen activator inhibitor-1
PDGF	platelet-derived growth factor
PDHK4	pyruvate dehydrogenase kinase 4
PEPCK	phosphoenolpyruvate carboxykinase
$PGF_{1\alpha}$	prostaglandin $F_{1\alpha}$
PI3K	phosphatidylinositol 3-kinase
PPAR	peroxisome proliferator–activated receptor
PPRE	PPAR response element
RAR	retinoic acid receptor
RXR	retinoid X receptor
SOD	superoxide dismutase
SR-B1	scavenger receptor class B type 1
STAT	signal transducer and activator of transcription
TNF	tumor necrosis factor
TR	triiodothyronine receptor
UCP	uncoupling protein
VCAM-1	vascular cell adhesion molecule-1
VEGF	vascular endothelial growth factor
VLDL	very-low-density lipoprotein

REFERENCES

1. Zhang X, Young HA. PPAR and the immune system—what do we know? Int Immunopharm 2002;2:1029-1044
2. Yki-Järvinen H. Thiazolidinediones. N Engl J Med 2004; 351:1106-1118
3. Issemann I, Green S. Activation of a member of the steroid hormone receptor superfamily by peroxisome proliferators. Nature 1990;347:645-650
4. Duval C, Chinetti G, Trottein F, et al. The role of PPARs in atherosclerosis. Trends Mol Med 2002;8:422-430
5. Berger J, Moller DE. The mechanisms of action of PPARs. Annu Rev Med 2002;53:409-435
6. Hauner H. The mode of action of thiazolidinediones. Diabetes Metab Res Rev 2002;18:S10-S15
7. Smith SA. Peroxisome proliferator–activated receptors and the regulation of mammalian lipid metabolism. Biochem Soc Trans 2002;30:1086-1090
8. Lim H, Dey S. Minireview: A novel pathway of prostacyclin signaling—hanging out with nuclear receptors. Endocrinology 2002;143:3207-3210
9. Desvergne B, Upenberg A, Devchand PR, Wahli W. The peroxisome proliferator–activated receptors at the crossroad of diet and hormonal signaling. J Steroid Biochem Mol Biol 1998;65:65-74
10. Etgen G, Oldham BA, Johnson WT, et al. A tailored therapy for the metabolic syndrome. The dual peroxisome proliferator–activated receptor-alpha/gamma agonist LY465608 ameliorates insulin resistance and diabetic hyperglycemia while improving cardiovascular risk factors in preclinical models. Diabetes 2002;51:1083-1087
11. Plutzky J. Peroxisome proliferator–activated receptors in vascular biology and atherosclerosis: emerging insights for evolving paradigms. Curr Atheroscler Rep 2000;2: 327-335
12. Jalouli M, Carlsson L, Ameen C, et al. Sex difference in hepatic peroxisome proliferator–activated receptor alpha expression: influence of pituitary and gonadal hormones. Endocrinology 2003;144:101-109
13. Fruchart J-C, Staels B, Duriez P. PPARs, metabolic disease and atherosclerosis. Pharmacol Res 2001;44:345-352
14. Iemitsu M, Miyauchi T, Maeda S, et al. Aging-induced decrease in the PPAR-alpha level in hearts is improved by exercise training. Am J Physiol Heart Circ Physiol 2002;283:H1750-H1760
15. Muoio DM, Way JM, Tanner CJ, et al. Peroxisome proliferator–activated receptor-alpha regulates fatty acid utilization in primary human skeletal muscle cells. Diabetes 2002;51:901-909
16. Guerre-Millo M, Rouault C, Poulain P, et al. PPAR-alpha–null mice are protected from high-fat diet–induced insulin resistance. Diabetes 2001;50:2809-2814

17. Fruchart J-C. Peroxisome proliferator–activated receptor-alpha activation and high-density lipoprotein metabolism. Am J Cardiol 2001;88(suppl):24N-29N
18. Ruotolo G, Howard BV. Dyslipidemia of the metabolic syndrome. Curr Cardiol Rep 2002;4:494-500
19. Diep QN, Amiri F, Touyz RM, et al. PPARalpha activator effects on Ang II–induced vascular oxidative stress and inflammation. Hypertension 2002;40:866-871
20. Kleemann R, Gervois PP, Verschuren L, et al. Fibrates down-regulate IL-1–stimulated C-reactive protein gene expression in hepatocytes by reducing nuclear p50–NFkappa B–C/EBP-beta complex formation. Blood 2003;101:545-551
21. Kleemann R, Verschuren L, De Rooij BJ, et al. Evidence for anti-inflammatory activity of statins and PPAR{alpha}-activators in human C-reactive protein transgenic mice in vivo and in cultured human hepatocytes in vitro. Blood 2004;103:4188-4194
22. Xu X, Otsuki M, Saito H, et al. PPARalpha and GR differentially down-regulate the expression of nuclear factor-kappaB–responsive genes in vascular endothelial cells. Endocrinology 2001;142:3332-3339
23. Jackson SM, Parhami F, Xi XP, et al. Peroxisome proliferator–activated receptor activators target human endothelial cells to inhibit leukocyte-endothelial cell interaction. Arterioscler Thromb Vasc Biol 1999;19: 2094-2104
24. Tham DM, Martin-McNulty B, Wang YX, et al. Angiotensin II is associated with activation of NF-kappaB–mediated genes and downregulation of PPARs. Physiol Genomics 2002;11:21-30
25. Iglarz M, Touyz RM, Amiri F, et al. Effect of peroxisome proliferator–activated receptor-alpha and -gamma activators on vascular remodeling in endothelin-dependent hypertension. Arterioscler Thromb Vasc Biol 2003;23: 45-51
26. Hermanowski-Vosatka A, Gerhold D, Mundt SS, et al. PPARalpha agonists reduce 11beta-hydroxysteroid dehydrogenase type 1 in the liver. Biochem Biophys Res Commun 2000;279:330-336
27. Evans JL, Goldfine ID, Maddux BA, Grodsky GM. Oxidative stress and stress-activated signaling pathways: a unifying hypothesis of type 2 diabetes. Endocr Rev 2002;23:599-622
28. Munday MR, Hemingway CJ. The regulation of acetyl-CoA carboxylase—a potential target for the action of hypolipidemic agents. Adv Enzyme Regul 1999;39: 205-234
29. Campbell FM, Kozak R, Wagner A, et al. A role for peroxisome proliferator–activated receptor alpha (PPARalpha) in the control of cardiac malonyl-CoA levels: reduced fatty acid oxidation rates and increased glucose oxidation rates in the hearts of mice lacking PPARalpha are associated with higher concentrations of malonyl-CoA and reduced expression of malonyl-CoA decarboxylase. J Biol Chem 2002;277:4098-4103
30. Lee GY, Kim NH, Zhao ZS, et al. Peroxisomal-proliferator–activated receptor alpha activates transcription of the rat hepatic malonyl-CoA decarboxylase gene: a key regulation of malonyl-CoA level. Biochem J 2004;378:983-990
31. Young ME, Goodwin GW, Ying J, et al. Regulation of cardiac and skeletal muscle malonyl-CoA decarboxylase by fatty acids. Am J Physiol Endocrinol Metab 2001;280: E471-E479
32. Barrero MJ, Camarero N, Marrero PF, Haro D. Control of human carnitine palmitoyltransferase II gene transcription by peroxisome proliferator–activated receptor through a partially conserved peroxisome proliferator–responsive element. Biochem J 2003;369:721-729
33. Lee HJ, Choi SS, Park MK, et al. Fenofibrate lowers abdominal and skeletal adiposity and improves insulin sensitivity in OLETF rats. Biochem Biophys Res Commun 2002;296:293-299
34. Marx N, Sukhova G, Murphy C, et al. Macrophages in human atheroma contain PPAR gamma: differentiation-dependent peroxisomal proliferator–activated receptor gamma (PPAR gamma) expression and reduction of MMP-9 activity through PPAR gamma activation in mononuclear phagocytes in vitro. Am J Pathol 1998;153: 17-23
35. Sewter C, Blows F, Considine R, et al. Differential effects of adiposity on peroxisomal proliferator–activated receptor gamma1 and gamma2 messenger ribonucleic acid expression in human adipocytes. J Clin Endocrinol Metab 2002;87:4203-4207
36. Berger J, Tanen M, Elbrecht A, et al.. Peroxisome proliferator–activated receptor-gamma ligands inhibit adipocyte 11beta-hydroxysteroid dehydrogenase type 1 expression and activity. J Biol Chem 2001;276: 12629-12635
37. Rossi A, Kapahi P, Natoli G, et al. Anti-inflammatory cyclopentanone prostaglandins are direct inhibitors of IκB kinase. Nature 2000;403:103-108
38. Plutzky J. The potential role of peroxisome proliferator–activated receptors on inflammation in type 2 diabetes mellitus and atherosclerosis. Am J Cardiol 2003; 92(suppl):34J-41J
39. Chawla A, Schwarz EJ, Dimaculangan DD, Lazar MA. Peroxisome-proliferator activated receptor (PPAR) gamma: adipose-predominant expression and induction early in adipocyte differentiation. Endocrinology 1994;135: 798-800
40. Chinetti G, Fruchart JC, Staels B. Peroxisome proliferator–activated receptors (PPARs): nuclear receptors with functions in the vascular wall. Z Kardiol 2001;90(suppl 3): 125-132
41. Debril MB, Renaud JP, Fajas L, Auwerx J. The pleiotropic functions of peroxisome proliferator–activated receptor gamma. J Mol Med 2001;79:30-47
42. Wakino S, Law RE, Hsueh WA. Vascular protective effects by activation of nuclear receptor PPARgamma. J Diabetes Complications 2002;16:46-49
43. Calnek DS, Mazzella L, Roser S, et al. Peroxisome proliferator–activated receptor gamma ligands increase release of nitric oxide from endothelial cells. Arterioscler Thromb Vasc Biol 2003;23:52-57
44. Hu E, Tontonoz P, Spiegelman BM. Transdifferentiation of myoblasts by the adipogenic transcription factors PPAR gamma and C/EBP alpha. Proc Natl Acad Sci U S A 1995;92:9856-9860
45. Kamon J, Yamauchi T, Terauchi Y, et al. The mechanisms by which PPARgamma and adiponectin regulate glucose and lipid metabolism. Nippon Yakurigaku Zasshi 2003;122:294-300
46. Michalik L, Desvergne B, Wahli W. Peroxisome proliferator–activated receptors β/δ: emerging roles for a previously neglected third family member. Curr Opin Lipidol 2003;14:129-135

Exercise and Meditation 13

Nonpharmacologic behavioral and lifestyle changes, including exercise and dietary modifications with weight loss, constitute the foundation for the management of metabolic syndrome and are the most cost-effective and physiologically attractive interventions for the prevention of

- insulin resistance,
- metabolic syndrome,
- cardiovascular disease, and
- type 2 diabetes mellitus (DM).

The aim of such therapeutic lifestyle changes should be

- normalization of endothelial function and
- reversal of insulin resistance and the metabolic derangements of the metabolic syndrome.

Lowering endogenous insulin concentrations is a key indicator of successful therapy directed at the underlying insulin resistance and can be accomplished in part with exercise. Exercise is a key component in the prevention of cardiovascular and metabolic disease.

Table 13-1. Cardiovascular, Skeletal Muscle, and General Impact of Long-Term Exercise Training

Cardiovascular

Lower myocardial oxygen demand for any workload
Increased stroke volume
Improved endothelial function
Lower sympathetic activation
Enhanced vagal tone
Antihypertensive effect

Skeletal Muscle

Increased type I, slow-twitch oxidative fibers
Increased muscle fiber mass
Increased mitochondrial biogenesis
Increased glycogen and fatty acid storage and turnover
Increased capillary density
Enhanced nutritive blood flow
Improved insulin- and non–insulin-dependent glucose uptake
Improved uptake of fatty acids
Higher oxidative capacity

Adipose Tissue

Decreased subcutaneous and visceral-omental adipose tissue
Decreased adipocyte size
Enhanced responsiveness to lipolysis

General

Decreased inflammatory activation
Antioxidant effects
Induction of peroxisome activator–proliferator receptor-alpha expression
Enhanced metabolic rate
Increased aerobic fitness
Improved lipid profile
Improved insulin sensitivity
Reduced manifestations of the metabolic syndrome and type 2 diabetes mellitus
Reduced cardiovascular and overall morbidity and mortality

CLINICAL BENEFIT OF EXERCISE TRAINING

Adiposity and a lack of physical conditioning are risk factors for mortality. The cardinal health benefit that derives from appropriate exercise conditioning is maintenance or improvement of cardiorespiratory fitness (Table 13-1). **Fitness improves the overall survival odds and is protective against the development of cardiovascular disease and the metabolic syndrome.** Ponce de Leon searched for the fountain of youth and may have found an aspect of it. His physical exertions, in effect, improved his conditioning, reduced his obesity, and thereby extended his vigor and potential life span.

A reduction in total and abdominal-visceral adiposity may be one of the means whereby cardiovascular fitness attenuates the health risks associated with obesity as determined by body mass index (BMI) and waist circumference. In the sample of 828 sedentary participants in the Health, Risk Factors, Exercise Training, and Genetics (HERITAGE) Family Study, for a given BMI or waist circumference, individuals of moderate fitness had lower levels of total fat mass and abdominal subcutaneous and visceral adiposity than did individuals with low fitness.[1]

Cardiovascular Benefit. Physical activity has a favorable impact on the course of cardiovascular disease. Increasing exercise-related energy expenditure progressively reduces the risk for cardiovascular events.[2,3]

Vascular Risk Factors and Myocardial Infarction. Exercise beneficially affects vascular health. Increased physical activity reduces

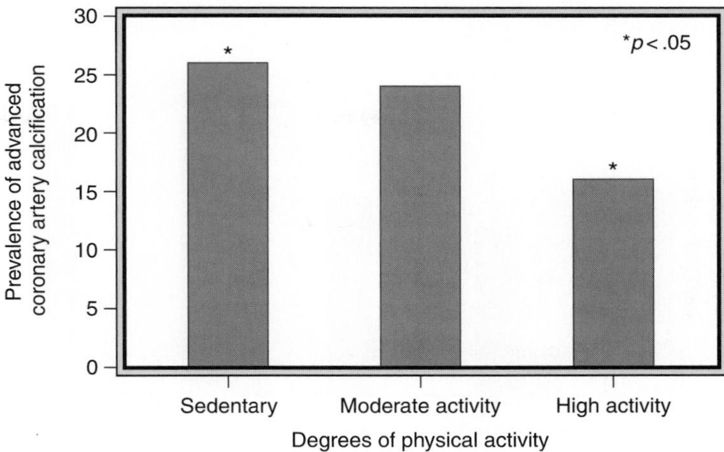

Figure 13–1.
Prevalence of advanced coronary artery calcification (>75th percentile for age and gender) as a function of different degrees of physical activity in 779 asymptomatic subjects with more than two metabolic risk factors. *(Modified from Desai MY, Nasir K, Rumberger JA, et al. Relation of degree of physical activity to coronary artery calcium score in asymptomatic individuals with multiple metabolic risk factors. Am J Cardiol 2004;94:729-732.)*

endothelial dysfunction in hypertension and hypercholesterolemia.[4] Exercise may have a modest, beneficial impact on hypertension.[5]

Physical activity is inversely related to the prevalence of coronary calcification. In 779 asymptomatic individuals with more than two metabolic risk factors, the median coronary calcium scores, as determined by electron beam tomography, were highest at a value of 24 in sedentary individuals, 18 in moderately active persons, and 11 in subjects engaging in long-duration moderate physical activity, $P < .002$ (Fig. 13-1).[6]

Cardiac rehabilitation decreases cardiac morbidity and the need for medications, emergency room visits, and hospitalization. Over 5 years, cardiac rehabilitation lowers the occurrence of nonfatal myocardial infarction.[7] In post–myocardial infarction patients, participation in cardiac rehabilitation lowers 3-year mortality by 25%,[8,9] and in patients with coronary heart disease (CHD), exercise decreases total mortality by 27%.[10]

Type of Physical Activity. There is an inverse association between the perceived rigor of exertion and the risk for CHD in older men.[11] Although any increase in physical activity is favorable, pursuit of leisure time physical activities may be associated with greater cardiovascular benefit than is the case with work-related physical stress. Whereas leisure time effort shows a strong, negative correlation with CHD, physical exertion at work in some instances has a strong, positive correlation with CHD, possibly because of the confounding effects of mental stress.[12]

Fitness versus Ponderosity and Cardiovascular Risk. Cardiovascular fitness appears to have greater impact on cardiovascular disease than do measures of obesity. According to data in older men, low cardiovascular fitness appears to be an independent predictor of cardiovascular events in all, both low and high, BMI groups later in life.[13] Among 906 women enrolled in the Women's Ischemia Syndrome Evaluation (WISE) study, fitness status was more important than obesity measures in predicting the presence of CHD. Lower scores on self-reported measures of physical fitness were more likely to be associated with CHD risk factors and obstructive CHD at baseline. Each 1–metabolic equivalent (met) increase in fitness measure was associated with an 8% decrease in the risk for major adverse cardiovascular events in follow-up. In contrast, neither BMI nor abdominal obesity gauges were significantly associated with obstructive CHD or adverse cardiovascular events after adjusting for other risk factors (Fig. 13-2).[14]

Metabolic Risk Reduction. The advantages of exercise extend beyond cardiovascular benefits. **Exercise improves all risk factors associated with the metabolic syndrome** (Table 13-2). Regular physical exercise improves

- endothelial dysfunction,
- blood pressure,
- whole-body glucose disposal,
- insulin sensitivity,
- caloric expenditure,

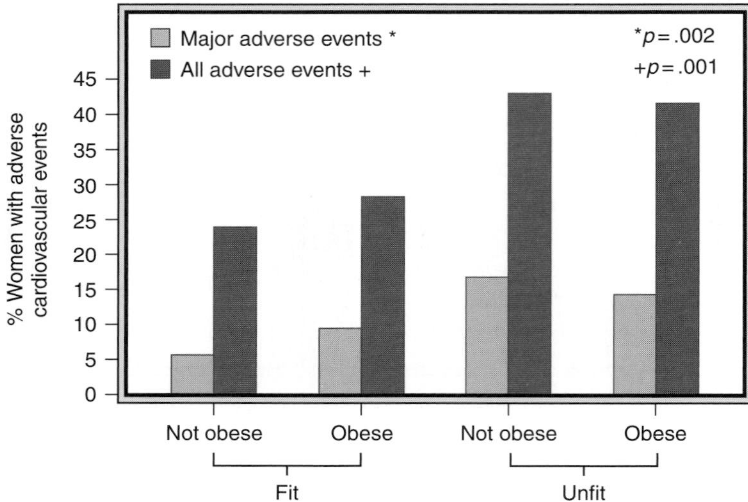

▸▸ **Figure 13–2.** Proportion of women with adverse cardiovascular events over 3.9 years of follow-up in the Women's Ischemia Syndrome Evaluation study by categories of obesity (body mass index >30) and self-scored fitness. *(Modified from Wessel TR, Arant CB, Olson MB, et al. Relationship of physical fitness vs body mass index with coronary artery disease and cardiovascular events in women. JAMA 2004;292:1179-1187.)*

- neurohormonal factors,
- body composition, and
- lipid metabolism

independently of weight loss.[15,16]

The prevalence of metabolic syndrome is inversely related to cardiorespiratory fitness levels. In 7104 women in the Aerobics Center Longitudinal Study (ACLS), there was a 19% prevalence of the metabolic syndrome in the lowest-fitness quintile as contrasted to a prevalence of 2.3% in the highest-fitness quintile (Fig. 13-3).[17] In the Nurse's Health Study, during 6 years of follow-up, a sedentary lifestyle, encompassing in particular television watching, was associated with a significantly elevated risk for type 2 DM. Even light to moderate regular physical activity substantially lowered the risk for DM.[18]

Current clinical evidence suggests that an increase in weekly physical activity up to 100 to 150 minutes, but preferably up to 150 to 300 minutes, with only modest reductions of 5% to 7% in current body weight may be sufficient to provide significant metabolic benefit and have a favorable impact on lipid disorders, glucose intolerance, and hypertension while reducing the onset of type 2 DM by 58% over a period of 3 years. Among persons older than 60 years, that risk reduction may reach 70%.[19,20]

The metabolic syndrome is associated with a higher incidence of cancer. **Exercise reduces the risk for breast and other cancers, and the longer the duration of exercise, the greater the benefit derived.**[21-24]

Table 13–2. Impact of Interventions on Dysfunctional Aspects of the Metabolic Syndrome

INTERVENTION	LIPIDS	BLOOD PRESSURE	VASCULATURE
Exercise	+	+	+
Weight loss	+	+	
Statins	+		+
Angiotensin-converting enzyme inhibitors		+	+
Angiotensin receptor blockers		+	+
Thiazolidinediones	+	+	+
Biguanides			+

+, Beneficial.
Adapted from Fonseca VA. Management of diabetes mellitus and insulin resistance in patients with cardiovascular disease. Am J Cardiol 2003;92(4A):50J-60J.

Mortality. Cardiorespiratory fitness substantially improves the odds of survival. Fitness lowers the all-cause mortality risk of excessive adiposity and, among men, appears to be more protective than the absence of ponderosity.

In an 8-year observational cohort study, 21,925 men aged 30 to 83 years underwent body composition assessment and a maximal treadmill exercise test to determine cardiorespiratory fitness. Lean men had increased longevity only if

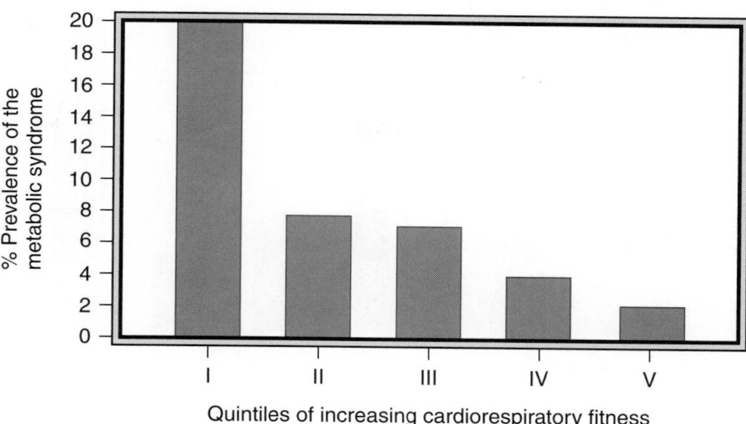

Figure 13–3. Age- and smoking-adjusted prevalence of the metabolic syndrome by quintile of cardiorespiratory fitness in 7104 women from the Aerobics Center Longitudinal Study, 1979 to 2000. *(Modified from Farrell SW, Cheng YJ, Blair SN. Prevalence of the metabolic syndrome across cardiorespiratory fitness levels in women. Obes Res 2004;12:824-830.)*

physically fit; after adjustment for multiple risk factors, unfit, lean men had twice the risk for all-cause mortality as fit, lean men, with a relative risk of 2.07, $P = .01$. Obese men who were fit did not have shorter survival; unfit, lean men had a greater risk for all-cause and CHD mortality than did fit, obese men. Fit men had greater longevity than unfit men did regardless of body composition or risk factor status. Similarly, unfit men with low waist girths (<87 cm) had greater all-cause mortality than did fit men with high waist girths (>99 cm), with all-cause mortality for large-waisted, fit men being similar to that of small-waisted, fit men.[25] Similarly, a longitudinal, prospective observational study at the University of North Carolina evaluated 2506 women and 2860 men with a mean age at baseline of 46.6 and 45.1 years, respectively, between 1972 and 1976.[26] Vital statistics were collected through 1998. Subjects were classified as fit—not fat, fit—fat, unfit—not fat, and unfit—fat. When compared with fit, not fat individuals, the adjusted hazard ratios for mortality from all causes and from cardiovascular disease were as follows[26]:

FOR WOMEN	FOR MEN
Fit—fat = 1.32	Fit—fat = 1.25
Unfit—not fat = 1.30	Unfit—not fat = 1.44
Unfit—fat = 1.57	Unfit—fat = 1.49

A fit and active way of life improves health and function and lowers mortality also in older individuals. A review of reports of prospective epidemiologic studies and clinical trials published in the peer-reviewed literature that included data from age groups of people 60 years and older supported a causal hypothesis of a steep, inverse dose-response relationship between activity or fitness categories and poor health outcomes. Active and fit elderly individuals were at much lower risk for morbidity, mortality, and loss of function than were sedentary, unfit persons.[27]

The survival benefits associated with increasing cardiovascular fitness also extend to individuals with the metabolic syndrome. In 19,000 men over 11 years of follow-up in the Kuopio Ischaemic Heart Disease Risk Factor Study, cardiovascular fitness was associated with a significantly lower relative risk for all-cause and cardiovascular mortality. Survival improved in parallel with fitness, even in men with the metabolic syndrome.[16] In 3757 men 20 to 83 years of age in the ACLS study with the metabolic syndrome, after adjusting for risk factors such as family history of CHD, age, BMI, and cigarette and alcohol consumption, a higher fitness level provided a protective effect against all-cause and cardiovascular mortality (Fig. 13-4).[28]

Even in the presence of documented DM, there is a steep, inverse relationship between fitness and mortality, independent of BMI. In a study of 2196 men with DM (average age, 49.3 ± 9.5 years) who underwent a maximal exercise test during 1970 to 1995, with mortality follow-up through the end of 1996, the risk for all-cause mortality was inversely related to fitness. In the fully adjusted model, the risk for mortality was 4.5, 2.8, and 1.6 for the first (lowest fitness), second, and third fitness quartiles, respectively, with the fourth quartile (highest fitness) being

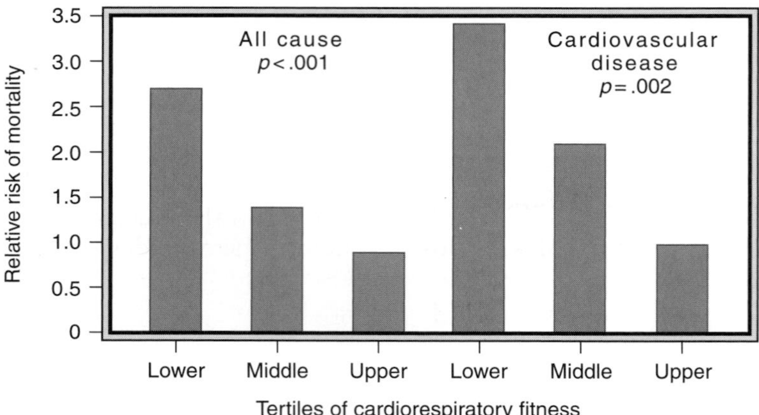

⏩ **Figure 13–4.**
Relative risk for all-cause and cardiovascular disease mortality in 3757 men aged 20 to 83 years with a diagnosis of metabolic syndrome across baseline tertiles of cardiorespiratory fitness from the Aerobics Center Longitudinal Study. Relative risks are adjusted for age, year of examination, smoking status, alcohol consumption, family history of cardiovascular disease, and body mass index. *P* values are for tests of linear trend across the fitness categories. *(Modified from Katzmarzyk PT, Church TS, Blair SN. Cardiorespiratory fitness attenuates the effects of the metabolic syndrome on all-cause and cardiovascular disease mortality in men. Arch Intern Med 2004;164:1092-1097.)*

the reference point (*P* for trend < .0001). In contrast, after adjustment for fitness, there was no significant trend across BMI categories for mortality. In fact, even for normal-weight men with DM, the relative risks for mortality were 6.6, 3.2, and 2.2 for the first, second, and third quartiles of fitness, respectively, as compared with the fittest fourth quartile (*P* for trend < .0001), with similar results found in the overweight and obese weight categories.[29]

Feasibility and Accessibility of Physical Training. Unfortunately, at present only a minority of people in the United States pursue physical exercise. Seventy-two percent of women and 65% of men do not engage in regular leisure time exercise, and between 40 and 50 million U.S. adults are completely sedentary.[30] Furthermore, most health care insurance does not routinely provide financial coverage for lifestyle counseling in the absence of an established diagnosis of type 2 DM. It is thus challenging to provide the population at risk for the metabolic syndrome with the incentive and the specific methods for implementing and sustaining the necessary lifestyle changes.

Because individuals with the metabolic syndrome may have concomitant occult or clinical CHD, adverse cardiovascular and physiologic responses during exercise training are possible. Individuals interested in exercise should be advised to obtain prior medical clearance with exercise stress testing before initiating a moderate-intensity exercise program. Stress testing may identify symptomatic and silent ischemia, ischemic thresholds, and arrhythmias. Furthermore, it provides data on heart rate and blood pressure responses to exercise to allow a tailored and appropriate exercise prescription. Untrained individuals should be oriented by qualified staff or by a personal trainer at a fitness or rehabilitation facility. Individuals should be advised to perform 5 to 10 minutes of warm-up and stretching exercises before an exercise protocol and to adequately cool down for 5 to 10 minutes after the workout.

However, realistically, the physical activity goals required to attain a moderate to high cardiorespiratory fitness level with substantial health benefits are readily achievable for most healthy individuals without special programs and training. In a questionnaire study of a clinic population of 13,444 men and 3972 women 20 to 87 years of age in which the physical activity patterns associated with low, moderate, and high cardiorespiratory fitness were examined, moderate to high levels of fitness were associated with an average leisure time energy expenditure of 525 to 1650 kcal/wk for men and 420 to 1260 kcal/wk for women. These levels of energy expenditure were achieved with a brisk walk of approximately 30 minutes on most days of the week, specifically, with men in the moderate and high fitness categories walking between 130 and 138 minutes per week and women in these categories walking between 148 and 167 minutes per week.[31]

EXERCISE AND MITOGEN-ACTIVATED PROTEIN KINASE

Exercise training is associated with significant physiologic adaptations involving changes in myocyte fiber type, muscle hypertrophy, and a variety of metabolic adaptations.

Physical exertion provides a significant stimulus for the regulation of multiple transcriptional processes and signaling cascades in skeletal muscle to effect these changes.[15] Every single bout of exercise can induce transient changes in myocyte gene transcription that contribute to the cumulative, chronic adaptations to repeated bouts of exercise.[32]

Mitogen-Activated Protein Kinase Function. Structural adaptations of skeletal muscle to exercise training may be mediated by mitogen-activated protein kinase (MAPK) signaling pathways.

The MAPK cascade comprises a series of several protein kinases, the structure of which is highly conserved between diverse organisms. MAPK pathways relay signals from the plasma membrane to targets in the cytoplasm and nucleus. They stimulate phosphorylation of transcription factors in response to extracellular stimuli such as growth factors, cytokines, stress-inducing agents, ultraviolet light, and physical tension or stretch. In the process, they frequently amplify the signal. MAPK cascades are involved in a multiplicity of signal transduction pathways, and the biologic responses associated with different signals are diverse.[33]

Exercise and Mitogen-Activated Protein Kinase Activation. The exercise-induced, adaptive changes in myocyte protein expression may be mediated via increased signal transduction through the MAPK signaling cascades. **Muscle contractile activity, acute physical exercise, and endurance training can activate three isoforms of the MAPK signaling pathways,** including

1. extracellular signal–regulated kinase 1 and 2 (ERK1/2) or p42/44 MAPK,
2. c-Jun NH_2-terminal kinase (JNK), and
3. the p38/Hog 1 MAPK,

to regulate transcriptional activity.[33]

MAPKs are phosphorylated and activated by MAPK/ERK kinases (MAPKKs), which in turn are phosphorylated and activated by MAPKK kinases (MAPKKKs). Acute exercise or endurance training increases downstream substrates of ERK and p38 MAPK such as p90 ribosomal S6 kinase (RSK2) activity and MAPK-activated protein kinase (MAPKAPK) 1 and 2, respectively.[34,35] Activation of the ERK pathway may also entail Ras-Raf associations.[34-36]

EXERCISE AND MUSCLE TYPE

The degree of physical activity over the long term has an impact on fiber type preponderance in skeletal muscle, with significant metabolic implications.

There are three categories of skeletal muscle fibers:

1. type I, or slow-twitch, oxidative fibers;
2. type IIa, or fast-twitch, oxidative and glycolytic fibers; and
3. type IIb, or fast-twitch, glycolytic fibers.

Type I skeletal muscle fibers, by definition, have relatively high oxidative enzyme capacities when compared with type II fibers. They are more fatigue resistant and have a greater number of mitochondria and mitochondrial enzymes, as well as higher fatty acid oxidative capacity. For the same amount of work, oxygen consumption by the efficient type I muscles is only 40% to 50% that of type II fibers.[37] **Type I fiber utilization with oxidative metabolism predominates at sustained, lower levels of exercise. Type II fiber utilization supervenes as exercise levels exceed the anaerobic threshold and is associated with an increase in lactate production.**[38]

Type I fibers have more glucose transporters (GLUT4s) than type II fibers do. Insulin-stimulated glucose transport is thus greater in type I oxidative fibers than in the other fiber types. **Whole-body glucose uptake is positively correlated with the abundance of type I muscles and negatively correlated with the quantity of type IIb muscles.**[39]

Whereas obesity and inactivity decrease type I fibers, thus lowering the anaerobic threshold and exercise capacity, exercise and

endurance training increase the proportion of slow-twitch, insulin-sensitive type I muscle fibers. Exercise-induced muscle hypertrophy actually reflects a higher proportion of type I, slow-twitch oxidative myofibers with increased capillary density, mitochondrial mass, and glycogen and fatty acid stores.[40]

EXERCISE AND AUTONOMIC FUNCTION

Exercise training accrues neurovegetative advantages. Although results have been inconsistent, sympathetic activity tends to decrease with exercise training and baroreflex sensitivity is restored.[41,42]

Parasympathetic Tone. Exercise enhances parasympathetic tone. Moderate-intensity endurance training enhances parasympathetic activity with increased aerobic power.

Heart rate variability (HRV) is a measure of autonomic control. There are two spectral components of HRV:

1. the high-frequency (HF) component (0.15 to 0.50 Hz) represents vagal efferent activity, and
2. the low-frequency (LF) component (0.05 to 0.15Hz) represents sympathetic activity.

Power spectral analysis of HRV with training demonstrates

- increases in HF (parasympathetic) components,
- declines in LF (sympathetic) components, and
- a fall in the LF/HF ratio

as a result of enhanced vagal and diminished sympathetic cardiac modulation because of conditioning.[41,42]

EXERCISE AND ENDOTHELIAL FUNCTION

A sedentary lifestyle is linked to endothelial dysfunction, increased oxidative stress, and elevated systemic markers of inflammation. Physical inactivity increases cardiovascular morbidity and mortality. In contrast, exercise has repeatedly been shown to improve endothelial vasomotor function and cardiovascular risk.

Physical Inactivity and Endothelial Dysfunction. A sedentary lifestyle impairs endothelial function in healthy individuals, even in the absence of other cardiovascular risk factors. Interestingly, such endothelial dysfunction is reversible. Five to 9 weeks of rest in young, healthy mice induced a specific impairment in endothelium-dependent vasodilation by reducing the vascular expression of endothelial nitric oxide synthase (eNOS). As sedentary mice commenced exercise, the expression of eNOS increased severalfold.[43] Correspondingly, during the 16-year follow-up of 12,138 men in the Multiple Risk Factor Intervention Trial (MRFIT), the incidence of cardiovascular deaths was higher in sedentary than in active men.[44]

Impact of Exercise on eNOS. Exercise training increases endothelium-dependent vasodilation, largely by increasing elaboration of nitric oxide (NO).

Effect of Shear Stress on eNOS. During exercise, the endothelial monolayer on the luminal surface of blood vessels is exposed to increased blood flow.[45-47] **Via acute or chronic increases in mechanical shear stress as a result of higher blood flow, exercise promotes endothelial NO release, smooth muscle cell relaxation, and vasodilation.** This effect has been observed in cultured cells and in isolated vessels.[48,49]

Exercise exerts a dual positive impact on vascular NO production:

1. **Within minutes, exercise enhances eNOS activity** by increasing the phosphorylation of eNOS at Ser1177. In a clinical study of CHD patients, 4 weeks of aerobic exercise training caused a threefold increase in Akt kinase–dependent phosphorylation of eNOS at Ser1177, which correlated with enhanced eNOS activity, greater elaboration of NO, and improved endothelial function in vivo.[50]
2. **Over the course of hours, exercise increases the protein expression of eNOS.** There is enhanced expression of the vascular, constitutive eNOS gene in the epicardial coronary arteries of chronically exercised dogs.[51] Similarly, in CHD patients, 4 weeks of aerobic exercise training increased eNOS messenger RNA (mRNA) expression

with a twofold rise in vascular eNOS protein content in the left internal mammary artery.[50]

Acetylcholine and eNOS. During exercise, in addition to the direct effects of shear stress, the enzymatic activity of eNOS is stimulated by the neurotransmitter acetylcholine, thus promoting endothelial NO release. With muscle contractions, acetylcholine from the neuromuscular junction diffuses to the vascular endothelium and activates muscarinic receptors. Acetylcholine activation of both M_2 and M_4 muscarinic receptors results in marked calcium-dependent activation of eNOS in a time- and concentration-dependent manner.[52,53]

Additional Factors Having an Impact on eNOS. There are additional mechanisms activated by exercise that enhance NO production:

- **Exercise induces adenosine 5′-monophosphate (AMP)-activated protein kinase (5′-AMPK or AMPK).** Activated AMPK may stimulate eNOS activity via Ser1177 phosphorylation and thereby raise NO production.[54,55]
- **Exercise increases bradykinin levels.** Exercise shear stress inhibits tissue angiotensin-converting enzyme (ACE). ACE inhibition, while decreasing the production of angiotensin II, inhibits degradation of bradykinin, with beneficial effects on eNOS activity.[56]

Impact of Exercise on Nitric Oxide Bioavailability. Exercise enhances the bioavailability of NO.

By lowering tissue angiotensin II levels, exercise reduces the generation of reactive oxygen species. At the same time, exercise induces the expression of superoxide dismutase, which lowers oxidant stress, thus diminishing the oxidative consumption of NO and enhancing NO bioavailability.[57]

Impact of Exercise on Systemic Endothelial Function. Increased NO bioavailability may be greatest in the specific vascular beds exposed to repetitive increases in blood flow during exercise. However, **higher NO bioavailability may not be restricted to the vascular bed of the trained muscle. Rather, exercise-enhanced vascular shear stress also increases eNOS function in the coronary circulation, in the aorta, and systemically as a result of changes in heart rate, pulse pressure, blood viscosity, and blood flow.** This effect has been observed in healthy individuals, in hypertensive patients, and in CHD and heart failure patients.[45-47]

The systemic effect of exercise training on endothelial function was demonstrated in a study of 10 patients with CHD and 10 controls after 8 weeks of lower limb aerobic and resistance training. Exercise significantly improved nonexercised brachial flow–mediated dilation in the CHD patients, as determined by vascular ultrasonography. Lower limb exercise training, in effect, improved upper limb, endothelium-dependent conduit vessel dilation, consistent with a generalized vascular effect rather than one limited to the vasculature of the exercising lower extremity musculature.[58]

Impact of Exercise Intensity on Endothelial Function. Exercise intensity modulates the effects of exercise on endothelial function.

In healthy young men, 12 weeks of moderate-intensity exercise at 50% maximal oxygen consumption (V_{O_2}max) augmented endothelium-dependent vasodilation.[59] Similarly, in a 12-week study of 18 men with CHD engaged in moderate exercise in the context of cardiac rehabilitation, training improved endothelial function, as measured by brachial artery flow–mediated dilation together with an increase in plasma nitrite and nitrate levels and superoxide dismutase activity and lowered oxidative stress.[60]

However, **the beneficial vascular effect of moderate exercise may not necessarily pertain to excessively mild or strenuous physical training at 25% and 75% V_{O_2}max, respectively.** Whereas mild exercise had no impact on endothelial function, high-intensity exercise increased indices of oxidative stress.[61] The major increase in oxygen uptake by skeletal muscle as a result of high-intensity training is, in fact, associated with increased free radical formation, which may mitigate the beneficial endothelial effects of exercise.[59]

eNOS-Independent Effects of Exercise on Endothelial Function. There are eNOS-independent mechanisms that may contribute to exercise-related, beneficial effects on the vasculature. Exercise-induced increases in prostaglandin release may have a vasculoprotective role.[62]

Akt Kinase. Physical training stimulates Akt kinase activity. **The close correlation between physical exercise and Akt kinase phosphorylation and activation not only translates into improved eNOS activity but also enhances vascular regenerative processes.** Akt kinase performs several NO-independent functions. It is instrumental for

- endothelial cell migration,
- endothelial cell proliferation, and
- the mobilization and functional activity of bone marrow–derived endothelial progenitor cells,

all critical features for vascular repair, angiogenesis, and neovascularization of ischemic tissue.[63]

Endothelial Progenitor Cells. Physical activity increases the production and circulating numbers of endothelial progenitor cells. Bone marrow–derived endothelial progenitor cells play a critical role in vascular repair and angiogenesis.

In mice exercised for 4 weeks on a running wheel at 5.1 ± 0.8 km/day, the number of endothelial progenitor cells increased by 280% ± 25%, when compared with controls, in peripheral blood and bone marrow, with a similar increase in endothelial progenitor cells expanded from spleen-derived mononuclear cells. In an NO-dependent fashion, exercise increased serum levels of vascular endothelial growth factor (VEGF) and reduced the rate of apoptosis in spleen-derived endothelial progenitor cells. Exercise significantly inhibited carotid neointima formation after vascular injury, but increased neoangiogenesis in a subcutaneous disk model when compared with controls.[64]

In 19 patients with stable CHD, moderate exercise training for 28 days similarly led to a significant increase in the number of circulating endothelial progenitor cells and a reduction in endothelial progenitor cell apoptosis.[64]

Vascular Effects of Exercise as a Function of Time. NO may play different roles in the short-term, intermediate, and long-term adaptations to exercise, with a time frame spanning a few weeks to years.

- Short-term adaptations to meet the metabolic demands of exercise may focus largely on vasodilation, mediated in part by NO.
- Longer-term adaptation entails vascular remodeling, whereby NO may be involved in a signaling cascade that subsequently triggers structural changes, such as an increase in vessel diameter.

These protracted adaptations contribute to the reduction in resting blood pressure that can be observed after as little as 4 weeks of training.[65]

Nitric Oxide and Metabolism. Adaptations in the skeletal muscle NO system contribute to some of the vascular and metabolic benefits of training.

NOS is constitutively expressed not only in endothelial cells but also in skeletal myocytes. Exercise enhances the synthesis of NO by NOS in both sites and engenders increased NO effects, not only in the vasculature but also in the musculature. The NO-mediated increase in blood flow and concomitant upgrade in fuel supply with exercise parallel and complement the increase in nutrient uptake and oxidative capacity implemented by the effects of NO in muscle.

Role of Nitric Oxide in Glucose Uptake. NO may function as a mediator of exercise-mediated glucose uptake.

Long-term exercise training increases the expression of eNOS in skeletal myocytes and the rate of NO release.[34] Modulation of the NO pathway in muscle by physical training improves glucose entry into skeletal muscle.[65]

Nitric Oxide and the Metabolic Rate. NO may enhance oxidative capacity and the metabolic rate.

An NO–cyclic guanosine 3′,5′-monophosphate (cGMP)-dependent pathway triggers mitochondrial biogenesis in diverse cell types and modulates the energy balance of the body. This process is dependent on the cGMP-mediated induction of peroxisome proliferator–activated receptor-gamma (PPAR-γ) coactivator-1α (PGC-1α), a master regulator of mitochondrial biogenesis. Correspondingly, eNOS-null (eNOS–/–) mutant mice have a marked reduction in mitochondrial biogenesis, associated with a lower metabolic rate and accelerated weight gain, when compared with wild-type mice.[66]

INFLAMMATION AND OXIDATIVE STRESS

Moderate-intensity exercise may reduce inflammation and oxidative stress. NO-related mechanisms appear to underlie some of these changes and, in a positive feedback mode, further enhance NO bioavailability.

Inflammatory Markers. Exercise has a systemic anti-inflammatory effect.

It modulates activation of the proinflammatory transcription factor nuclear factor kappaB (NFκB).[67] In rats, regular exercise decreased the content of the p50 and p65 subunits of NFκB, thereby attenuating activation of NFκB with a corresponding rise in the content of inhibitory factor κB.[68] Exercise inhibition of tissue ACE also mitigates the inflammatory pathways associated with the production of angiotensin II.[56] **Moderate physical training lowers markers of inflammation,** and levels of proinflammatory cytokines such as

- C-reactive protein (CRP),
- serum amyloid A,
- interleukin-6 (IL-6), and
- soluble intercellular adhesion molecule-1 (ICAM-1)

are inversely and independently associated with leisure time physical activity.[12]

In the Cardiovascular Health Study, higher physical activity was associated with lower levels of several proinflammatory markers, independent of gender, age, race, cigarette use, BMI, hypertension, cardiovascular disease, and DM.[69] In the National Health and Nutrition Examination Survey (NHANES) III, individuals who regularly jogged or pursued aerobic dancing were less likely to have elevated proinflammatory markers, independent of gender, age, race, BMI, cigarette use, and health status.[70] CRP levels were reduced in long-distance runners after 9 months of training, but not in sedentary controls.[71]

In healthy, albeit obese women, a year-long program encompassing a low-fat diet and exercise reduced plasma levels of tumor necrosis factor-alpha (TNF-α), IL-6, soluble ICAM-1, and soluble vascular cell adhesion molecule-1 (VCAM-1). Endothelial function improved as reflected by the degree of blood pressure lowering after an infusion

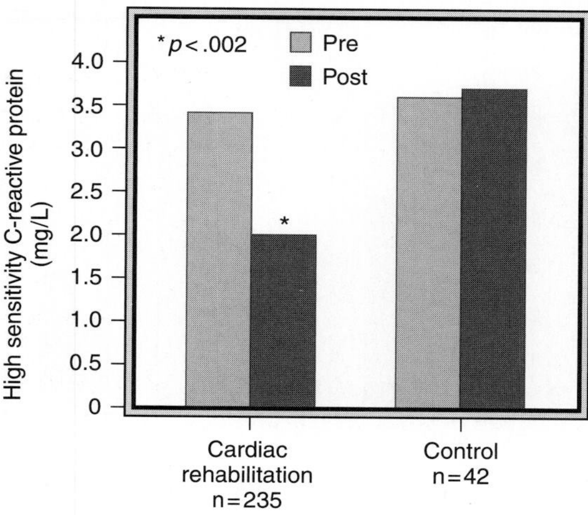

Figure 13–5.
Median changes in high-sensitivity C-reactive protein with cardiac rehabilitation in coronary heart disease patients. *(Modifed from Milani RV, Lavie CJ, Mehra MR. Reduction in C-reactive protein through cardiac rehabilitation and exercise training. J Am Coll Cardiol 2004; 43:1056-1061.)*

of L-arginine.[72] A randomized, controlled, 2-year intervention trial of exercise and weight loss in premenopausal, obese women significantly lowered levels of IL-6, IL-18, and CRP.[73]

In 277 CHD patients, 3 months of formal phase II cardiac rehabilitation and exercise training programs significantly lowered CRP by 41% (P = .002) when compared with nonexercising CHD controls (Fig. 13-5).[74] Inflammatory markers were reduced in patients with peripheral arterial disease after 6 months of a walking program, which also improved symptoms of claudication.[75]

Exercise mitigates the chronic inflammatory state of the metabolic syndrome. In a study of 1640 individuals with fitness assessed via exercise stress testing, subjects with the metabolic syndrome who maintained a high fitness level had markedly lower CRP levels than did those with a low fitness level (Fig. 13-6). Fitness modulated CRP concentrations independent of components of the metabolic syndrome. Furthermore, the effect of physical fitness on individuals with the metabolic syndrome was more pronounced than that in subjects without metabolic abnormalities.[76]

Oxidative Stress. Moderate exercise exerts antioxidant effects by lowering the elaboration

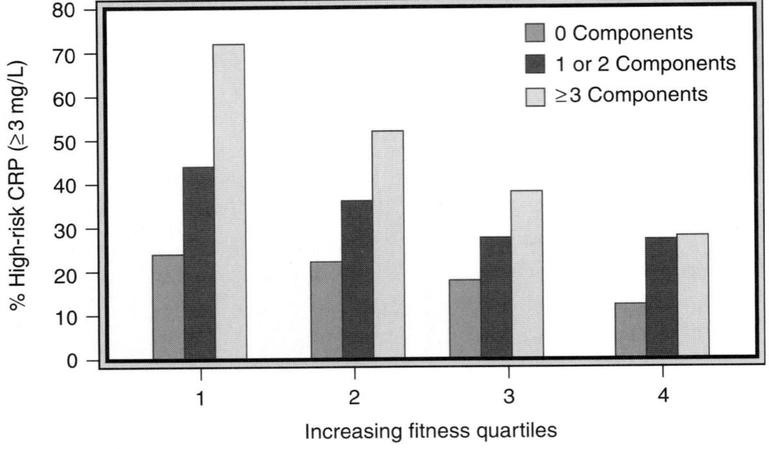

Figure 13–6.
Frequency of high-risk C-reactive protein (≥3.0 mg/L) as a function of fitness quartiles (lowest = 1) and the number of components of the metabolic syndrome. *(Modified from Aronson D, Sella R, Sheikh-Ahmad M, et al. The association between cardiorespiratory fitness and C-reactive protein in subjects with the metabolic syndrome. J Am Coll Cardiol 2004;44:2003-2007.)*

of pro-oxidant species and raising the expression of endogenous antioxidants.

Regular physical exercise attenuates potentially harmful oxidative damage.[77] The increased expression of endogenous antioxidants with moderate physical training thwarts oxidant-mediated NO inactivation, thereby increasing NO bioavailability to the vasculature and subjacent tissues. As exercise increases eNOS expression and NO production, it enhances the expression of extracellular superoxide dismutase in vascular smooth muscle in a cGMP/cGMP-dependent protein kinase (cGK)-dependent fashion.[78] Exercise shear stress also augments glutathione peroxidase as an endogenous antioxidant[62] and lowers angiotensin II–mediated generation of oxidant stress via inhibition of tissue ACE.[56]

EXERCISE AND ADENOSINE 5′-MONOPHOSPHATE–ACTIVATED PROTEIN KINASE

Physical exercise is a significant stimulus for the regulation of multiple metabolic processes in skeletal muscle. A single bout of exercise can alter rates of protein metabolism in skeletal myocytes by inducing transient changes in gene transcription as an adaptive mechanism.[32] In this respect, **AMPK appears to be an important sensor of energy status and modulator of cellular processes by matching myocyte energy supply with demand.**

Stimulation of AMPK. AMPK is activated by an incipient deficit in high-energy phosphate production in the cell. It is stimulated by a rise in cytoplasmic AMP and a fall in creatine phosphate. High-intensity exercise can robustly increase the activity of AMPK. Exercise-stimulated AMPK activity is dependent on the energy demands engendered by muscle contraction, as reflected by

- force development and
- stimulation frequency.[79]

Activated AMPK phosphorylates target proteins. ERK and atypical protein kinase C (PKC) increase and ultimately lead to greater transcription of the GLUT4 gene and hexokinase activity.[35,80]

Exercise and AMPK Isoforms. AMPK has two isoforms, α1 and α2. The AMPK-α2 complex is more important in regulating exercise-mediated muscle metabolism than α1 is. In fact, with exercise the α1 isoform does not change.

The increased activity of the AMPK-α2 isoform is a function of aerobic exercise intensity. Low- to moderate-intensity aerobic exercise induces an intensity-dependent increase in AMPK-α2.[35] With acute, intense exercise at 75% peak $\dot{V}O_2$, a threefold to fourfold increase in activation of the AMPK-α2 isoform ensues, which reverses 3 hours after exercise.[81] Even in type 2 diabetic patients, 45 minutes of bicycle exercise at 70% $\dot{V}O_2$max increased AMPK-α2 activity 2.7-fold, again with no change in α1.[35]

Exercise and AMPK Metabolic Effects. Exercise activation of AMPK up-regulates both glucose and lipid metabolism in skeletal muscle in order to meet the higher energy demand of working myocytes.

Glucose Metabolism. Exercise leads to an insulin-independent increase in glucose transport and skeletal muscle glycogen content, mediated in part by AMPK.

Acute activation of AMPK by exercise increases GLUT4 translocation to the sarcolemma for increased glucose uptake. Chronic exposure of muscle to exercise initiates AMPK-mediated alterations in the transcriptional regulation of GLUT4 and hexokinase II.[35,79,82]

Fatty Acid Metabolism and Metabolic Rate. Stimulation of AMPK by exercise increases the metabolic rate and fatty acid oxidation.

AMPK raises the activity of uncoupling protein-3.[35] Activation of AMPK by exercise also lowers the concentration of malonyl coenzyme A (CoA) via beta phosphorylation of acetyl CoA carboxylase (ACC), thereby enhancing fatty acid oxidation.

Specifically, ACC beta phosphorylation is tightly coupled to AMPK signaling and is especially sensitive to exercise intensity. ACC catalyzes the synthesis of malonyl CoA. Malonyl CoA is a potent allosteric inhibitor of carnitine palmitoyltransferase I (CPT-I), the enzyme that controls the transfer of fatty acyl CoA into the mitochondria for oxidation.[83] With ACC inactivation, the concentration of malonyl CoA decreases, and thus the malonyl CoA–dependent inhibition of CPT-I is mitigated.

In a study of eight men cycling for 20 minutes at each of three sequential intensities, calculated fat oxidation increased in parallel with ACC beta phosphorylation, until it declined during the highest-intensity exercise.[84]

EXERCISE AND PEROXISOME PROLIFERATOR–ACTIVATED RECEPTORS

PPARs are lipid-activated nuclear receptors that mediate the pleiotropic effects encompassing the control of metabolism and inflammation by controlling the transcription of target genes. Of the PPAR isoforms, **there is only little expression of PPAR-γ and greater expression of PPAR-α in skeletal muscle.**

PPAR-γ. Exercise up-regulates the expression of PPAR-γ. PPAR-γ plays a key role in

- adipogenesis,
- insulin sensitivity, and
- control of inflammatory processes.

It activates the transcription of genes involved in lipogenesis, adipocyte differentiation, and fatty acid esterification. In a 16-week, chronic exercise study of fructose-fed, spontaneously hypertensive rats running at 20 m/min, 0% grade, 60 min/day, 5 days/wk, exercise training significantly up-regulated PPAR-γ expression in fat, as well as in skeletal muscle.[85]

PPAR-α. PPAR-α, moderately expressed in skeletal muscle, plays an important role regulating pathways of free fatty acid metabolism in myocytes. PPAR-α increases mitochondrial beta oxidation and degradation of fatty acids, thereby providing energy for the contractile activity of cardiac and skeletal myocytes while decreasing the esterification of free fatty acids into myocyte triglycerides, or triacylglycerols.[86,87]

PPAR-α expression is greater in type I than in type II fibers and rises with exercise training. After 6 weeks of endurance training in healthy men, PPAR-α increased 3-fold and 1½-fold in type I and type II fibers, respectively, $P < .001$.[88] Twelve weeks of endurance training in women induced a twofold induction of skeletal muscle PPAR-α protein content.[89]

The mRNA and protein expression of PPAR-α decreases with inactivity and old age. Exercise intervention, however, reverses the aging-related decline in expression of PPAR-α, thus restoring skeletal and cardiac muscle metabolic capacity.[87]

EXERCISE AND SUBSTRATE OXIDATION

Increased expression of skeletal muscle NOS, the PPARs, AMPK, and other gene products with physical exercise increases carbohydrate and fatty acid substrate utilization.

Carbohydrate Metabolism. Endurance training enhances the oxidative capacity of skeletal muscle for carbohydrate metabolism. Exercise increases the mRNA and protein expression of GLUT4 and other key proteins that regulate glucose metabolism.[90,91] Thus, muscle biopsy 22 hours after an acute, 1-hour cycling session at 65% peak Vo_2 showed that induction of GLUT4 protein increased by 32% to 51%.[92]

Fatty Acid Oxidation. Chronic exercise and endurance training enhance the gene expression of key enzymes for fat metabolism, as well as the oxidative capacity of skeletal muscle for fatty acids.

Mitochondria. Exercise increases the mRNA of transcriptional coactivators for mitochondrial biogenesis, thereby engendering an adaptive increase in the number of mitochondria.[90,91]

Lipoprotein Lipase. To increase fat oxidation, physical activity facilitates myocyte uptake of fatty acid. Correspondingly, there is an increase in lipoprotein lipase (LPL).

After an acute, 1-hour exercise session of cycling at 65% peak Vo_2, LPL activity increased over 24 hours. Muscle biopsy 22 hours after exercise showed increased induction of LPL protein by 170% to 240%, which was not related to activation of β-adrenergic receptors.[92] Chronic, 3-month, low-intensity training at 40% of peak Vo_2 resulted in an increase in total fat oxidation during exercise, as marked by a rise in LPL mRNA.[93] Simple walking and standing activities are important in maintaining high levels of LPL activity in the slow-twitch, oxidative muscles that posturally support the skeleton. Intensive exercise training additionally increases LPL activity in the fast-twitch, glycolytic muscles.[94] Aging is associated with a loss of skeletal muscle LPL activity and protein, especially in the weight-bearing, postural skeletal muscle. With increasing age, this loss is associated with a reduction in triglyceride metabolism that results in postprandial as well as fasting hypertriglyceridemia. In contrast, endurance-trained, older individuals have a favorable triglyceride metabolism, comparable to that of young subjects.[95]

Fatty Acid Transport and Oxidation. Exercise enhances the expression of genes involved in fatty acid uptake across the sarcolemma and mitochondrial membranes and beta oxidation of fatty acids.

Fatty acid transport proteins such as the sarcolemmal fatty acid transporter fatty acid binding protein ($FABP_{PM}$), fatty acid translocase (FAT/CD36), the rate-limiting mitochondrial fatty acid transporter CPT-I (Fig. 13-7), and β-hydroxyacyl-CoA dehydrogenase (β-HAD), a key enzyme of beta oxidation, are all increased with exercise, as is the expression and activity of muscle cytochrome-*c* oxidase (Fig. 13-8).[90,91]

LIPIDS

Exercise has a modest effect on plasma lipid levels as a result of its modulation of fatty acid metabolism. The beneficial impact of exercise on plasma lipids is drastically enhanced by concomitant dietary intervention.[96]

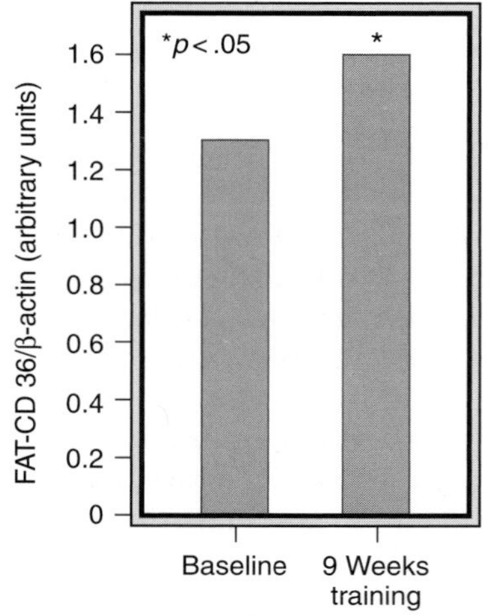

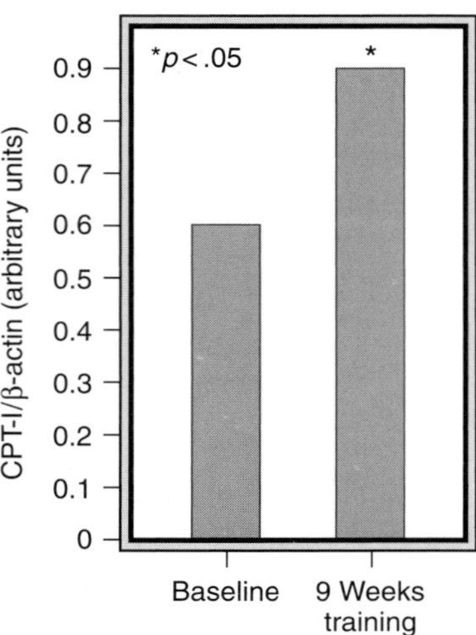

Figure 13–7. Effect of 9-week cycle training on gene expression of fatty acid translocase (FAT)/CD36 and carnitine palmitoyltransferase I (CPT-I) in humans. *(Modified from Tunstall RJ, Mehan KA, Wadley GD, et al. Exercise training increases lipid metabolism gene expression in human skeletal muscle. Am J Physiol Endocrinol Metab 2002;283:E66-E72.)*

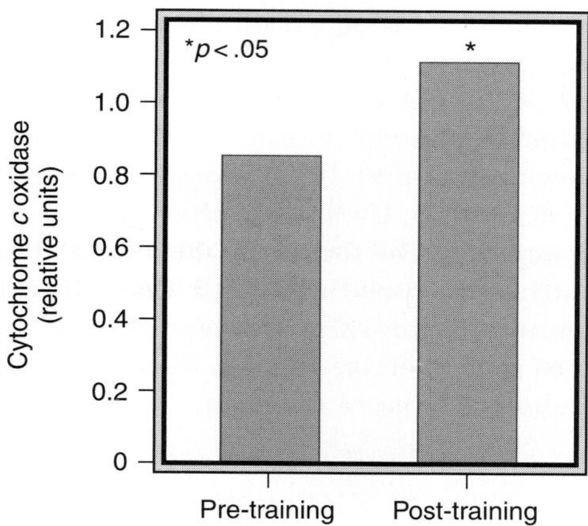

Figure 13–8.
Seven-day human exercise training effect on the mitochondrial marker enzyme cytochrome-*c* oxidase in skeletal muscle. *(Modified from Youngren JF, Keen S, Kulp JL, et al. Enhanced muscle insulin receptor autophosphorylation with short-term aerobic exercise training. Am J Physiol Endocrinol Metab 2001;280:E528-E533.)*

Low-Density Lipoproteins. Low-density lipoprotein (LDL) levels are not generally affected by physical training.[97] **However, exercise does seem to improve the LDL subfraction profile with a decrease in small, dense LDL particles.** The amount of training, rather than the intensity of exercise, may be a more important determinant of lipoprotein particle size.[98] In a series of reports on the HERITAGE Family Study, a 20-week bicycle-training course reduced levels of total cholesterol as well as apolipoprotein B-100.[99]

Triglycerides. Exercise lowers triglyceride levels. In the HERITAGE Family Study, 20 weeks of bicycle exercise reduced triglyceride levels.[99] With exercise training, triglycerides in excess of 250 mg/dL decline by 20%.[97]

Endothelial function is impaired after fat ingestion, in part related to a rise in circulating triglyceride concentrations. **Preprandial exercise reduces postprandial triglyceride concentrations and thus improves postprandial vascular function.** Ten lean (waist <90 cm) and 10 centrally obese (waist >100 cm) middle-aged men ingested a high-fat meal containing 80 g fat and 70 g carbohydrate with or without a preprandial 90-minute treadmill exercise. Exercise reduced fasting and postprandial triglyceride concentrations by 25% in both the lean and centrally obese groups ($P < .0005$). For all subjects, postpran-dial endothelium-dependent and endothelium-independent functions were 15% and 20% higher (both $P < .05$), respectively, in the exercise relative to the control trial.[100]

LPL activity may contribute to the hypotriglyceridemic effect of moderate exercise, although other mechanisms may play a role.[94] **The NO/cGMP signaling pathway, activated by exercise, modulates hepatic fatty acid metabolism and may contribute to a lowering of hepatic very-low-density lipoprotein (VLDL) secretion, in conjunction with PPAR-α and AMPK activation.** In a rat hepatocyte model, NO, in a signaling cascade involving the activation of soluble guanylate cyclase, cGMP, and cGK, inhibited fatty acid synthesis but enhanced fatty acid oxidation, an effect mediated in part by the inhibition of calcium release from the endoplasmic reticulum. NO and cGMP stimulate fatty acid oxidation via two different mechanisms:

1. inhibition of ACC activity, which lowers levels of malonyl CoA and thereby increases CPT-I and fatty acid beta oxidation, and
2. malonyl CoA–independent stimulation of CPT-I.[101]

High-Density Lipoproteins. Activation of PPAR-α and PPAR-γ by exercise may favorably enhance the expression of genes encoding proteins involved in high-density lipoprotein (HDL) metabolism.[85,102] As a result of these changes and the reduction in triglyceride-rich lipoprotein concentration, **HDL levels increase by 8% to 10% with exercise training.**[97] In the HERITAGE Family Study series, 20 weeks of bicycle exercise raised HDL2 and HDL3, apolipoprotein A-I levels, and LPL activity. The change in HDL was found to be proportional to the reduction in visceral fat and inversely related to baseline HDL and baseline triglyceride.[99] Cholesterol ester transfer protein (CETP) genotype differences may contribute to the interindividual differences in the magnitude of plasma HDL changes occurring with endurance exercise training.[103]

EFFECTS OF EXERCISE ON METABOLISM IN OVERWEIGHT

There is a strong, 30% to 50% heritability factor for genotype involvement in the

adipogenic response to overfeeding.[104] **Interestingly, this genetic relationship is mitigated by exercise training.**[105] As physical exercise increases fatty acid and carbohydrate substrate utilization and metabolism, there is a resultant reduction in body fat mass and weight. In particular, **exercise enhances the impact of dietary efforts at weight loss by favorably modulating metabolic activity.**

Although the amount of weight lost with exercise efforts alone is not impressive, in the absence of exercise, overweight, middle-aged individuals may experience a 2-lb weight gain per year.[106]

Acute Response. Even one bout of exercise can alter the metabolic responses to food. A bout of glycogen-depleting exercise, followed by a 60% fat meal, can result in fat oxidation matching fat intake, with no net fat storage.[107,108] In obese individuals, 2 hours of moderate exercise increases spontaneous and β-receptor–mediated lipolysis.[109]

Chronic Response. With chronic exercise training, sympathetic tone decreases and circulating catecholamine levels are lower.[41,42] As a result, catecholamine receptor sensitivity, in particular, visceral-omental adipocyte β-receptor sensitivity, is increased. **Chronic exercise conditioning enhances lipolysis in association with an overall increment in fatty acid oxidation.** These changes tend to be greater in men than women, but they are lost after only 4 days of inactivity.[110]

Long-term exercise conditioning reduces total-body fat. Six months of endurance training resulted in a reduction in total-body fat and weight loss.[103] In an 8-month exercise program, nondieting, overweight men and women lost weight and fat mass in a dose-responsive manner as a function of exercise frequency and intensity.[106] A 12-month-long, moderate-intensity sports/recreational activity program in overweight, postmenopausal women, when compared with stretch-placebo controls, reduced body weight and body fat significantly. A significant dose response for greater body fat loss was observed with increasing duration of exercise.[111] In a 16-month, controlled efficacy trial involving 131 participants randomized to exercise or control from two Midwestern universities, exercise prevented weight gain in women and produced weight loss of 5.2 ± 4.7 kg in men, whereas controls showed significant increases in BMI, weight, and fat mass.[112]

Adipocyte Change with Exercise. Exercise has a favorable impact on adipocyte response to lipolytic stimuli. Ordinarily, **after weight loss, adipocytes of the formerly obese remain less sensitive to lipolytic stimuli than do those from normal controls. However, even the pursuit of mild exercise renders these adipocytes metabolically more dynamic.**[113]

EFFECTS OF EXERCISE ON NORMAL GLUCOSE AND INSULIN METABOLISM

Exercise increases insulin-independent skeletal muscle glucose uptake in order to enhance ongoing fuel supply to the working myocytes while ambient insulin levels are low. After exercise, the insulin-dependent rates of both glucose uptake and glycogen synthesis rise to replenish myocyte energy stores.

Insulin-Independent Glucose Uptake during Exercise. Muscle glucose uptake during exercise has to occur largely via insulin-independent mechanisms because the anabolic insulin pathways, geared toward fuel storage, are down-regulated.[114] **An acute bout of exercise improves insulin-independent glucose uptake.**

The immediate effects of acute exercise occur at the level of the GLUT4 isoform of muscle glucose transporters. Exercise increases glucose uptake capacity in skeletal muscle with an increase in GLUT4 translocation to the plasma membrane. Exercise-induced glucose transport activity can be entirely accounted for by the degree of GLUT4 translocation to the plasma membrane.[34] For example, 30 to 60 minutes of aerobic exercise at 60% to 70% peak Vo_2 can decrease glucose concentrations, even in insulin-resistant muscle, via contraction-induced stimulation of GLUT4 translocation. Exercise causes enhanced disappearance of glucose during a glucose tolerance test.[115]

With chronic conditioning, an increase in GLUT4 mRNA precedes a rise in total GLUT4 content, which may double.[116]

The direct effects of exercise on glucose transport and insulin signaling are not entirely understood and remain controversial. There are several potential mechanisms:

- There appears to be at least a partial dependence on cytoplasmic levels of 5′-AMP and activation of AMPK.
- Contraction-associated calcium release may play a role.[34]
- NO may be a mediator of exercise-mediated glucose signaling.[34,65]
- Exercise may enhance an insulin-independent increase in glucose transport via MAPK signaling pathways by regulating transcriptional activity.[35]

Insulin Action after Exercise. The normal molecular mechanisms for the activation of insulin signal transduction pathways after exercise training entail the following events. At physiologic concentrations, normal insulin signaling in skeletal muscle activates insulin receptor tyrosine kinase activity, which results in insulin receptor substrate-1 (IRS-1) tyrosine phosphorylation and IRS-1–associated phosphatidylinositol 3-kinase (PI3K) activity. Akt-1/protein kinase B (PKB) is a downstream effector of PI3K and a potential mediator of insulin-mediated glucose uptake.[117]

Exercise enhances insulin sensitivity. The enhanced insulin sensitivity in skeletal muscle is generally not systemic but restricted to the muscle group that is actually performing the work.[118] Improved sensitivity to insulin signaling contributes to the restoration or overcompensation of glycogen stores for the exercised muscle, such that an endurance-trained muscle commands higher glycogen stores than an untrained muscle does.

Although aerobic training has traditionally been considered the premier mode for enhancing skeletal muscle insulin metabolism, resistance training confers a similar benefit. Resistance training does not just quantitatively increase lean body mass. Like aerobic training, resistance work also elevates skeletal muscle GLUT4 concentrations and enhances insulin sensitivity (Fig. 13-9).[119]

Time Course of the Skeletal Muscle Insulin Response. Plasma insulin concentrations actually decrease during exercise. Immediately after exercise, insulin action is in fact compromised,

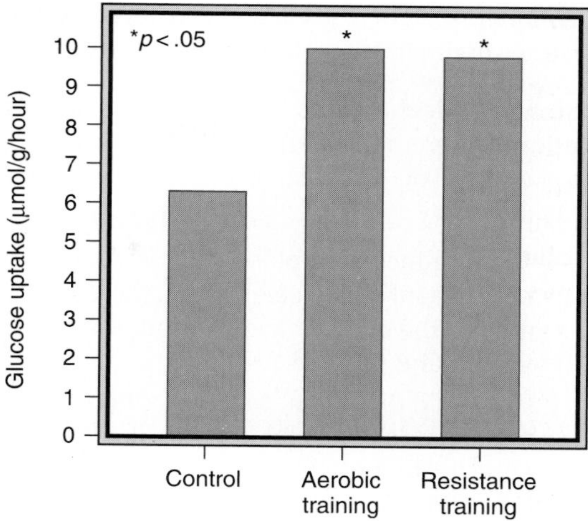

Figure 13–9.
Glucose uptake in the hind limbs of aerobically and resistance-trained rats. *(Modified from Yaspelkis BB, Singh MK, Trevino B, et al. Resistance training increases glucose uptake and transport in rat skeletal muscle. Acta Physiol Scand 2002;175:315-323.)*

possibly because of the elevated levels of circulating catecholamines and free fatty acids with exercise.[114]

The training-induced enhancement of the metabolic action of insulin, based primarily in the previously exercised muscles, occurs several hours after training, upon recovery from exercise.[114] Even a single bout of exercise will improve insulin action in the affected muscle. Insulin signal transduction at the level of the insulin receptor, IRS1 and IRS2, as well as PI3K, is enhanced in the exercised myocyte.[35,120]

After 1 week of physical training, there is a 33% increase in insulin sensitivity in skeletal muscle, and insulin signal transduction is enhanced at different molecular levels:

- a 40% increase in insulin receptor autophosphorylation,
- a twofold enhancement of insulin-induced IRS-1 and IRS-2 phosphorylation,
- a twofold increase in IRS-1/2 association with PI3K,
- a twofold rise in PI3K activity, and
- a twofold enhancement of serine phosphorylation and activation of Akt-1/PKB.[35]

Sensitization to insulin may last up to 48 hours after exercise.[118] Carbohydrate deprivation after exercise prolongs the sensitization to insulin. In contrast, postexercise carbohydrate loading, conducive to glycogen resynthesis, results in faster normalization of insulin sensitivity.[121]

Potential Mechanisms of Enhanced Insulin Action. Different mechanisms may contribute to the effects of chronic training on insulin sensitivity:

- Training increases blood flow and capillary recruitment in skeletal muscle, thereby promoting the delivery and distribution of both insulin and glucose.[114]
- Fatty acid oxidation, together with exercise depletion of skeletal muscle lipid stores, appears to be a metabolic construct that raises insulin sensitivity.[114] PPAR-α, NOS, and AMPK mechanisms may be involved.
- The degree of glycogen depletion during exercise is a major stimulant for the enhanced insulin-mediated glucose transport and glycogen synthase activity in the recovery period.[121] The molecular mechanisms linking glycogen content to insulin action may involve greater Akt kinase and AMPK activation.[114]
- The amplified insulin-stimulated glucose uptake after exercise training arises, in part, from the heightened mRNA and protein expression, as well as function of the insulin receptor, IRS-1, PI3K, and ERK1.[33,118]

EXERCISE AND INSULIN RESISTANCE

Insulin sensitivity is related to the degree of physical activity and fitness and is controlled by the chronic exposure of muscle to exercise.[122] **Insensitivity to insulin develops with inactivity, as may occur after several days of bed rest.**

The reduced insulin sensitivity of aging is, in fact, largely due to physical inactivity.[116] Mitochondrial function, muscle fat oxidative capacity, and insulin sensitivity are all closely correlated and are not necessarily impaired by age, but by physical inactivity. Thus, in an exercise study examining the effects of age versus conditioning, measures of insulin sensitivity were higher in trained than in untrained individuals but were similar between age groups. In stepwise regression, among body composition, VO_2max, and muscle biochemical characteristics, muscle fat oxidative capacity was the main predictor of insulin sensitivity ($r = .60$, $P < .001$).[123]

Derangements in Insulin-Resistant Skeletal Muscle. With insulin resistance, insulin-mediated glucose uptake is impaired in skeletal muscle.

GLUT4 translocation to the sarcolemma for glucose uptake appears to be inadequate.[124] With obesity and a sedentary lifestyle, insulin-resistant muscles have a lower percentage of type I fibers and a lower density of GLUT4 protein in type I fibers. Type II fast-twitch, glycolytic, insulin-insensitive muscle fibers are preferentially expressed. Insulin-resistant skeletal muscle has lower oxidative capacity and lower rates of fatty acid oxidation as measured by enzyme activity.[125] Endothelial dysfunction and a diminution in skeletal muscle blood flow with compromised nutritional perfusion are associated with insulin resistance. The insensitivity of myocytes to insulin may in part be due to impaired insulin-mediated capillary recruitment.[124]

Exercise Intervention in Insulin Resistance. Both an acute session of exercise and chronic endurance training have beneficial effects on insulin resistance by affecting insulin-dependent and insulin-independent pathways. **Resistance and aerobic exercise training improve insulin-mediated glucose uptake by skeletal muscle.** However, metabolic training adaptations are primarily restricted to the muscles recruited for the exercise performance.[126,127]

Evidence for the benefits of exercise on insulin action derives from studies in trained athletes and from cross-sectional and longitudinal studies.[120] **Even in insulin-resistant persons, participation in regular exercise programs can lead to improved glucose tolerance and insulin action, as well as better health outcomes.**[128]

Chronic exercise enhances insulin sensitivity. Ten weeks of training significantly improved skeletal muscle glucose extraction and whole-body glucose uptake in aged healthy individuals and in individuals with type 2 DM.[129] One year of chronic intensive exercise training, 5 days a week with 40 to 60 minutes of running, dramatically improved or normalized both insulin and glucose responses to a glucose tolerance test.[130] Less intensive chronic exercise training achieved lesser benefits.[131] A 2-year intervention of exercise and weight loss in obese women significantly improved adiponectin levels and insulin sensitivity.[73] Each 500-kcal increment in weekly exercise activity lowered the incidence of type 2 DM in college alumni by 6%.[132]

Mechanism of Exercise Improvement in Metabolic Insulin Signaling. With insulin resistance, exercise can improve whole-body insulin-mediated glucose disposal and metabolism.[126,127] A number of exercise mechanisms that mediate improved postexercise insulin sensitivity with normal metabolism apply to insulin resistance. The improvement in insulin sensitivity occurs multifactorially.

Insulin Signaling Molecules. With insulin resistance, the increased protein expression and function of IRS-1, GLUT4, and other insulin signaling molecules upon exercise training enhance insulin signaling efficacy for

- glucose transport,
- glycogen synthase activation and glycogen synthesis, and
- amino acid transport.[34]

Muscle Fiber Metabolism. There is a preponderance of type II muscle fibers with insulin resistance. **Exercise increases the proportion of slow-twitch, insulin-sensitive, type I oxidative muscle fibers** and engenders hypertrophy of such insulin-sensitive muscle. Mitochondrial biogenesis is enhanced in myocytes, with resultant improvement in fatty acid oxidative capacity (Fig. 13-10).[90,91,133]

Adipocyte Size. Enlarged adipocytes, arising from an antiadipogenic milieu, are associated with insulin resistance. **With exercise, there is a beneficial reduction in adipocyte size,** especially in the visceral-omental location, and such reduction renders adipocytes potentially more sensitive to insulin. These changes tend to be greater in men than in women.[110]

Endothelial Function. Insulin resistance is associated with endothelial dysfunction. **Exercise may improve insulin sensitivity by increasing endothelial function.** Higher eNOS expression and activity, via NO/cGMP/cGK signaling, directly improve insulin signaling. Additionally, greater skeletal muscle perfusion and insulin-mediated capillary recruitment enhance the delivery of insulin and fuel substrates to target tissues.[65]

Visceral Adiposity. Visceral adiposity is associated with insulin resistance and hyperinsulinemia. **There is a strong genetic component to the increase in visceral fat as a response to overfeeding, which is allayed by exercise training.**[104] **The regular pursuit of exercise may, in fact, prevail over genotype in this regard.**[105] **Because visceral fat functions as a "first-response" source of fuel, exercise causes a preferential mobilization of abdominal visceral fat.**[134] As physical exercise increases fatty acid and carbohydrate substrate utilization, there is a resultant reduction in visceral fat with beneficial physiologic consequences. Specifically, with exercise, fasting insulin levels fall and glucose

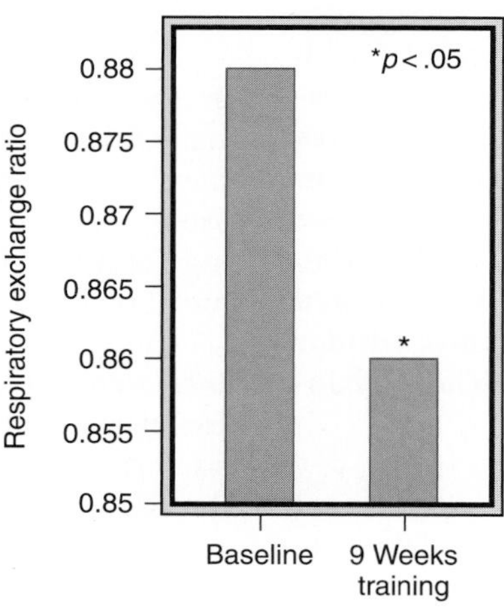

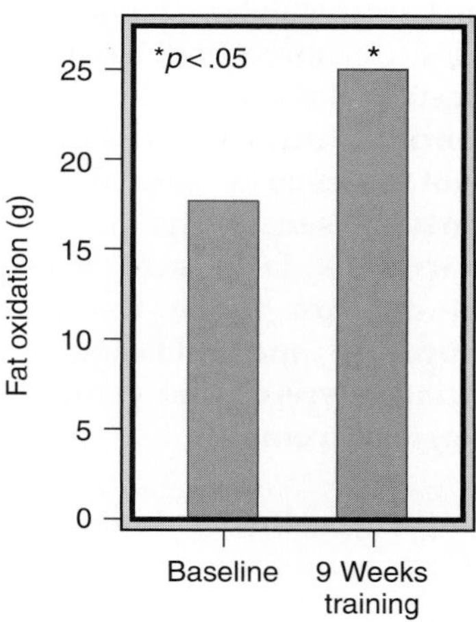

Figure 13–10. Respiratory exchange ratio and total fat oxidized during 60 minutes of exercise after 9 days of cycle training in humans. *(Modified from Tunstall RJ, Mehan KA, Wadley GD, et al. Exercise training increases lipid metabolism gene expression in human skeletal muscle. Am J Physiol Endocrinol Metab 2002;283:E66-E72.)*

disposal is enhanced as a function of the decline in visceral fat.[105]

Exercise decreases the degree of visceral ponderosity irrespective of weight loss. In the absence of weight loss, there is nevertheless a reduction in visceral fat with regular exercise.[135]

Visceral fat is reduced in proportion to fat loss. Obese men who lost weight via exercise lost similar proportions of subcutaneous and visceral fat.[135] In the series of reports on the Minnesota HERITAGE Family Study, a 20-week bicycle-training course was found to reduce visceral fat and adiposity in general.[99] Six-month endurance training resulted in a reduction in total-body and intra-abdominal fat together with a loss of weight.[103] A randomized, 12-month-long, moderate-intensity sports program trial in sedentary, overweight, postmenopausal women achieved significant reductions in intra-abdominal and subcutaneous abdominal fat. Specifically, there was a 4.2% loss of total-body fat and a 6.9% loss of intra-abdominal visceral fat. A significant dose response for greater body fat loss was observed with increasing duration of exercise. Walking was the activity reported most frequently.[111] Obese, nondiabetic women performing moderate-intensity aerobic exercise four to five times a week for 14 months increased fitness and decreased body fat mass, with a greater loss of abdominal fat than mid-thigh fat.[136] In the 16-month, controlled efficacy trial of 131 participants randomized to exercise or control from two Midwestern universities, exercising men or women all demonstrated significant reductions in visceral fat.[112]

Enhanced Fatty Acid Beta Oxidation of Intramyocellular Lipid. Ectopic accumulation of intramyocellular fat is associated with insulin resistance. However, **the mere presence of intramyocellular triacylglycerol does not necessarily have detrimental effects on insulin sensitivity.**[137] **As physical exercise increases fatty acid substrate utilization, it appears to be the resultant increased turnover and oxidation of intramyocellular triacylglycerol that confer beneficial physiologic outcomes.**[105]

Intramyocellular Lipid as a Source of Contractile Energy. Although plasma free fatty acids, present in micromolar concentrations, are a major lipid energy source for skeletal muscle, circulating VLDL triglycerides, as well as the intramyocellular lipid depot, constitute other potential venues for fatty acids. During prolonged exercise of moderate intensity, non–plasma-derived fatty acids play an increasingly significant role as an energy source. Intramyocellular lipids located within skeletal myocytes are considered to be a major source of these fatty acids.[137] During moderate-intensity exercise, circulating free fatty acids and intramyocellular lipid provide roughly equal proportions of fatty acid for oxidation.[138]

Increase in Intramyocellular Fat with Training. Intramyocellular lipid actually increases with exercise training. This increase is a very early response to training. Two weeks of bicycle training in nine untrained men (23.3 ± 3.2 years of age, BMI of 22.6 ± 2.6 kg/m^2) significantly raised intramyocellular fat content by 42% ± 14%, as determined by proton magnetic resonance spectroscopy, before a significant rise in fat oxidation or insulin sensitivity.[137]

Training-Induced Increases in PPAR-α and Enzymes for Intramyocellular Fat Catabolism. Training induces significant selective increases in the mRNA levels of key enzymes involved in the metabolism of intramyocellular lipid. Specifically, there was up-regulation of the mRNA of enzymes such as

- hormone-sensitive lipase, involved in lipolytic mobilization of fatty acids from intramyocellular lipid stores,
- FABP3, engaged in intramyocellular fatty acid transport, and
- cytochrome-*c* oxidase I, implicated in oxidative phosphorylation

in the tibialis anterior muscle of endurance-trained versus untrained subjects. Furthermore, there was coregulation of the transcript level for these enzymes with the level of mRNA encoding for PPAR-α, the master regulator of lipid metabolism.[139]

Increased Myocellular Fat Hydrolysis with Exercise. Intramyocellular triacylglycerol hydrolysis increases during exercise to accommodate the rise in fatty acid oxidation. In fact, even the contraction of isolated muscles can stimulate the hydrolysis and oxidation of intramyocellular lipid in the absence of hormonal or neural input.[138] After 120 minutes of moderate-intensity exercise in eight individuals, muscle biopsy showed an increase in fatty acid oxidation rates during exercise.[140] In exercising, young healthy men, intramyocellular fat content decreased significantly during cycling.[137] In 18 moderately active, 18- to 38-year-old men ($n = 9$) and women ($n = 9$), intramyocellular lipid decreased significantly with exercise (by 11.5% to 28.5% for men and 17.1% to 21.7% for women; $P < .05$).[141] After 120 minutes of moderate-intensity exercise at 60% VO_2max in eight subjects, muscle biopsy revealed a 62% ± 7% net decline in muscle lipid content in oxidative type I fibers only, with no subsequent change during recovery.[140] Slow recovery of myocellular fat stores was also seen in a magnetic resonance spectroscopy study of nine moderately trained subjects after 45 minutes of interval cycling. Immediately after exercise, myocellular fat was 38% lower than pre-exercise levels ($P < .05$) and remained reduced by 30% through the 60-minute recovery.[142]

However, whereas moderate-intensity aerobic exercise at 60% to 70% VO_2max markedly reduced intramyocellular lipid in a time-dependent fashion, as assessed by magnetic resonance spectroscopy, exercise of similar duration at higher workloads exceeding 80% VO_2max did not reduce myocellular fat.[143]

Causes of Increased Intramyocellular Lipid Turnover. Enhanced fatty acid beta oxidation in myocytes with increased turnover of intramyocellular lipid stores exerts an insulin-sensitizing effect.[144] Exercise activates a number of factors that enhance the metabolic rate and fatty acid oxidation and thus may promote insulin signaling in insulin-resistant individuals:

- **NOS.** Exercise increases skeletal muscle NOS activity and expression. The NO/cGMP signaling pathway may enhance the metabolic rate and fatty acid catabolism.[66,101]
- **PPAR-α.** The exercise-mediated increase in skeletal muscle PPAR-α decreases fatty acid esterification into myocyte triacylglycerol while promoting muscle lipid catabolism and intramyocellular fat turnover.[85-87,145,146]
- **Leptin.** Obesity and insulin resistance are associated with hyperleptinemia and leptin resistance. Exercise reduces leptin levels, probably because of a training-induced change in body fat mass.[147] This reduction in the plasma levels of leptin may have a favorable impact on the sensitivity to leptin signaling with beneficial metabolic effects. In rats, 4 weeks of exercise caused a reduction of leptin in mesenteric and subcutaneous adipose tissue.[148]
- **Adiponectin.** Adiponectin is an adipose tissue–derived adipokine. Plasma adiponectin levels are inversely related to obesity and insulin resistance. Chronic exercise training in normal, nonobese subjects does not increase adiponectin.

However, **exercise training in overweight, insulin-resistant subjects may increase plasma adiponectin levels with an insulin-sensitizing effect.** In 24 insulin-resistant, obese individuals with varying degrees of glucose tolerance, a 6-month program of a hypocaloric diet, combined with moderate physical activity, caused a 6.9 ± 0.1-kg weight loss with a significant improvement in the insulin sensitivity index. Adiponectin increased significantly only in the diabetic subjects.[149] A short-term exercise intervention in 26 sedentary, overweight men similarly increased circulating adiponectin levels, with an improvement in insulin sensitivity.[150]

Adiponectin may improve insulin sensitivity via AMPK activation in skeletal muscle and the liver.[151]

- **AMPK.** Insulin resistance impairs the activation of AMPK-α1 in response to contraction, but it has no effect on AMPK-α2.[152] The metabolic effect of AMPK stimulation by exercise is enhancement of alternative, non–insulin-dependent glucose transport. By increasing fatty acid oxidation and the metabolic rate, activation of AMPK by exercise probably contributes to insulin sensitization.[35,151]

Intramyocellular Fat, Oxidative Capacity, and Insulin Resistance. Magnetic resonance spectroscopic documentation of intramyocellular lipid accumulation, more than extramyocellular and total-body fat, correlates with insulin resistance in humans. It would thus appear paradoxical that endurance-trained athletes should have elevated stores of intramyocellular lipid.

However, in contrast to sedentary, insulin-resistant subjects, such athletes have very high oxidative capacity in type I fibers with an increased number of mitochondria that engender greater turnover of intramyocellular lipid. As a result, their skeletal muscles are remarkably insulin sensitive.[153]

Enhanced fatty acid beta oxidation in myocytes exerts an insulin-sensitizing effect independent of the presence of intramyocellular lipid or changes in the amount of such lipid. L6 myotubes, transduced with adenoviruses encoded with CPT-I isoforms, proportionally increased oxidation of the long-chain fatty acids palmitate and oleate coincident with an increase in insulin-stimulated glucose incorporation into glycogen and insulin-stimulated phosphorylation of p38 MAPK. In this instance, insulin sensitization with CPT-I overexpression and accelerated beta oxidation occurred in the absence of a reduction in intracellular triacylglycerol, diacylglycerol, ceramide, or long-chain acyl CoA.[144]

There is a significant relationship between the oxidative capacity of skeletal muscle and insulin sensitivity. In a muscle biopsy study of type 2 diabetic patients versus trained and untrained nondiabetic controls, skeletal muscle oxidative capacity was a better predictor of insulin sensitivity than either the intramyocellular triacylglycerol concentration or long-chain fatty acyl CoA content was.[154]

Insulin sensitivity and muscle fat oxidative capacity are coregulated by the level of physical conditioning, independent of intramyocellular lipid. In eight sedentary, elderly subjects (63.5 ± 3.3 years old), muscle fat oxidative capacity and insulin sensitivity improved in parallel after 8 weeks of endurance training ($r = .79, P < .01$).[123] In overweight and obese sedentary men, an increase in insulin sensitivity with moderate-intensity exercise was similarly predicted by improvements in the fat oxidation rate and aerobic capacity, independent of myocyte triacylglycerol. Specifically, 18 nondiabetic, sedentary, overweight to obese men aged 37.4 ± 1.3 years with a BMI of 30.9 ± 0.7 kg/m^2 at baseline trained at 55% to 70% of Vo_2max for 40 minutes per session four times weekly for 10 weeks and were studied by magnetic resonance spectroscopy. Although myocyte lipid levels 24 to 36 hours after the last bout of exercise remained unchanged, central abdominal fat decreased 5% at program end. Coincident with a significant rise in mean whole-body, insulin-stimulated glucose uptake of 16% was an increase in mean aerobic capacity of 11%, as well as a significant increment in the basal fat oxidation rate of 41%.[155]

Reciprocal Relationship of Oxidative Capacity and Insulin Action. Sensitivity to insulin's anabolic action is related to the oxidative capacity of skeletal muscle inasmuch as insulin also appears to be a major regulating factor of mitochondrial oxidative phosphorylation in human skeletal muscle.[156] **In reciprocal fashion, not only does higher oxidative capacity increase myocyte sensitivity to insulin signaling, but with insulin sensitivity, insulin also increases the mitochondrial capacity for oxidative phosphorylation.** In insulin-sensitive human skeletal muscle, mitochondrial protein synthesis was increased via insulin infusion by 20% to 25% together with a rise in oxidative capacity, as measured by higher activity of the mitochondrial oxidative enzymes citrate synthase and cyclooxygenase (COX) and the greater mitochondrial adenosine 5′-triphosphate (ATP) production rate. In contrast, in insulin-resistant type 2 DM patients, insulin did not increase skeletal muscle mitochondrial ATP production.[125]

MEDITATIVE MINDFULNESS AND EXERCISE

Stress experiences are pervasive. In Western civilization, stress is omnipresent in modern-day life. Relentless, daily exposure to chronic stress engenders a multitude of adverse physiologic sequelae.

Western relaxation pursuits are compartmentalized to infrequent interludes of vacations or spa visits. Certain sedentary, inactive relaxation venues may, ironically, themselves engender endothelial dysfunction, insulin resistance, and ultimately, physiologic stress. Tools are needed to manage stress in real time to lessen its detrimental, long-term, physiologic impact.

Whereas conventional exercise has no mindful component, mind-body exercises encompass muscular activity together with an internally directed focus to achieve a temporary self-contemplative, meditative state. This is of significant mental and physical value inasmuch as it improves self-care and potentially lowers health care needs. Ideally, stress relaxation techniques should be incorporated in everyday life to modulate stress responses at their inception.

Meditative Breathing. Slow, diaphragmatic breathing with a slowing of the heart rate is one of the fastest ways to trigger a relaxation response. Shallow, chest breathing is widespread and common, and breathing becomes increasingly shallow or is briefly arrested with stress exposure.

Technique. Meditative techniques with rhythmic, deep diaphragmatic breathing can be corralled to alleviate the physiology of stress. Inhalation should be through the nose, exhalation through the mouth. With diaphragmatic breathing, a person may focus either on tracking breathing, on a mantra (i.e., a repeated word or phrase), or on an object to be contemplated. Such focused attention, aiming to clear the mind from the usual, persistent, chaotic stream of consciousness, is termed mindfulness.[157,158]

Physiologic and Psychological Effects. Meditative techniques with proper relaxation may evoke a physiologic relaxation response characterized by a reduction in

- heart rate,
- respiratory rate, and
- oxygen uptake

that may effectively mitigate stress responses.[157,159,160]

Meditative breathing and mindfulness may influence neuronal pathways in the brainstem and have an effect on the respiratory center and thalamic levels, where numerous cell groups function to gate sensory input and influence autonomic nervous system output.[157,158]

Meditation may improve emotional contentment. Electrical brain activity in the left frontal area, as measured via electroencephalography and brain imaging techniques, is associated with a sense of happiness and calmness, whereas increased activity on the right is associated with feelings of sadness, anxiety, and worry. An 8-week pursuit of meditative techniques in novice meditators, when compared with controls, significantly increased activity in the left side of the brain's frontal area. The subjects correspondingly experienced more positive emotions and demonstrated an improved immune response with an enhanced antibody response to an influenza vaccination.[161] Meditation may have a favorable impact on anxiety.[162]

Meditative techniques may also be of benefit in lowering systemic hypertension.[163]

Mind-Body Activities. Mind-body activities combine exercise routines with rhythmic, slow, deep, diaphragmatic breathing in order to set into motion physiologic mechanisms that trigger the relaxation response, the antithesis to the fright-flight-fight response.

Yoga. Yoga is rooted in East Indian philosophy and has been practiced for thousands of years. The term derives from the Sanskrit word *yuj*, which means "join" or "unitive discipline." The aim of yoga practice is to bring the mind and body into a balance so that the individual is united with the universal self. Physical postures, or *asanas*, are performed in a seated, lying, or standing position. Such postures are maintained with *pranayama*, or controlled breathing. Some yoga types are performed in a warm environment to facilitate muscle stretches. There are different types of yoga: Bikram yoga, Vinyasa yoga, Kundalini yoga, Hatha yoga, Iyengar yoga, Viniyoga, Integral yoga, and Ashtanga yoga.[164]

In a 7-day trial using yoga for asthma therapy, pulmonary function improved by relaxation of the inspiratory and expiratory muscles. After yoga training, there were reductions in

- the heart rate, with the rate dropping on average from 89 to 76 beats per minute,
- diastolic blood pressure, and
- sympathetic reactivity,

with no change in parasympathetic activity.[165]

Martial Arts. Martial arts can be defined as a discipline of self-defense and combat. The origins of martial arts are subject to controversy. However, the traditions can be traced thousands of years. Over the past decade, sport- and health-promoting outlooks, such as cardiovascular fitness, have superseded the self-defense aspects.[166]

Martial arts are divided into two classes:

1. Soft martial arts focus on redirecting an opponent's attack and using more, albeit less powerful punches and kicks. Tai Chi Chuan is such an example.

2. Hard martial arts such as the Korean Tae Kwon Do use powerful blocks and punches that can destroy an opponent's body parts. Fewer movements are involved, but they are performed with greater force.[166]

Hard and soft martial arts are purported to have great health benefits for the practitioner, but most reports are anecdotal.

Qigong. Chi Kung or Qigong is a tradition of spiritual, martial, and health exercises developed in China nearly 3000 years ago. Qigong comprises two concepts:

1. *Qi*, the vital energy of the body, and
2. *gong*, the skill of working with the qi.

Postures and movements are coordinated with diaphragmatic, deep breathing.[164]

Qigong meditative breathing techniques reduce the

- heart rate,
- respiratory rate,
- systemic blood pressure, and
- rate-pressure product

in participants.[167]

Qigong training may stabilize the autonomic nervous system by modulating parasympathetic tone. Qigong augments HRV by increasing HF (parasympathetic) power and decreasing the LF/HF power ratio, suggestive of an increase in cardiac parasympathetic tone.[168]

Tai Chi Chuan. Tai Chi Chuan, also known as taiji or taijiquan, is a style of Chinese martial art. It is a soft, nonimpact form related to Qigong. Tai Chi Chuan may have been established by Chinese hermit monks approximately 3000 years ago. Since the 17th century, it has further evolved in China as a method of meditation, exercise, and self-defense. It is characterized by slow, supple movements that are coordinated with controlled, diaphragmatic breathing and mental concentration to attain tranquility of mind. Tai Chi Chuan forms are derived from studying movements of animate and inanimate nature, representing all the cardinal directions and the basic elements.[169,170]

The tradition of Tai Chi Chuan is deeply rooted in Taoism and Confucianism. A central doctrine of Taoism is the union of opposites called "yin" and "yang."

EXAMPLES OF "YIN"	EXAMPLES OF "YANG"
Earth	Heaven
Night	Day
Femininity	Masculinity
Veins	Arteries
Inhalation	Exhalation
Rest	Movement

Tai Chi applies the yin and yang principles of opposites via rest and movement, inhalation and exhalation, with the goal of attaining longevity and good health by meditation and lifestyle modification.[169]

There are many styles of Tai Chi:

- the Chen style is oldest. It has fast and slow, large movements;
- the Yang style is the most popular and has 108 forms with slow, large movements;
- the Wu style is moderately paced with compact movements;
- the Sun style has fast compact forms; and
- Tai Chi Chih is a simplified version of Tai Chi with only 20 simple movements that are readily learned.[169,170]

Metabolic Demand. Tai Chi Chuan is a moderately intense aerobic exercise. Oxygen uptake during Tai Chi practice is approximately 55% of peak oxygen uptake. The heart rate during Tai Chi is 53% to 58% of the predicted maximal heart rate at 4.1 to 4.6 mets.[171]

Tai Chi–Qigong is an aerobic exercise of low to moderate intensity potentially suitable for cardiopulmonary rehabilitation. It has 54 motions. The exercise intensity of each motion is about 3 mets, and the energy expenditure of each set is about 60 kcal. The estimated intensity of Tai Chi–Qigong in elderly individuals approximates 50% to 60% of peak oxygen uptake at 58% of the predicted maximum heart rate.[172]

Physiologic Effects. Tai Chi training has beneficial effects on cardiopulmonary function and fitness. Aerobic capacity and peak VO_2 may improve by up to 34%.[173]

Tai Chi Chuan may increase HRV. There is an increase in total variance (TV), in intervals between adjacent RR complexes (RRI), and in the standard deviation of all normal-to-normal QRS complexes

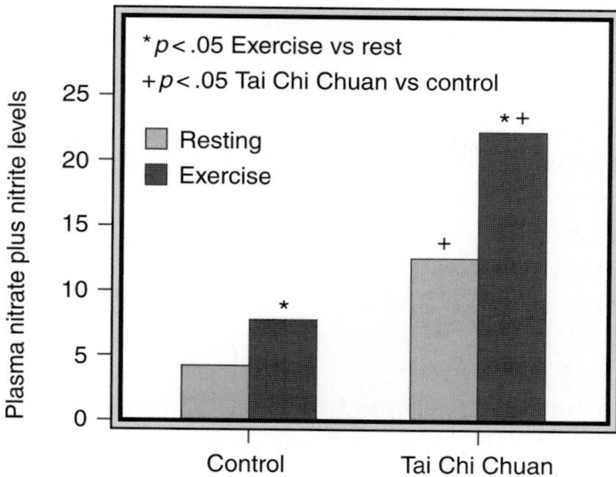

Figure 13–11.
Effect of strenuous exercise on nitric oxide metabolites in control exercise and Tai Chi Chuan–trained elderly men. *(Modified from Wang J-S, Lan C, Wong M-K. Tai Chi Chuan training to enhance microcirculatory function in healthy elderly men. Arch Phys Med Rehabil 2001;82:1176-1180.)*

(SDNNI), suggestive of an augmentation in cardiac autonomic activity.[172,174]

Tai Chi Chuan may improve peripheral endothelial function.[175] It is associated with increased endothelium-dependent dilation of the skin vasculature and microcirculation. In a study of the elderly, rest and exercise skin blood flow was increased, with an improvement in skin conductance and temperature. Plasma NO metabolites, nitrite plus nitrate, were higher (Fig. 13-11).[173,176]

Tai Chi has been explored as a mode of cardiac rehabilitation in small patient groups. The practice of Tai Chi may lower systemic blood pressure, heart rate, and catecholamine levels. When compared with controls, there was a significant increase in HDL levels and the HDL/total cholesterol ratio.[173,177] After an 8-week course of Tai Chi by post–myocardial infarction patients, blood pressure was lower and compliance with practice was higher (82%) in the Tai Chi cohort than in the regular cardiac rehabilitation (73%) or the support group (4%).[169] Low-risk, post–coronary bypass patients tolerate Tai Chi. When compared with a home-based exercise program as control, participation was greater, and patients achieved a significantly higher peak Vo_2 and anaerobic threshold.[178]

Tai Chi has been used in the elderly with a variety of benefits. The age-related decline in physical function may be attenuated and long-term adherence to practice may be enhanced by mind-body integration. There is a significant loss of body fat. Training in the elderly enhances endurance, balance, strength, and flexibility. The incidence of falls is decreased.[169,170] The practice of Tai Chi may improve immune function. In a study of 36 men and women 60 to 80 years old, 45 minutes of Tai Chi three times weekly for 15 weeks significantly improved measures of immunity to herpes zoster by 50%.[179,180]

Psychological Effects. Application of Tai Chi after a stressful situation elicits stress reduction. In general, there is improvement in a participant's psychological profile with reductions in perceived stress, anger, fatigue, and confusion. Salivary cortisol levels decrease, suggestive of a reduction in tension, depression, and anxiety.[169,170]

Tae Kwon Do. Tae Kwon Do is the practice of ancient Korean hard martial arts. Tae Kwon Do training involves basic patterns, forms, and simulated and free sparring. Basic techniques such as punching, kicking, and blocking are performed individually in stationary positions or as part of body movements in formal stances. Compositions of basic patterns are termed "forms." Free sparring is a performance of offensive and defensive techniques against an opponent. Tae Kwon Do practice is pursued in a dynamic and persistent manner.[181]

Tae Kwon Do is conducive to cardiovascular conditioning and is of benefit for improvement in coordination, weight control, and fat loss. Twenty minutes of practice achieves a mean 88% to 92% of the predicted maximum heart rate, a mean oxygen consumption at 68% to 72% peak Vo_2, and a total caloric consumption of approximately 200 kcal for women and 300 kcal for men.[181] In a study of Tae Kwon Do, 85% of class attendees were able to increase the number of push-ups, improve trunk flexion, and lengthen one-leg stance balance times. Interest among the participants continued to be high, and the dropout rate was low.[166]

ADJUNCTS TO EXERCISE

A rise in regional and systemic blood flow is a hallmark of exercise training. A number of other relaxation modalities may share some of the benefits of exercise with less personal effort.

Sauna. Sauna is a thermal therapy that has been in use for thousands of years. A sauna is typically a wood-paneled room with wooden benches, heated by a rock-filled electric heater to a temperature between 80° C and 100° C at the level of the sauna user's head. Humidity is generated in the sauna as water, tossed against the hot rocks, evaporates. Sauna use typically lasts for 5 to 20 minutes per session.[182]

The physiologic responses to sauna therapy are triggered by a rise in skin temperature up to 40° C. With exposure to heat in the sauna, skin blood flow increases from 5% to 10% to a value of 50% to 70% of cardiac output with some reduction in renal, splanchnic, and skeletal muscle blood flow. While stroke volume remains unchanged, the heart rate increases to 100 to 150 beats per minute and cardiac output increases from 5 to 6 L/min to 9 to 10 L/min. The blood pressure response is variable.[182]

Repeated thermal therapy improves endothelial function by up-regulating eNOS expression in the arterial endothelium. In hamsters, within 1 week of sauna treatment, a 40-fold increase in eNOS mRNA was observed.[183] Two weeks of daily sauna therapy in men with coronary risk factors and abnormal endothelial function significantly improved brachial flow–mediated dilation.[184] In infants with congestive heart failure as a result of a ventricular septal defect, sauna therapy improved hemodynamics concomitant with a rise in urine nitrate/nitrite levels (Fig. 13-12).[185]

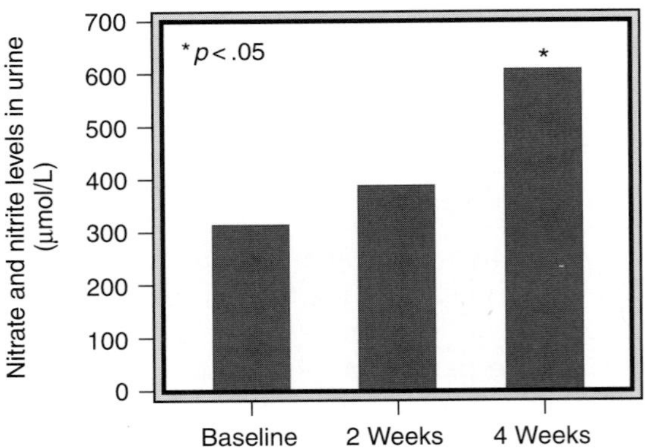

Figure 13–12.
Effect of sauna therapy on urine nitrate/nitrite levels in infants with congestive heart failure. *(Modified from Sugahara Y, Ishii M, Muta H, et al. Efficacy and safety of thermal vasodilation therapy by sauna in infants with severe congestive heart failure secondary to ventricular septal defect. Am J Cardiol 2003;92:109-113.)*

In adult patients with congestive heart failure, a single sauna bathing session improved hemodynamics. Repeated sauna sessions at 60° C lasting 15 minutes daily for a duration of 2 weeks led to improvements in cardiac function, a reduction in heart failure symptoms, lowering of brain natriuretic factor (BNP), and an improvement in endothelial function as measured by flow-mediated dilation. The percent change in BNP correlated with the percent change in flow-mediated dilation.[186]

Sauna therapy may not be tolerated by patients taking β-blockers or short-acting nitroglycerin. Sauna is contraindicated for patients with severe aortic stenosis, unstable angina, recent myocardial infarction, decompensated heart failure, and cardiac arrhythmias. Similarly, the ingestion of alcohol while using the sauna is not recommended.[182]

Massage. Therapeutic massage has been considered beneficial for relaxation and for stress reduction. An increasing number of small studies have suggested that massage reduces the heart rate, lowers blood pressure, increases blood and lymphatic flow, relaxes muscles, improves range of motion, and releases endorphins. Massage is reported to relieve stress and may be of benefit in a variety of musculoskeletal and functional disorders.[187]

Sleep. What appears to be the opposite of exercise, namely, sufficient, regular sleep, may also be important for the prevention of insulin resistance. Sleep does not increase blood flow. However, **adequate sleep, like exercise, reduces sympathetic activation, is conducive to weight control, and benefits insulin sensitivity.**

A century ago, average Americans slept approximately 9 hours per night.[188] Over the past 40 years, self-reported sleep duration in the United States has decreased by almost 2 hours. Thirty-three percent of U.S. adults sleep less than 6.5 hours a night, and that number reaches 49% among shift workers.[189] The increasing demands of modern society have limited the duration of sleep in children as well.[190]

There appear to be neural interconnections linking sleep and metabolic homeostasis. Overlapping molecular components of sleep and metabolic pathways suggest a coordination between periods of fasting and sleep and periods of wakefulness, food seeking, and energy storage.

Sleep deprivation may perturb the homeostatic correlation between these pathways and trigger energy conservation with increased energy intake and decreased energy expenditure. The anorexigenic hormone leptin appears to play a role because it has an impact not only on metabolic pathways but also on the quality of consolidated sleep.[190]

Sleep deprivation in rodents and humans is associated with increased stress activation and hyperphagia. In a randomized clinical study of 12 healthy, young, normal-weight men, sleep restriction was associated with an average 18% reduction in leptin ($P = .04$), a 28% elevation in the orexigenic factor ghrelin ($P < .04$), and a 24% and 23% increase in hunger and appetite, respectively ($P = .01$), especially for calorie-dense foods of high carbohydrate content.[191] In a study of varying sleep duration (4 versus 8 versus 12 hours per night), the decrease in leptin levels with sleep restriction was quantitatively associated with increased sympathovagal imbalance, altered cortisol and thyroid-stimulating hormone profiles, and higher insulin resistance.[192]

In a prospective study of 924 individuals aged 18 to 91 years from four primary care practices, there was a significant, nearly linear inverse relationship between total sleep time and increasing overweight and obesity. However, this relationship did not pertain to extremely obese persons (BMI of 40 to 85 kg/m^2), possibly because of the confounding effects of soporific, proinflammatory cytokines such as IL-6 and TNF-α.[193]

CONCLUSION

Although our species may call itself "homo sapiens," our physiology is structurally and functionally defined by the bulk of our skeletal musculature, which is intended to secure our locomotion, food procurement, defense, and escape.

In skeletal muscle, exercise, NOS activity, and insulin signaling are linked not only on the molecular and vascular but also on the metabolic level. Increased NO bioavailability does not solely raise blood flow and nutrient supply. It also increases mitochondrial biogenesis, the metabolic rate, and fatty acid oxidation, all effects that enhance sensitivity to insulin signaling. This linkage makes sense teleologically. The greater metabolic demand of working muscle is met by a higher blood flow supply and greater uptake of fuels with more efficient metabolic processing during contractions and by storage during the recovery period.

There are other relationships that similarly link working muscle with enhanced metabolic activity and insulin sensitivity. As a result, exercise has a positive impact on insulin resistance in a multifactorial way. Physical conditioning improves insulin sensitivity inasmuch as it

- changes muscle fiber type, thereby improving muscle oxidative metabolism and efficiency;
- activates AMPK-α2, PPAR-α, and NOS to up-regulate glucose metabolism and fatty acid oxidation; and
- decreases the visceral fat depot, lowers adipocyte size, and enhances the turnover of intramyocellular lipid as fatty acids are consumed as fuel.

In this respect, interestingly, with preserved insulin signaling, insulin itself boosts oxidative capacity. In short, exercise partitions fatty acid in working muscle from storage to oxidative consumption, in the process also enhancing sensitivity to the necessary, restorative anabolic effects of insulin.

As part of this mechanism, exercise also modulates the physiologic impact of certain phenomena:

- Unbalanced lipolysis may, as with inflammation, increase circulating free fatty acids, with injurious side effects. Exercise augments lipolysis, albeit with a concomitant up-regulation of free fatty acid beta oxidation effecting their appropriate disposal, with a favorable outcome.
- Ectopic intramyocellular lipid has been observed with insulin resistance. Its ultimate impact is, however, a function of its derivation, site, and turnover. The intramyocellular lipid in type II fibers of sedentary individuals, derived in a proinflammatory state from adipocyte lipolysis and a decline in fatty acid oxidation, has negative health implications. Intramyocellular lipid in the type I fibers of athletes, engendered in the setting of increased fatty acid oxidation and turnover, is associated with heightened sensitivity to insulin signaling.

Although the insulin-sensitizing effects of physical training are confined to the muscle groups exercised, a systemic sensitization to insulin is expected to arise from long-term conditioning.

Table 13-3. Diverse Effects of Selected Activities

ACTIVITY	ANTIOXIDANT	ANTI-INFLAMMATORY	ENDOTHELIAL PROTECTIVE	ANTI-HYPERTENSIVE	AMPK ACTIVATION	PPAR-γ
Aerobic exercise	+	+	+	+	+	+
Resistance training	N/A	N/A	+	N/A	+	N/A
Meditation	N/A	N/A	N/A	+	N/A	N/A
Yoga	N/A	N/A	N/A	+	N/A	N/A
Qigong	N/A	N/A	N/A	+	N/A	N/A
Tai Chi Chuan	N/A	N/A	+	+	N/A	N/A
Tae Kwon Do	N/A	N/A	N/A	N/A	N/A	N/A
Sauna	N/A	N/A	+	N/A	N/A	N/A
Massage	N/A	N/A	N/A	+	N/A	N/A
Sleep	N/A	N/A	N/A	N/A	N/A	N/A

+, Beneficial effect; N/A, data not available.

Exercise-induced improvements in endothelial function, in indices of inflammation and oxidative stress, in fatty acid oxidative consumption, and in the status of visceral fat and intramyocellular lipid would all be expected to enhance systemic insulin sensitivity (Table 13-3).

Unfortunately, the benefits of exercise, irrespective of the degree of conditioning attained, are evanescent and remain in place only with ongoing physical activity. After only a few days of idling, our bodies, in a "use it or lose it" construct, gradually deteriorate. With inactivity, the endothelium, not needed to supply blood flow to working muscle, becomes dysfunctional. Nonworking skeletal muscle atrophies. A sedentary lifestyle impairs constitutional NOS, AMPK, and PPAR-α expression and signaling, thereby economizing on energy production. Metabolically inefficient, glycolytic type II fibers are predominantly expressed, which further compromises myocyte mechanical performance and aerobic capacity. There is a resultant reduction in fatty acid oxidative consumption and the metabolic rate that allows the accumulation of intramyocellular lipid. In the absence of an anabolic stimulus, metabolism is defined by catabolism and resistance to insulin signaling. The resulting perturbations eventually lead to the manifestations of the metabolic syndrome, type 2 DM, cardiovascular disease, acute ischemic syndromes, morbidity, and mortality. Ultimately, an inactive organism that is no longer engaged in physical effort effectively self-destructs.

Skeletal muscle is, however, flexible in its regenerative reserve. As a result, physical fitness and insulin sensitivity are dynamic, not static states. Although inactivity begets insulin resistance, insulin resistance can repeatedly be reversed through the resumption of exercise conditioning. With the increasing U.S. and global epidemic of sedentary obesity eventuating in insulin resistance and the metabolic syndrome, exercise training thus empowers afflicted individuals with a potent self-care tool for preventing or reversing that pathophysiology. Exercise training prevails over the genetic underpinnings to visceral adiposity and insulin resistance and is of benefit even in the absence of weight loss. It also comes as a relief for ordinary individuals that it is moderate exercise, not extreme athletic training, that engenders beneficial anti-inflammatory and antioxidative effects with improvements in endothelial function.

Exercise training enhances insulin sensitivity by decreasing inflammation, improving endothelial function, and augmenting myocyte fatty acid oxidation. The fatty acid oxidative capacity of skeletal muscle relates to aerobic capacity, which in turn defines fitness, thus effectively relating

PPAR-α	METABOLIC RATE	BENEFICIAL LIPID EFFECTS	VISCERAL ADIPOSITY	ECTOPIC FAT	WEIGHT LOSS	CARDIOVASCULAR EVENTS	INSULIN SENSITIVITY
+	+	+	+	+	+	+	+
							+
N/A	N/A	N/A	N/A	N/A	N/A	N/A	N/A
N/A	N/A	N/A	N/A	N/A	N/A	N/A	N/A
N/A	N/A	N/A	N/A	N/A	N/A	N/A	N/A
N/A	N/A	N/A	N/A	N/A	N/A	N/A	N/A
N/A	N/A	N/A	N/A	N/A	+	N/A	N/A
N/A	N/A	N/A	N/A	N/A	+	N/A	N/A
N/A	N/A	N/A	N/A	N/A	N/A	N/A	N/A
N/A	N/A	N/A	N/A	N/A	N/A	N/A	N/A
N/A	?+	N/A	N/A	N/A	?+	N/A	+

physical fitness to insulin sensitivity. Physical fitness, more than the absence of ponderosity or other factors, is the major determinant of cardiovascular and metabolic risk and long-term, disease-free survival, in effect linking health span to life span. It is obviously in every individual's interest to assume the responsibility for his or her own health and embrace this extremely effective, safe, and inexpensive prevention and treatment modality. As is true for the mind, it is truly a "use it or lose it" paradigm for muscle, body, and life.

GLOSSARY

ACC	acetyl-CoA carboxylase
ACE	angiotensin-converting enzyme
ACLS	Aerobics Center Longitudinal Study
AMP	adenosine 5′-monophosphate
AMPK	5′-AMP–activated protein kinase
ATP	adenosine 5′-triphosphate
BMI	body mass index
BNP	brain natriuretic factor
CETP	cholesterol ester transfer protein
cGK	cGMP-dependent protein kinase
cGMP	cyclic guanosine 3′,5′-monophosphate
CHD	coronary heart disease
CoA	coenzyme A
COX	cyclooxygenase
CPT-I	carnitine palmitoyltransferase I
CRP	C-reactive protein
DM	diabetes mellitus
eNOS	endothelial nitric oxide synthase
ERK	extracellular signal–regulated kinase
FABP	fatty acid binding protein
FAT	fatty acid translocase
GLUT	glucose transporter
β-HAD	β-hydroxyacyl-CoA dehydrogenase
HDL	high-density lipoprotein
HERITAGE	Health, Risk Factors, Exercise Training, and Genetics Family Study
HF	high frequency
HRV	heart rate variability
ICAM-1	intracellular adhesion molecule-1
IL	interleukin
IRS	insulin receptor substrate
JNK	c-Jun NH_2-terminal kinase
LDL	low-density lipoprotein
LF	low frequency
LPL	lipoprotein lipase
MAPK	mitogen-activated protein kinase
MAPKK	MAPK kinase
MAPKKK	MAPKK kinase
MAPKAPK	MAPK-activated protein kinase

met	metabolic equivalent
MRFIT	Multiple Risk Factor Intervention Trial
NFκB	nuclear factor kappaB
NO	nitric oxide
NOS	nitric oxide synthase
PGC-1α	PPAR-γ coactivator-1α
PI3K	phosphatidylinositol 3-kinase
PKB	protein kinase B
PKC	protein kinase C
PPAR	peroxisome proliferator–activated receptor
RRI	interval between adjacent RR complexes
RSK2	p90 ribosomal S6 kinase
SDNNI	standard deviation of all normal-to-normal QRS complexes
TNF	tumor necrosis factor
TV	total variance
VCAM-1	vascular cell adhesion molecule-1
VEGF	vascular endothelial growth factor
VLDL	very-low-density lipoprotein
$\dot{V}O_2$	oxygen consumption
$\dot{V}O_2max$	maximal oxygen consumption
WISE	Women's Ischemia Syndrome Evaluation

REFERENCES

1. Janssen I, Katzmarzyk PT, Ross R, et al. Fitness alters the associations of BMI and waist circumference with total and abdominal fat. Obes Res 2004;12:525-537
2. Manson JE, Greenland P, LaCroix AZ, et al. Walking compared with vigorous exercise for the prevention of cardiovascular events in women. N Engl J Med 2002; 347:716-725
3. Tanasescu M, Leitzmann MF, Rimm EB, et al. Exercise type and intensity in relation to coronary heart disease in men. JAMA 2002;288:1994-2000
4. Ballady G (guest ed). Crawford MH (ed). Exercise in Secondary Prevention and Cardiac Rehabilitation. Philadelphia, WB Saunders, 2001, p 19
5. Rogers M, Probst M, Gruber J, et al. Differential effects of exercise training intensity on blood pressure and cardiovascular responses to stress in borderline hypertensive humans. J Hypertens 1996;11:1369-1375
6. Desai MY, Nasir K, Rumberger JA, et al. Relation of degree of physical activity to coronary artery calcium score in asymptomatic individuals with multiple metabolic risk factors. Am J Cardiol 2004;94:729-732
7. Hedback B, Perk J, Wodlin P. Long-term reduction of cardiac mortality after myocardial infarction: 10-year results of a comprehensive rehabilitation programme. Eur Heart J 1993;14:831-835
8. Oldridge NB, Guyatt JE, Fischer ME, et al. Cardiac rehabilitation after myocardial infarction: combined experience of randomized clinical trials. JAMA 1988;260:945-950
9. O'Connor GT, Buring JE, Yusuf S, et al. An overview of randomized trials of rehabilitation with exercise after myocardial infarction. Circulation 1989;80:234-244
10. Joliffe J, Rees K, Taylor R, et al. Exercise-based rehabilitation for coronary heart disease. Cochrane Database Syst Rev 2001(1):CD001800
11. Lee I-M, Sesso HD, Oguma Y, Paffenbarger RS Jr. Relative risk of physical activity and risk of coronary heart disease. Circulation 2003;107:1110-1116
12. Rothenbacher D, Hoffmeister A, Brenner H, Koenig W. Physical activity, coronary heart disease, and inflammatory response. Arch Intern Med 2003;163:1200-1205
13. Wei M, Kampert JB, Barlow CE, et al. Relationship between low cardiorespiratory fitness and mortality in normal-weight, overweight, and obese men. JAMA 1999;282:1547-1553
14. Wessel TR, Arant CB, Olson MB, et al. Relationship of physical fitness vs body mass index with coronary artery disease and cardiovascular events in women. JAMA 2004;292:1179-1187
15. Benefits and recommendations for physical activity programs for all Americans: a statement for health professionals by the Committee on Exercise and Cardiac Rehabilitation of the Council on Clinical Cardiology, American Heart Association. Circulation 1993;86:340-344
16. Laaksonen DE, Lakka HM, Niskanen LK, et al. Low levels of leisure-time physical activity and cardiorespiratory fitness predict development of the metabolic syndrome. Diabetes Care 2002;25:1612-1618
17. Farrell SW, Cheng YJ, Blair SN. Prevalence of the metabolic syndrome across cardiorespiratory fitness levels in women. Obes Res 2004;12:824-830
18. Hu FB, Li TY, Colditz GA, et al. Television watching and other sedentary behaviors in relation to risk of obesity and type 2 diabetes mellitus in women. JAMA 2003; 289:1785-1791
19. Diabetes Prevention Program Research Group. Reduction of the incidence of type 2 diabetes with lifestyle intervention or metformin. N Engl J Med 2002;346:393-403
20. Tuomilehto J, Lindstrom J, Eriksson JG, et al. Prevention of type 2 diabetes mellitus by changes in lifestyle among subjects with impaired glucose tolerance. N Engl J Med 2001;344:1343-1350
21. Breslow RA, Ballard-Barbash R, Munoz K, Graubard BI. Long-term recreational physical activity and breast cancer in the National Health and Nutrition Examination Survey I epidemiologic follow-up study. Cancer Epidemiol Biomarkers Prev 2001;10:805-808
22. Lee IM, Rexrode KM, Cook NR, et al. Physical activity and breast cancer risk: the Women's Health Study (United States). Cancer Causes Control 2001;12:137-145
23. Lee IM, Sesso HD, Paffenbarger RS Jr. A prospective cohort study of physical activity and body size in relation to prostate cancer risk (United States). Cancer Causes Control 2001;12:187-193.
24. McTiernan A, Kooperberg C, White E, et al. Recreational physical activity and the risk of breast cancer in postmenopausal women: the Women's Health Initiative Cohort Study. JAMA 2003;290:1331-1336

25. Lee CD, Blair SN, Jackson AS. Cardiorespiratory fitness, body composition, and all-cause and cardiovascular disease mortality in men. Am J Clin Nutr 1999;69:373-380
26. Stevens J, Cai J, Evenson KR, Thomas R. Fitness and fatness as predictors of mortality from all causes and from cardiovascular disease in men and women in the lipid research clinics study. Am J Epidemiol 2002;156: 832-841
27. Blair SN, Wei M. Sedentary habits, health, and function in older women and men. Am J Health Promot 2000; 15:1-8
28. Katzmarzyk PT, Church TS, Blair SN. Cardiorespiratory fitness attenuates the effects of the metabolic syndrome on all-cause and cardiovascular disease mortality in men. Arch Intern Med 2004;164:1092-1097
29. Church TS, Cheng YJ, Earnest CP, et al. Exercise capacity and body composition as predictors of mortality among men with diabetes. Diabetes Care 2004;27:83-88
30. Food and Nutrition Board, Institute of Medicine. Dietary References, Intakes of Energy, Carbohydrates, Fiber, Fat, Protein, and Amino Acids (Macronutrients). Washington, DC, National Academy Press, 2002
31. Stofan JR, DiPietro L, Davis D, et al. Physical activity patterns associated with cardiorespiratory fitness and reduced mortality: the Aerobics Center Longitudinal Study. Am J Public Health 1998;88:1807-1813
32. Sakamoto K, Goodyear LJ. Invited review: Intracellular signaling in contracting skeletal muscle. J Appl Physiol 2002;93:369-383
33. Henriksen EJ. Exercise effects of muscle insulin signaling and action. Invited review: Effects of acute exercise and exercise training on insulin resistance. J Appl Physiol 2002;93:788-796
34. Ryder JW, Chibalin AV, Zierath JR. Intracellular mechanisms underlying increases in glucose uptake in response to insulin or exercise in skeletal muscle. Acta Physiol Scand 2001;171:249-257
35. Zierath JR. Invited review: Exercise training–induced changes in insulin signaling in skeletal muscle. J Appl Physiol 2002;93:773-781
36. Osman AA, Hancock J, Hunt DG, et al. Exercise training increases ERK2 activity in skeletal muscle of obese Zucker rats. J Appl Physiol 2001;90:454-460
37. Coyle EF, Sidossis LS, Horowitz JF, Beltz JD. Cycling efficiency is related to the percentage of type I muscle fibers. Med Sci Sports Exerc 1992;24:782-788
38. Segal SS, Kurjiaka DT. Coordination of blood flow control in the resistance vasculature of skeletal muscle. Med Sci Sports Exerc 1995;27:1158-1164
39. Song XM, Ryder JW, Kawano Y, et al. Muscle fiber type specificity in insulin signal transduction. Am J Physiol 1999;277:R1690-R1696
40. Ryder JW, Gilbert M, Zierath JR. Skeletal muscle and insulin sensitivity: pathophysiological alterations. Front Biosci 2001;6:154-163
41. Smith ML, Hudson DL, Graitzer HM, et al. Exercise training bradycardia: the role of autonomic balance. Med Sci Sports Exerc 1989;21:40-44
42. Goldsmith RL, Bigger JT Jr, Bloomfield DM, et al. Physical fitness as a determinant of vagal modulation. Med Sci Sports Exerc 1997;29:812-817
43. Suvorava T, Lauer N, Kojda G. Physical inactivity causes endothelial dysfunction in healthy young mice. J Am Coll Cardiol 2004;44:1320-1327
44. Leon AS, Myers MJ, Connett J. Leisure time physical activity and the 16-year risks of mortality from coronary heart disease and all-causes in the Multiple Risk Factor Intervention Trial (MRFIT). Int J Sports Med 1997;18 (suppl 3):S208-S215
45. Paffenbarger RS, Hyde RT, Wing AL, et al. The association of changes in physical-activity level and other lifestyle characteristics with mortality among men. N Engl J Med 1993;328:538-545
46. Green DJ, Cabel T, Fox C, et al. Modification of forearm resistance vessels by exercise training in young men. J Appl Physiol 1994;77:1829-1833
47. Hambrecht R, Wolf A, Gielen S, et al. Effect of exercise on coronary endothelial function in patients with coronary artery disease. N Engl J Med 2000;342:454-460
48. Miller VM, Vanhoutte PM. Enhanced release of endothelium-derived factors by chronic increases in blood flow. Am J Physiol 1988;255:H446-H451
49. Uematsu M, Ohara Y, Navas JP, et al. Regulation of endothelial cell nitric oxide synthase mRNA expression by shear stress. Am J Physiol 1995;269:C1371-C1378
50. Hambrecht R, Adams V, Erbs S, et al. Regular physical activity improves endothelial function in patients with coronary artery disease by increasing phosphorylation of endothelial nitric oxide synthase. Circulation 2003; 107:3152-3158
51. Sessa WC, Pritchard K, Seyedi N, et al. Chronic exercise in dogs increases coronary vascular nitric oxide production and endothelial cell nitric oxide synthase gene expression. Circ Res 1994;74:349-353
52. Waid DK, Chell M, El-Fakahany EE. M(2) and M(4) muscarinic receptor subtypes couple to activation of endothelial nitric oxide synthase. Pharmacology 2000; 61:37-42
53. Schnyder B, Pittet M, Durand J, Schnyder-Candrian S. Rapid effects of glucose on the insulin signaling of endothelial NO generation and epithelial Na transport. Am J Physiol Endocrinol Metab 2001;282:E87-E94
54. Fryer LG, Hajduch E, Rencurel F, et al. Activation of glucose transport by AMP-activated protein kinase via stimulation of nitric oxide synthase. Diabetes 2000; 49:1978-1985
55. Morrow VA, Foufelle F, Connell JM, et al. Direct activation of AMP-activated protein kinase stimulates nitric-oxide synthesis in human aortic endothelial cells. J Biol Chem 2003;278:31629-31639
56. Rieder M, Carmona R, Krieger J, et al. Suppression of angiotensin-converting enzyme expression and activity by shear stress. Circ Res 1997;80:312-319
57. Fukai T, Siegfried MR, Ushio-Fukai M; et al. Regulation of the extracellular superoxide dismutase by nitric oxide and exercise training. J Clin Invest 2000;105:1631-1639
58. Walsh JH, Bilsborough W, Maiorana A, et al. Exercise training improves conduit vessel function in patients with coronary artery disease. J Appl Physiol 2003;95:20-25
59. Davies KJA, Quintanilha AT, Brooks GA, et al. Free radicals and tissue damage produced by exercise. Biochem Biophys Res Commun 1982;107:1198-1205
60. Edwards DG, Schofield RS, Lennon SL, et al. Effect of exercise training on endothelial function in men with coronary artery disease. Am J Cardiol 2004;93: 617-620
61. Goto C, Higashi Y, Kimura M, et al. Effect of different intensities of exercise on endothelium-dependent vasodilation in humans: role of endothelium-dependent nitric oxide and oxidative stress. Circulation 2003;108:530-535
62. Ades PA, Green NM, Coello CE. Effects of exercise and cardiac rehabilitation on cardiovascular outcomes. Cardiol Clin 2003;21:435-448
63. Dimmeler S, Zeiher AM. Exercise and cardiovascular health: Get active to "AKTivate" your endothelial nitric oxide synthase. Circulation 2003;107:3118-3120
64. Laufs U, Werner N, Link A, et al. Physical training increases endothelial progenitor cells, inhibits neointima

formation, and enhances angiogenesis. Circulation 2004;109:220-226
65. Kingwell BA. Nitric oxide–mediated metabolic regulation during exercise: effects of training in health and cardiovascular disease. FASEB J 2000;14:1685-1696
66. Nisoli E, Clementi E, Paolucci C, et al. Mitochondrial biogenesis in mammals: the role of endogenous nitric oxide. Science 2003;299:896-899
67. Pastva A, Estell K, Schoeb TR, et al. Aerobic exercise attenuates airway inflammatory responses in a mouse model of atopic asthma. J Immunol 2004;172:4520-4526
68. Radak Z, Chung HY, Naito H, et al. Age-associated increase in oxidative stress and nuclear factor kappaB activation are attenuated in rat liver by regular exercise. FASEB J 2004;18:749-750
69. Geffken D, Cushman M, Burke G, et al. Association between physical activity and markers of inflammation in a healthy elderly population. Am J Epidemiol 2001; 153:242-250
70. King DE, Carek P, Mainous AG, Pearson WS. Inflammatory markers and exercise: differences related to exercise type. Med Sci Sports Exerc 2003;35:575-581
71. Mattusch F, Dufaux B, Heine O, et al. Reduction of the plasma concentration of C-reactive protein following nine months of endurance training. Int J Sports Med 2000;21:21-24
72. Ziccardi P, Nappo F, Giugliano G, et al. Reduction of inflammatory cytokine concentrations and improvement of endothelial functions in obese women after weight loss over one year. Circulation 2002;105:804-809
73. Esposito K, Pontillo A, Di Palo C, et al. Effect of weight loss and lifestyle changes on vascular inflammatory markers in obese women: a randomized trial. JAMA 2003; 289:1799-1804
74. Milani RV, Lavie CJ, Mehra MR. Reduction in C-reactive protein through cardiac rehabilitation and exercise training. J Am Coll Cardiol 2004;43:1056-1061
75. Tisi PV, Hulse M, Chulakadabba A, et al. Exercise training for intermittent claudication: does it adversely affect biochemical markers of the exercise-induced inflammatory response? Eur J Vasc Endovasc Surg 1997;14:344-350
76. Aronson D, Sella R, Sheikh-Ahmad M, et al. The association between cardiorespiratory fitness and C-reactive protein in subjects with the metabolic syndrome. J Am Coll Cardiol 2004;44:2003-2007
77. Goto S, Radak Z, Nyakas C, et al. Regular exercise: an effective means to reduce oxidative stress in old rats. Ann NY Acad Sci 2004;1019:471-474
78. Harrison DG, Cai H. Endothelial control of vasomotion and nitric oxide production. Cardiol Clin 2003;21: 289-302
79. Litherland GJ, Hajduch E, Hundai HS. Intracellular signalling mechanisms regulating glucose transport in insulin-sensitive tissues. Mol Membr Biol 2001;18:195-204
80. Farese RV. Function and dysfunction of aPKC isoforms for glucose transport in insulin-sensitive and insulin-resistant states. Am J Physiol Endocrinol Metab 2002; 283:E1-E11
81. Wojtaszewski JF, Nielsen P, Hansen BF, et al. Isoform-specific and exercise intensity–dependent activation of 5′-AMP–activated protein kinase in human skeletal muscle. J Physiol 2000;528:221-226
82. Holmes BF, Kurth-Kracek EJ, Winder WW. Chronic activation of 5′-AMP–activated protein kinase increases GLUT-4, hexokinase, and glycogen in muscle. J Appl Physiol 1999;87:1990-1995
83. Saha AK, Ruderman NB. Malonyl-CoA and AMP-activated protein kinase: an expanding partnership. Mol Cell Biochem 2003;253:65-70
84. Chen ZP, Stephens TJ, Murthy S, et al. Effect of exercise intensity on skeletal muscle AMPK signaling in humans. Diabetes 2003;52:2205-2212
85. Kawamura T, Yoshida K, Sugawara A, et al. Regulation of skeletal muscle peroxisome proliferator–activated receptor gamma expression by exercise and angiotensin-converting enzyme inhibition in fructose-fed hypertensive rats. Hypertens Res 2004;27:61-70
86. Guerre-Millo M, Rouault C, Poulain P, et al. PPAR-alpha–null mice are protected from high-fat diet–induced insulin resistance. Diabetes 2001;50:2809-2814
87. Iemitsu M, Miyauchi T, Maeda S, et al. Aging-induced decrease in the PPAR-alpha level in hearts is improved by exercise training. Am J Physiol Heart Circ Physiol 2002;283:H1750-H1760
88. Russell AP, Feilchenfeldt J, Schreiber S, et al. Endurance training in humans leads to fiber type-specific increases in levels of peroxisome proliferator–activated receptor-gamma coactivator-1 and peroxisome proliferator–activated receptor-alpha in skeletal muscle. Diabetes 2003;52:2874-2881
89. Horowitz JF, Leone TC, Feng W, et al. Effect of endurance training on lipid metabolism in women: a potential role for PPAR-alpha in the metabolic response to training. Am J Physiol Endocrinol Metab 2000;279: E348-E355
90. Ibrahimi A, Bonen A, Blinn WE, et al. Muscle-specific overexpression of FAT/CD36 enhances fatty acid oxidation by contracting muscle, reduces plasma triglycerides and fatty acids, and increases plasma glucose and insulin. J Biol Chem 1999;26761-26766
91. Tunstall RJ, Mehan KA, Wadley GD, et al. Exercise training increases lipid metabolism gene expression in human skeletal muscle. Am J Physiol Endocrinol Metab 2002;283:E66-E72
92. Greiwe JS, Holloszy JO, Semenkovich CF. Exercise induces lipoprotein lipase and GLUT-4 protein in muscle independent of adrenergic-receptor signaling. J Appl Physiol 2000;89:176-181
93. Schrauwen P, van Aggel-Leijssen DP, Hul G, et al. The effect of a 3-month low-intensity endurance training program on fat oxidation and acetyl-CoA carboxylase-2 expression. Diabetes 2002;51:2220-2226
94. Gill JMR, Herd SL, Vora V, Hardman AE. Effects of a brisk walk on lipoprotein lipase activity and plasma triglyceride concentrations in the fasted and postprandial states. Eur J Appl Physiol 2003;89:184-190
95. Hamilton MT, Areiqat E, Hamilton DG, Bey L. Plasma triglyceride metabolism in humans and rats during aging and physical inactivity. Int J Sport Nutr Exerc Metab 2001;11(suppl):S97-S104
96. Schuler G, Hambrecht R, Schlierf G, et al. Regular physical exercise and low-fat diets: effects on progression of coronary artery disease. Circulation 1992; 86:1-11
97. Brochu M, Poehlman E, Savage P, et al. Modest effects of exercise training alone on coronary risk factors and body composition in coronary patients. J Cardiopulm Rehabil 2000;20:180-188
98. Kraus WE, Houmard JA, Duscha BD, et al. Effects of the amount and intensity of exercise on plasma lipoproteins. N Engl J Med 2002;347:1483-1492
99. Leon AS, Gaskill SE, Rice T, et al. Variability in the response of HDL cholesterol to exercise training in the HERITAGE Family Study. Int J Sports Med 2002; 23:1-9
100. Gill JMR, Al-Mamari A, Ferrell WR, et al. Exercise and cardiovascular function. Effects of prior moderate exercise on postprandial metabolism and vascular function

in lean and centrally obese men. J Am Coll Cardiol 2004;44:2375-2382
101. Garcia-Villafranca J, Guillen A, Castro J. Involvement of nitric oxide/cyclic GMP signaling pathway in the regulation of fatty acid metabolism in rat hepatocytes. Biochem Pharmacol 2003;65:807-812
102. Fruchart J-C. Peroxisome proliferator–activated receptor-alpha activation and high-density lipoprotein metabolism. Am J Cardiol 2001;88(suppl):24N-29N
103. Wilund KR, Ferrell RE, Phares DA, et al. Changes in high-density lipoprotein-cholesterol subfractions with exercise training may be dependent on cholesteryl ester transfer protein (CETP) genotype. Metabolism 2002; 51:774-778
104. Levine JA, Eberhardt NL, Jensen MD. Role of nonexercise activity thermogenesis in resistance to fat gain in humans. Science 1999;283:212-214
105. Oppert JM, Nadeau A, Tremblay A, et al. Negative energy balance with exercise in identical twins: plasma glucose and insulin responses. Am J Physiol 1997;272: E248-E254
106. Slentz CA, Duscha A, Johnson JL, et al. Effects of the amount of exercise on body weight, body composition, and measures of central obesity. Arch Intern Med 2004; 164:31-39
107. Schrauwen P, van Marken Lichtenbelt WD, Saris WH, Westerterp KR. The adaptation of nutrient oxidation to nutrient intake on a high-fat diet. Z Ernahrungswiss 1997;36:306-309
108. Schrauwen P, Lichtenbelt WD, Saris WH, Westerterp KR. Fat balance in obese subjects: role of glycogen stores. Am J Physiol 1998;274:E1027-E1033
109. Harant I, Marion-Latard F, Crampes F, et al. Effect of a long-duration physical exercise on fat cell lipolytic responsiveness to adrenergic agents and insulin in obese men. Int J Obes Relat Metab Disord 2002; 26:1373-1378
110. Martin WH 3rd, Dalsky GP, Hurley BF, et al. Effect of endurance training on plasma free fatty acid turnover and oxidation during exercise. Am J Physiol 1993;265: E708-E714
111. Irwin ML, Yasui Y, Ulrich CM, et al. Effect of exercise on total and intra-abdominal body fat in postmenopausal women: a randomized controlled trial. JAMA 2003;289: 323-330
112. Donnelly JE, Hill JO, Jacobsen DJ, et al. Effects of a 16-month randomized controlled exercise trial on body weight and composition in young, overweight men and women. The Midwest Exercise Trial. Arch Intern Med 2003;163:1343-1350
113. Nicklas BJ, Rogus EM, Goldberg AP. Exercise blunts declines in lipolysis and fat oxidation after dietary-induced weight loss in obese older women. Am J Physiol 1997;36:E149-E155
114. Wojtaszewski JFP, Nielsen JN, Richter EA. Invited review: Effect of acute exercise on insulin signaling and action in humans. J Appl Physiol 2002;93:384-392
115. Hughes VA, Fiatarone MA, Fielding RA, et al. Exercise increases muscle GLUT4 levels and insulin action in subjects with impaired glucose tolerance. Am J Physiol Endocrinol Metab 1993;264:E855-E862
116. Winder WW. AMP-activated protein kinase: possible target for treatment of type 2 diabetes. Diabetes Technol Ther 2000;2:441-448
117. Klippel A, Kavanaugh WM, Pot D, Williams LT. A specific product of phosphatidylinositol 3-kinase directly activates the protein kinase Akt through its pleckstrin homology domain. Mol Cell Biol 1997;17: 338-344
118. Luciano E, Carneiro EM, Carvalho CRO, et al. Endurance training improves responsiveness to insulin and modulates insulin signal transduction through the phosphatidylinositol 3-kinase/Akt-1 pathway. Eur J Endocrinol 2002;147:149-157
119. Yaspelkis BB, Singh MK, Trevino B, et al. Resistance training increases glucose uptake and transport in rat skeletal muscle. Acta Physiol Scand 2002;175: 315-323
120. Youngren JF, Keen S, Kulp JL, et al. Enhanced muscle insulin receptor autophosphorylation with short-term aerobic exercise training. Am J Physiol Endocrinol Metab 2001;280:E528-E533
121. Richter EA, Derave W, Wojtaszewski JF. Glucose, exercise and insulin: emerging concepts. J Physiol 2001;535: 313-322
122. Seals DR, Hagberg JM, Allen WK, et al. Glucose tolerance in young and older athletes and sedentary men. J Appl Physiol 1984;56:1521-1525
123. Rimbert V, Boirie Y, Bedu M, et al. Muscle fat oxidative capacity is not impaired by age but by physical inactivity: association with insulin sensitivity. FASEB J 2004;18: 737-739
124. Clark MG, Wallis MG, Barrett EJ, et al. Blood flow and muscle metabolism: a focus on insulin action. Am J Physiol Endocrinol Metab 2003;284:E241-E258
125. Stump CS, Short KR, Bigelow ML, et al. Effect of insulin on human skeletal muscle mitochondrial ATP production, protein synthesis, and mRNA transcripts. Proc Natl Acad Sci U S A 2003;100:7996-8001
126. Dela F, Larsen JJ, Mikines KJ, et al. Insulin-stimulated muscle glucose clearance in patients with NIDDM. Effects of one-legged physical training. Diabetes 1995; 44:1010-1020
127. Kelley DE, Goodpaster BH. Effects of physical activity on insulin action and glucose tolerance in obesity. Med Sci Sports Exerc 1999;31(suppl):S619-S623
128. Rodgers MA, Yamamoto C, King DS, et al. Improvement in glucose tolerance after 1 week of exercise in patients with mild NIDDM. Diabetes Care 1988;11:613-618
129. Dela F, Mikines KJ, Larsen JJ, Galbo H. Glucose clearance in aged trained skeletal muscle during maximal insulin with superimposed exercise. J Appl Physiol 1999;87:2059-2067
130. Holloszy JO, Schultz J, Kusnierkiewicz J, et al. Effects of exercise on glucose tolerance and insulin resistance. Acta Med Scand 1986;711(suppl):55-65
131. Ivy JL. Role of exercise training in the prevention and treatment of insulin resistance and non–insulin-dependent diabetes mellitus. Sports Med 1997;24: 321-336
132. Helmrich SP, Ragland DR, Leung RW, Paffenbarger RS. Physical activity and reduced occurrence of non–insulin dependent diabetes mellitus. N Engl J Med 1991;325: 147-152
133. McFarlane SI, Kumar A, Sowers JR. Mechanisms by which angiotensin-converting enzyme inhibitors prevent diabetes and cardiovascular disease. Am J Cardiol 2003;91(suppl):30H-37H
134. Schwartz RS, Shuman WP, Larson V, et al. The effect of intensive endurance exercise training on body fat distribution in young and older men. Metabolism 1991; 40:545-551
135. Ross R, Dagnone D, Jones PJ, et al. Reduction in obesity and related comorbid conditions after diet-induced weight loss or exercise-induced weight loss in men. A randomized, controlled trial. Ann Intern Med 2000; 133:92-103

136. Despres JP, Pouliot MC, Moorjani S, et al. Loss of abdominal fat and metabolic response to exercise training in obese women. Am J Physiol 1991;261:E159-E167
137. Schrauwen-Hinderling VB, Schrauwen P, Hesselink MK, et al. The increase in intramyocellular lipid content is a very early response to training. J Clin Endocrinol Metab 2003;88:1610-1616
138. Jensen MD. Fate of fatty acids at rest and during exercise: regulatory mechanisms. Acta Physiol Scand 2003;178: 385-390
139. Schmitt B, Fluck M, Decombaz J, et al. Transcriptional adaptations of lipid metabolism in tibialis anterior muscle of endurance-trained athletes. Physiol Genomics 2003;15:148-157
140. van Loon LJ, Koopman R, Stegen JH, et al. Intramyocellular lipids form an important substrate source during moderate intensity exercise in endurance-trained males in a fasted state. J Physiol 2003;553:611-625
141. White LJ, Ferguson MA, McCoy SC, Kim H. Intramyocellular lipid changes in men and women during aerobic exercise: a (1)H-magnetic resonance spectroscopy study. J Clin Endocrinol Metab 2003;88: 5638-5643
142. White LJ, Robergs RA, Sibbitt WL Jr, et al. Effects of intermittent cycle exercise on intramyocellular lipid use and recovery. Lipids 2003;38:9-13
143. Brechtel K, Niess AM, Machann J, et al. Utilisation of intramyocellular lipids (IMCLs) during exercise as assessed by proton magnetic resonance spectroscopy (^{1}H-MRS). Horm Metab Res 2001;33:63-66
144. Perdomo G, Commerford SR, Richard AM, et al. Increased beta-oxidation in muscle cells enhances insulin-stimulated glucose metabolism and protects against fatty acid induced insulin resistance despite intramyocellular lipid accumulation. J Biol Chem 2004; 279:27177-27186
145. Ye JM, Doyle PJ, Iglesias MA, et al. Peroxisome proliferator–activated receptor (PPAR)-alpha activation lowers muscle lipids and improves insulin sensitivity in high fat–fed rats: comparison with PPAR-gamma activation. Diabetes 2001;50:411-417
146. Muoio DM, Way JM, Tanner CJ, et al. Peroxisome proliferator–activated receptor-alpha regulates fatty acid utilization in primary human skeletal muscle cells. Diabetes 2002;51:901-909
147. Halle M, Berg A, Northoff H, Keul J. Importance of TNF-alpha and leptin in obesity and insulin resistance: a hypothesis on the impact of physical exercise. Exercise Immunol Rev 1998;4:77-94
148. Baha T, Kanda T, Yoshida A, et al. Reciprocal changes in leptin and tumor necrosis factor-alpha with exercise in insulin resistant rats. Res Commun Mol Pathol Pharmacol 2000;108:133-143
149. Monzillo LU, Hamdy O, Horton ES, et al. Effect of lifestyle modification on adipokine levels in obese subjects with insulin resistance. Obes Res 2003;11:1048-1054
150. Kriketos AD, Gan SK, Poynten AM, et al. Exercise increases adiponectin levels and insulin sensitivity in humans. Diabetes Care 2004;27:629-630
151. Yamauchi T, Kamon J, Minokoshi Y, et al. Adiponectin stimulates glucose utilization and fatty-acid oxidation by activating AMP-activated protein kinase. Nat Med 2002;8:1288-1295
152. Winder WW, Hardie DG. AMP-activated protein kinase, a metabolic master switch: possible roles in type 2 diabetes. Am J Physiol 1999;277:E1-E10
153. Pulawa LK, Eckel RH. Overexpression of muscle lipoprotein lipase and insulin sensitivity. Curr Opin Clin Nutr Metab Care 2002;5:569-574
154. Bruce CR, Anderson MJ, Carey AL, et al. Muscle oxidative capacity is a better predictor of insulin sensitivity than lipid status. J Clin Endocrinol Metab 2003;88:5444-5451
155. Gan SK, Kriketos AD, Ellis BA, et al. Changes in aerobic capacity and visceral fat but not myocyte lipid levels predict increased insulin action after exercise in overweight and obese men. Diabetes Care 2003;26:1706-1713
156. Boirie Y. Insulin regulation of mitochondrial proteins and oxidative phosphorylation in human muscle. Trends Endocrinol Metab 2003;14:393-394
157. Wallace RK. Physiological effects of transcendental meditation. Science 1970;167:1751-1754
158. Liu G, Cui R, Li G, Huang G. Changes in brainstem and cortical auditory potentials during Qi-Gong meditation. Am J Chin Med 1990;23:95-103
159. Wallace RK, Benson H, Wilson A. Wakeful hypometabolic state. Am J Physiol 1971;221:795-799
160. Wallace RK, Benson H. The physiology of meditation. Sci Am 1972;7:46-47
161. Davidson RJ, Kabat-Zinn J, Schumacher J, et al. Alterations in brain and immune function produced by mindfulness meditation. Psychosom Med 2003;65: 564-570.
162. Eppley KR, Abrams AI, Shear J. Differential effects of relaxation techniques on trait anxiety: a meta-analysis. J Clin Psychol 1990;45:957-974
163. Schneider RH, Staggers F, Alexander CN, et al. A randomized controlled trial of stress reduction for hypertension in older African Americans. Hypertension 1995;26:820-827
164. LaForge R. Mind-body fitness: encouraging prospects for primary and secondary prevention. J Cardiovasc Nurs 1997;11:53-65
165. Khanam AA, Sachdeva U, Guleria R, Deepak KK. Study of pulmonary and autonomic functions of asthma patients after yoga training. Indian J Physiol Pharmacol 1996;40:318-324
166. Brudnack MA, Dundero D, Van Hecke FM. Are the "hard" martial arts, such as the Korean martial art, Tae Kwon-Do, of benefit to senior citizens? Med Hypotheses 2002;59:485-491
167. Lee MS, Kim BG, Huh HJ, et al. Effect of Qi-training on blood pressure, heart rate, and respiration. Clin Physiol 1999;20:3:173-176
168. Lee MS, Huh HJ, Kim BG, et al. Effects of Qi-training on heart rate variability. Am J Chin Med 2002;30:463-470
169. Lan C, Lai J-S, Chen S-Y. Tai Chi Chuan. An ancient wisdom on exercise and health promotion. Sports Med 2002;32:217-224
170. Taylor-Piliae RE. Tai Chi as an adjunct to cardiac rehabilitation exercise training. J Cardiopulm Rehabil 2003;23: 90-96
171. Lan C, Chen SY, Lai JS, et al. Heart rate responses and oxygen consumption during Tai Chi Chuan practice. Am J Chin Med 2001;29:403-410
172. Chao YFC, Chen SY, Lan C, Lai JS. The cardiorespiratory response and energy expenditure of Tai-Chi-Qui-Gong. Am J Chin Med 2002;30:451-461
173. Lan C, Lai JS, Chen SY, et al. 12-month Tai Chi training in the elderly: its effects on health fitness. Med Sci Sports Exerc 1998;30:345-351
174. Vaananen J, Xusheng S, Wang S, et al. Taichiquan acutely increases heart rate variability. Clin Physiol Funct Imaging 2002;22:2-3
175. Wang JS, Lan C, Chen SY, Wong MK. Tai Chi Chuan training is associated with enhanced endothelium-dependent dilation in skin vasculature of healthy older men. J Am Geriatr Soc 2002;50: 1024-1030

176. Wang J-S, Lan C, Wong M-K. Tai Chi Chuan training to enhance microcirculatory function in healthy elderly men. Arch Phys Med Rehabil 2001;82:1176-1180
177. Channer KS, Barrow D, Barrow R, et al. Changes in haemodynamic parameters following Tai Chi Chuan and aerobic exercise in patients recovering from acute myocardial infarction. Postgrad Med J 1996;72: 349-351
178. Lan C, Chen S-Y, Lai J-S, Wong M-K. The effect of Tai Chi on cardiorespiratory function in patients with coronary artery bypass surgery. Med Sci Sports Exerc 1999; 31:634-638
179. Rundle RL. Adults performing Tai Chi Chih boost immunity to shingles. Wall St J 2003;September 22:B4
180. Irwin MR, Pike JL, Cole JC, Oxman MN. Effects of a behavioral intervention, Tai Chi Chih, on varicella-zoster virus specific immunity and health functioning in older adults. J Psychosom Med 2003;65:824-830.
181. Toskovic NN, Blessing D, Williford HN. The effect of experience and gender on cardiovascular and metabolic responses with dynamic Tae Kwon Do exercise. J Strength Cond Res 2002;16:278-285
182. Nguyen Y, Naseer N, Frishman WH. Sauna as a therapeutic option for cardiovascular disease. Cardiol Rev 2004;12:321-324
183. Ikeda Y, Biro S, Kamogawa Y, et al. Repeated thermal therapy upregulates arterial endothelial nitric oxide synthase expression in Syrian golden hamsters. Jpn Circ J 2001;65:434-438
184. Imamura M, Biro S, Kihara T, et al. Repeated thermal therapy improves impaired vascular endothelial function in patients with coronary risk factors. J Am Coll Cardiol 2001;38:1083-1088
185. Sugahara Y, Ishii M, Muta H, et al. Efficacy and safety of thermal vasodilation therapy by sauna in infants with severe congestive heart failure secondary to ventricular septal defect. Am J Cardiol 2003;92: 109-113
186. Kihara T, Biro S, Imamura M, et al. Repeated sauna treatment improves vascular endothelial and cardiac function in patients with chronic heart failure. J Am Coll Cardiol 2002;39:754-759
187. Massage Therapy Facts for Physicians. Alternative Medicine Alert 2003;6:S1-S2
188. Webb WB, Agnew HW. Are we chronically sleep deprived? Bull Psychon Soc 1975;6:47-48
189. National Sleep Foundation. National Sleep Foundation 2000 Omnibus "Sleep in America" Poll. http://www.sleepfoundation.org/publications/2000poll.cfm
190. Bass J, Turek FW. Sleepless in America. A pathway to obesity and the metabolic syndrome? Arch Intern Med 2005;165:15-16
191. Spiegel K, Tasali E, Penev P, Van Cauter E. Brief communication: sleep curtailment in healthy young men is associated with decreased leptin levels, elevated ghrelin levels, and increased hunger and appetite. Ann Intern Med 2004;141:846-850
192. Spiegel K, Leproult R, L'Hermite-Baleriaux M, et al. Leptin levels are dependent on sleep duration: relationships with sympathovagal balance, carbohydrate regulation, cortisol, and thyrotropin. J Clin Endocrinol Metab 2004;89:5762-5771
193. Vorona RD, Winn MP, Babineau TW, et al. Overweight and obese patients in a primary care population report less sleep than patients with a normal body mass index. Arch Intern Med 2005;165:25-30

Weight Loss 14

According to epidemiologic and animal experimental studies, leanness and weight control may be associated with an extended life span.[1] However, **the typical U.S. adult gains about three fourths of a pound per year.**[2] **In the absence of exercise, overweight middle-aged individuals may experience a 2-lb yearly weight gain.**[3] Correspondingly, there is an increasing epidemic of overweight and obesity in this country, as well as globally.

Morbid obesity is a chronic metabolic disorder and a serious health concern associated with increased morbidity and mortality. With obesity there is an increased risk for coronary heart disease (CHD), stroke, hypertension, type 2 diabetes mellitus (DM), dyslipidemia, and all-cause mortality. A body mass index (BMI) greater than 35 kg/m^2 increases insulin resistance, hyperinsulinemia, and hyperglycemia and leads to an increased risk for DM by greater than 60-fold in women and 42-fold in men. Mortality rates from all causes, especially CHD, are increased by 50% to 100%.[4,5]

One mechanism linking adiposity with insulin resistance and cardiovascular disease appears to be the enhanced production of adipokines, such as interleukin-6 (IL-6) and tumor necrosis factor-alpha (TNF-α). Elevated levels of C-reactive protein (CRP) and IL-6, indicative of chronic, subclinical inflammation, are associated with insulin resistance and incident cardiovascular disease, including myocardial infarction, stroke, and peripheral vascular disease.[4]

The majority of cases of metabolic syndrome occur in overweight individuals. Weight control is a widely recommended clinical goal in patients with obesity and the metabolic syndrome. **Weight loss reverses many, albeit not all, of the features of the metabolic syndrome.** Lowering endogenous insulin concentrations, a key feature of successful therapy reflecting improved sensitivity to insulin, can be accomplished with weight reduction. There is, in fact, strong evidence that weight loss in overweight and obese individuals improves risk factors for DM and cardiovascular disease.[4,5]

Regular physical activity and cardiorespiratory fitness are core components of successful weight loss programs and are

critical to the long-term maintenance of weight control. Data regarding the benefits of weight loss in combination with exercise training have been addressed in detail in the preceding chapter, "Exercise and Meditation." Specific dietary approaches are covered in the next chapter, "Diet and Supplements," and anorexigenics are discussed in the final chapter, "Pharmacology."

HOMEOSTATIC RESPONSES TO WEIGHT GAIN AND WEIGHT LOSS

Hunger and appetite play essential roles in the regulation of food-seeking behavior. Eating is an extremely important, basic human drive that is critical for survival of the individual and the species. Hunger and appetite are physiologically highly regulated through complex biochemical signaling.

Weight Gain. With an accretion of excess body weight, there are minimal physiologic signals to stimulate the reversal of weight gain. In fact, the highest weight attained tends to be preserved by an organism. Weight gain induces no compensatory loss of appetite, no increase in the metabolic rate, and no drive to raise energy expenditure via physical activity. Rather, physical activity tends to decline with weight gain.[6]

Weight Loss. The body conserves its fat stores at the maximal level achieved, thereby effectively resetting its "settling point." Efforts at weight loss via dietary measures are thwarted by powerful physiologic signals deriving from numerous genetic, behavioral, environmental, and nutritional factors that seek to restore the highest body weight.[7] Thus, efforts at dietary weight loss do not have a lasting effect and are plagued by high rates of recidivism.

The greater the weight loss, the more intense the neurohormonally driven, primal hunger urge to overcome the conscious decision to lose weight. The homeostatic neurohormonal system regulating energy balance creates behavioral and metabolic challenges to the maintenance of weight loss that may be impossible to overcome.[8] An increase in the hunger drive, a reduction in resting energy expenditure, down-regulation in reproductive and growth functions, and a step-up in adipose tissue fat uptake conspire to render the long-term maintenance of dietary weight loss a daunting challenge. The neurohormonal adaptations are complex and encompass changes in the activity of thyroid, growth, and sex hormones.[7] Additionally, other factors play a role.

Ghrelin. Although obese humans actually have lower ghrelin levels than normal-weight controls do, **diet-induced weight loss causes a rebound rise in ghrelin levels.** Because ghrelin appears to act centrally on receptors in the arcuate nucleus to enhance appetite via activation of the neuropeptide Y/agouti-related peptide pathway, elevated plasma levels will undermine weight loss efforts by intensely augmenting hunger and food-seeking behavior.[1]

Leptin. Leptin, secreted by adipocytes, is an important factor for the adaptive response to fasting and for the neuroendocrine alterations with caloric restriction.[9] **Because the reduction in body fat decreases the production of leptin, lower leptin plasma levels, in the absence of leptin resistance, increase food intake and lower metabolic energy expenditures via central mechanisms.** To ensure maintenance of weight loss, the lower metabolic rate after dieting would necessitate the continuation of very low energy intake.[8]

Lipoprotein Lipase. Lipoprotein lipase (LPL), located on the luminal surface of the capillary endothelium near muscle and adipose tissue, is the rate-limiting enzyme for the hydrolysis and clearance of circulating triglyceride. Free fatty acids derived from the hydrolyzed triglyceride are readily available for transport into subjacent tissues for oxidation or storage. Because there is a direct relationship between adipose tissue LPL activity and fatty acid uptake, the relative activity of the enzyme determines fatty acid availability to adipose tissue and adipose tissue fat storage. LPL also influences the composition and concentration of lipoprotein lipids.[10]

Adipose tissue LPL activity in humans responds to acute and chronic changes in energy balance. During feeding in normal subjects, adipose tissue LPL activity increases to direct fuel toward storage in adipose tissue. During fasting and periods of low energy intake, adipose tissue LPL activity decreases in order to preserve free fatty acid availability as a fuel source for working tissues.[10]

Obese individuals have higher adipose tissue LPL activity than lean persons do, even when expressed relative to fat cell size. After weight loss and a period of weight maintenance at a reduced body weight, there are variable changes in adipose tissue LPL activity. LPL may increase, remain unchanged, or decrease in the weight-reduced state. Subjects who have a low initial LPL activity are more likely to increase their adipose tissue LPL activity with weight loss. **An increase in LPL activity may adversely affect changes in body fat storage and lipid metabolism and thereby thwart efforts at maintenance of weight loss by enhancing the ability of adipocytes to take up nutrients for storage.**[10] Additionally, greater tonic inhibition of basal lipolysis by endogenous adenosine may increase the activity of adipose tissue LPL after weight loss and predispose to recurrent adiposity.[11]

Beyond Weight Loss—Sustained Caloric Restriction. Chronic caloric restriction increases the life span of many types of animals. The anti-aging effects of caloric restriction may derive from the adaptive response of the neuroendocrine and metabolic response systems to maximize survival during periods of food shortage.[9]

Although activation of adenosine 5′-monophosphate–activated protein kinase (AMPK) plays a central role in allowing cells to adapt to nutrient deprivation in vitro, AMPK does not appear to play a role in the metabolic adaptation to acute and chronic nutritional stress in vivo. In mice, 4 months of caloric restriction–induced weight loss did not increase AMPK activity; however, the amount of phosphorylated acetyl CoA carboxylase (ACC) was dramatically decreased because of decreased protein expression.[12]

On the other hand, **adiponectin may play an important role in the beneficial effects of long-term caloric restriction** by affecting the expression of transcription factors involved in fatty acid oxidation and energy utilization. Rats maintained on long-term caloric restriction for up to 20 months showed a significant increase in plasma adiponectin and insulin sensitivity. Triacylglycerol levels in the liver and skeletal muscle fell significantly below those observed in rats fed ad libitum. Elevated concentrations of plasma adiponectin in long-term, calorically restricted rats were associated with increased expression of transcription factor messenger RNA (mRNA) for peroxisome proliferator–activated receptor-alpha (PPAR-α), PPAR-γ, and PPAR-δ, but decreased expression of sterol regulatory element binding protein-1c (SREBP-1c), which caused down-regulation of cholesterol and low-density lipoprotein (LDL) receptor synthesis.[13]

WEIGHT LOSS EFFECTS ON ADIPOSE TISSUE

Obesity invariably implies an excessive expansion of white adipose tissue. Adipose tissue can increase in mass by more than twice the lean body weight. Adipose tissue mass, aside from stromal tissue, represents the product of adipocyte number and volume. It is the only organ in the body capable of such impressive plasticity.[14]

Role of Normal Adipose Tissue. Adipose tissue in fit, normal-weight individuals serves an important function as insulator and mechanical shock absorber for essential organs, as a storage site for energy-dense fuel, and as one nexus in the network modulating the nutritional, hormonal, immune, and metabolic status of the organism. In this latter function, **adipose tissue assumes the function of an endocrine and immune organ.**

Role of Adipose Tissue in Obesity. With hypertrophy and hyperplasia of adipose tissue, the metabolic and immune functions of adipose tissue can be drastically amplified and distorted. Particularly with the "stress effects" of an inactive, sedentary lifestyle or in the presence of a chronic inflammatory nidus, the hyperplastic adipose tissue of obesity can turn into a highly active endocrine and immune organ "tumor" whose hormonal and cytokine output amplifies a systemic proinflammatory state while shifting metabolic homeostasis to catabolism with insulin resistance.

Weight Loss Effects on Adipose Depots. Weight loss implies a negative energy balance, a mismatch wherein energy output chronically exceeds energy intake. With a chronic, negative energy balance, the organism needs to mobilize and deplete endogenous fuel sources, largely from the ample triacylglycerol reservoirs.

Mobilization plus consumption of excess fat stores gives rise to conditions that have a favorable impact on metabolism.

Adipose Mass and Adipocyte Size. The mass of adipose tissue and adipocyte size partly determine the level of circulating hormonal and proinflammatory adipokines. **Lipolysis, in the setting of a negative energy balance, mobilizes lipid stores from adipocytes. The resulting weight reduction is accompanied by decreased adipose tissue mass and adipocyte volume, thereby lessening the circulating levels of mediators of inflammation and insulin resistance.**[15]

Visceral/Omental Fat. Visceral-omental adiposity is a major factor in insulin resistance. With enlargement, the visceral-omental fat depot becomes metabolically very active and participates in the proinflammatory, catabolic state of insulin resistance.

Visceral-omental adipose tissue functions essentially as a "first-responder" fat depot to allow ready mobilization of its fat as fuel. There is consequently regional variability in adipocyte triglyceride turnover with caloric restriction such that lipid mobilization from visceral fat depots is favored over mobilization from peripheral subcutaneous sites. In particular, catecholamine-induced lipolysis is enhanced in visceral fat but decreased in subcutaneous fat.[4] **A sustained negative energy balance with weight reduction diminishes the visceral-omental adipose tissue mass and thus minimizes its metabolic impact.**

The visceral-omental fat depot is reduced in proportion to systemic fat loss with weight reduction. Obese men who lose weight via diet or exercise lose equivalent proportions of subcutaneous and visceral fat.[16]

Ectopic Fat. Ectopic, nonadipose tissue deposition of fat is associated with insulin resistance. **As weight loss depletes ectopic sites of intrahepatocellular and intramyocellular lipid storage, the negative metabolic impact of that pathophysiology abates.** The reduction in ectopic intracellular fat storage, rather than a change in total-body fat or extramyocellular lipid, predicts a reversal in insulin resistance.[17]

Free Fatty Acids. Weight loss causes a reduction in free fatty acid levels. Although adipose tissue lipolysis releases free fatty acids, a negative energy balance entails the consumption of circulating free fatty acids as fuel by metabolically active organs, thus undermining any negative impact that free fatty acids may have on endothelial function and insulin signaling.

ANTI-INFLAMMATORY AND VASCULOPROTECTIVE EFFECTS OF WEIGHT LOSS

Because of the reduction in the mass and cell size of metabolically active adipose tissue, weight loss via caloric restriction or malabsorptive gastric surgery has beneficial metabolic effects.

Anti-inflammatory Effects. Obesity, in particular visceral adiposity, is associated with elevated circulating markers of inflammation. **Weight loss via caloric restriction or malabsorptive gastric surgery has an anti-inflammatory effect whereby levels of proinflammatory cytokines and adhesion molecules are lowered.** Weight loss leads to a reduction in the levels of

- TNF-α,
- IL-6,
- CRP,
- adhesion molecules, and
- plasminogen activator inhibitor-1 (PAI-1).[5,18-20]

In 56 healthy premenopausal obese women (age range, 25 to 44 years; BMI, 37.2 ± 2.2 kg/m^2), after 1 year of 9.8 ± 1.5-kg weight reduction with exercise and counseling, sustained weight loss was associated with a reduction in TNF-α, IL-6, P-selectin, intercellular adhesion molecule-1 (ICAM-1), and vascular adhesion molecule-1 (VCAM-1).[18] Similarly, IL-18 levels, associated with body weight and abdominal fat deposition, were reduced with weight loss.[21]

Parasympathetic Tone. Obesity is associated with autonomic dysfunction and lower parasympathetic tone.[22] **With weight loss, norepinephrine levels decline, neurohormonal**

activation is lessened, and parasympathetic tone rises. The increment in cardiac vagal tone correlates significantly with decreases in body weight, fat mass, abdominal fat, waist circumference, serum insulin, and heart rate.[23]

Increased vagal tone may not be maintained long-term if body weight is regained. In long-term follow-up over 1 year, the increase in parasympathetic tone was gradually attenuated during a year of attempted weight maintenance.[24]

Endothelial Function. Obesity, in particular visceral adiposity, is associated with endothelial dysfunction. **By down-regulating the inflammatory state, dietary weight loss ameliorates endothelial dysfunction.**

In healthy, premenopausal, obese women (BMI, 37.2 ± 2.2 kg/m^2), sustained weight loss after 1 year of weight reduction with exercise was associated with a reduction in cytokine and adhesion molecule levels together with an improvement in vascular responses to L-arginine.[18] Similar findings were obtained when dietary weight loss was augmented by liposuction.[25]

IMPACT OF WEIGHT LOSS ON THE METABOLIC SYNDROME

The reduction in visceral adiposity, ectopic fat, adipocyte volume, and free fatty acids with weight loss is highly correlated with an improvement in systemic insulin resistance, dyslipidemia, and the risk for development of type 2 DM.[26-29]

Insulin Resistance. The insulin-sensitizing effect of weight reduction is well documented. **Weight loss is accompanied by a reduction in indicators of systemic insulin resistance and the risk for development of type 2 DM.**[30,31] Weight loss is thus one of the cornerstones of the therapeutic lifestyle changes for the metabolic syndrome. **Even modest weight loss of 5 to 10 kg, or 5% to 7% of body weight, has a favorable impact on many of the metabolic disturbances and cardiovascular risk factors of the metabolic syndrome,** such as

- insulin resistance,
- hyperinsulinemia,
- atherogenic dyslipidemia,
- hypertension, and
- left ventricular hypertrophy in normotensive and hypertensive obesity.[32-34]

Interventions leading to weight loss or prevention of weight gain with increased exercise are lifestyle changes that have been reported to achieve a 42% to 58% reduction in the progression to type 2 DM.[35,36]

In addition to the effects on lipid depots, a number of other factors contribute to the improvement in insulin resistance with weight loss.

PPAR-α and PPAR-γ. Weight loss induces the expression of PPAR-α and PPAR-γ. Increased activation of these PPARs may be a key mechanism for improving cardiovascular and metabolic risk.

Mice with combined leptin and LDL receptor deficiency, relative to lean mice, are prone to obesity, insulin resistance, hypertriglyceridemia, hypertension, impaired left ventricular function, and accelerated atherosclerosis. Expression of PPAR-α and PPAR-γ is down-regulated in such double-knockout mice. Diet restriction in these obese mice caused a 45% weight loss accompanied by an up-regulation of PPAR-α and PPAR-γ with changes in the expression of genes regulating oxidative stress, inflammation, glucose transport, lipid metabolism, and insulin signaling. These weight loss–induced changes in gene expression engendered increased insulin sensitivity, decreased hypertriglyceridemia, reduced blood pressure and heart rate, increased left ventricular ejection fraction, and reduced atherosclerosis. Increased PPAR-α and PPAR-γ expression was inversely related to plaque volume and to oxidized LDL content in atheromatous plaque.[37]

Inflammatory Cytokines. Improvements in glucose metabolism with weight loss programs are independently associated with decreases in cytokine concentrations, which suggests that **a reduction in inflammation is a potential mechanism that mediates the enhancement of insulin sensitivity.**

The decrement in TNF-α is proportional to the increase in muscle glucose transporter-4 (GLUT4) and glucose uptake with weight loss.[19] In abdominally obese male subjects, elevated plasma levels of IL-8 and IL-6 were correlated with measures of insulin resistance. After 24 weeks of caloric restriction and a 30% reduction in fat mass, there were significant reductions in the proinflammatory cytokines IL-6, IL-8, and TNF-α; fasting insulin levels; and homeostasis model assessment (HOMA) measures of insulin resistance.[38] In obese individuals, dietary weight loss in excess of 10% body weight significantly reduced the markedly elevated plasma levels of TNF-α with an improvement in insulin sensitivity.[39] Six months of weight loss in women induced by diet and exercise resulted in significant reductions in visceral adiposity and IL-6, which were both independent predictors of improvement in insulin sensitivity.[40]

Leptin. The increase in insulin action after weight loss may be related to the decrease in leptin levels mediated by the loss of body fat.

With sustained weight loss exceeding 7% of body mass, plasma leptin concentrations decreased in parallel with plasma insulin.[41] In obese, postmenopausal women, elevated plasma leptin levels correlated with basal hyperinsulinemia and with the impaired insulin response to hyperglycemia. After 4 months of dietary weight loss with resistive training, the improvement in insulin response to a glucose load paralleled the decline in leptin levels.[42]

Adiponectin. Insulin sensitivity may increase in response to a rise in adiponectin levels as a result of weight loss. The increment in adiponectin concentration probably occurs because of a reduction in fat mass and concomitant attenuation of the autocrine/paracrine suppressive effects of TNF-α and IL-6. It is positively correlated with insulin sensitivity and with the anti-inflammatory and vasculoprotective effects of weight loss.[43,44]

Weight loss of 10% or more, achieved through a low-energy Mediterranean-style diet and higher physical activity in obese women over a period of 2 years, induced a significant reduction in free fatty acid levels with a significant rise in adiponectin, both of which were independently associated with enhancement of insulin sensitivity.[45]

Dyslipidemia. The enhancement in insulin sensitivity after weight loss is accompanied by a reduction in atherogenic dyslipidemia.[30,31]

In a 15-week weight-reducing program involving 32 obese men and premenopausal women aged 36 to 50 years with a daily 500- to 800-kcal energy deficit below the subjects' estimated sedentary energy expenditure, weight loss promoted significant reductions in plasma triglyceride and LDL concentrations in all subjects.[46]

Antihypertensive and Diuretic Effects. Hypertension is an aspect of the metabolic syndrome. **Weight loss and the associated diuresis reduce blood pressure in both hypertensive and nonhypertensive overweight individuals.**[4]

Blood pressure in obese patients is sensitive to the intake of sodium. Adipocytes express natriuretic clearance receptors that engender an effective deficit of natriuretic peptides in obesity and cause sodium retention and volume expansion. Fasting and weight loss lower the expression of adipocyte natriuretic peptide clearance receptors and thereby increase the availability of natriuretic peptide to enhance sodium excretion.[47]

Hyperinsulinemia and heightened renal sympathetic nerve activity similarly stimulate enhanced renal tubular sodium reabsorption with insulin resistance in obesity, effects that are relieved by weight loss.

Mortality. The metabolic syndrome is associated with increased mortality, and **weight loss improves the odds for survival.** In a large study of 43,457 overweight women, a 12-year follow-up study showed that at least 9 kg of intentional weight loss caused a 53% reduction in obesity-related deaths.[48]

INTERVENTIONS FOR WEIGHT LOSS

A proinflammatory state, such as underlies insulin resistance, by its very nature is antiadipogenic and mitigates further weight gain. It represents a mild version of the more advanced stage of cachexia in end-stage heart failure or malignancy.

Ironically, it is the antiadipogenic effects of caloric restriction, via dietary curtailment or malabsorptive surgery, that can reverse the negative impact of inflammation-linked catabolism in overweight individuals.

Rational Dietary Approach. Dietary weight loss is difficult to initiate and harder yet to sustain because of psychological and behavioral issues and the powerful physiologic responses that seek to reestablish the highest body weight. Dietary weight loss needs to be approached rationally, prudently, with understanding, with a long-term view in mind, with patience, and with modest expectations.

Metabolic Rate. To achieve weight loss, caloric intake should be lower than the person's metabolic rate. The metabolic rate is a measure of the number of calories the body consumes per day. The majority of a day's caloric consumption is determined by the resting metabolic rate, or the energy required to maintain basal physiologic functions. Determinants of a person's metabolic rate are multifactorial and are a function of genetics, gender, age, height, weight, body composition, muscle composition, general activity level, and any pathologic or pharmacologic factors that may have an impact on thermogenesis.

A person's metabolic rate may be estimated by formulas. However, such formulas are inadequate, especially those for women or for overweight individuals. The metabolic rate can be quantitatively assessed via metabolic testing, measuring oxygen uptake and carbon dioxide production, a "metabolic rest test" in lieu of a "metabolic stress test." Hand-held devices are available for office testing. Conceivably, direct assessment of a person's metabolic rate may assist in individually tailoring guidelines for daily caloric intake.[49]

Weight Loss Goal. It generally takes years to become overweight or obese. Accordingly, dietary weight loss requires time and perseverance to reach the proposed target. Without attention to the resulting disturbances in biochemical signaling, crash diets, albeit successful in the short term, rarely achieve sustained, long-term weight loss. Serial crash diets with recurrent cycles of weight loss, followed by recrudescent weight gain, may be physiologically more harmful than sustained ponderosity.

To succeed in weight control, there should be two aims:

1. **avoid further weight gain** and
2. **have a realistic aim of losing, e.g., 10% of current weight over a period of 6 to 12 months.** Specifically, the clinician and patient should aim for a weight loss pattern of not more than 0.5 to 1 pound per week to avoid an excessive, neurohormonal reaction to the disturbed homeostatic physiologic balance.[4]

The lifestyle changes undertaken should focus on modifying eating habits and increasing physical activity. They need to be realistic, doable, and sustainable, with education and support.[6]

Individuals who successfully lose weight and sustain weight loss share a number of characteristics. They

- assiduously monitor caloric intake, physical activity, and body weight,
- consume 1300 to 1400 kcal/day,
- eat breakfast,
- consume less than 25% of their diet as fat, and
- walk the equivalent of more than 4 miles per day.[50]

National Heart, Lung and Blood Institute guidelines recommend weight loss with a 500- to 1000-kcal/day caloric deficit.[51] The generous consumption of at least 8 to 12 cups of water per day may be of benefit. One helpful strategy to limit caloric intake may be the incorporation of calorie- and portion-controlled meal replacement products in the diet.[52]

Surgical Intervention. Diet-induced weight loss improves the metabolic complications of abdominal obesity. However, successful long-term weight management is difficult to achieve, and the majority of obese persons who lose weight by implementing lifestyle changes regain their lost weight over time. The lack of efficacy of current medical obesity therapies has led to interventional approaches such as liposuction and bariatric surgery. The number of bariatric surgical procedures has increased drastically over the past several years. In 2003, more than 100,000 procedures were performed.[53]

Interestingly, the mere surgical reduction of adipose tissue mass does not convey a metabolic advantage. It appears critical for the achievement of metabolic benefits with surgically induced weight loss that the reduction in fat mass be associated with the induction of a negative energy balance. In the absence of lifestyle measures that impart a negative energy balance, simple procedural removal of even large amounts of fat, as via liposuction, is of little metabolic merit and has no impact on the visceral-omental fat mass, on adipocyte size, and on ectopic fat stores and free fatty acid fluxes.[54]

Liposuction. Liposuction, also known as lipoplasty or suction-assisted lipectomy, is the most common aesthetic surgical procedure performed in the United States and is overall one of the more common elective surgical procedures. Nearly 400,000 procedures are performed annually. Recent advances in liposuction techniques allow the removal of a considerable mass of subcutaneous adipose tissue.[54]

Studies of the metabolic effects of liposuction have yielded varied results, possibly because of differences in subjects' baseline weight and insulin sensitivity, the assessment of insulin sensitivity, subjects' lifestyle and weight changes after liposuction, or variations in the site and volume of adipose tissue removed.[54]

In some instances, liposuction may be associated with amelioration of insulin resistance and reduction of circulating proinflammatory markers. Thirty healthy premenopausal obese women with a BMI between 30 and 45 kg/m^2 had a net lipid loss of 2.7 ± 0.7 kg 6 months after liposuction and significantly reduced concentrations of IL-6, IL-18, TNF-α, and CRP with significantly increased serum levels of adiponectin and high-density lipoprotein (HDL). The amount of fat aspirate correlated with changes in insulin sensitivity, as measured by HOMA, with the decrease in TNF-α, and with the increase in adiponectin.[55]

Contrasting findings have been obtained in other studies, in which abdominal liposuction of subcutaneous adipose tissue did not significantly improve obesity-associated metabolic abnormalities and did not achieve the metabolic benefits of dietary weight loss. Liposuction in 15 obese women, after decreasing the volume of subcutaneous abdominal adipose tissue by 28% to 44% and effecting a 9- to 10-kg loss of fat or 18% to 19% of total-body fat, did not significantly alter the insulin sensitivity of muscle, liver, or adipose tissue as assessed by stimulation of glucose disposal, suppression of glucose production, and suppression of lipolysis, respectively. There were no significant alterations in plasma concentrations of CRP, IL-6, TNF-α, and adiponectin or in blood pressure, insulin homeostasis, or lipid profile.[54]

Gastric Pacing. The implantable gastric stimulator, a pacemaker-like device, has been found to be safe and effective for the induction and maintenance of weight loss.

Implantable gastric stimulation electrically stimulates the stomach with a pacemaker-like device. The device is implanted in a minimally invasive procedure. Investigation in over 500 patients globally has shown it to be safe and seemingly free of long-term sequelae.[56] In two trials of 133 patients, loss of excess weight approached 20% after 20 months of follow-up.[57] In the Laparoscopic Obesity Stimulation Survey trial, 69 patients with a mean age of 41 years underwent implantation of a gastric stimulator between January 2002 and December 2003. Their mean BMI was 41 kg/m^2 with a mean weight of 115.0 kg. At 15 months, 21% of the excessive weight was lost. Appetite was reduced and postprandial and interprandial satiety was increased after implantation without a rise in ghrelin levels.[58] In 10 years' experience with gastric stimulation in 65 patients, there was significant weight loss without side effects. Blood pressure improved significantly and rapidly. Almost all patients with symptomatic gastroesophageal reflux reported relief of symptoms during gastric pacing. At 7 months after the procedure, there was an improvement in insulin resistance.[59]

Bariatric Surgery. Bariatric surgery may currently be the most effective approach to achieve sustained weight loss with metabolic benefit. It is the most efficacious intervention for the actual reversal of type 2 DM. With respect to food intake, bariatric surgery can be classified as

1. restrictive,
2. mixed restrictive-malabsorptive, and
3. predominantly malabsorptive.

According to the National Institutes of Health established guidelines, bariatric surgery can be considered for high-risk patients with

- BMI >40 kg/m^2 or
- BMI >35 kg/m^2 and comorbid conditions

in whom dietary restrictions and physical therapy have failed.[60]

Types of Bariatric Surgery. Purely restrictive interventions are

- vertically banded gastroplasty and
- gastric banding with adjustable and nonadjustable bands,

whereby a small gastric pouch is created, which then empties through a narrow outlet into the rest of the stomach. Predominantly malabsorptive procedures include

- biliopancreatic diversion and
- duodenal switch.

Mixed malabsorptive-restrictive interventions encompass

- Roux-en-Y gastric bypass or gastric jejunoileal bypass and
- gastric bypass with biliopancreatic diversion.

The restrictive-malabsorptive Roux-en-Y gastric bypass currently accounts for over 90% of bariatric surgery procedures. With gastric bypass, a small 10- to 30-mL portion of the upper part of the stomach is connected directly to the jejunum. This gastric jejunoileal bypass causes weight loss via physical restriction and malabsorption of food intake.[31,61]

Anticipated Weight Loss. With bariatric surgery, one third of the excess body weight is lost by 12 to 18 months postoperatively, and 48% to 74% of the excess weight is lost after 5 years. Weight loss is more effective with malabsorptive and mixed malabsorptive-restrictive interventions than with purely restrictive gastroplasty or gastric banding procedures.[31,61]

Bariatric surgery appears to result in long-term weight loss. In the prospective, controlled Swedish Obese Subjects Study, obese subjects with a mean age of 48 years and a mean BMI of 41 kg/m^2 who underwent gastric surgery were contemporaneously matched with conventionally treated obese control subjects and analyzed after a follow-up of at least 2 years (4047 subjects) or 10 years (1703 subjects). After 2 years, weight had increased by 0.1% in the control group and had decreased by 23.4% in the surgery group ($P < .001$). After 10 years, the weight increase was 1.6% and loss was 16.1%, respectively ($P < .001$).[62]

Comorbidities and Inflammatory Markers. In the majority of patients, there is improvement or resolution of obesity-related comorbid conditions. Efficacy on all counts is higher for malabsorptive and mixed malabsorptive-restrictive interventions than for restrictive gastric procedures. Asthma and obstructive sleep apnea are improved or resolved in 85.7% of individuals. Dyslipidemia improves in 70%, and hypertension is resolved in 61.7% and ameliorated in 70% of surgical patients. Eighty-five percent of patients experience partial or complete resolution of type 2 DM. Significant improvements in pancreatic beta cell function may occur. Resolution of DM may be seen within days of bariatric surgery, before the achievement of profound weight loss.[44,63]

Bariatric surgery appears to result in long-term improvement in lifestyle and amelioration of metabolic and cardiovascular risk factors. In the Swedish Obese Subjects Study, energy intake was lower and the proportion of physically active subjects higher in the surgery group than in the control group at 2 and 10 years. Throughout this observation period, rates of recovery from DM, dyslipidemia, hypertension, and hyperuricemia were more favorable in the surgery group than in the control group, with lower 2- and 10-year incidence rates for DM, hypertriglyceridemia, and hyperuricemia after surgery.[62]

The metabolic improvements are associated with reductions in proinflammatory cytokines. Reductions in levels of CRP and IL-6 and an increase in adiponectin levels correlate with enhanced or restored sensitivity to insulin signaling.[5,44]

Survival. Successful bariatric surgery may be associated with improved longevity. At 9 years, 2010 gastric bypass patients in the Swedish Obese Subjects Study, when compared with 2037 nonsurgical, obese, medically managed subjects, had a 9% versus 28% mortality rate, with an 80% decline in annual mortality.[64] In 1035 bariatric surgery patients at 5-year follow-up, there was an absolute 5.49% and relative 89% reduction in mortality risk when compared with 5746 nonsurgical, obese controls, $P < .001$.[44,65]

Bariatric surgery may lower mortality even for diabetic patients. For every 9 years of follow-up, surgically treated diabetic patients had a 1% mortality as opposed to the 9% mortality for medically treated diabetic patients.

Gut Hormones. In contrast to other weight loss interventions, malabsorptive-restrictive gastric bypass causes favorable alterations in gut-related hormones. Alterations in the balance of gut hormones differ for the diverse surgical interventions and appear to be a function of whether partial gastrectomy is performed, the distal part of the stomach is bypassed, and the enteric contents are separated from the biliopancreatic effluent.[44] With gastric jejunoileal bypass, elevated peptide YY3-36 (PYY) levels and a reduction in ghrelin levels result in a sharp decline in appetite, thereby enhancing weight loss and avoiding the risk of rebound weight gain. Additionally, levels of leptin, resistin, acylation-stimulating protein, enteroglucagon, cholecystokinin, and other gastrointestinal satiety mediators may be affected.[1,66]

Risks and Side Effects. Thirty-day operative mortality ranges from 0.1% for restrictive procedures, 0.5% for gastric bypass, to 1.1% for the biliopancreatic diversion or duodenal switch procedure.[44] Aside from the inconvenience of dietary restrictions associated with bariatric surgery, impaired absorption may cause deficient levels of vitamin B_{12}, folate, iron, and calcium. Cholelithiasis develops in a third of bypass patients. Stomal stenosis or marginal ulcers may develop in 5% to 15% of patients.[67] After massive weight loss, many individuals may opt for further, at times extensive plastic surgery to remove redundant skin folds.

Exercise as an Adjunct to Weight Loss. Exercise should complement any dietary or surgical weight loss approach. Exercise will mitigate the loss of lean body mass as a result of a sustained negative energy balance. Exercise will also favorably increase fatty acid oxidative consumption and the metabolic rate,[68,69] thus supporting the efforts at weight loss and counteracting some of the adipostatic responses that may be incurred in follow-up.

Exercise, when combined with a structured weight reduction program, may

- potentiate weight loss,
- increase visceral and subcutaneous fat loss,
- protect from the loss of lean muscle mass,
- improve features of the metabolic syndrome, and
- enhance weight loss maintenance.

After weight loss, in most instances adipocytes from the formerly obese remain less sensitive to lipolytic stimuli than do those from normal controls. However, even the pursuit of mild exercise renders these adipocytes metabolically more dynamic.[70]

When added to weight loss, higher-intensity exercise may lower or prevent the loss of lean muscle mass and more efficaciously improve physical fitness and risk factors for CHD when compared with low-intensity or no exercise training. In a study of 99 obese women focusing on diet only, diet plus low-intensity walking, and diet plus high-intensity aerobic dance approaches to weight loss, weight loss plus aerobic dance, when compared with the other options, more significantly helped preserve fat-free and bone-free body mass. That group had significantly greater improvements in strength, exercise capacity, LDL, and fasting glucose than did the low-intensity or no-exercise groups.[71]

Exercise and weight loss have complementary effects on reducing aspects of the metabolic syndrome. In a 6-month study, 53 obese men and women with hyperinsulinemia, dyslipidemia, and hypertension characteristic of the metabolic syndrome were randomly assigned to either aerobic exercise only, exercise with weight loss, or no intervention. Hyperinsulinemic responses

Table 14-1. Diverse Effects of Selected Weight Loss Approaches

DIET/NUTRITION	ANTIOXIDANT	ANTI-INFLAMMATORY	ENDOTHELIAL PROTECTIVE	ANTIHYPERTENSIVE	PPAR-γ	PPAR-α
Calorie restriction	N/A	+	+	+	+	+
Liposuction	N/A	0	0	0	N/A	N/A
Bariatric surgery	N/A	+	N/A	+	N/A	N/A

+, Beneficial effect; 0, neutral effect; N/A, data not available.

to glucose challenge were significantly reduced in both the exercise and exercise–weight loss intervention groups. Individuals with the largest amount of weight loss showed the greatest reduction in abnormal insulin responses. Diastolic blood pressure was significantly reduced only in the combined exercise and weight loss group.[72]

CONCLUSION

It is striking that there is no physiologic check and balance to limit weight gain and ponderosity. As the difficulty in losing weight and maintaining weight loss attests, the body appears to reset its weight maintenance barometer to the highest weight attained. This would make teleologic sense for organisms that have sought to survive in an environment generally characterized by episodic deprivation.

In many instances, ponderosity is associated with a proinflammatory state. Excessive consumption of calories and fats induces hypertrophy and expansion of fat tissue, which effectively creates a hormone- and cytokine-producing adipose tumor capable of massively amplifying ambient inflammatory processes and engendering insulin resistance. Circulating free fatty acids, endothelial dysfunction, and ectopic intracellular fat deposition evoke secondary insulin resistance mechanisms, the metabolic syndrome, and an abundance of cardiovascular, metabolic, and oncologic risk factors.

From this perspective, caloric restriction would be expected to diminish the mechanisms boosting inflammation and insulin resistance. Because of resetting of the body weight settling point with weight gain, dietary loss of massive amounts of weight is unsustainable in the long term. However, a mere 7% to 10% weight reduction appears sufficient to effect significant normalization of metabolic, inflammatory, vascular, and hemodynamic parameters. In view of the physiologic resistance to weight loss, it is even questionable whether more substantial weight loss is desirable or healthy.

Fitness lowers the all-cause mortality risk of excessive adiposity and, among men, appears to be more protective than the absence of ponderosity. A fit, fat man's prognosis is nearly as good as a fit, not fat man's, and unfit, not fat men have a greater risk for all-cause and CHD mortality than do fit, fat men.[73,74] Although there is no question that it would be better not to have gained weight in the first place, once overweight is reached, weight loss, beyond a modest reduction, is no longer a goal in and of itself. It is of greater importance to create an anti-inflammatory milieu with preserved endothelial function and cardiorespiratory fitness via the pursuit of a physically very active lifestyle.

Exercise, just like dietary observance, implies effort on the part of the individual and may be unattractive. In this respect, surgical intervention might appear to be a relatively painless way to remove the offending adipose load. However, here again, the truism "no pain—no gain" applies. Unfortunately, the mere surgical removal of even massive amounts of subcutaneous fat via liposuction, in the absence of an exercise program, may not improve obesity-associated metabolic abnormalities because it has no impact on visceral-omental fat, adipocyte size, ectopic intracellular fat stores, and fatty acid fluxes. A negative energy balance appears to be essential for achieving the metabolic benefits of weight loss (Table 14-1). Even bariatric surgery, to be effective, entails the creation of a chronic caloric deficit via malabsorption.

Ultimately, barring pharmacologic intervention, free fatty acids appear to be a central metabolic predicament that needs to be dealt with

METABOLIC RATE	BENEFICIAL LIPID EFFECTS	VISCERAL ADIPOSITY	ECTOPIC FAT	ADIPONECTIN	CARDIOVASCULAR EVENTS	INSULIN SENSITIVITY
+	+	+	+	+	+	+
N/A	0	0	0	N/A	N/A	0
N/A	+	N/A	N/A	+	+	+

"painfully"—one way or the other—either through deliberate relative starvation and caloric restriction, exercise training and conditioning, or through surgically induced malabsorption—partitioning fatty acids toward oxidation and consumption rather than storage.

In light of the current obesity epidemic, treatment models are needed that achieve modest weight loss or at least prevent further weight gain. Long-term, regular, moderate-intensity exercise needs to be a part of normal life for everyone, in all age groups, especially for overweight and moderately obese men and women on ad libitum diets. For individuals incapable of incorporating regular physical activity, safe and effective pharmacotherapy for obesity would be of benefit, with surgical intervention truly a last resort, when all other options have failed.

GLOSSARY

ACC	acetyl CoA carboxylase
AMPK	adenosine 5′-monophosphate–activated protein kinase
BMI	body mass index
CHD	coronary heart disease
CoA	coenzyme A
CRP	C-reactive protein
DM	diabetes mellitus
GLUT	glucose transporter
HDL	high-density lipoprotein
HOMA	homeostasis model assessment
ICAM-1	intercellular adhesion molecule-1
IL	interleukin
LDL	low-density lipoprotein
LPL	lipoprotein lipase
PAI-1	plasminogen activator inhibitor-1
PPAR	peroxisome proliferator–activated receptor
PYY	peptide YY3-36
SREBP	sterol regulatory element binding protein
TNF-α	tumor necrosis factor-α
VCAM-1	vascular adhesion molecule-1

REFERENCES

1. Marx J. Cellular warriors at the Battle of the Bulge. Science 2003;299:846-849
2. Parker-Pope T. The cheese and yoghurt diet: assessing the dairy industry's weight-loss claim. Wall St J 2004; June 8:D1
3. Slentz CA, Duscha A, Johnson JL, et al. Effects of the amount of exercise on body weight, body composition, and measures of central obesity. Arch Intern Med 2004; 164:31-39
4. Poirier P, Despres JP. Exercise in weight management of obesity. Cardiol Clin 2001;19:459-470
5. Kopp HP, Kopp CW, Festa A, et al. Impact of weight loss on inflammatory proteins and their association with the insulin resistance syndrome. Arterioscler Thromb Vasc Biol 2003;23:1042-1047
6. Pi-Sunyer X. A clinical view of the obesity problem. Science 2003;299:859-860
7. Pereira MA, Swain J, Goldfine AB, et al. Effects of a low-glycemic load diet on resting energy expenditure and heart disease risk factors during weight loss. JAMA 2004;292:2482-2490
8. Friedman JM. A war on obesity, not the obese. Science 2003;299:856-858
9. Chiba T, Yamaza H, Higami Y, Shimokawa I. Anti-aging effects of caloric restriction: involvement of neuroendocrine adaptation by peripheral signaling. Microsc Res Tech 2002;59:317-324
10. Nicklas BJ, Rogus EM, Berman DM, et al. Responses of adipose tissue lipoprotein lipase to weight loss affect lipid levels and weight regain in women. Am J Physiol Endocrinol Metab 2000;279:E1012-E1019
11. Berman DM, Nicklas BJ, Ryan AS, et al. Regulation of lipolysis and lipoprotein lipase after weight loss in obese, postmenopausal women. Obes Res 2004;12:32-39
12. Gonzalez AA, Kumar R, Mulligan JD, et al. Metabolic adaptations to fasting and chronic caloric restriction in heart, muscle, and liver do not include changes in AMPK activity. Am J Physiol Endocrinol Metab 2004;287: E1032-E1037
13. Zhu M, Miura J, Lu LX, et al. Circulating adiponectin levels increase in rats on caloric restriction: the potential for insulin sensitization. Exp Gerontol 2004;39:1049-1059
14. Li J, Yu X, Pan W, Unger RH. Gene expression profile of rat adipose tissue at the onset of high-fat-diet obesity. Am J Physiol Metab 2002;282:E1334-E1341
15. Hsueh WA, Law R. The central role of fat and effect of peroxisome proliferator–activated receptor-gamma on progression of insulin resistance and cardiovascular disease. Am J Cardiol 2003;92(suppl):3J-9J
16. Ross R, Dagnone D, Jones PJ, et al. Reduction in obesity and related comorbid conditions after diet-induced weight loss or exercise-induced weight loss in men. A randomized, controlled trial. Ann Intern Med 2000;133:92-103
17. Greco AV, Mingrone G, Giancaterini A, et al. Insulin resistance in morbid obesity: reversal with intramyocellular fat depletion. Diabetes 2002;51:144-151
18. Ziccardi P, Nappo F, Giugliano G, et al. Reduction of inflammatory cytokine concentrations and improvement of endothelial functions in obese women after weight loss over one year. Circulation 2002;105:804-809
19. Calles-Escandon J, Ballor D, Harvey-Berino J, et al. Amelioration of the inhibition of fibrinolysis in elderly,

obese subjects by moderate energy intake restriction. Am J Clin Nutr 1996;64:7-11
20. Tchernof A, Nolan A, Sites CK, et al. Weight loss reduces C-reactive protein levels in obese postmenopausal women. Circulation 2002;105:564-569
21. Esposito K, Pontillo A, Ciotola M, et al. Weight loss reduces interleukin-18 levels in obese women. J Clin Endocrinol Metab 2002;87:3864-3866
22. Martini G, Riva P, Rabbia F, et al. Heart rate variability in childhood obesity. Clin Auton Res 2001;11:87-91
23. Rissanen P, Franssila-Kallunki A, Rissanen A. Cardiac parasympathetic activity is increased by weight loss in healthy obese women. Obes Res 2001;9:637-643
24. Laaksonen DE, Laitinen T, Schonberg J, et al. Weight loss and weight maintenance, ambulatory blood pressure and cardiac autonomic tone in obese persons with the metabolic syndrome. J Hypertens 2003;21:371-378
25. Nicoletti G, Giugliano G, Pontillo A, et al. Effect of a multidisciplinary program of weight reduction on endothelial functions in obese women. J Endocrinol Invest 2003;26:RC5-RC8
26. Schneider BS, Faust IM, Hemmes R, Hirsch J. Effects of altered adipose tissue morphology on plasma insulin levels in the rat. Am J Physiol 1981;240:E358-E362
27. Weyer C, Wolford JK, Hanson RL, et al. Subcutaneous abdominal adipocyte size, a predictor of type 2 diabetes, is linked to chromosome 1q21-q23 and is associated with a common polymorphism in LMNA in Pima Indians. Mol Genet Metab 2001;72:231-238
28. Weyer C, Foley JE, Bogardus C, et al. Enlarged subcutaneous abdominal adipocyte size, but not obesity itself, predicts type II diabetes independent of insulin resistance. Diabetologia 2000;43:1498-1506
29. Stern JS, Batchelor BR, Hollander N, et al. Adipose-cell size and immunoreactive insulin levels in obese and normal-weight adults. Lancet 1972;2:948-951
30. Jimenez J, Zuniga-Guajardo S, Zinman B, Angel A. Effects of weight loss in massive obesity on insulin and C-peptide dynamics: sequential changes in insulin production, clearance, and sensitivity. J Clin Endocrinol Metab 1987;64:661-668
31. Kral JG, Bjorntorp P, Schersten T, Sjostrom L. Body composition and adipose tissue cellularity before and after jejuno-ileostomy in severely obese subjects. Eur J Clin Invest 1977;7:413-419
32. Owen K, Haas T, Svacina S, Matoulek M. Weight reduction and aspects of the metabolic syndrome. Sb Lek 2001;102:385-393
33. Van Gaal LF, Wauters MA, De Leeuw IH. The beneficial effects of modest weight loss on cardiovascular risk factors. Int J Obes 1997;21(suppl 1):S5-S9
34. Himeno E, Nishino K, Nakashima Y, et al. Weight reduction regresses left ventricular mass regardless of blood pressure level in obese subjects. Am Heart J 1996;131: 313-319
35. Diabetes Prevention Program Research Group. Reduction of the incidence of type 2 diabetes with lifestyle intervention or metformin. N Engl J Med 2002;346:393-403
36. Tuomilehto J, Lindstrom J, Eriksson JG, et al. Prevention of type 2 diabetes mellitus by changes in lifestyle among subjects with impaired glucose tolerance. N Engl J Med 2001;344:1343-1350
37. Verreth W, Keyzer D, Pelat M, et al. Weight loss-associated induction of peroxisome proliferator–activated receptor-α and peroxisome proliferator–activated receptor-γ correlate with reduced atherosclerosis and improved cardiovascular function in obese insulin-resistant mice. Circulation 2004;110:3259-3269
38. Bruun JM, Verdich C, Toubro S, et al. Association between measures of insulin sensitivity and circulating levels of interleukin-8, interleukin-6 and tumor necrosis factor-alpha. Effect of weight loss in obese men. Eur J Endocrinol 2003;148:535-542
39. Dandona P, Weinstock R, Thusu K, et al. Tumor necrosis factor-alpha in sera of obese patients: fall with weight loss. J Clin Endocrinol Metab 1998;83:2907-2910
40. Ryan AS, Nicklas BJ. Reductions in plasma cytokine levels with weight loss improve insulin sensitivity in overweight and obese postmenopausal women. Diabetes Care 2004;27:1699-1705
41. Havel PJ, Kasim-Karakas S, Mueller W, et al. Relationship of plasma leptin to plasma insulin and adiposity in normal weight and overweight women: effects of dietary fat content and sustained weight loss. J Clin Endocrinol Metab 1996;81:4406-4413
42. Ryan AS, Pratley RE, Elahi D, Goldberg AP. Changes in plasma leptin and insulin action with resistive training in postmenopausal women. Int J Obes Relat Metab Disord 2000;24:27-32
43. Stumvoll M, Haering H-U. Glitazones: clinical effects and molecular mechanisms. Ann Med 2002;34:217-224
44. Buchwald H, Avidor Y, Braunwald E, et al. Bariatric surgery. A systematic review and meta-analysis. JAMA 2004;292:1724-1737
45. Esposito K, Pontillo A, Di Palo C, et al. Effect of weight loss and lifestyle changes on vascular inflammatory markers in obese women: a randomized trial. JAMA 2003;289:1799-1804
46. Imbeault P, Almeras N, Richard D, et al. Effect of a moderate weight loss on adipose tissue lipoprotein lipase activity and expression: existence of sexual variation and regional differences. Int J Obes Relat Metab Disord 1999;23:957-965
47. Mehra MR, Uber PA, Park MH, et al. Obesity and suppressed B-type natriuretic peptide levels in heart failure. J Am Coll Cardiol 2004;43:1590-1595
48. Williamson DF, Pamuk E, Thun M, et al. Prospective study of intentional weight loss and mortality in never-smoking overweight white US women aged 40-64 years. Am J Epidemiol 1995;141:1128-1141
49. Parker-Pope T. How to find out exactly what you can eat and still lose weight. Wall St J 2003;September 16:D1
50. Klein S, Wadden T, Sugerman HJ. AGA technical review on obesity. Gastroenterology 2002;123:882-932
51. Freedman MR, King J, Kennedy E. Popular diets: a scientific review. Obes Res 2001;9(suppl 1):1S-40S
52. Bowerman S. The role of meal replacements in weight control. In Bessenen DH, Kushner R (eds): Evaluation and Management of Obesity. Philadelphia, Hanley & Belfus, 2002, pp 53-58
53. Steinbrook R. Surgery for severe obesity. N Engl J Med 2004;350:1075-1079
54. Klein S, Fontana L, Young VL, et al. Absence of an effect of liposuction on insulin action and risk factors for coronary heart disease. N Engl J Med 2004;350: 2549-2557
55. Giugliano G, Nicoletti G, Grella E, et al. Effect of liposuction on insulin resistance and vascular inflammatory markers in obese women. Br J Plast Surg 2004;57: 190-194
56. Shikora SA. Implantable gastric stimulation for the treatment of severe obesity. Obes Surg 2004;14:545-548
57. Shikora SA. "What are the yanks doing?" the U.S. experience with implantable gastric stimulation (IGS) for the treatment of obesity—update on the ongoing clinical trials. Obes Surg 2004;14(Suppl 1):S40-S48

58. De Luca M, Segato G, Busetto L, et al. Progress in implantable gastric stimulation: summary of results of the European multi-center study. Obes Surg 2004; 14(Suppl 1):S33-S39
59. Cigaina V. Long-term follow-up of gastric stimulation for obesity: the Mestre 8-year experience. Obes Surg 2004;14(Suppl 1):S14-S22
60. National Institutes of Health Consensus Development Panel. Gastrointestinal surgery for severe obesity. Ann Intern Med 1991;115:956-961
61. Stone NJ, Kushner R. Effects of dietary modification to reduce vascular risks and treatment of obesity. Cardiol Clin 2003;21:415-433
62. Sjöström L, Lindroos A-K, Peltonen M, et al, for the Swedish Obese Subjects Study Scientific Group. Lifestyle, diabetes, and cardiovascular risk factors 10 years after bariatric surgery. N Engl J Med 2004;351:2683-2693
63. MacNeil JS. Gastric bypass surgery can erase the metabolic syndrome. Cardiol News April 2004:11
64. Sjostrom CD, Lissner L, Wedel H, Sjostrom L. Reduction in incidence of diabetes, hypertension, and lipid disturbances after intentional weight loss induced by bariatric surgery: the SOS Intervention Study. Obes Res 1999;7: 477-484
65. Christou NV, Sampalis JS, Lieberman M, et al. Surgery decreases long-term mortality, morbidity, and health care use in morbidly obese patients. Ann Surg 2004;240: 416-423
66. Batterham RL, Cohen MA, Ellis SM, et al. Inhibition of food intake in obese subjects by peptide YY3-36. N Engl J Med 2003;349:941-948
67. National Heart, Lung, and Blood Institute and North American Association for the Study of Obesity: The Practical Guide: Identification, Evaluation, and Treatment of Overweight and Obesity in Adults. October 2000. www.nhlbi.nih.gov/guidelines/obesity/practgde.htm
68. Schrauwen P, van Marken Lichtenbelt WD, Saris WH, Westerterp KR. The adaptation of nutrient oxidation to nutrient intake on a high-fat diet. Z Ernahrungswiss 1997;36:306-309
69. Schrauwen P, Lichtenbelt WD, Saris WH, Westerterp KR. Fat balance in obese subjects: role of glycogen stores. Am J Physiol 1998;274:E1027-E1033
70. Nicklas BJ, Rogus EM, Goldberg AP. Exercise blunts declines in lipolysis and fat oxidation after dietary-induced weight loss in obese older women. Am J Physiol 1997;36:E149-E155
71. Okura T, NakataY, Tanaka K. Effects of exercise intensity on physical fitness and risk factors for coronary heart disease. Obes Res 2003;11:1131-1139
72. Watkins LL, Sherwood A, Feinglos M, et al. Effects of exercise and weight loss on cardiac risk factors associated with syndrome X. Arch Intern Med 2003;163: 1889-1895
73. Stevens J, Cai J, Evenson KR, Thomas R. Fitness and fatness as predictors of mortality from all causes and from cardiovascular disease in men and women in the lipid research clinics study. Am J Epidemiol 2002;156: 832-841
74. Lee CD, Blair SN, Jackson AS. Cardiorespiratory fitness, body composition, and all-cause and cardiovascular disease mortality in men. Am J Clin Nutr 1999;69:373-380

Diet and Supplements 15

There are significant interactions among gene expression, diet, and risk for disease. Depending on genetic makeup, a certain dietary approach may be hazardous to one's health or neutral. Thus, whereas type 2 diabetes mellitus (DM) is rampant among the Pima Indians of Arizona exposed to a modern American lifestyle and diet, there is no significant increase in the incidence of DM among the Mexican Pima Indians, who pursue a more active lifestyle on a traditional diet. Conversely, although the inhabitants of Singapore share a similar diet, lifestyle, and prosperity, the incidence of coronary heart disease (CHD) varies among residents of Chinese, Indian, and Malaysian descent.[1]

Strictly controlled dietary interventions in animal models have moved the focus from macronutrient proportions to an understanding of the unique effects of individual subtypes of fats, carbohydrates, and proteins on insulin action.[2] **Informed lifestyle approaches involving changes in diet and physical activity are essential and attractive tools for the prevention and management of insulin resistance because of their low cost, minimal risk, and patient empowerment.**

BACKGROUND

Over the past several decades, a number of developments in the food industry have encouraged weight gain in the United States.

High-Fructose Corn Syrup. In the 1970s, surpluses in agricultural corn production led to the development of high-fructose corn syrup. High-fructose corn syrup is made by converting cornstarch into a liquid. Exposure of this liquid to enzymatic processing generates highly concentrated fructose as an inexpensive sweetener that can be more cheaply produced than refined cane sugar. High-fructose corn syrup has been quickly adopted as a sweetener by the food and beverage industry. It is used in a wide array of prepared foods ranging from baby meals, salad dressings, and juices to soft drinks, ice cream, and energy bars.[3]

In contrast to the fructose found in fruit, as the name implies, high-fructose corn syrup contains high concentrations of fructose not naturally encountered. Fructose appears to be absorbed and processed differently from other sugars and may be readily converted to triglycerides by the liver.[3]

Highly Saturated Oils. The food industry also readily adopted cheap imports of the highly saturated palm and palm kernel oil. Like fructose, palm oil and palm kernel oil have been implicated in engendering insulin resistance. Their *trans*–fatty acid derivatives pose significant CHD risks.[3]

Food Portion Size. With the greater ease and affordability of convenience and snack food manufacture came a proliferation of inexpensive, high-calorie products and giant serving sizes. Furthermore, there has been an increasing accommodation of large body size by the industry. For example, the size of clothes has inflated—what is now a size 8 may have been a size 10 or 12, and "medium" may have been "large" in the past; such mislabeling affords the wearer the illusion of continued shapeliness. There are now easy- or baggy-fit clothes, elastic waistlines, an expansion of available XXX-large clothing sizes, and more accommodating scales, furniture, and coffins, all compounded by a convenient lifestyle that minimizes physical exertion and deemphasizes the need for rigorous physical exercise.

THE TRADITIONAL FOOD PYRAMID

The classic diet-heart hypothesis postulates that dietary saturated fat and cholesterol are causally related to obesity and CHD. Correspondingly, nutritional recommendations from the government and the medical profession have advised the avoidance of saturated fats and have recommended the food pyramid as a dietary guide.

The traditional food pyramid diet encourages the liberal consumption of carbohydrates, such as rice, bread, cereals, and pasta (Fig. 15-1). Fresh fruits and vegetables are recommended next, followed by meat and dairy products, and most sparingly, fats and oils.[4-6] Common, preventive medicine practice restricts dietary fat to less than 30% of the total energy intake.

The data to support such intervention are lacking. Simply lowering the percentage of energy from total fat in the diet is unlikely to improve lipid profiles or reduce the incidence

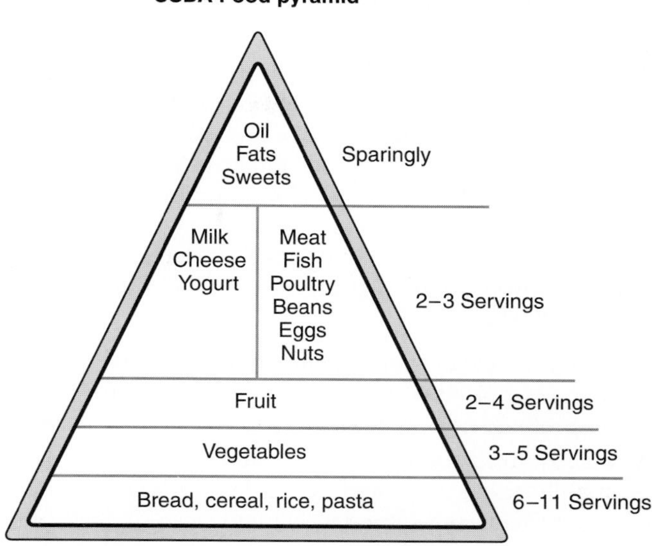

Figure 15–1. Daily servings of food groups as recommended by the traditional U.S. Department of Agriculture food pyramid. *(Modified from http://www.pueblo.gsa.gov/cic_text/food/food-pyramid/main.htm.)*

of CHD. In fact, high carbohydrate intake may raise triglyceride levels, thus lowering protective high-density lipoprotein (HDL) levels.

Another problem that appears to have arisen with this approach is that no distinction is made between refined and unprocessed carbohydrates. In contrast to unrefined carbohydrates, refined carbohydrates, as are widely used in the manufacture of white bread, white rice, and pasta, are quickly digested. In the process, they rapidly release glucose into the circulation, which stimulates a surge of insulin release to absorb and store the calories. High insulin levels derived from a high-carbohydrate diet may also impede fatty acid oxidation, instead enhancing fat storage. After the uptake of glucose, the ensuing relative decline in plasma glucose has been thought to trigger recurrent hunger, thereby encouraging snack food intake and contributing to ponderosity as a result of overeating. Of greater concern, diets high in simple sugars, in particular fructose, lead to insulin resistance.[2]

Revision of the Traditional Food Pyramid. In 2004, the U.S. Dietary Guidelines Advisory Committee submitted new dietary guidelines to the Departments of Agriculture and Health and Human Services. An overhauling of the 1992 graphic food pyramid is in the process to reflect the new recommendations in which fewer servings of grain, but more of fruits and vegetables, dairy products, and fish are encouraged.[7]

Food Consumption Guidelines for a 2200-Calorie Diet: Number of Daily Servings

FOOD GROUP	SERVING SIZE	2000	2004
Fruits	½ Cup	3	4
Vegetables	½ Cup	4	6
Grains	Slice of bread	9	7 (whole grain, 3)
Meat and beans	Ounces	6	6
Milk	Cup	2-3	3
Oils	Gram	NA	27
Discretionary daily calories		NA	235

NA, not available.
Adapted from Zamiska N. New diet guide: fewer grains, more veggies. Wall St J 2004;August 30:B1

Weekly Variety of Vegetables on a 2200-Calorie Diet

CUPS PER WEEK	FOOD COLOR, TYPE, AND EXAMPLE
3	Dark green: broccoli, spinach
2	Orange: carrot, squash
3	Legumes: lentil, kidney bean, tofu
6	Starchy: potato, corn, green pea
7	Other: tomato, lettuce, onion

Adapted from Zamiska N. New diet guide: fewer grains, more veggies. Wall St J 2004;August 30:B1

ALTERNATIVE DIETARY APPROACHES

Many dietary approaches have sought the avoidance of ponderosity and CHD. Effective dietary means to lower the magnitude of diurnal insulin secretion focus on the increased intake of soluble fiber and chromium as occurs in low-carbohydrate or low–glycemic index diets.

Specifically, strategies that may be associated with improved weight management and a lower risk for CHD are

- high intake of fruit, vegetables, nuts, whole grains, and fiber while curtailing the intake of refined carbohydrates;
- substitution of monounsaturated and especially polyunsaturated fatty acids for *trans*–fatty acids and saturated fat; and
- increases in ω-3 fatty acids from fish oil or plant sources.

Numerous dietary venues pursue these aims.

The Dietary Approaches to Stop Hypertension Diet. The Dietary Approaches to Stop Hypertension (DASH) diet is primarily designed to lower blood pressure. The diet focuses on

- high intake of fruit, vegetables, and nuts (nine servings per day),
- low-fat dairy products, and
- reduced-fat foods.

This diet is lower in total fat, saturated fat, and cholesterol. It is replete with nutrients associated with improved insulin sensitivity, including magnesium, calcium, and protein. It has higher levels of potassium and fiber than the typical American diet does. The nutrient content of the DASH diet appears to be instrumental in reducing blood pressure. **Besides lowering blood pressure, the DASH diet also appears to reduce plasma lipids, the incidence of gout, and insulin resistance.**[8-10]

The Mediterranean Diet. The traditional Mediterranean diet has been championed for the prevention of CHD. The traditional dietary patterns of Crete, Greece, and southern Italy have been considered to be responsible for the longevity and cardiovascular health of local populations despite their high intake of fat.[11] Although at least 16 countries border the Mediterranean with varying cultures and traditions and diverse dietary habits, the traditional diets have been characterized by a number of common features:

- high fiber;
- abundant fruits and vegetables;
- whole-grain plant foods such as cereals, nuts, and legumes;
- olive oil as the principal fat source;
- low to moderate amounts of fish and poultry;
- low quantity of red meat; and
- moderate wine use with meals (Fig. 15-2).[12]

Permutations of a Mediterranean Diet. A variety of dietary permutations, such as the Indo-Mediterranean diet, which includes the use of mustard and soybean oil, can be as effective as the Mediterranean diet. In effect, imitation Mediterranean diets should derive the major food groups from the following sources:

- protein—nuts, soybeans, legumes, poultry, fish;
- fat—monounsaturated and ω-3 fatty acids: nuts, fish, flax, purslane, olive, and rapeseed;

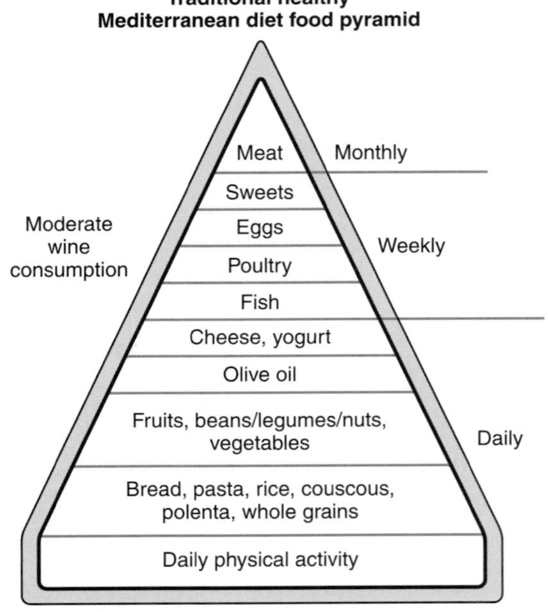

›› **Figure 15–2.**
Daily servings of food groups in a traditional Mediterranean diet food pyramid. *(Modified from Hu FB. The Mediterranean diet and mortality—olive oil and beyond. N Engl J Med 2003;348:2595-2596.)*

saturated and *trans*–fatty acids should be eliminated; and
- carbohydrates—low glycemic loads with abundant soluble fiber: whole unrefined grains, fruits, and vegetables, including leafy greens, with small amounts of alcohol (<5 g/day).[12]

Inflammatory Markers and the Metabolic Syndrome. Adherence to the traditional Mediterranean diet is associated with a reduction in the concentration of markers of inflammation and coagulation. It improves endothelial function and lowers insulin resistance.

From 2001 to 2002, 3042 individuals from Greece, 18 to 87 years old, were evaluated regarding their adherence to the Mediterranean diet. Individuals in the highest tertile of dietary observance had 20% lower C-reactive protein (CRP) levels ($P = .015$), 17% lower interleukin-6 (IL-6) levels ($P = .025$), 15% lower homocysteine levels ($P = .031$), 14% lower white blood cell counts ($P = .001$), and 6% lower fibrinogen levels ($P = .025$) than did those in the lowest tertile.[13] Similar findings were obtained in a 2-year prospective, controlled study of the Mediterranean diet in 180 individuals with the metabolic syndrome, as defined by the Adult Treatment Panel (ATP) III. Subjects on the diet had significantly lower levels of CRP ($P = .01$) and IL-6 ($P = .04$), with a lower measure of insulin resistance ($P < .001$) and improvement in endothelial function ($P < .001$). More than half the patients in the dietary intervention group had no further features of the metabolic syndrome in follow-up, in contrast to the "prudent diet" control group, where the majority had persistent features of the metabolic syndrome ($P < .001$).[14]

Cardiovascular Events and Mortality. Regular consumption of a Mediterranean diet lowers cardiovascular events and mortality.

A 44-month prospective study of 22,043 healthy Greek adults found that a higher degree of adherence to the traditional Mediterranean diet was associated with a significant reduction in total mortality and mortality from cardiovascular disease and cancer (Fig. 15-3).[15] The Lyon Diet Heart Study of 605 patients after myocardial infarction (MI) compared an American Heart Association (AHA) Step I diet with a Mediterranean diet. There was a 73% reduction in the combined end points of cardiac death and nonfatal MI and a 70% reduction in cardiac mortality in the Mediterranean diet group.[16] A trial of an Indo-Mediterranean diet in 1000 CHD patients in India similarly resulted in a significant decrease in all cardiac end points, sudden cardiac death, and nonfatal MI relative to Step I diet subjects.[17]

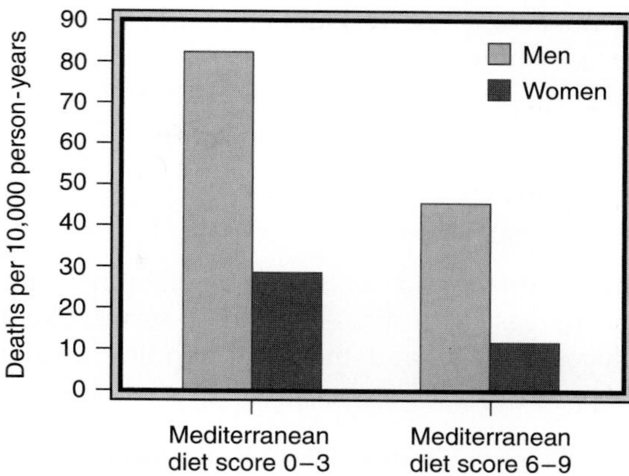

Figure 15–3.
Impact of low (score of 0 to 3) versus high (score of 6 to 9) adherence to a traditional Mediterranean diet on overall mortality for men and women. *(Modified from Trichopoulou A, Costacou T, Bamia C, Trichopoulos D. Adherence to a Mediterranean diet and survival in a Greek population. N Engl J Med 2003;348:2599-2608.)*

Mediterranean Diet in Conjunction with Other Measures. The Mediterranean diet is a useful adjunct to other lifestyle or pharmacologic interventions.

In conjunction with regular, modest physical activity in individuals aged 70 to 90 years, the Mediterranean diet was associated with a more than 50% lower rate of all-cause and cause-specific mortality.[18] The combination of dietary intervention with the Mediterranean diet and statin treatment (fluvastatin, 40 mg/day) for 12 months in 131 consecutive patients with documented CHD and a mean serum cholesterol level of 193 mg/dL improved endothelial function, as reflected by flow-mediated dilation in the brachial artery, to a greater degree than did statin treatment alone. This dietary intervention was also associated with a significantly greater decline in triglyceride levels.[19]

Low–Glycemic Index Diet. Carbohydrates are structurally diverse. The different chemical compositions and physical structures of dietary carbohydrates, such as

- sugars,
- oligosaccharides,
- starches, and
- nonstarch polysaccharides,

are digested and absorbed at different rates by the gastrointestinal tract. As a result, blood glucose levels—and the corresponding insulin responses—differ for diverse carbohydrates.

The Glycemic Index. The varied blood sugar responses to the ingestion of diverse carbohydrates have been standardized as the glycemic index. Specifically, the glycemic index compares the plasma glucose response to the ingestion of 50-g portions of carbohydrates to be tested with the normal glucose response elicited by a 50-g oral glucose standard.[20]

Another scale related to the glycemic index is the glycemic load, which is potentially more pertinent. The glycemic load (glycemic index × carbohydrate amount) measures the increase in plasma glucose engendered by a typical serving size of a particular food item.[21] Ratings for different foods can be found on websites such as www.glycemicindex.com.

High–Glycemic Index Intake and Plasma Lipids. Higher dietary glycemic loads exert adverse effects on blood lipids and are associated with an increased risk for CHD.

When matched for carbohydrate content, consumption of higher–glycemic index foods induce larger elevations in fasting triglyceride levels with greater suppression of HDL levels than do low–glycemic index foods.[12,22]

The fructose-fed rat, maintained exclusively on a high-glycemic diet, is a well-established animal model of hypertriglyceridemia. After only 2 weeks of fructose feeding, these rats have reduced expression of peroxisome proliferator–activated receptor-alpha (PPAR-α). Hepatic lipogenesis is induced, and fatty acid oxidative consumption is diminished, suggestive of the early phases of the metabolic syndrome.[20]

The adverse metabolic impact of an elevated dietary glycemic load is most pronounced in overweight individuals. In the Nurses' cohort study, women with a body mass index (BMI) greater than 25 kg/m^2, whose dietary consumption fell into the highest glycemic load quintile, had higher mean triglyceride levels than did women following the same diet with a BMI of 25 kg/m^2 or less.[23]

Chromium. Chromium plays a role in modulating the sensitivity to insulin signaling. Specifically, insulin receptor kinase activity is enhanced by chromium. Ample postprandial hyperglycemic responses increase the renal excretion of chromium. Chronic chromium loss as a result of the persistent consumption of high–glycemic index meals may have an adverse impact on insulin receptor sensitivity.[20]

Metabolic Effects of a Low–Glycemic Index Diet. Low–glycemic index diets rich in slowly digested/resistant carbohydrates may have long-term beneficial effects on lipid metabolism. Low-glycemic foods may reduce insulin resistance and improve the metabolic syndrome.[24]

Consumption of a high-fiber/low-glycemic diet containing dairy products and a higher amount of unsaturated fats than currently recommended may be instrumental in the prevention of DM and cardiovascular complications.[2,25]

Low–glycemic index diets result in

- lower levels of postprandial free fatty acids,
- reduced synthesis of very-low-density lipoprotein (VLDL),
- reduced numbers of small, dense low-density lipoprotein (LDL), and
- increased HDL concentrations.[20]

In healthy, overweight men, a 5-week low– versus high–glycemic index diet

- lowered postprandial glucose and insulin curves;
- lowered postprandial triglyceride levels;
- decreased total-body adipose tissue by 700 g without a change in body weight;
- decreased RNA levels for leptin, lipoprotein lipase, and hormone-sensitive lipase in subcutaneous abdominal adipose tissue; and
- increased total lean body mass.[26]

Weight loss on a low–glycemic load diet favorably affects the physiologic adaptations to weight loss and may be of benefit in weight loss maintenance. In a parallel-design, restricted-energy weight loss study, 39 overweight and obese individuals 18 to 40 years old were randomized to either a low–glycemic load versus a low-fat diet and monitored until 10% of body weight was lost. After achievement of the weight loss goal, subjects in the low-glycemic group differed significantly from those in the low-fat group in that they had a smaller decline in resting energy expenditure by 80 kcal/day, reported less hunger, had less insulin resistance, and had lower serum triglyceride and CRP levels and blood pressure measures despite similar body compositions.[27]

Vegetarian Diet. Vegetarian diets may improve lipid profiles. If such diets incorporate elements known to be lipid lowering, a vegetarian approach may mimic low doses of statin therapy in efficacy. Examples of foods that may potentially contribute to lipid lowering are

- soy protein foods,
- high-fiber oat and barley products,
- almonds and other tree nuts,
- olive oil,
- shiitake mushrooms,
- garlic,
- chili peppers,
- plant sterols, and
- green tea.

Such are the findings of a small study comparing a low-fat, vegetarian diet (8% drop in LDL) with the same diet plus lovastatin (31% reduction in LDL) versus a vegetarian diet rich in lipid-lowering food groups (29% reduction in LDL).[28] In a comparison between Chinese vegetarians and omnivores, vegetarians were more insulin sensitive than their omnivore counterparts. The degree of insulin sensitivity appeared to be correlated with years on a vegetarian diet.[29]

High–Dietary Fiber Diet. Water-insoluble dietary fiber accelerates intestinal transit and may be of benefit because potential carcinogens are more rapidly excreted.

A diet rich in water-soluble fiber may have beneficial effects on lipid and glucose homeostasis and cardiovascular health. Viscous, soluble fiber derives from

- cereal grains,
- fruit,
- vegetables,
- dried beans,
- peas,
- legumes,
- guar gum,
- mucilage, and
- psyllium.[30]

A potential mechanism for the observed metabolic benefit of soluble fiber revolves around the delayed absorption of glucose, fat, and cholesterol from the intestines. Soluble fiber forms a gel-like material in the gastrointestinal tract with absorptive properties for micronutrients, and greater fiber viscosity achieves a greater effect. The alterations in intestinal handling of nutrients may have an impact on the secretion of incretins. A lower insulin response partitions less fat toward storage, and excessive food intake is avoided. Over time, there is a resultant increase in insulin sensitivity at the cellular level with significantly higher plasma membrane glucose transporter 4 (GLUT4) content in skeletal muscle and a rise in hepatic insulin extraction. Binding of bile acids is also enhanced by soluble fiber. Altered bile acid metabolism in the gastrointestinal tract contributes to lowering of cholesterol synthesis.[30]

Inflammation. A higher intake of dietary fiber modulates systemic inflammation and lowers levels of proinflammatory cytokines.

In a study of 4900 adults in the 1999 to 2000 National Health and Nutrition Examination Survey (NHANES 99-00), after controlling for demographic factors, BMI, smoking, alcohol consumption, exercise, and total caloric intake, subjects in the third and fourth highest quartiles of fiber consumption had a lower risk for elevated CRP (odds ratio, 0.64 and 0.58, respectively) than did the lowest quartile.[31]

Cardiovascular Disease. Higher intake of dietary water-soluble fiber is linked to a lower incidence of cardiovascular disease.

A 10-g daily increment in fiber intake corresponds to a 19% reduction in the risk for CHD.[32] In the NHANES I Epidemiologic Follow-up Study, 9776 adults free of cardiovascular disease at baseline were monitored for an average of 19 years. When compared with the lowest quartile of dietary fiber intake (median, 5.9 g/day), participants in the highest quartile (median, 20.7 g/day) had an adjusted relative risk of 0.88 for CHD events and 0.89 for cardiovascular events.[33]

Metabolic Impact. High dietary fiber has a beneficial impact on carbohydrate and lipid metabolism. The inclusion of sufficient dietary fiber, such as psyllium, in a meal (20 to 35 g/day) flattens the postprandial glycemic and insulinemic excursions and favorably influences plasma lipid levels in type 2 DM patients.[30]

Low-Carbohydrate Diets. Low carbohydrate intake entails a diet rich in protein or fat content, or in both. High–glycemic index carbohydrate diets elicit hormonal changes that limit the availability of nutrients to be used as fuel in the postprandial period, thereby stimulating hunger and further voluntary food-seeking behavior.[34] The premise of a low-carbohydrate dietary approach rests on suppressing an excessive postprandial insulin response that would impede fatty acid oxidation and favor triacylglycerol storage. There is also the expectation that avoidance of carbohydrates will improve a sense of satiety and mitigate hunger-driven snacking and thus curtail excessive caloric intake. Although protein, when coingested with carbohydrates, as occurs in typical Western diets, markedly potentiates the insulin response, animal dietary protein by itself causes little insulin release.

High-Protein, High-Fat Diets. Low-carbohydrate, high-protein, high-fat diets have become increasing popular.[35,36] The Atkins diet, proposed first in 1973, with follow-up publications in 1992 and 2002, is the best known of these diets.[37]

Impact on Weight Loss and Lipid Profile. Over a period of 6 to 12 months, low-carbohydrate diets appear to effect moderate weight loss with beneficial changes in the lipid profile.

A 1-year study of a low-carbohydrate, high-protein/fat diet, when compared with a standard low-fat/high-carbohydrate diet, was more efficacious in achieving weight loss and caused a larger increase in HDL, a greater decline in triglyceride, and a smaller insulin response to a glucose load (Fig. 15-4).[38] Similar findings, specifically, greater weight loss, greater improvement in insulin sensitivity, and greater triglyceride reduction, were obtained in a 6-month, low-carbohydrate versus low-fat dietary comparison in severely obese individuals (Fig. 15-5).[39] In a randomized controlled trial of an Atkins-style diet, 120 healthy study participants aged 18 to 65 years with a BMI of 30 to 60 kg/m^2 were assigned either to a low-carbohydrate, high-protein or to a low-fat, low-cholesterol, low-calorie diet. At 6 months, dietary compliance was higher in the low-carbohydrate than in the low-fat group (76% versus 57%, respectively; P = .02), with greater weight loss in the low-carbohydrate than the low-fat group (–12.9% versus –6.7%, respectively; $P < .001$), a greater decrease in serum triglyceride levels

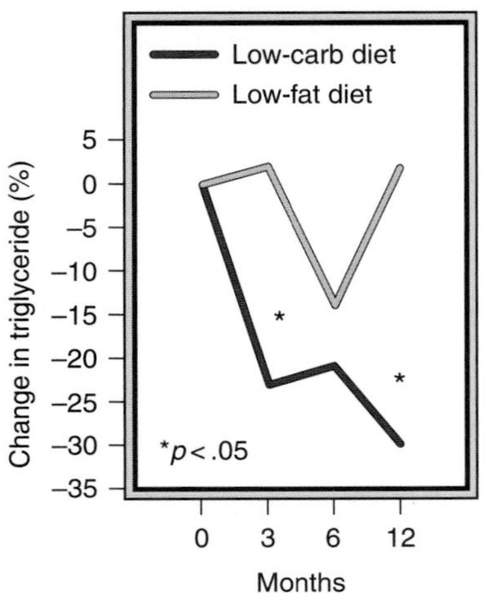

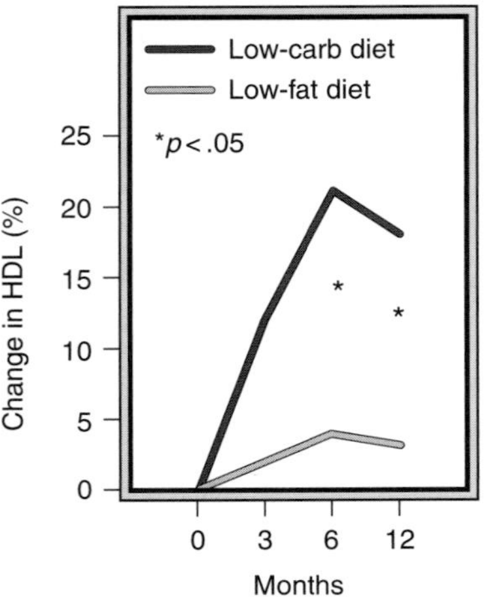

▸▸ **Figure 15–4.** Percent change in plasma levels of triglyceride and high-density lipoprotein (HDL) during a 1-year low-carbohydrate versus low-fat diet. *(Modified from Foster GD, Wyatt HR, Hill JO, et al. A randomized trial of a low-carbohydrate diet for obesity. N Engl J Med 2003;348:2082-2090.)*

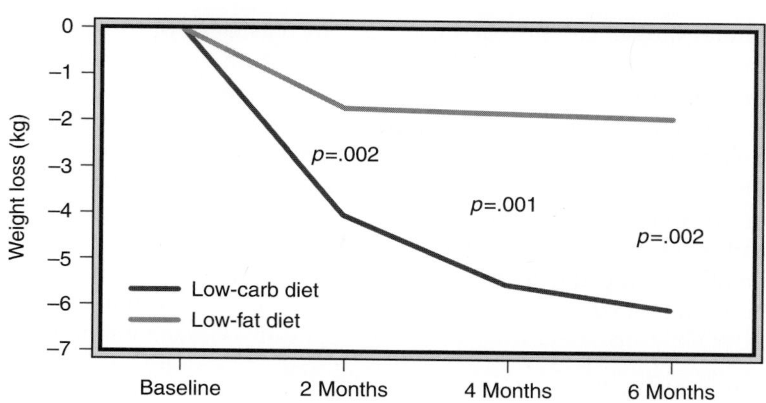

Figure 15–5. Mean weight loss over a 6-month period for subjects maintained on a low-carbohydrate versus low-fat diet. *(Modified from Samaha FF, Iqbal N, Seshadri P, et al. A low-carbohydrate as compared with a low-fat diet in severe obesity. N Engl J Med 2003; 348:2074-2081.)*

(change, −74.2 mg/dL versus −27.9 mg/dL; $P = .004$), and a greater increase in HDL levels (+5.5 mg/dL versus −1.6 mg/dL, $P < .001$).[40] In a 12-month study comparing a low-carbohydrate with a conventional diet for a BMI of 35 kg/m^2 or greater, with 83% of the participants having DM or the metabolic syndrome, the low-carbohydrate diet showed similar weight loss but a better lipid profile (greater decrease in triglyceride levels [$P = .044$] and less decrease in HDL cholesterol levels [$P = .025$]).[41]

Modified Low-Carbohydrate Approaches. The liberal consumption of animal fat and protein has raised concern about the proinflammatory potential of the low-carbohydrate diet as originally proposed. There is also the suspicion that over the long term, unbalanced low-carbohydrate diets may raise the risk of overtaxing renal function because of the high protein loads. There might be a risk for osteoporosis and nephrolithiasis. High-protein diets may be deficient in important nutrients such as vitamins A and E, folate, calcium, iron, potassium, dietary fiber, and other protective constituents of fruits and vegetables. There may ultimately be a higher associated incidence of cardiovascular disease and cancer.

In the Nurses' Health Study, when compared with disease-free controls, the women in whom type 2 DM developed were more likely to consume higher amounts of heme iron, *trans*–fatty acids, and red and processed meats and lower amounts of cereal fiber and magnesium. This group had higher levels of plasma CRP, fasting insulin, hemoglobin, ferritin, and glycated hemoglobin A (HbA_{1C}), the relative risk for DM rising linearly with ferritin levels.[42] In a different analysis of the same study over 14 years of follow-up, the increased intake of red and especially other processed meat was positively associated with the development of type 2 DM.[43]

Modifications of the low-carbohydrate approach emphasize the use of lean meat as a protein source, monounsaturated fat and nuts as a fat source, low–glycemic index starch, and fiber, with unrestricted vegetable consumption. Such diets compare favorably with low-fat dietary approaches. In a recent study of a modified approach to high-fat, low-carbohydrate diets, 60 participants were randomized for 12 weeks to one of two calorie-restricted diets (1300 kcal/day for women, 1600 kcal/day for men): the U.S. National Cholesterol Education Program (NCEP) diet versus a modified low-carbohydrate diet. Diet composition in the final 8 weeks was as follows:

NUTRIENT CATEGORY	NCEP DIET	MODIFIED LOW-CARBOHYDRATE DIET
Fat	30% 10%-15% monounsaturated	39% 13% monounsaturated
Carbohydrate	55%	28%, mainly complex
Protein	15%	33%

Weight loss was significantly higher by 6.1 lb in the modified diet, which alone caused significant reductions in the levels of total cholesterol and triglycerides with an increase in the size of LDL particles.[44]

Protein Subtypes. Although common nutritional advice argues against excessive protein intake, under certain circumstances, increased intake of protein, particularly as derived from plant or fish sources, may lower blood pressure and reduce the risk for cardiovascular disease. Select protein sources may exert their beneficial effects via an increased intake of biologically active amino acids, peptides, or highly correlated nutrients. However, the data are not yet sufficiently compelling to advocate increased consumption of such protein sources.[45]

Soy Protein. Soy protein may have vasculoprotective and lipid-lowering effects.

Soy protein is absorbed more slowly than animal protein. Soy is a major source of the isoflavone class of phytoestrogens, principally daidzein and genistein. These isoflavones act as weak selective estrogen receptor modulators and reversibly bind with greater affinity to the β-isoform than to the α-isoform of the estrogen receptor. β-Isoforms of the estrogen receptor are preferentially expressed in

- the central nervous system,
- the cardiovascular system,
- bone, and
- skin.

The α-isoforms predominate in

- the uterus and
- breast tissue.

Soy stimulates glucagon secretion and may thus actually enhance fat oxidation. Soy isoflavones may improve plasma lipids in normocholesterolemic, postmenopausal women.[46] In a nutritional study comparing the consumption of soy protein (25 to 50 g/day) containing isoflavones with animal protein consumption, significant reductions in levels of total cholesterol, LDL, and triglycerides occurred with soy but not with animal protein, the most profound effects occurring in individuals with the highest baseline lipid values.[47,48] Daily consumption of soy protein has a favorable impact on vascular reactivity and improves endothelial function regardless of any changes in plasma lipoproteins.[48-50] Consumption of 25 g/day of isoflavone-containing soy protein is considered part of a heart-healthy diet, when consumed as a substitute for animal products and highly processed foods.[51] Ethanol-washed soy products should be avoided because of the depletion of isoflavones and other bioactive compounds that occurs in the process.[52]

Flaxseed Meal. Flaxseed meal supplementation has marked cholesterol- and triglyceride-lowering effects and may provide a therapeutic strategy to reduce hypertriglyceridemia and hepatic steatosis.

SHR/N-cp rats, a genetic model of obesity, insulin resistance, and type 2 DM, placed on diets containing 20% of energy from flaxseed meal for 6 months rather than from casein (control) or soy protein concentrate, had significant reductions in total cholesterol (–41%), LDL, and HDL when compared with casein-fed rats. Flaxseed meal feeding in this animal model also significantly lowered plasma triglycerides and decreased fat deposition in the liver when compared with casein feeding.[53]

Fish Protein. Fish protein appears to prevent the development of insulin resistance in skeletal muscle through a direct action of amino acids on insulin-stimulated glucose uptake in skeletal myocytes.[54]

Cod protein is a natural insulin-sensitizing agent that may prevent obesity-linked insulin resistance in skeletal muscle by normalizing insulin activation of the phosphatidylinositol 3-kinase (PI3K)/Akt pathway and by selectively improving GLUT4 translocation to the T tubules. In high-fat–fed rats consuming casein or soy protein for 4 weeks, insulin receptor substrate-1 (IRS-1)-associated PI3K activity and activation of the downstream kinase Akt/protein kinase B (PKB) by insulin were severely impaired. A cod protein diet fully prevented the deleterious effects of fat feeding on insulin signaling, with improved translocation of GLUT4 to the T tubules but not to the plasma membrane.[55] The beneficial effects of cod protein occurred without any reductions in body weight gain, adipose tissue accretion, or expression of tumor necrosis factor-alpha (TNF-α) in fat and muscle.[54]

GENERAL IMPACT OF FATS ON METABOLISM

Fatty acids consumed in the diet have a multiplicity of roles. They are used as

- fuel;
- structural components of cells;

- triglyceride and phospholipid precursors to signaling messengers;
- precursors to the biosynthesis of eicosanoids such as prostaglandins, prostacyclins, thromboxanes, leukotrienes, and lipoxins;
- regulators of immune and inflammatory responses; and
- modulators of gene expression via activation of PPAR and other transcription factors.[56]

Utilization of Fat Calories. Fat is an energy-dense fuel source for cellular metabolism. The efficiency of nutrient utilization is highest for fats, lower for carbohydrates, and lowest for protein. Postprandial fuel selection favors the oxidation of dietary protein and carbohydrates. In contrast, fats are preferentially stored as triglyceride (i.e., triacylglycerol) in adipose tissue. Alcohol further increases dietary fat storage by inhibiting lipid oxidation.[57]

High-fat diets are conducive to overconsumption. Fat-induced feedback control of appetite appears to be weak or too delayed to prevent excessive food intake.[57]

Differential Fat Oxidation Rates and Obesity. The intake of saturated fats is strongly linked to the development of obesity. Saturated fats

- are poorly oxidized for energy,
- are readily stored,
- are ineffectively mobilized by lipolytic stimuli,
- impair membrane function, and
- increase the expression of genes associated with adipocyte proliferation.[2]

Postprandial fat oxidation rates are higher after meals enriched with monounsaturated fatty acids than with saturated fats.

A simple change from saturated to monounsaturated dietary fat may have a beneficial impact on weight control in men with a large waist circumference who are consuming a relatively high-fat diet. In 14 men aged 24 to 49 years with a BMI in the range of 20 to 32 kg/m^2, within the 5 hours after a monounsaturated fatty acid breakfast, there was a significantly greater postprandial fat oxidation rate and lower postprandial carbohydrate oxidation rate than after a saturated fat breakfast. The thermic effect of a monounsaturated fat meal was significantly higher in large-waisted than in narrow-waisted men.[58]

Impact of Fats on Immune Function. Aside from their role as a source of fuel, **fatty acids function as signals that modulate immune and inflammatory responses.** Dietary fatty acids are thus of major import in the newly emerging area of diet–gene expression interactions.

Fatty acids participate in many intracellular signaling pathways. They

- act as ligands for nuclear receptors, such as the PPARs, regulating a host of cell responses,
- influence the stability of plasmalemmal lipid rafts,
- modulate eicosanoid metabolism in the cells of the immune system, and
- modulate T-lymphocyte activation.

Some or all of these mechanisms may be involved in the modulation of immune function by fatty acids.[59]

Dietary Fat and Inflammation. Nutritional fat may have an effect on systemic inflammatory activity and may thus be linked to metabolic and cardiovascular disease. In general, a higher intake of saturated fat is proinflammatory and increases systemic markers of inflammation such as TNF-α.[60]

A high-fat evening meal induces a proinflammatory and hypofibrinolytic state. In individuals with type 2 DM, a fatty meal increases plasma levels of CRP and plasminogen activator inhibitor-1 (PAI-1) activity. Postprandial lipidemia also induces oxidative stress.[61] In the NHANES 99-00 survey, after controlling for demographic and risk factors, the third and fourth quartiles of highest saturated fat consumption were associated with an elevation in plasma CRP.[31]

Fatty Acids as Modulators of Transcription Factors. Depending on the cell-specific context and the target gene, fatty acids can take very different routes to alter transcription.[62]

In rats, a high-fat diet early in life consisting of a 60% fat cafeteria fare led to early modification of the expression of nuclear receptors in the liver and in white adipocytes.[60]

Peroxisome Proliferator–Activated Receptors. PPARs are transcription factors that regulate an extensive network of genes involved in glucose and lipid metabolism and immune regulation. PPARs use fatty acids as endogenous receptor ligands. As PPAR subtypes bind to fatty acids, their conformation shifts to the active configuration to allow coactivator recruitment to the receptor, a requisite event for ligand-mediated gene activation. Fatty acids between 14 and 20 carbons in length can stably bind to PPAR.[63]

Non-PPAR Transcription Factors. PPARs are not the sole transcription factor involved in mediating fatty acid effects on gene transcription. In addition to the PPAR family, **several other transcription factors have been identified as targets for fatty acid regulation,** including

- hepatic nuclear factor-4,
- the sterol regulatory element binding protein-1c (SREBP-1c),
- the liver X receptor (LXR),
- the retinoid X receptor (RXR), and
- nuclear factor kappaB (NFκB).[63]

Dietary Fat and Endothelial Function. High intake of saturated and *trans*–fat adversely affects vascular function. A single, high-fat meal transiently impairs endothelial function for up to 4 hours because of the impact of high free fatty acid levels and postprandial triglyceride-rich lipoproteins. In general, the typical Western diet with three meals per day induces postprandial lipidemia for up to 12 hours daily. Because postprandial hypertriglyceridemia is an independent risk factor for cardiovascular disease, the resultant, prolonged perturbations in endothelial function are probably contributors to the pathogenesis of vascular disease.[61]

Fat Impact on Insulin Resistance. There may be a causal relationship between dietary fat and insulin action, an assumption supported by recent dietary intervention studies. It is, however, the type of fat,

- saturated versus unsaturated versus partially hydrogenated and
- animal versus plant fat,

rather than the total percentage of fat in the diet that better predicts the risk for insulin resistance. **A higher intake of saturated animal fat and *trans*-fat negatively affects glucose metabolism and is strongly linked to the development of insulin resistance.**[2,64]

The composition of fatty acids found circulating in plasma or stored in muscle reflects not only physical activity, genetics, and fetal nutrition, but also ongoing dietary intake. Insulin resistance is associated with a fatty acid pattern in plasma characterized by an increased proportion of palmitic (16:0) and palmitoleic acids (16:1 n-7) and a low proportion of linoleic (18:2 n-6) acids. Increased saturation of sarcolemmal fatty acids is also associated with insulin resistance. Similarly, the composition of phospholipids in skeletal muscle is closely related to the insulin sensitivity of skeletal muscle.[65]

TYPES OF FAT

Lipid Classification. Lipids are classified into simple and complex categories. The simple lipids,

- terpenes,
- steroids, and
- prostaglandins,

contain no molecular backbone or fatty acid components and are not saponifiable. The complex lipids have distinctive backbones:

LIPID	MOLECULAR BACKBONE
Acylglycerols	Glycerol
Phosphoglycerides	Glycerol 3-phosphate
Sphingolipids	Sphingosine
Waxes	High-molecular-weight nonpolar alcohols

They all contain fatty acid components and are consequently saponifiable.[66]

Triglycerides and Dietary Fats. Vegetable cooking oil and animal fat consist mainly of triacylglycerols, or triglycerides. Triglycerides are chemical compounds formed from one molecule of glycerol with three fatty acid molecules.

Glycerol and Fatty Acid Esters. Glycerol combinations with fatty acids form esters termed acylglycerols, or glycerides.

Glycerol is a trihydric alcohol containing three hydroxyl groups (–OH). Activated fatty acids, or fatty acyl coenzyme A (CoA) formed by the action of acyl CoA synthases on fatty acids, acylate the alcohol hydroxyl groups (–OH):

$$\underset{\textit{Fatty acyl CoA}}{-\overset{\overset{\displaystyle O}{\|}}{C}-S-CoA} + \underset{\textit{Glycerol hydroxyl group}}{-CH_2OH} \longrightarrow \underset{\textit{Acyl glycerol}}{-\overset{\overset{\displaystyle O}{\|}}{C}OCH_2-} + \underset{\textit{CoA}}{CoA-SH}$$

Fatty acids may combine with any of the three hydroxyl groups of glycerol to create a wide variety of compounds.

GLYCEROL PLUS	YIELDS -ACYLGLYCEROL OR -GLYCERIDE
One fatty acid	Monoacylglycerol, or monoglyceride
Two fatty acids	Diacylglycerol, or diglyceride
Three fatty acids	Triacylglycerol, or triglyceride

Thus, a typical triglyceride of olive oil consists of two radicals of oleic acid and one of palmitic acid attached to glycerol.[67]

Triglycerides in edible fat are constituted from diverse fatty acids. Even animal fat sources contain unsaturated fatty acids, and animal fat triglycerides rarely incorporate in excess of 70% saturated fatty acids. For example, lard has 54% unsaturated fatty acid radicals (Table 15-1):[67]

Diacylglycerol. Diacylglycerol oils might be of benefit in managing aspects of the metabolic syndrome.

Diacylglycerol is an intermediate product of triacylglycerol hydrolysis and accounts for up to 10% of glycerides in plant-derived, edible fats and oils. Recent developments in oil chemistry have led to the commercial availability of a novel diacylglycerol oil. Oil containing 70% diacylglycerol has metabolic characteristics distinct from those of oils with triacylglycerol of similar fatty acid composition. Specifically, diacylglycerol-enriched

Table 15-1. Percentage of Total Fatty Acid Composition of Edible Fats*

	Saturated					Monopolyunsaturated		
FAT	CAPRIC ACID C10:0	LAURIC ACID C12:0	MYRISTIC ACID C14:0	PALMITIC ACID C16:0	STEARIC ACID C18:0	OLEIC ACID C18:1	LINOLEIC ACID C18:2	α-LINOLENIC ACID C18:3
Beef tallow	—	—	3	24	19	43	3	1
Butterfat (cow)	3	3	11	27	12	29	2	1
Butterfat (human)	2	5	8	25	8	35	9	1
Canola oil	—	—	—	4	2	62	22	10
Cocoa butter	—	—	—	25	38	32	3	—
Cod liver oil	—	—	8	17	—	22	5	—
Coconut oil	6	47	18	9	3	6	2	—
Corn oil (maize oil)	—	—	—	11	2	28	58	1
Cottonseed oil	—	—	1	22	3	19	54	1
Flaxseed oil	—	—	—	3	7	21	16	53
Grape seed oil	—	—	—	8	4	15	73	—
Lard (pork fat)	—	—	2	26	14	44	10	—
Olive oil	—	—	—	13	3	71	10	1
Palm oil	—	—	1	45	4	40	10	—
Palm kernel oil	4	48	16	8	3	15	2	—
Peanut oil	—	—	—	11	2	48	32	—
Safflower oil	—	—	—	7	2	13	78	—
Sesame oil	—	—	—	9	4	41	45	—
Soybean oil	—	—	—	11	4	24	54	7
Sunflower oil	—	—	—	7	5	19	68	1
Walnut oil	—	—	—	11	5	28	51	5

*Percentages may not add to 100% because of rounding up and other constituents not listed.
Adapted from http://www.scientificpsychic.com/fitness/fattyacids.html.

oils lower plasma triglyceride, decrease postprandial lipidemia, and reduce body fat mass when compared with triacylglycerol oils.[68]

Fatty Acids—Cell Uptake. Many different kinds of dietary fatty acids are derived from animal, plant, and microorganism sources. Nonesterified fatty acids enter cells via fatty acid transporters and are rapidly activated via conversion to fatty acyl CoA thioesters by acyl CoA synthases. Fatty acyl CoAs are substrates for the synthesis of neutral lipids such as triglycerides and cholesterol esters and the synthesis of polar lipids such as phospholipids, sphingolipids, and plasmalogens. They serve as substrates for elongation, desaturation, oxidation, and protein acylation reactions.[63]

Fatty Acid Classification. Fatty acids are long carbohydrate chains with a proximal methyl (CH_3–) and a terminal carboxyl (–COOH) group. Fatty acids are designated via three characteristics:

1. the number of carbons constituting the chain length,
2. the number of unsaturated carbon-carbon double bonds, and
3. the location, starting from the methyl end, of the first double bond.

Thus, linoleic acid is designated as 18:2 n-6 for an 18-carbon fatty acid with two double bonds, the first one located between carbons 6 and 7.[66]

Omega Nomenclature. These fatty acids also use the Greek alphabet (α, β, γ, ... ω) to identify the location of the double bonds. In this designation,

- the "alpha" (α) carbon is the carbon closest to the carboxyl (–COOH) group, and
- the "omega" (ω) carbon is the carbon of the methyl group (CH_3–) of the chain because ω is the last letter of the Greek alphabet.

In this nomenclature, n-6 linoleic acid is an ω-6 fatty acid because it has a double bond six carbons away from the "omega" carbon. Similarly, n-3 linolenic acid is an ω-3 fatty acid because of its double bond three carbons away from the "omega" carbon.

Saturated Fatty Acids. In saturated fatty acids, the carbohydrate chain is fully saturated with no double bonds. Examples of saturated fatty acids are

- n-dodecanoic or lauric acid (12:0),
- n-tetradecanoic or myristic acid (14:0),
- n-hexadecanoic or palmitic acid (16:0),
- n-octadecanoic or stearic acid (18:0), and
- n-eicosanoic or arachidic acid (20:0).

The second number, in this case "0," indicates the absence of unsaturated double bonds. Melting points for all fatty acids listed are above room temperature and increase with the length of the carbon chain. These fatty acids are thus usually solid at room temperature.[66] Saturated fats derive principally from animal sources. Saturated fats obtained from plant sources are palm, palm kernel, coconut, and peanut oils.

Unsaturated Fatty Acids. Unsaturated fatty acids predominate over saturated ones in higher plants and in animals living at low temperatures; they have lower melting points than saturated fatty acids do for the same chain length.

Monounsaturated Fatty Acids. Monounsaturated fatty acids have one unsaturated double bond, typically between carbons 9 and 10, in *cis*-conformation. The double bond of unsaturated fatty acids in *cis*-alignment is nonrotating and rigidly angulated at about 30 degrees. Examples of monounsaturated fatty acids are

- palmitoleic acid (16:1 n-9), a 16-carbon fatty acid with one double bond located between carbons 9 and 10, and
- oleic acid (18:1 n-9).

As a result of the natural *cis*-configuration, oleic acid appears like a boomerang, a flattened "V."

Polyunsaturated Fatty Acids. Polyunsaturated fatty acids (PUFAs) have more than one unsaturated double bond, all in *cis*-configuration. Typically, as in monounsaturated fats, one double bond is located between carbon atoms 9 and 10. Some of the additional ones may be positioned between the methyl origin of the chain and this carbon 9-10 double bond. Examples are

- linoleic acid (18:2 n-6),
- linolenic acid (18:3 n-3), an 18-carbon fatty acid with three double bonds, the

first one located between carbons 3 and 4, and
- arachidonic acid (20:4 n-6).

For n-3 PUFAs such as linolenic acid, the first double bond occurs between carbons 3 and 4. The longer the chain and the higher the number of *cis*-double bonds, the less linear the molecular conformation and the lower the melting point of the fatty acid because of less potential for close molecular "cordwood-like" stacking.

Cis- and Trans-Conformation. Unsaturated fatty acids in *trans*-configuration are very rare in nature and are generally synthetically created.[66] The terms

- *cis* means "on this side" of the double bond (e.g., "cisalpina," on this side of the Alps), and
- *trans* means "on the other side" of the double bond (e.g., "transalpina," on the other side of the Alps).

In terms of chemical bonds, the respective configurations are

C C / H H (*cis*)   C H / H C (*trans*)

HEALTH EFFECTS OF SPECIFIC FATTY ACID SUBTYPES

Although consumption of anything more than the minimally recommended amounts of dietary fat in the past had been considered to be a risk factor for vascular health, it has become increasingly apparent that disparate lipids can have drastically different and even beneficial effects on cardiovascular and metabolic health.

A large array of structurally distinct fatty acids are encountered in vegetable and animal sources of dietary fat (Table 15-2):

Saturated Fatty Acids. The consumption of saturated fats is associated with a substantial risk for cardiovascular diseases, and saturated fatty acids such as palm oil and palm kernel oil are implicated in the generation of insulin resistance. However, certain saturated fats do appear to have beneficial biologic effects. Medium-chain fatty acids, such as lauric and capric acid, play an important role in supporting the immune system. Such observations might, in fact, prompt a reexamination of the physiologic effects of the highly saturated coconut and palm kernel oils and other natural oils.[67]

Table 15-2. Dietary Fatty Acids Commonly Encountered in Fats

FAT	COMMON NAME	SCIENTIFIC NAME	CARBONS	DOUBLE BONDS
Butter	Butyric acid	Butanoic acid	4	0
	Caproic acid	Hexanoic acid	6	0
Animal fat	Palmitoleic acid	9-Hexadecanoic acid	16	1
	Stearic acid	Octadecanoic acid	18	0
Palm kernel oil	Myristic acid	Tetradecanoic acid	14	0
Coconut oil	Caprylic acid	Octanoic acid	8	0
	Capric acid	Decanoic acid	10	0
	Lauric acid	Dodecanoic acid	12	0
Palm oil	Palmitic acid	Hexadecanoic acid	16	0
Corn oil	Linoleic acid	9,12-Octadecadienoic acid	18	2
Rapeseed/canola oil	Behenic acid	Docosanoic acid	22	0
	Erucic acid	13-Docosenoic acid	22	1
Borage oil	γ-Linolenic acid (GLA)	6,9,12-Octadecatrienoic acid	18	3
Olive oil	Oleic acid	9-Octadecanoic acid	18	1
Flaxseed oil	α-Linolenic acid (ALA)	9,12,15-Octadecatrienoic acid	18	3
Peanut oil	Arachidic acid	Eicosanoic acid	20	0
Fish oil	Gadoleic acid	9-Eicosenoic acid	20	1
	EPA	5,8,11,14,17-Eicosapentaenoic acid	20	5
	DHA	4,7,10,13,16,19-Docosahexaenoic acid	22	6

Adapted from http://www.scientificpsychic.com/fitness/fattyacids.html.

Partially Hydrogenated Fatty Acids. Saturated and unsaturated fatty acids have different conformations. The most probable, minimal energy conformation of saturated fatty acids is straight and fully extended. The ability of these carbon chain molecules to be stacked like cordwood partly accounts for their increasingly higher melting points with increasing length of the carbon chain.

Correspondingly, the nonlinear, naturally *cis*-configured PUFAs have low melting points and are liquid at room temperature. PUFAs are readily oxidized at the site of their double bonds, which induces rancidity. These double bonds can be hydrogenated and thus saturated, thereby straightening the molecules, raising melting points, and increasing the resistance of the fat to oxidation.[67]

In the hydrogenation process, unsaturated fatty acids are heated with metal catalysts in the presence of pressurized hydrogen gas. Hydrogen is incorporated into the fatty acid double bonds, fully saturating them with hydrogen. The fully saturated fats are actually too waxy and solid for use as food additives. Consequently, PUFA oils are only partially hydrogenated by interrupting the saturation process when the desired consistency is achieved.[67]

Even with partial hydrogenation, the reduction in the number of available double bonds renders unsaturated fatty acids less susceptible to oxidation or rancidity, thereby increasing product shelf life. As their conformation straightens, "partially hydrogenated" oils attain higher melting points and may be solid at room temperature.[67]

***Trans*-Fats.** *Trans*–fatty acids are present mainly in partially hydrogenated oils. As PUFAs are partially hydrogenated at high temperatures with metal catalysts and pressurized hydrogen, the ensuing chemical reactions may, as a side effect, change a large percentage of the naturally *cis*-configured fatty acid double bonds to the *trans*-conformation.[67]

The *trans*-conformation of unsaturated fatty acids is less angulated and straighter than the natural *cis*-form. Because the straighter conformation of *trans*-isomers, just like that of saturated fats, allows for tighter packing, *trans*-isomers of fatty acids have much higher melting points than the natural *cis*-forms do. Like saturated fats, *trans*-fats can thus assume a solid state at room temperature, and vegetable oils may thus be fashioned into solid vegetable shortening.[66]

Elaidic acid (18:1 n-9 *trans*) is the *trans*-isomer of oleic acid (18:1 n-9) and is the most common *trans*-fat used in the United States. Though not naturally occurring, it is found in the lipids of human tissues as a result of the consumption of commercially hydrogenated products.[66] *Trans*-fat is widely used in margarine, pastries, French fries, and other foods.

Commercial *trans*-fat production began in the early 20th century and increased steadily as processed vegetable fats displaced animal fats. Currently, 2% to 4% of dietary energy consumption derives from *trans*–fatty acids.[30]

Adverse Health Impact of *Trans*–Fatty Acids. Although saturated fats are implicated in the generation of insulin resistance, *trans*–fatty acid derivatives pose even larger risks for CHD and insulin resistance. Except for commercial practicality, *trans*-fats have no redeeming physiologic benefit but are unmitigatingly hazardous to metabolic and cardiovascular health.

Naturally *cis*-configured, long-chain PUFAs have distinctive molecular conformations and are implicated in the modulation of many metabolic, immunologic, and inflammatory pathways. However, upon *trans*-reconfiguration and forfeiture of the distinctive *cis*-shapes, partially saturated *trans*–fatty acids assume nonfunctional shapes that cannot be recognized by enzymes or transcription factors. The incorporation of large amounts of *trans*–fatty acids into cell membranes may have an adverse impact on membrane structure, function, and signaling.[67]

Trans–fatty acids have adverse effects on the lipoprotein profile. Although the underlying mechanisms are unclear, *trans*–fatty acid consumption increases serum levels of LDL while decreasing levels of HDL. In the observational, prospective Nurses' Health Study, stable consumption of a diet high in *trans*–fatty acids contributed to the incidence of CHD.[69]

Trans–fatty acids have additional, adverse metabolic effects. They interfere with the normal metabolism of essential fatty acids by disrupting the production of various hormones and clotting factors. Experimental and epidemiologic data suggest that *trans*–fatty acids may increase the risk for obesity and may trigger insulin resistance and type 2 DM. *Trans*–fatty acids disrupt the fluidity of cell membranes, thereby interfering with the normal signal transduction of insulin receptors.[70]

In their dietary guidelines, the AHA and U.S. Department of Agriculture recommend curtailment of *trans*–fatty acid consumption.[70]

Monounsaturated Fatty Acids, Olive Oil. Healthy, monounsaturated fatty acids may be derived from

- olive oil,
- rapeseed/canola oil,
- nuts, and
- avocados.

Olive oil has been treasured in Mediterranean countries for centuries for its healing and nutritional properties. Olive oil may be implicated in the prevention of CHD and some types of cancer because of its high levels of

- monounsaturated fatty acids such as oleic acid (18:1 n-9),
- n-3 PUFAs, and
- polyphenolic compounds.

Monounsaturated fatty acids have beneficial effects on blood lipids and oxidative stress. The U.S. Food and Drug Administration (FDA) has allowed olive oil and foods containing olive oil to bear labels stating that consumption of 2 tablespoons, or 23 g, daily of these products may help reduce the risk for CHD.[12]

Essential Fatty Acids. Mammals can synthesize saturated and monounsaturated fatty acids from other precursors but are unable to synthesize certain PUFAs because they can only desaturate carbon bonds starting at n-9 and higher. In the absence of certain n-3 and n-6 PUFAs, organisms fail to thrive and ultimately die. **This renders the n-3 and n-6 series of PUFAs "essential," and such essential PUFAs must be derived from dietary sources.** Linoleic (18:2 n-6) and linolenic (18:3 n-3) fatty acids are examples of essential fatty acids:

- n-6 linoleic acid is the predominant plant-derived dietary PUFA, a precursor for arachidonic acid (20:4 n-6) and eicosanoids;
- n-3 linolenic acid is the predominant plant-derived dietary n-3 PUFA, a precursor for
  - eicosapentaenoic acid (EPA) (20:5 n-3) and
  - docosahexaenoic acid (DHA) (22:6 n-3).

Linoleic acid, arachidonic acid, and DHA are prominent PUFAs among cellular phospholipids. Linoleic acid is the most abundant essential fatty acid and is found in 10% to 20% of mammalian triacylglycerols and phosphoglycerides.[63,66]

Essential fatty acids are grouped into two families,

1. the n-6 fatty acids and
2. the n-3 fatty acids.

n-6 Fatty Acids. Vegetable oils are the principal source of n-6 PUFAs and contain a high proportion of linoleic acid (18:2 n-6).

- Corn oil,
- sesame oil,
- safflower oil,
- sunflower oil,
- canola oil, and
- soy oil

are common examples of predominantly n-6 vegetable oils.

n-6 versus n-3 Polyunsaturated Fatty Acid Intake. Though still controversial, n-6 PUFAs may best be consumed in a 4:1 ratio with n-3 oils.[71] If n-6 PUFAs are the predominant substrate for fatty acid chain elongation, there is a resultant increase in the availability of arachidonic acid, which can engender the production of proinflammatory, vasoconstrictive, and prothrombotic eicosanoids such as thromboxane.[72]

The ratio of α-linolenic acid (ALA) (18:3 n-3) to linoleic acid (18:2 n-6) in human plasma and blood cell membranes is 1:100. Because enzymes involved in fatty acid chain elongation and desaturation have much higher affinity for ALA than for linoleic acid, even small increases in dietary ALA intake may have a significant impact on fatty acid incorporation into membranes. A diet-dependent incorporation of ALA into red blood cell membranes has been shown.[72]

n-3 Fatty Acids. n-3 Fatty acids are principally found in

- marine plankton and
- fatty fish.

Nonmarine sources of n-3 fatty acids are primarily

- walnuts and
- flaxseed.

The main component of flaxseed and walnut oil is ALA (18:3 n-3), which can be converted to EPA (20:5 n-3) and DHA (22:6 n-3), the predominant fatty acids of fatty fish and fish oil.

Lesser, nonmarine sources of n-3 fatty acids are

- rapeseed/canola oil,
- olive and mixed-seed oil,
- hemp seed, and
- rabbit meat.[71]

Even smaller amounts of n-3 PUFAs occur in soybeans and sea vegetables such as nori and arame.

n-3 α-Linolenic Acid. The regular consumption of coldwater fish, and thus long-chain n-3 fatty acids such as EPA and DHA, has substantial health benefits. Given fish exposure to mercury and other toxins, which may attenuate the beneficial effects of fish, and the increasing exhaustion of natural fishery resources, nonmarine sources of n-3 PUFAs are of increasing interest.[72]

α-Linolenic Acid Dietary Sources. ALA (18:3 n-3) may be a suitable alternative to marine fatty acids. ALA is mainly procured from plants and is a principal component of flaxseed, walnuts, and walnut oil. ALA is also derived from nonhydrogenated vegetable oils, beans, broccoli, and green leafy vegetables. In addition, it is found in cheese, particularly alpine cheese. Milk products from linseed-supplemented cows appear to have higher ALA content.[72]

Cardioprotective Effects of α-Linolenic Acid. **A diet rich in ALA appears to be protective against fatal cardiovascular events.** The evidence for a cardioprotective effect of ALA derives from epidemiologic data, basic science studies, animal models, and primary and secondary prevention trials. Substitution of nutrients low in ALA content with foods high in ALA content and diets containing a relatively high amount of ALA are desirable. The minimal amount of ALA required is a subject of debate. According to the 2003 guidelines of the AHA, an intake of 1.5 to 3 g/day appears to be of benefit.[72]

ALA may reduce cardiac arrhythmias and the incidence of MI. It decreases the beating rate of isolated rat cardiac myocytes and suppresses arrhythmias. In a clinical study, the content of adipose tissue ALA and nonfatal MI were inversely correlated.[72]

There may be a dosing effect for ALA protection. The Nurses' Health Study suggested a dose-dependent decrease in fatal cardiac disease, in particular, sudden death. There was a 45% reduction in relative risk for sudden cardiac death with a daily dietary intake of 1.36 g of ALA (fifth and highest quintile) when compared with an intake of 0.71 g/day in the first and lowest quintile.[72]

Two secondary prevention trials for CHD via nutritional intervention, the Lyon Diet Heart Study and the Indo-Mediterranean Diet Heart Study, demonstrated a significant reduction in cardiovascular deaths. This effect was ascribed primarily to the cardioprotective effects associated with the increased consumption of ALA.[72]

Conjugated Linoleic Acid. Conjugated linoleic acid (CLA) is a naturally occurring dietary fatty acid. It is synthesized in vivo from linoleic acid or ALA by rumen bacteria, such as the anaerobic bacterium *Butyrivibrio fibrisolvens*, which convert ALA and linoleic acid into vaccenic and rumenic acid. It may also be produced during heat processing of animal-derived foods such as cooked meats, pasteurized dairy products, and processed cheese, particularly alpine cheese.[72,73]

CLA has anti-inflammatory properties. It reduces the messenger RNA (mRNA) expression of cyclooxygenase-2 (COX-2), inducible nitric oxide synthase (iNOS), and TNF-α in macrophages. It decreases the production of prostaglandin E_2 (PGE_2), TNF-α, and inflammatory nitric oxide (NO), IL-1β, and IL-6 (Fig. 15-6). The anti-inflammatory properties of CLA may be mediated in part via CLA ligand activation of PPAR-γ.[73]

CLA has been found to have antiatherogenic effects. It lowers circulating LDL and triglyceride levels. CLA increases lean body mass and reduces visceral and body fat mass. It improves glucose tolerance, is antidiabetic, and has anticarcinogenic effects.[72,73]

Supplementation with CLA, either as free fatty acid or as triacylglycerol, lowers body fat mass.

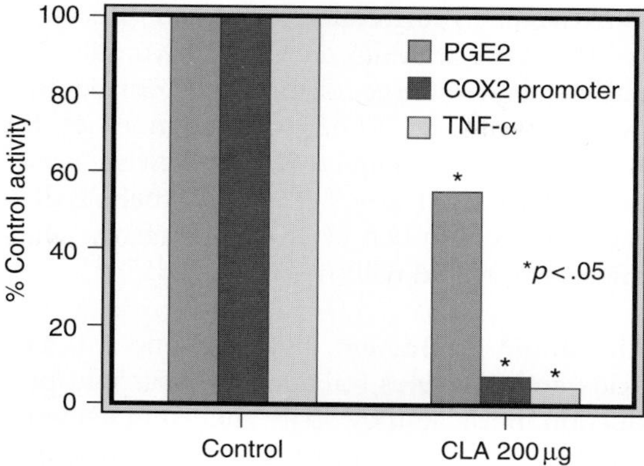

Figure 15–6.
Decreased activity of inflammatory mediators in mouse macrophage cells on exposure to conjugated linoleic acid (CLA). COX2, cyclooxygenase-2; PGE2, prostaglandin E_2; TNF, tumor necrosis factor. *(Modified from Yu Y, Correll JP, Heuvel V. Conjugated linoleic acid decreases production of proinflammatory products in macrophages: evidence for a PPAR-gamma–dependent mechanism. Biochim Biophys Acta 2002:1581:89-99.)*

In a randomized, double-blind, placebo-controlled trial of 180 healthy male and female individuals with a BMI ranging from 25 to 30 kg/m², subjects were divided into three study arms and assigned to receive 4.5 g/day of olive oil as placebo, CLA free fatty acid, or CLA triacylglycerol. By 12 months, body weight and BMI decreased significantly for the CLA triacylglycerol group, with no change in the subjects who received placebo. In both CLA groups, body fat mass was significantly lower and lean body mass higher at 12 months.[74]

Fish Oil. The consumption of fish oil substantially lowers cardiovascular morbidity and mortality. It is associated with a reduction in the incidence of MI, stroke, sudden death, and overall mortality. The low incidence of heart disease among Greenland Inuit, Icelanders, and Japanese is attributed to their high dietary intake of fish containing n-3 PUFA marine oil.[75]

After ingestion, dietary n-3 PUFAs are widely distributed to virtually every cell in the body with effects on

- membrane composition and function,
- receptor signaling,
- eicosanoid synthesis, and
- regulation of gene expression.

n-3 PUFAs affect diverse physiologic processes such as the regulation of plasma lipids and neuronal and visual function. There is growing evidence that the n-3 PUFA marine oils, in particular, EPA and DHA, have beneficial antiplatelet, immunomodulating, and antiarrhythmic effects. EPA and DHA play an important role in the prevention and treatment of inflammatory metabolic and cardiovascular pathology, including

- insulin resistance,
- atherosclerosis,
- thrombosis,
- stroke, and
- hypertension;

other inflammatory conditions such as

- asthma,
- arthritis,
- migraine headache,
- psoriasis,
- depression, and
- dementia; and

carcinomas such as

- breast,
- colon, and
- prostate cancer.[63,76]

Structural Formulas of n-3 Polyunsaturated Fatty Acids. The beneficial n-3 PUFAs are all long-chain fatty acids with multiple unsaturated carbon-carbon bonds. Specifically, the chemical formulas of the principal n-3 PUFAs are as follows:

Formula		
CH_3-CH_2-(CH=CH-CH_2)$_3$-(CH_2)$_6$-COOH	18:3 n-3	Linolenic acid
CH_3-CH_2-(CH=CH-CH_2)$_4$-(CH_2)$_3$-COOH	18:4 n-3	Octadecatetraenoic acid
CH_3-CH_2-(CH=CH-CH_2)$_5$-(CH2)$_2$-COOH	20:5 n-3	Eicosapentaenoic acid (EPA)
CH_3-CH_2-(CH=CH-CH_2)$_6$-CH_2-COOH	22:6 n-3	Docosahexaenoic acid (DHA)

Adapted from Botham KM, Zheng X, Napolitano M, et al. The effects of dietary n-3 polyunsaturated fatty acids delivered in chylomicron remnants on the transcription of genes regulating synthesis and secretion of very-low-density lipoprotein by the liver: modulation by cellular oxidative state. Exp Biol Med (Maywood) 2003;228:143-151.

Algae as Sources of Fatty Acids. Marine oils derive ultimately from microalgae. Microalgae contain a wide range of fatty acids in their lipids. Of particular importance is the presence of significant quantities of the essential PUFAs

- n-6 linolenic acid (18:2) and
- n-3 linolenic acid (18:3)

and the highly polyunsaturated n-3 fatty acids

- octadecatetraenoic acid (18:4 n-3),
- EPA (20:5 n-3), and
- DHA (22:6 n-3)

in their membranes.[76]

The best known algal classes of marine microalgae, or phytoplankton, present in the ocean populations are the

- diatoms (Bacillariophyta),
- dinoflagellates (Dinophyta),
- green algae (Chlorophyta), and
- blue-green algae (Cyanophyta).

Marine microalgae constitute the food base that supports the entire animal population of the oceans. Microalgae are thus the primary source of EPA and DHA for fish. Humans obtain their marine n-3 PUFA supplies indirectly via dietary consumption of oily fish. Declining fish stocks may ultimately dictate the use of alternative derivations for EPA and DHA. Microalgae may be a good source of n-3 PUFAs to fill this gap.[76]

Anti-inflammatory Effects. PUFA consumption has anti-inflammatory effects and lowers systemic markers of inflammation.

In a cross-sectional dietary study of n-3 and n-6 fatty acid consumption and inflammatory markers in 859 healthy men and women, there were statistically significant inverse associations between the intake of EPA and DHA and plasma levels of soluble TNF receptors 1 and 2, with weaker inverse associations for CRP. At high levels of n-3 fatty acid intake, the combination of n-3 and n-6 fatty acids was related to the lowest levels of inflammation.[77]

There are numerous mechanisms by which high intake of EPA and DHA may reduce inflammatory mediators.

Peroxisome Proliferator–Activated Receptor. n-3 PUFAs, such as EPA, are highly polyunsaturated and readily undergo oxidation. Oxidized EPA potently activates PPAR-α, a member of the nuclear receptor family. DHA likewise serves as a PPAR-α activator.[78] It is likely that PPAR-α mediates a number of the anti-inflammatory effects associated with n-3 fatty acids.[79]

Eicosanoid Production. Both n-3 and n-6 fatty acids are substrates for human eicosanoid production. Because they share the same enzymes for the synthesis of prostaglandins and leukotrienes, n-3 PUFAs compete with arachidonic acid (20:4 n-6) in the creation of eicosanoids (Fig. 15-7). The biologic activity of n-3 PUFA-derived eicosanoids differs from that of arachidonic acid derivatives, thereby causing an anti-inflammatory effect.

Specifically, arachidonic acid serves as a substrate for several enzymatic, proinflammatory pathways:

- cyclooxygenases, such as COX-1, a constitutive enzyme, or COX-2, an inducible enzyme: COX products of arachidonic acid give rise to prostanoids and thromboxanes and modulate thromboregulatory, inflammatory, and chemotactic responses;
- lipoxygenases (5-, 12-, or 15-LOX): the LOX pathway catalyzes the insertion of molecular oxygen into arachidonic acid as the first

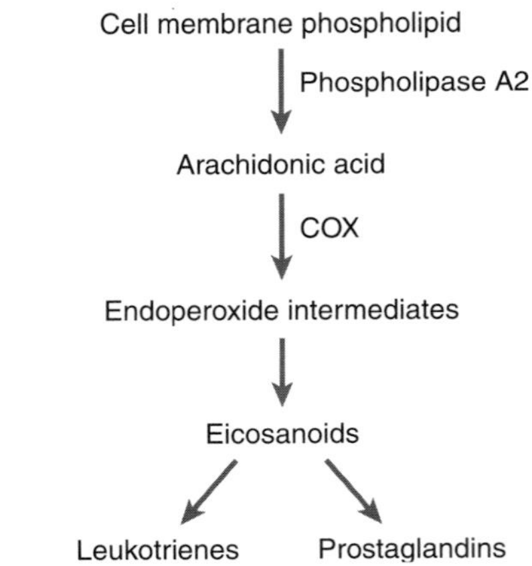

Figure 15–7.
Synthesis of eicosanoids from arachidonic acid. COX, cyclooxygenase. *(Modified from Zhang X, Young HA. PPAR and the immune system—what do we know? Int Immunopharm 2002;2:1029-1044.)*

step in the formation of leukotrienes and hydroxyeicosatetraenoic acids. LOX products are involved in mediating vascular permeability, vasoconstriction, and bronchoconstriction; and

- cytochrome P-450 monooxygenases: the microsomal cytochrome P-450–linked monooxygenases catalyze the nicotinamide adenine dinucleotide phosphate oxidase (NADH/NADPH)-dependent oxidation of fatty acids to yield a variety of eicosanoids, a mechanism important in cells such as hepatocytes with little COX or LOX activity.[63]

Nonesterified PUFAs, released from the sn-2 position of membrane phospholipids via the action of specific phospholipases (phospholipase A_2), compete with arachidonic acid as substrates for these enzymatic, inflammatory pathways. Part of the anti-inflammatory properties of marine oils derives from their modulation of eicosanoid signaling by affecting the synthesis, bioactivity, and metabolic clearance of COX and LOX eicosanoid products:

- synthesis: when compared with arachidonic acid, EPA and DHA are conformationally poor substrates for the COX and LOX reactions because their oxygenation efficiency is significantly lower than that of arachidonic acid;
- bioactivity: most n-3 fatty acid–derived eicosanoids have significantly lower bioactivity and fewer inflammatory properties than the arachidonic acid product does; and
- clearance: n-3 PUFAs also enhance eicosanoid catabolism via peroxisomal degradation.[63,77]

Inhibition of T-Cell Activation. The immunomodulatory role of PUFAs occurs in part via inhibition of T-cell activation. Because a variety of T-cell signaling proteins are located in plasmalemmal lipid rafts, the physicochemical integrity of lipid raft membranes is essential for T-cell signal transduction. PUFAs inhibit T-cell activation by altering the fatty acyl composition of the cell membranes, thereby displacing acylated signaling proteins from membrane lipid rafts.

Specifically, within lipid rafts, the cytoplasmic leaflet of the plasma membrane is enriched in lipids containing saturated fatty acyl groups. Under physiologic conditions, signaling proteins, acylated with saturated fatty acyl residues, partition with high affinity into the lipid environment of such rafts. In EPA-treated T cells, the PUFA-altered fatty acyl composition of raft lipids engenders the selective displacement of palmitoylated proteins from lipid rafts. Thus, treatment of Jurkat T cells with polyunsaturated EPA resulted in marked enrichment of raft lipids with PUFAs, and PUFAs were significantly incorporated into phosphatidylethanolamine, which predominantly resides in the cytoplasmic leaflet of the membrane lipid bilayer.[80] In mice, dietary n-3 PUFAs were selectively incorporated into T-cell raft and soluble membrane phospholipids. Phosphatidylserine and glycerophosphoethanolamine, highly localized to the inner cytoplasmic leaflet, were enriched to a greater extent with PUFAs than were sphingomyelin, phosphatidylinositol, and glycerophosphocholine in the exoplasmic leaflet of the plasma membrane bilayer.[81]

Cytokines, Chemokines, and Oxidative Stress. n-3 PUFAs reduce the production of TNF-α.[60] n-3 PUFAs modulate cytokine production and the release of the soluble TNF receptors by influencing

- eicosanoid-independent pathways,
- physicochemical membrane characteristics,
- signal transduction processes, and
- nuclear receptors such as the PPARs or NFκB.[77]

DHA decreases NADH/NADPH oxidase activity, thereby lowering oxidative stress. It decreases the expression of intercellular adhesion molecule (ICAM) and vascular cell adhesion molecule-1 (VCAM-1).[78]

Oxidized EPA, but not the native, unoxidized PUFA, significantly inhibits human neutrophil and monocyte adhesion to endothelial cells in vitro. In the process, EPA inhibits expression of the endothelial adhesion receptor and markedly reduces leukocyte rolling and adhesion to the endothelium, activities associated with decreased inflammation in the vascular wall.[79]

Vascular Dysfunction, Coronary Heart Disease, and Mortality. n-3 PUFAs have a favorable

impact on hemodynamic parameters. A diet high in n-3 fatty acids (i.e., fish oil) may

- **improve endothelium-dependent vasodilation and**
- **lower systemic blood pressure.**[82]

In a cross-sectional analysis of 9758 men aged 50 to 59 years without CHD in France and Ireland from 1991 to 1993, systolic and diastolic blood pressure was lower in consumers than in nonconsumers of fish.[83]

n-3 PUFAs favorably affect cardiovascular disease. In patients with established CHD, fish oil can reduce the incidence of new CHD events. PUFAs are readily incorporated into atheromatous plaque with beneficial effects. Whereas increased consumption of n-6 PUFAs does not affect the fatty acid composition or the stability of plaque over time, n-3 PUFA ingestion enhances the stability of atheromata.[84]

Plaque stabilization may contribute to the reduction in nonfatal and fatal cardiovascular events associated with increased n-3 PUFA intake.[84] Among primary prevention studies, the Nurses' Health Study involving 84,000 women participants showed a negative relationship between fish intake and the risk for CHD.[85] The United States Physicians' Health Study involving 20,551 men showed a 52% reduction in sudden death with the regular consumption of one or more fish servings per week.[86] Among secondary prevention studies, the Gruppo Italiano per lo Studio della Sopravvivenza nell'Infarto Miocardico Prevenzione Trial with 11,324 post-MI patients showed supplementation with 1 g/day of n-3 PUFA over a period of 3.5 years to be associated with a significant 15% reduction in the rates of all-cause mortality, nonfatal MI, and nonfatal stroke.[87] A significant decline in sudden death with n-3 PUFA intake was apparent at 4 months.[88] In a meta-analysis of prospective cohort studies, there was a consistently inverse association between fish consumption and CHD mortality rates, with an apparent dose-response relationship between fish consumption and risk for CHD mortality. An increment of 20 g/day of fish intake lowered CHD mortality rates by 7%, and once-weekly fish consumption significantly reduced death from CHD by 15%. The inverse association was more apparent in studies with follow-up periods extending over 12 years or longer.[89]

Marine Oil and Obesity. The intake of n-3 PUFAs is not linked to the development of obesity. n-3 PUFAs are readily oxidized for energy and are thus consumed rather than stored. They

- are less readily incorporated into storage triacylglycerol,
- are easily mobilized by lipolytic stimuli, and
- lower the expression of genes associated with adipocyte proliferation.

Increased PUFA intake in animal models is associated with reduced adiposity.[2,63]

n-3 Fatty Acids and Insulin Resistance. Fish oil may lower insulin resistance. Increased n-3 PUFA intake in animal models is associated with improved insulin action.[2,63] PUFAs have a significant, beneficial effect on insulin sensitivity in various tissues, particularly skeletal muscle.[12,16]

Especially after the achievement of some weight loss, dietary n-3 PUFAs may further enhance insulin sensitivity. In an obese rat dietary model of insulin and leptin resistance, diet supplementation with fish oil, with chromium, or with both lowered plasma glucose while improving both insulin and leptin sensitivity when compared with the high-fat diet control group.[90]

The beneficial anti-inflammatory and vascular effects of fish consumption enhance insulin sensitivity. Additionally, n-3 PUFA interaction with the PPARs and with SREBP-1c contribute to the insulin-sensitizing impact of marine oil.

Peroxisome Proliferator–Activated Receptors. Activation of PPAR-α and PPAR-γ enhances insulin sensitivity in skeletal muscle and adipose tissue. Fatty acids that are slowly or poorly incorporated into storage lipids appear to more effectively activate PPAR, and EPA thus appears to be a preferred endogenous ligand for the PPARs.

PPARs can bind many fatty acids, for example, binding oleic acid and EPA with nearly equivalent affinity. Differential lipid metabolism imposes a physiologic discrimination at the cellular level that favors EPA as a PPAR ligand over oleic acid: in the synthesis of triacylglycerol, when compared with oleic acid CoA, EPA CoA is a poor substrate for the enzyme diacylglycerol acyltransferase. EPA is therefore assimilated into neutral storage lipids less effectively than oleic acid is. The residual higher, nonused intracellular EPA levels are thus more available to preferentially activate the PPARs.[63]

From a structural perspective, EPA (20:5 n-3) is a suitable endogenous ligand for the PPARs. Because DHA has more than 20 carbons, activation of PPARs by DHA (22:6 n-3) probably requires prior retroconversion to EPA, a process that entails peroxisomal oxidation.[63]

Sterol Regulatory Element Binding Protein-1c. n-3 PUFA action on insulin responsiveness in the liver may extend beyond its activation of PPAR activity and entail inhibition of SREBP-1c as well.

SREBP-1c is a transcription factor required for the insulin-mediated induction of hepatic fatty acid and of triacylglycerol synthesis. n-3 PUFAs restrict the gene expression and nuclear content of SREBP-1c in hepatocytes, thereby suppressing hepatic lipogenesis. In the process, dietary PUFAs suppress the transcription of many genes involved in de novo lipogenesis, including

- fatty acid synthase,
- stearoyl CoA desaturase-1,
- L-pyruvate kinase, and
- S14 protein.

Coupling this action with the n-3 PUFA–mediated induction of PPAR-regulated genes shifts hepatic metabolism away from lipid synthesis and storage to lipid oxidation. This mechanism prevents the ectopic intrahepatocellular lipid overload and hepatic lipotoxicity associated with insulin resistance.[62,63]

Plasma Lipids. Consumption of n-3 PUFAs may improve plasma lipids, in part by interfering with the mechanisms that engender hepatic steatosis associated with insulin resistance.[62,63]

Triglycerides. Fish oil may lower triglyceride levels by 19%.[91] n-3 PUFAs impair VLDL assembly and secretion.

In rats, n-3 PUFA delivery to hepatocytes via n-3 PUFA–enriched chylomicron remnants, in contrast to n-6 PUFA or absent enrichment, down-regulated the mRNA expression for acyl CoA:cholesterol acyltransferase 2 (ACAT2), which may play a role in inhibiting VLDL secretion.[76] In a clinical case report, n-3 PUFAs, at doses ranging from 1 to 6 g/day, decreased triglyceride levels to a similar degree as conventional pharmacologic measures. Specifically, fish oil can reduce elevated plasma triglycerides by an average of 30% to 52% in subjects with borderline-high (150 to 199 mg/dL) to high (200 to 499 mg/dL) triglycerides. Although fish oil has not been reported to induce hepatotoxicity, an increase in transaminases may be experienced while undergoing fish oil therapy.[92] For severe hypertriglyceridemia, with triglycerides higher than 1000 mg/dL, 6 to 8 g of fish oil per day may be a useful adjunct to diet, exercise, and drug therapy with fibrates or niacin.[30]

High-Density Lipoprotein. By reducing circulating triglyceride levels, n-3 PUFAs favorably affect HDL levels.

In a cross-sectional analysis of men aged 50 to 59 years without CHD, triglycerides were lower and HDL levels higher in fish consumers than in nonconsumers.[83] n-3 PUFAs may induce a 16% increase in HDL, suggestive of a reduction in cardiovascular risk factors. A sustained fish diet can also lower lipoprotein(a) (Lp[a]).[91]

Arrhythmia and Sudden Death. n-3 PUFAs from fish oil supplementation are readily incorporated into cell membranes with stabilizing electrophysiologic effects. Fish intake may decrease the risk for atrial fibrillation and lower the risk for sudden death.

Atrial Fibrillation. Among elderly adults, consumption of broiled or baked fish is associated with a lower incidence of atrial fibrillation.

In a prospective, population-based, multivariate analysis of 4815 adults aged 65 years, consumption of tuna and other broiled or baked fish was inversely associated with the incidence of atrial fibrillation during 12 years of follow-up. There was a 28% lower risk for atrial fibrillation with fish intake one to four times per week ($P = .005$) and a 31% lower risk with fish consumption five times per week ($P = .008$) when compared with fish intake less than once per month.[93]

Ventricular Tachycardia. n-3 PUFAs may raise the threshold for the development of ventricular tachycardia. In a clinical pilot study, the intravenous infusion of n-3 PUFAs was well tolerated by patients, did not induce arrhythmias, but resulted in a reduction of sustained ventricular tachycardia.[94]

Heart Rate and Sudden Death. Fish oil consumption is associated with slowing of the heart rate and a reduction in the incidence of sudden death.

Among fish consumers in a cross-sectional analysis of men aged 50 to 59 years without CHD, heart rates were statistically lower than in nonconsumers across the quantitative categories of fish intake. The DHA content of erythrocyte phospholipids was inversely correlated with the heart rate ($P < .03$). Because the heart rate is positively associated with the risk for sudden death, this association may in part underlie the lower risk for sudden death observed in fish consumers.[83] A high-fish diet results in the substitution of myocardial membrane arachidonic acid for EPA, which decreases myocyte excitability and may be responsible for the reduction in sudden death seen with fish consumption.[95]

Chronic Diseases. n-3 PUFAs improve the prognosis of other chronic inflammatory diseases:

- Fish oil intake may ameliorate rheumatoid arthritis, osteoarthritis, asthma, psoriasis, Raynaud's disease, ulcerative colitis, Crohn's disease, and possibly, multiple sclerosis.[96]
- In a 4-year prospective study of 815 persons aged 65 to 94 years, participants who consumed fish or long-chain n-3 PUFAs and DHA once a week had a 60% lower risk for Alzheimer's disease than did those who rarely or never consumed fish.[97]
- The consumption of salmon may diminish the risk for prostate cancer and have a favorable impact on mood disturbances.

Dietary Guidelines for Fish Oil Consumption. Fish oil consumption has been officially endorsed to improve public health outcomes.

The U.S. National Institutes of Health (NIH) recommends a total daily intake of 650 mg/day of EPA and DHA, 2.22 g/day of ALA, and 4.44 g/day of linoleic acid. The FDA has announced that labels of foods containing n-3 PUFAs can state that consumption of these products may help reduce the risk for CHD. The AHA has endorsed new fish oil guidelines for patients with documented CHD. Ideally, CHD patients should derive their daily fish oil from an approximately 3-oz serving of fatty fish such as salmon, herring, trout, mackerel, or sardines. At least two fish servings a week would be of benefit. Somewhat leaner fish, such as canned tuna, halibut, and flounder, are also acceptable but need to be consumed in larger portions.

Because fish oil capsules provide similar benefit, the AHA also allows n-3 fatty acids to be taken as a supplement. Of the widely marketed 1-g fish oil capsules containing 180 mg EPA and 120 mg DHA, three capsules a day can assume the place of a fish serving. If fasting triglyceride levels exceed 200 mg/dL, 2 to 4 g of n-3 PUFAs per day may be consumed.

Fish intake can have some deleterious effects because of methyl-mercury contamination and the accumulation of other toxins. Shark, swordfish, king mackerel, and tilefish may have high levels of mercury and should be avoided.

ω-3 Fatty Acid Content and Methyl-Mercury Level in Commonly Consumed Fish

FISH	ω-3 FATTY ACID OUNCES PER 3 OUNCES OF FISH	METHYL-MERCURY LEVEL
Salmon	0.68-1.83	Low
Sardines	0.98-1.70	Low
Oyster	0.37-1.17	Low
Halibut	0.40-1.00	Medium
Shark	0.90	High
Tilefish	0.80	High
White tuna, canned	0.73	Medium
Swordfish	0.70	High
Lobster	0.007-0.41	Medium
Crabs	0.34-0.40	Low-medium
Pollack	0.46	Low
Mackerel	0.34	High
Shrimp	0.27	Low
Clams	0.24	Low
Light tuna, canned	0.26	Low
Scallops	0.17	Low

Adapted from Neergaard L. Don't be scared off fish by mercury warnings. Pittsburgh Tribune 2003;Thursday, December 25:A13.

NUTS AND PEANUTS

Nuts contain primarily unsaturated fatty acids (monounsaturated and polyunsaturated), as well as magnesium, vitamins, minerals, and antioxidants. Nuts are a good source of soluble and insoluble fiber. They are rich in L-arginine and are an excellent source of vitamin E. Epidemiologic studies suggest that nut consumption has favorable effects on plasma lipids and CHD.

Different Nut Varieties. Not all nuts are equivalent. Macadamia nuts and cashews contain higher levels of saturated fatty acids than do other varieties and may not share the same health benefits. For example, cashews have 3 g of saturated fatty acid per ounce versus 2 g of saturated fatty acid per ounce for peanuts, which are actually more properly described as legumes. Peanuts contain the flavonoid resveratrol, which is also found in red wine and may be vasculoprotective. Almonds have the highest level of vitamin E and calcium. Walnuts have the highest level of n-3 PUFAs, specifically ALA.[99]

Impact on Plasma Lipids. Nuts may improve the lipid profile.

In hyperlipidemic individuals, almond and walnut consumption significantly reduced levels of total cholesterol, LDL, oxidized LDL, Lp(a), and apolipoprotein B-100 while increasing HDL. The effect was dose dependent.[100]

Endothelial Function. Consumption of walnuts may improve endothelial function.

In 20 hypercholesterolemic men and women 55 years old on average, the substitution of walnuts for monounsaturated fat in the Mediterranean diet had a beneficial lipid-lowering effect and significantly improved endothelium-dependent vasodilation with a significant reduction in the level of VCAM-1.[101]

Type 2 Diabetes Mellitus. The consumption of nuts lowers the incidence of DM.

The Nurses' Health Study ($N = 121{,}700$ women) investigated the relationship between nut consumption and type 2 DM. The study found that women in the highest quartile of nut ingestion, at least five times weekly, demonstrated an age-adjusted relative risk of 0.55 for type 2 DM when compared with the quartile of women who hardly ever consumed nuts. A similar comparison pertained for the consumption of peanut butter, with a relative risk of 0.79 for type 2 DM when comparing the highest and lowest peanut butter consumers.[102]

Weight Considerations. Nuts are high in fat and rank high in caloric density. There is the concern that increasing nut consumption might worsen weight management. However, in the Nurses' Health Study, the ingestion of nuts in the highest quartile was not associated with a significantly greater weight gain than lower nut consumption was.[102]

Dietary Guidelines for Nut Consumption. One to 2 oz/day of a variety of nuts as part of a healthy diet may provide a health benefit. There is FDA approval for walnut packages to carry a health claim regarding a reduction in CHD risk with the consumption of 1.5 oz of walnuts per day.

TEA

Tea is second only to water as the world's most popular beverage. Tea has been consumed in Asia for millennia, and its consumption has been growing in Western countries as its health benefits have come to be more widely appreciated.[103]

Tea Varieties. White, green, oolong, and black teas are prepared from the tender, new leaves of the shrub *Camellia sinensis*. The distinct tea types derive from differences in the preparation of tea leaves:

- Green tea is prepared from steamed, dried, unfermented tea leaves in a process that preserves polyphenols.
- Young tea leaves undergo even less processing in the preparation of white tea.
- Oolong tea is partially fermented.
- For the preparation of black tea, the tea leaves are fully fermented, cured, and thus auto-oxidized. This process intensifies the flavor of tea, but may break down some of the beneficial chemicals in tea.

Black tea may thus lack some of the health benefits of white, green, or oolong tea. In fact, catechins constitute greater than 80% of the flavonoids in green tea, but only 20% to 30% in black tea.[104] It is unclear whether the decaffeination process compromises the catechin content of decaffeinated tea.

Antioxidant and Anti-inflammatory Properties. The most widely known benefits of green tea relate to its antioxidant and anti-inflammatory properties, attributable mainly to its high levels of polyphenolic flavonoids. Tea polyphenols, also termed catechins, are up to eight times more potent in antioxidant efficacy than vitamin C, as measured by radical scavenging activity. Antioxidants may help repair or prevent the damage caused by free radicals.[105]

Epigallocatechin-3-gallate (Fig. 15-8) is the major active polyphenol in tea. The effects of epigallocatechin-3-gallate observed in laboratory studies include

- inhibition of NFκB activation, thus reducing the inflammatory response,[105]
- improvements in antioxidant potential,
- repression of reactive oxygen species activity,
- inhibition of apoptosis of activated neutrophils,
- inhibition of TNF-α gene expression, and
- pronounced suppression of chemokine-induced neutrophil chemotaxis.[106]

Weight Loss Effects. Long-term consumption of tea catechins may be beneficial for the suppression of diet-induced obesity. Green tea may promote weight loss via several potential mechanisms of action:

- Green tea inhibits gastric and pancreatic lipases. It thus interferes with the breakdown of dietary triglyceride and fatty acid absorption into the small intestine, which can potentially limit weight gain.
- Green tea catechins significantly increase fatty acid beta oxidation activity in the liver.
- Catechol *O*-methyltransferase (COMT) is an enzyme that decreases thermogenesis in adipose tissue. Green tea catechins may inhibit the enzyme, thus enhancing adipose tissue thermogenesis and fat metabolism.[107-110]

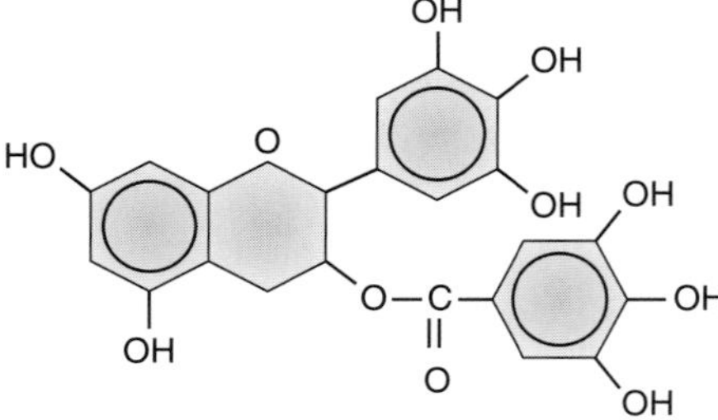

▸▸ **Figure 15–8.**
Chemical structure of epigallocatechin-3-gallate.

In animal studies, supplementation with tea catechins significantly reduced high-fat diet–induced body weight gain, visceral and hepatic fat accumulation, and the development of hyperinsulinemia and hyperleptinemia.[111]

Clinical studies using green tea extract with 250 to 270 mg epigallocatechin-3-gallate demonstrated

- increased energy expenditure,
- higher fat oxidation,
- greater weight loss, and
- decreased waist circumference

when compared with placebo. Effects were seen by 2 to 4 weeks, with a 4.6% reduction in weight and 4.5% reduction in waist circumference by 3 months.[107]

Vasculoprotective Effects. The consumption of tea is of benefit for cardiovascular health.

Endothelial Function. Tea consumption may reverse endothelial vasomotor dysfunction and protect vascular health.

In a study of 50 patients with CHD, endothelium-dependent, flow-mediated dilation of the brachial artery improved after short-term (2 hours) and long-term (4 weeks) consumption of black tea.[112]

Hypertension. Habitual consumption of tea may, in some populations, reduce the risk for the development of hypertension.

In a cross-sectional study of 1507 normotensive Taiwanese subjects aged 20 years or older in 1996, habitual tea drinkers consuming 120 to 599 mL/day of green or oolong tea had a 46% lower risk for the development of hypertension than did nonhabitual tea drinkers, independent of socioeconomic, dietary, or risk factors.[113]

Atherogenesis. The intake of tea interferes with aspects of evolving atherogenesis.

Epigallocatechin-3-gallate reduced evolving atherosclerotic lesions in hypercholesterolemic, apolipoprotein E–null mice without influencing established atherosclerosis.[114] Catechins present in tea blocked LDL oxidation and inhibited the migration of vascular smooth muscle cells from the tunica media to the subendothelial region, a key event in the development and progression of atherosclerosis.[115] Tea may inhibit platelet aggregation and thereby decrease the occurrence of thromboembolic events.[116,117]

Coronary Heart Disease Events. Black and green tea intake lowers the occurrence of CHD morbidity and mortality.

Black and green tea intake of one or more cups per day is inversely associated with the occurrence of MI with an odds ratio of 0.56 to 0.58.[116,117] In the population-based Rotterdam Study of 4807 subjects without a history of MI over a 5.6-year period, tea drinkers had a relative risk of 0.57 for incident MI when compared with non–tea drinkers. This inverse association was stronger for fatal than for nonfatal events.[118] In a prospective cohort study of 1900 patients hospitalized for acute MI—part of the Determinants of Myocardial Infarction Onset Study—both total mortality and cardiovascular mortality were lower in moderate and heavy tea drinkers than in tea abstainers.[119]

Insulin-Sensitizing Effects. Because of its antioxidant and anti-inflammatory potency and its effects on fat metabolism, thermogenesis, and vascular function, tea has insulin-sensitizing effects. The chronic consumption of tea catechins may be beneficial for the prevention of insulin resistance.

Most of the insulin-potentiating activity for green and oolong tea is due to epigallocatechin-3-gallate. For black tea, epigallocatechin-3-gallate is active, as well as tannins, theaflavins, and other compounds. The efficacy of tea is impaired by the addition of milk, nondairy creamers, or soymilk, whereas the addition of lemon is neutral in effect.

Tea, as normally taken, increased insulin activity more than 15-fold in an in vitro epididymal fat cell assay.[120] Green tea polyphenols in a diabetic rat model reduced glucose levels and raised glucose tolerance significantly. In diabetic individuals, 4 weeks of daily consumption of 50 oz of strong oolong tea reduced average pretreatment plasma glucose levels from 220 to 162 mg/dL after treatment, with no effect seen in the water consumption control group.[121]

Lipid-Lowering Effects. The effects of tea on thermogenesis, fat oxidation, and insulin sensitivity contribute to the favorable impact that green tea has on circulating lipids.

Green tea may reduce cholesterol and triglyceride levels in mildly hyperlipidemic adults. When compared with caffeinated placebo, 3 weeks of five daily servings of tea significantly lowered levels of total and LDL cholesterol, apolipoprotein B, and Lp(a).[122]

Other Effects. Green tea has been found to have antibacterial, antiviral, anticarcinogenic, antiangiogenic, and antimutagenic activities. In a mouse model, green tea was found to inhibit breast cancer cell proliferation. Green tea contains L-theanine, an amino acid that is implicated in promoting relaxation.

ALCOHOL AND WINE

Alcoholic beverages have been consumed by numerous societies for thousands of years. The earliest wine consumers were noted to be better nourished and less prone to sickness. The ancient Israelites and Greeks valued the medicinal properties of wine, and wine has been used in religious ritual. The 16th century German physician Paracelsus stated that "whether wine is a nourishment, a medicine, or a poison is a matter of dosage."[123]

The French paradox, ascribed to the protective effects of wine imbibition, relates to the observation that mortality rates from CHD are unexpectedly lower in France than in the United Kingdom or the United States despite diets similarly rich in saturated fatty acids.[124] Similar observations have been made in other countries.[125]

Excessive alcohol consumption is associated with hypertension, left ventricular hypertrophy, cardiomyopathy, atrial fibrillation, hemorrhagic stroke, and many noncardiovascular diseases. Alcohol is abused by up to 10% of middle-aged men.[126]

Antioxidant Effects. Wine, particularly red wine, has antioxidant properties that confer health benefits over and above those attributable to alcohol.[127] Wine has an abundance of phenolic acids, polyphenols, and flavonoids such as resveratrol and gallic acid. Polyphenols are derivatives of diphenylpyrans, which are found in the skins, seeds, and stems of purple grapes. Phenolic compounds imbue wine with its taste and bouquet. They are potent antioxidants that allow wines to age.[128]

In a study of cultured vascular smooth muscle cells, short-term and long-term treatment with red wine polyphenolic compounds markedly reduced the platelet-derived growth factor (PDGF) AB–induced production of reactive oxygen species and interfered with phosphorylation of p38 mitogen-activated protein kinase (MAPK), thus preventing the redox-sensitive activation of the p38 MAPK pathway.[129] Wine decreases the oxidation of LDL.[130]

Anti-inflammatory Effects. Alcohol has anti-inflammatory effects.

Alcohol reduces the increase in NFκB, which is responsible for the expression of several inflammatory genes. CRP is a nonspecific marker for inflammation, but is increasingly being recognized as an independent and significant risk factor for CHD. Moderate alcohol consumption may lower CRP by up to 35%.[131,132] Light alcohol consumption is associated with lower levels of IL-6 and CRP in elderly, well-functioning men and women.[133] CRP has a U-shaped relationship with alcohol consumption, the lowest plasma level being associated with the intake of two to four drinks daily.[134] Data from the recent NHANES III study, which included a complete evaluation of 11,572 U.S. adults, found that CRP levels were significantly higher in alcohol abstainers, regardless of the level of alcohol ingestion.[135]

Vasculoprotective Properties. Alcohol, and wine in particular, have vasculoprotective properties.

In fact, in cirrhotic patients the vascular intima of the coronary circulation is spared from atheromatous disease. The protective, vascular effects of wine are complemented by an attendant increase in HDL, a reduction in fibrinogen, and lower platelet reactivity and aggregability.[136]

Endothelial Function. Wine enhances endothelial function.[128] It improves endothelium-dependent vasodilation.

Red wine up-regulates the endothelial nitric oxide synthase (eNOS) gene in human endothelial cells. It is likely that the polyphenol content of red wine is responsible for the up-regulation of eNOS. The enhanced mRNA and protein expression of eNOS results in the increased production of bioactive NO.[137] Wine polyphenols also inhibit the endothelial synthesis of endothelin-1,[138] and flow-mediated vessel dilation is enhanced by red wine.[139]

Atherogenesis. Red wine polyphenolic compounds may have antiangiogenic and antiatherosclerotic properties. Moderate wine consumption with meals appears to be more cardioprotective than at other times because it reduces the postprandial endothelial dysfunction caused by high-fat meals.

Resveratrol, a red wine polyphenol, inhibits a number of proatherogenic responses of inflammatory and vascular smooth muscle cells in early atherosclerosis. Red wine

- reduces the expression of monocyte chemotactic protein-1 (MCP-1),
- lowers the expression of intracellular adhesion molecules,
- decreases foam cell formation,
- decreases the abnormal expression of intracellular tissue factor,
- reduces the expression of vascular endothelial growth factor (VEGF),
- has antiproliferative effects,
- lowers neointimal hyperplasia, and
- decreases smooth muscle cell migration.[140]

The consumption of up to two alcoholic drinks per day is inversely associated with extensive coronary calcification. The risk for severe coronary calcification is 50% lower in individuals who consume one to two alcoholic beverages per day than in nondrinkers.[141]

In a cross-sectional study using data from the population-based Rotterdam Coronary Calcification Study, data on alcohol consumption were available for 1795 individuals without known CHD, aged on average 71 years. Coronary calcification was quantified via electron beam computed tomography. When compared with nondrinkers, the odds ratio of extensive coronary calcification was 0.60 for those who consumed one drink or less daily, 0.51 for those who consumed one to two drinks daily, but 0.90 for those who consumed in excess of two drinks a day.[141]

Antithrombotic Effects. Alcohol has antithrombotic and fibrinolytic effects. It decreases fibrinogen levels, platelet activation, and platelet aggregability and adhesion while increasing levels of plasminogen and tissue plasminogen activator (tPA).[142]

Moderate red wine intake significantly reduces platelet deposition triggered by damage to the vessel wall, in part as a result of inhibition of RhoA translocation to the platelet membrane. An experimental porcine model of diet-induced hyperlipidemia was fed a Western-type, proatherogenic diet for a hundred days. Three doses of red wine were studied (20, 30, and 40 g of red wine per day) and compared with placebo-control pigs not imbibing any wine. Mural platelet deposition was significantly reduced in animals consuming red wine with their menu. Although total cholesterol levels were not significantly different among groups, expression of inactive RhoA in the platelet cytoplasm was increased, and the mRNA expression of tissue factor in lipopolysaccharide-stimulated monocytes was reduced in wine-drinking animals.[143]

Cardiovascular Disease. The ingestion of alcohol is associated with a low prevalence of cardiovascular disease.

Alcohol ingestion is inversely associated with the risk for fatal and nonfatal MI. Men who consume less than one drink per week have higher rates of MI than do men who consume alcohol on 3 to 7 days per week. The daily consumption of moderate amounts of wine is associated with lower mortality from cardiovascular, cerebrovascular, and other causes.[142] Alcohol consumption is associated with a reduced risk for percutaneous and surgical revascularization, and the multivariate relative risk for CHD is 0.55 (confidence interval, 0.39 to 0.77) for men who drink two drinks per day and 0.4 (confidence interval, 0.2 to 0.8) for women who drink two drinks per day when compared with teetotalers.[144,145] At 150 mL/day of wine consumption, there is a significant reduction in all vascular end points. Maximal risk reduction occurs at 750 mL/day of wine consumption.[146]

Plasma Lipids. Moderate ethanol intake from any type of beverage improves lipoprotein metabolism. Alcohol

- raises plasma HDL by 10% to 15%, possibly by increasing apolipoprotein A-I and A-II transport rates or production without changing HDL catabolism. Both larger and smaller HDL particle size fractions are increased;
- reduces LDL modestly;
- decreases Lp(a); and
- increases triglycerides.

The alcohol-related increase in HDL constitutes only 50% of the cardioprotective effect.[147]

Lipoprotein(a). Serum Lp(a) is a powerful predictor of CHD in patients. Serum Lp(a) is inversely and dose-dependently related to alcohol intake in patients with hypertension, and this relationship is independent of the size distribution of Lp(a) isoforms. The reduction in Lp(a) concentrations via regular consumption of alcohol has a favorable impact on the CHD risk profile of hypertensive patients and lowers their cardiovascular morbidity.[148]

Impact on Lipoprotein Metabolism. Alcohol affects not only the actual levels of circulating lipoproteins. It also alters the functionality of lipoproteins and enzymes involved in lipid metabolism.

Alcohol changes the composition of lipoproteins. It lowers the sialic acid content of the HDL apolipoproteins E and J. Alcohol effects an acetaldehyde modification of apolipoproteins. "Abnormal" lipids, such as phosphatidylethanol and fatty acid ethyl esters, arise in the presence of alcohol and associate with plasma lipoproteins. Alcohol modulates the interactions of lipoproteins with endothelial and smooth muscle cells, monocytes, and macrophages.[149]

Alcohol also changes plasma proteins and enzymes associated with lipoprotein metabolism, such as

- cholesteryl ester transfer protein (CETP),
- phospholipid transfer protein (PLTP),
- lecithin-cholesterol acyltransferase (LCAT),
- lipoprotein lipase (LPL),
- hepatic lipase (HL),

- paraoxonase-1, and
- phospholipases.[149]

Insulin Resistance. Alcohol enhances the sensitivity to insulin action.

Although the acute effects of alcohol induce a state of insulin resistance after a glucose load, long-term exposure to alcohol is associated with an improvement in insulin sensitivity. Consumers of moderate amounts of alcohol have less insulin resistance and a reduced risk for type 2 DM.

A substantial number of prospective studies suggest that regular, light to moderate, chronic alcohol intake is protective against the development of type 2 DM, as well as against the onset of CHD in diabetic subjects.[150] Moderate alcohol consumption of 30 g of alcohol, or two drinks, per day by postmenopausal, nondiabetic women improves insulin sensitivity by 7% and reduces the fasting insulin concentration by 19%. In the prospective cohort Nurses' Health Study with 116,671 participants, moderate alcohol consumption, when adjusted for multiple covariates, was inversely related to HbA_{1C} levels.[151]

Alcohol has antioxidant, anti-inflammatory, and vasculoprotective effects and would thus be expected to have a favorable impact on insulin resistance. In addition, a number of other factors may play a role:

- Alcohol may reduce hepatic gluconeogenesis.
- Alcohol increases insulin binding factors.
- Alcohol may increase plasma leptin levels, thereby decreasing appetite and food intake.[151]
- Moderate alcohol intake increases levels of adiponectin, an adipocyte-derived plasma protein positively associated with insulin sensitivity. In 23 healthy, middle-aged male subjects consuming four glasses of whisky (40 g of ethanol) or tap water daily with dinner for 17 days, the plasma adiponectin level increased by 11% (P = .0002). In an insulin-resistant subgroup, there was a concomitant increase in the index for insulin sensitivity that positively correlated with the alcohol-induced, relative rise in plasma adiponectin levels (r = .73, P = .02).[152]

Total Mortality. The beneficial and detrimental effects of alcohol may be described by a U-shaped relationship between alcohol consumption and total mortality. The minimum all-cause mortality for middle-aged and older individuals occurs at one to three drinks per day on 3 or more days per week. Individuals with a genetic polymorphism associated with slower alcohol metabolism derive more cardioprotection per drink than do those with a faster metabolism.[142]

COCOA AND CHOCOLATES

Flavonoids, or plant polyphenols, are major constituents of cocoa solids in dark chocolate. **Cocoa actually contains more flavonoids than wine or tea does.** Flavonoid bioavailability is greater for high-quality, dark chocolate than for milk chocolate because the addition of milk to lighten chocolate may inhibit gastrointestinal flavonoid absorption.

Cocoa flavonoids may be responsible for the vasculoprotective properties of dark chocolate. Dark chocolate consumption is associated with favorable blood pressure effects, with lowering of both systolic and diastolic blood pressure. It increases plasma antioxidant capacity in humans. Cocoa butter may have a beneficial impact on cholesterol levels. The acute ingestion of chocolate improves endothelial function as measured by flow-mediated dilation of the brachial artery, an effect that lasts for approximately 3 hours.[153]

FLAVONOIDS

There is an apparent low prevalence of CHD in populations that consume dietary sources rich in flavonoids. Consumption of a diet rich in flavonoids, such as red wine and tea, is associated with decreased cardiovascular risk and is of benefit as part of the overall strategy for improving vascular health. A better understanding of the pharmacokinetics and bioavailability of individual isoflavones is needed for definitive dietary recommendations.

Structure and Subtypes of Flavonoids. Several thousand flavonoids have been identified. They serve as plant pigments, many of which are metabolically active with beneficial health effects.

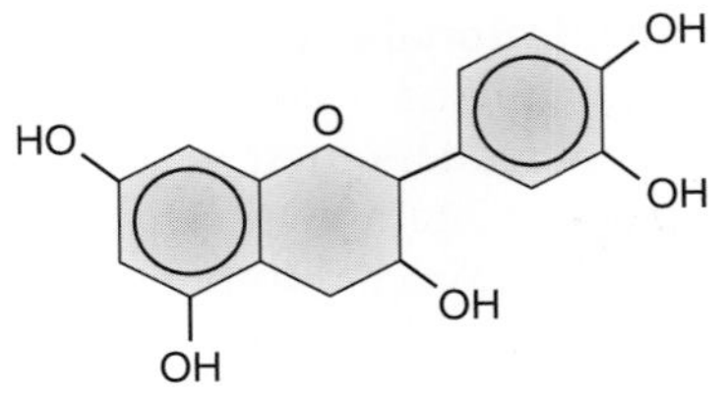

HO O OH OH OH OH

Epicatechin

Figure 15–9.
Two phenol rings linked by a three-carbon group compose part of a heterocyclic ring in the chemical structure of the simple flavonoid epicatechin.

Isoflavones or flavonoids are a subclass of polyphenols. They generally consist of two aromatic rings, each containing at least one hydroxyl group. The aromatic rings are connected through a three-carbon segment forming part of a six-member heterocyclic ring (Fig. 15-9). The flavonoids are further divided into subclasses based on the connection of an aromatic ring to the heterocyclic ring, as well as the oxidation state and functional groups of the heterocyclic ring. Within each subclass, individual compounds are characterized by specific hydroxylation and conjugation patterns.[154]

Many flavonoids in foods also occur as large molecules, or tannins, that are naturally present or generated during food handling. In the process, monomers are connected through specific carbon-carbon and ether linkages to form polymers. Catechins are simple flavonoids that are abundant in green tea. Proanthocyanidins are condensed tannins that are composed of smaller units, including catechins and epicatechins. They serve as precursors to anthocyanidins. Anthocyanidins are a type of complex flavonoid that produces blue, purple, or red food colors. Resveratrol is abundant in red grape skins and red wine. Quercetin is ubiquitous in higher plants, especially in red grapes and onions. Limonene is a flavonoid substance found in citrus rinds. Lycopene is present in tomatoes and watermelons. Derived tannins are formed during the fermentation and processing of black and oolong tea.[154]

Some flavonoids have estrogenic activity. Their similarity to steroidal estrogens has stimulated research into their potential to confer a cardiovascular benefit related to improved vascular function.[155]

Antioxidant Activity. Flavonoids have very potent antioxidant activity. They are water-soluble antioxidants that work in concert with the lipid-soluble carotene antioxidants to protect plants from free radical injury. Consumption of flavonoids may decrease lipid peroxidation.[156]

Anti-inflammatory Activity. Flavonoids have anti-inflammatory activity.

Curcumin selectively inhibits thromboxane production while sparing prostacyclin.[157] Flavonoids such as apigenin, chrysin, and kaempferol are all significant stimulators of PPAR-γ. Upon binding, they activate PPAR-γ via allosteric, conformational changes, thus reducing the inflammatory response by decreasing both inducible COX and iNOS.[155]

Gallic acid, one of the most abundant polyphenols in red wine, has antioxidant, anti-inflammatory, cardioprotective, and anticarcinogenic activity. Gallic acid is abundantly available not only in grape wine but also in green tea and chocolate. The total gallic acid content in various red wines ranges from 35 to 70 mg/L and is 2.2 mg/mL in green tea. Per serving, cocoa contains higher total gallate levels than green tea or red wine does (611 versus 165 and 340 mg per serving, respectively). Gallic acid can potently interfere with P-selectin function, an adhesion molecule that is implicated in atherothrombosis and malignancy. P-selectin mediates leukocyte-endothelium, leukocyte-platelet, and platelet-platelet interactions via the initial rolling of monocytes along the inflamed endothelium. It enhances platelet cohesion and platelet-leukocyte aggregation. P-selectin also plays a role in metastasis by promoting tumor growth and metastatic seeding. In effects not attributable to its antioxidant activity, gallic acid, at concentrations readily achieved after moderate wine, green tea, or cocoa consumption, inhibits P-selectin–mediated inflammation both in vitro and in vivo by binding and antagonizing P-selectin.[158]

Vascular Protection and Prevention of Coronary Heart Disease. Isoflavones have a favorable impact on several parameters of arterial function, such as improved

- endothelial function,
- arterial compliance, and
- vasodilatory effects of the microcirculation.

Endothelial dysfunction is reversed after the intake of flavonoid-containing beverages, including green tea, grape juice, and red wine.[159]

Flavonoid intake is associated with a reduced incidence of CHD events. In the Dutch Zutphen Study, cohorts of 550 to 800 men, monitored for 10 to 15 years, had strong inverse associations between the amount of flavonoid intake and CHD, stroke, and mortality from ischemic heart disease.[160,161] The 25-year Seven Countries Study of 12,763 men also demonstrated an inverse correlation between flavonoid intake and CHD mortality.[162]

Dietary Sources of Flavonoids. Flavonoids are widely distributed in nature. However, their distribution is not uniform, thus rendering only specific foods rich sources for one or more subclasses of these polyphenols. Isoflavones are also sold as nutriceuticals. The polyphenolic structure of flavonoids and tannins renders them quite sensitive to oxidative enzymes and cooking conditions.

Foods Rich in Biologically Active Flavonoids

FOOD GROUP	FOOD TYPE
Grape products	Red wine, red/purple grapes
Berries	Blueberries, cranberries, blackberries, cherries
Fruits	Cocoa, pomegranates, apricots, citrus fruits, tomatoes
Vegetables	Carrots, squash, onions, beets, purple cabbage
Legumes	Soy
Spices	Garlic, turmeric
Tea	White, green, oolong, black tea

Adapted from http://exchange.healthwell.com/nutritionsciencenews/nsn_backs/Aug_99/cancer.cfm.

ANTIOXIDANTS

Low levels of reactive oxygen and nitrogen species are byproducts of regular oxidative metabolism. These oxidant species participate in immunologic host defense and may function as signaling molecules. However, high levels of oxidant species, in the absence of appropriate compensatory, endogenous antioxidant responses, are potentially damaging to cellular macromolecules, lead to the activation of stress-sensitive signaling pathways, and are implicated in the pathogenesis of insulin resistance. Furthermore, oxidized LDL is the most atherogenic form of LDL.[105]

Antioxidant Rationale. Epidemiologic studies suggest that increased intake of a diet enriched in antioxidants reduces the risk for CHD. Conceptually, appropriate and effective antioxidant intake would be expected to prevent or reverse the activation of destructive oxidant pathways and LDL oxidation, thereby favorably affecting insulin sensitivity and vascular health.[105]

Antioxidants, Nitric Oxide, and eNOS. Dietary antioxidants improve the endothelial function of coronary and peripheral vessels via several mechanisms:

- Antioxidants may scavenge free radicals, thereby preventing NO oxidation and thus lengthening the half-life of NO.
- Antioxidants decrease the activation of redox-transcription factors, reduce free radical–induced inflammatory responses, and increase eNOS expression in human endothelial cells.[163]
- Antioxidants may also enhance the activity of NOS by preserving the NOS cofactor tetrahydrobiopterin (BH_4).[164]

Antioxidants mitigate the deleterious effect of high fat intake on endothelial function. Dietary antioxidant pretreatment via ingestion of dark leafy vegetables, red wine, or purple grape juice before or with a fatty meal can prevent fatty acid–induced endothelial dysfunction.[165,166] Interestingly, a prolonged, 4-week antioxidant food-phytochemical supplementation, not administered at the time of a meal, had a similar protective effect on vascular function and significantly increased NO metabolites consistent with increased NO bioactivity (Fig. 15-10).[167]

Lipid-Soluble Antioxidants—Vitamin E. Vitamin E is a potent lipid-soluble, chain-breaking antioxidant. There are eight naturally occurring tocopherols. Natural α-tocopherol (5,7,8-trimethyltocol) accounts for 90% of tocopherols in animal tissue and displays the greatest biologic activity in most bioassays. It is structurally related to a member of the coenzyme Q group and possesses similar biologic activity. The *d*-optical isomer is twice as active as the *l*-form, and natural *d*-α-tocopherol, derived from soybean oil, is twice as potent as the synthetic *dl*-version of vitamin E, synthesized from petroleum. γ-Tocopherol is another beneficial form of

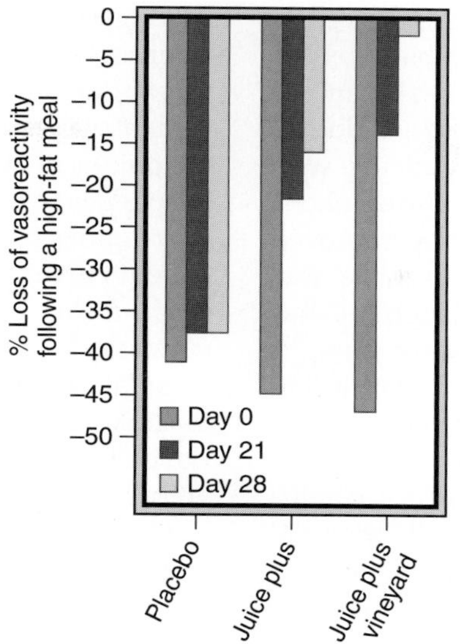

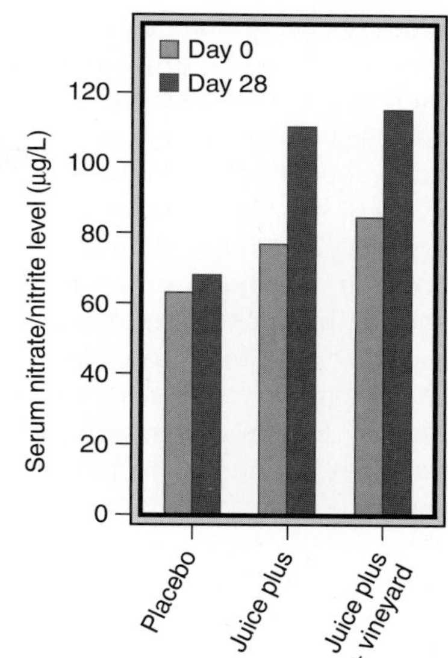

Figure 15–10. Impact of regular phytochemical antioxidant supplementation for 3 and 4 weeks on brachial artery vasoreactivity after a high-fat meal and on serum levels of nitrate/nitrite. *(Modified from Plotnick GD, Corretti MC, Vogel RA, et al. Effect of supplemental phytonutrients on impairment of the flow-mediated brachial artery vasoreactivity after a single high-fat meal. J Am Coll Cardiol 2003;41:1744-1749.)*

vitamin E found in nuts, vegetable oils, whole grains, and leafy vegetables.[168,169]

The data for vitamin E are inconsistent. Whereas vitamin E improves endothelial function in patients with multiple risk factors, such as cigarette smoking, a number of other studies have shown no benefit,[170] including the large-scale, randomized Heart Outcomes Prevention Evaluation (HOPE) trial, which failed to demonstrate any effect of vitamin E on CHD events.[171]

Excessive vitamin E supplementation may actually be harmful. In a meta-analysis of 19 placebo-controlled studies comprising 136,967 subjects who were taking 16.5 to 2000 IU/day of vitamin E, those taking 400 IU/day or more had 5% higher mortality in follow-up than control subjects did. Doses of 150 mg/day or less had no increased risk. Adverse effects may have been due to the displacement or inhibition of other endogenous antioxidants by high doses of vitamin E and thereby disrupting the natural balance of antioxidant activity. Vitamin E may, in fact, have pro-oxidant effects at high doses and contribute to lipoprotein peroxidation. Vitamin E confers an increased risk for bleeding because of its anticoagulant properties attributable to interference with vitamin K–dependent coagulation.[172]

Vitamin E Interdependence with Vitamin C. Lipid-soluble vitamin E is thought to require water-soluble vitamin C for effective antioxidant action. As vitamin E is oxidized by oxidant exposure, it needs to be reduced to regain its antioxidant efficacy. In order to export oxidant stress beyond the lipid milieu of cell membranes, vitamin E resorts to water-soluble, circulating vitamin C to regenerate the reduced form of α-tocopherol, which is capable of renewed antioxidant, intracellular engagement.

Vitamins E and C, working in concert, may inhibit the oxidation of LDL; lower levels of PAI-1, CRP, and IL-6; and restore endothelial function. Vitamins E and C protected against the elevations in PAI-1 and CRP induced by an evening high-fat meal.[61] Supplementation with antioxidant vitamins E and C also restored endothelial function in hyperlipidemic children.[163]

However, other studies of combinations of vitamins C and E have been disappointing, some showing increased mortality.[172,173] The Heart Protection Study examined such a combination in 20,536 individuals with CHD, type 2 DM, or peripheral vascular disease and demonstrated no impact on cardiovascular events.[174]

Water-Soluble Antioxidants—Vitamin C. Vitamin C is the main water-soluble antioxidant in human plasma. Epidemiologic studies suggest that individuals with low or deficient levels of vitamin C have increased cardiovascular risk.[175] Vitamin C may stabilize the NOS cofactor BH_4 and thus enhance endothelial NO synthesis. Ascorbate recycles the radical trihydrobiopterin back to BH_4, thereby increasing its availability.[163,176] Vitamin C administration consistently improves endothelium-dependent vasodilation in patients with CHD.[170] In hypertensives and cigarette smokers, 2 years of 2000 mg vitamin C per day improved vascular function, although no response was seen in hypercholesterolemics.[177] Vitamin C has an inhibitory effect on platelet aggregation.[178] In a prospective study of 85,118 women in the Nurses' Health Study, after adjusting for other variables, women who took vitamin C supplements of 360 mg/day or greater had a significant, 28% lower risk for incident CHD than did women who did not take such supplements. Vitamin C from dietary sources alone was not associated with risk reduction.[179]

α-Lipoic Acid. α-Lipoic acid is a naturally occurring antioxidant and a cofactor in the pyruvate dehydrogenase complex (Fig. 15-11). Supplementation decreases oxidative stress and restores the active, reduced forms of other endogenous antioxidants in vivo. α-Lipoic acid raises intracellular levels of glutathione.[66,180]

α-Lipoic acid and dihydrolipoic acid function as a redox couple. With a low redox potential of −0.32 V, α-lipoic acid is a powerful antioxidant in its reduced form. α-Lipoic acid

- exhibits direct free radical–scavenging properties,
- prevents singlet oxygen–induced DNA damage,
- reduces lipid peroxidation,
- prevents serum albumin glycation, and
- reduces NFκB activation in vitro as well as in patients with type 2 DM.

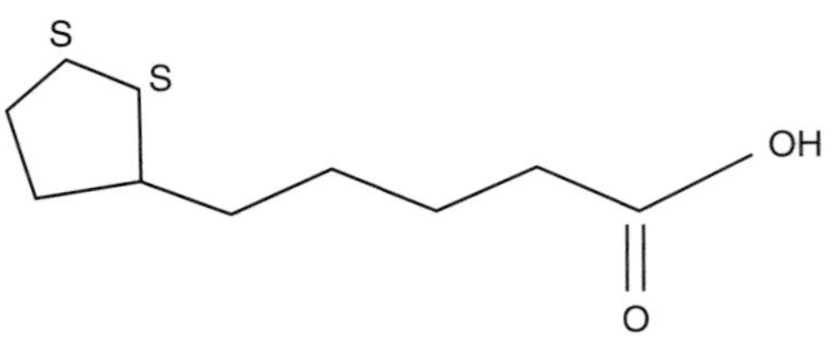

▸▸ **Figure 15–11.**
Chemical structure of α-lipoic acid.

α-Lipoic acid enhances not only antioxidant defenses but also endothelial cell function. Because insulin resistance is associated with excessive oxidant stress and dysfunctional endothelium, α-lipoic acid has been suggested as a dietary supplement for insulin-resistant states.[181]

α-Lipoic acid improves insulin sensitivity in patients with type 2 DM, possibly by protecting cells from oxidant stress–induced insulin resistance.[105] Muscle is the major site of insulin-stimulated glucose disposal. In diabetic patients, α-lipoic acid improves glucose transport in skeletal muscle and thereby results in enhanced glucose disposal.[182]

Oxidative stress causes rapid activation of the stress-sensitive p38 MAPK. In insulin resistance, the effects of α-lipoic acid may also be mediated by preventing the stress-induced activation of p38, coincident with the restoration of insulin signaling near the point of Akt/PKB phosphorylation, thus protecting insulin action.[182,183]

N-acetyl-L-cysteine is a positively charged analogue of α-lipoic acid. It functions as a reduced thiol donor with antioxidant properties and can also block the NFκB signaling cascade.[105]

Grape Seeds. Grape seeds contain antioxidant components that may be vasculoprotective. Procyanidins from *Vitis vinifera L.* grape seeds layer on the surface of endothelial cells. They dose-dependently inhibit extracellular oxidation and quench exogenous harmful radicals. They prevent endothelin-1–mediated vasoconstriction and dose-dependently relax vascular smooth muscle by stimulating prostacyclin release.[184]

Antioxidant Controversy. Despite the compelling rationale in favor of antioxidant therapy and some supportive experimental data, the protective role of antioxidants is only partially established by human studies. Observational and epidemiologic data, as well as randomized trials, have generated mixed results on the protective role of antioxidants against cardiovascular disease.

The antioxidant vitamins E and C can both exert pro-oxidant effects in vitro. They are incompletely effective at suppressing elevated levels of oxidative biomarkers in humans. Oral intake of vitamin E only modestly increases its plasma and tissue levels, and its slow rate of reaction with reactive oxygen species implies that vitamin E, at the concentrations reached in tissue, is unlikely to affect biologic outcomes. Myeloperoxidase has emerged as a major source of pro-oxidant radical generation in inflammatory syndromes; however, myeloperoxidase-catalyzed lipid peroxidation is resistant to inhibition by vitamin E.[185]

None of the major antioxidant trials to date has systematically measured markers of oxidative stress in order to ensure intervention in an appropriate treatment group and to document the efficacy of antioxidant therapy. The background antioxidant status of trial participants may have obscured a beneficial effect. In addition, the antioxidants studied may have had insufficient activity against the relevant oxidants. Moreover, different antioxidant strategies may have varied impact on diverse sources of oxidant stress. Failure of antioxidants in clinical trials may be due to the initiation of such therapy once a disease process has become established, whereas the benefits observed in animal models may derive from antioxidant intervention during the early phase of disease evolution.[114] Discrepant study findings may also be due to varying dietary vitamin content; suboptimal doses, formulations, and combinations of vitamins; or noncompliance and inadequate follow-up to detect a benefit.[186] Additionally, antioxidant supplements may have failed to cull the specific composite of antioxidants that render the consumption of fruits and vegetables so salubrious.

Although studies on antioxidant supplementation have been disappointing, recent data do reinforce the concept that regular intake of nutrients rich in dietary antioxidants is protective of vascular health.[187]

Foods Rich in Antioxidants

Asparagus	Chili peppers	Onion
Avocado	Collard greens	Oranges
Barley	Cranberries	Parsley
Bell peppers	Elderberries	Plums
Bilberries	Ginger	Spinach
Blueberries	Grapefruit	Strawberries
Broccoli	Kiwi	Tomatoes
Brussels sprouts	Lecithin	Watermelons
Cabbage	Melons	Yams
Carrots	Nuts	

Adapted from http://www.naturalways.com/medValFd.htm.

FOLIC ACID

Folic acid is a water-soluble B vitamin. It has a beneficial impact on cardiovascular disease, neurodegenerative disorders, neural tube defects, and cancer. Methyltetrahydrofolate, the active form of folic acid, functions as an electron donor, a hydrogen donor, and a methyl donor.

Folic acid helps restore endothelium-dependent vasodilation by maintaining the essential eNOS cofactor BH_4 and by lowering homocysteine levels:

1. A necessary cofactor for eNOS, BH_4 is essential for coupling of the eNOS reaction. Specifically, BH_4 mediates the coupling of L-arginine to the NADH/NADPH oxidase enzyme for L-arginine to be oxidized to NO and L-citrulline. Folic acid restores BH_4 by supplying both hydrogen and electrons to BH_2 and BH_3 (Fig. 15-12). In the absence of such coupling, the uncoupled eNOS reaction generates superoxide.[188,189]
2. By decreasing dimethylarginine dimethylaminohydrolase (DDAH) levels, homocysteine raises plasma levels of asymmetric dimethylarginine (ADMA), a competitive antagonist to L-arginine.[190] Homocysteine also impairs endothelium-derived hyperpolarizing factor–mediated small vessel dilation.[191] Folic acid remethylates homocysteine to methionine, thus lowering homocysteine levels.[192] The lowering of homocysteine effectively improves large and small vessel endothelial function.

Foods Rich in Folic Acid

Green vegetables	Broccoli, spinach, Brussels sprouts, cauliflower, asparagus
Legumes	Green, yellow, baked, pinto, and kidney beans; peas; lentils; peanuts
Fruits	Oranges, cantaloupes, strawberries
Nuts and seeds	Sunflower seeds
Whole-grain breads and cereals	Bran cereal, whole-wheat bread, wheat germ, quinoa

L-ARGININE

L-Arginine may have a beneficial impact on vascular function and sensitivity to insulin signaling.

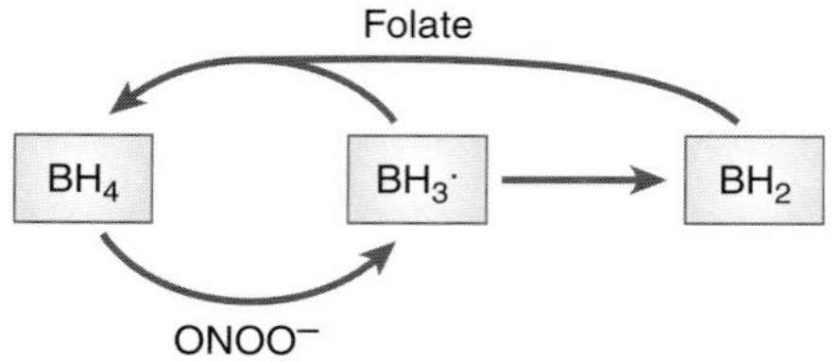

▸▸ **Figure 15–12.**
Folate-mediated restoration of tetrahydrobiopterin (BH_4) after its oxidation by peroxynitrite ($ONOO^-$), with generation of an intermediate radical and dihydrobiopterin (BH_2).

Dietary antioxidant intake and L-arginine supplementation may have synergistic effects with moderate exercise in increasing vascular protection. In hypercholesterolemic mice consuming a high-cholesterol diet with or without an exercise program and randomized to no supplements, to vitamins C and E, or to vitamins C and E and L-arginine, those receiving vitamins C and E and L-arginine had significant reductions in markers of oxidative stress. Additionally, in exercising, hypercholesterolemic mice, the effect of antioxidant and L-arginine supplementation was to further reduce the number of foam cells and the progression of atherosclerotic lesions when compared with exercise-only mice. The reduction in atherosclerotic lesion areas in exercised mice receiving antioxidants and L-arginine correlated with an increase in the expression of eNOS.[193]

High-dose L-arginine treatment appears to improve, but not completely normalize endothelial function and peripheral and hepatic insulin sensitivity in type 2 diabetic individuals. In 12 lean, type 2 diabetic subjects, 3 g of L-arginine was administered three times daily for 1 month. As eNOS substrate, L-arginine, acting through improvement in the NO/cyclic guanosine-3′, 5′-monophosphate (cGMP) pathway, normalized basal cGMP levels. L-Arginine significantly increased forearm blood flow by 36% and lowered systolic blood pressure by 14%. It increased glucose disposal during euglycemic-hyperinsulinemic clamp by 34% and decreased endogenous glucose production by 29% (Table 15-3).[194]

Table 15–3. Foods Rich in L-Arginine

Plant products	Carob, chocolate, coconut, hummus, soybeans, tofu, black beans
Dairy products	Milk, cheese, cottage cheese
Nuts	Peanuts, peanut butter, pecans, walnuts, almonds, Brazil nuts, cashews, filberts, pignoli nuts
Grains	White and whole wheat flour, oats, edible seeds
Meats and animal products	Gelatin, meat (venison, turkey, beef, chicken, pork), eggs
Sea products	Whelk (sea snail), dried spirulina (seaweed), fish (tuna, salmon, bass), spiny lobster, Alaskan king crab, crayfish, clams, octopus

CALCIUM AND DAIRY PRODUCTS

Increased calcium (Ca^{2+}) intake is related to reductions in body fat mass. Ca^{2+} plays a substantial role in reducing the incidence of obesity and the prevalence of insulin resistance. The impact of Ca^{2+} intake on weight loss, or on prevention of weight gain, has been demonstrated in a wide age range of white and African American individuals of both genders.[195]

Low-Calcium Diets. Low-calcium diets promote adiposity. Calcitriol, produced in response to low-Ca^{2+} diets, stimulates Ca^{2+} influx into human adipocytes. Intracellular Ca^{2+} plays a key role in the regulation of adipocyte lipid metabolism and triacylglycerol storage. Increased intracellular Ca^{2+} results in

- stimulation of lipogenic gene expression,
- stimulation of lipogenesis, and
- suppression of lipolysis,

thereby effecting adipocyte hypertrophy and increased adiposity.[196]

High-Calcium Diets. In contrast, high dietary Ca^{2+} contributes to the prevention of obesity. By suppressing calcitriol and a rise in intracellular Ca^{2+} levels, high-calcium diets attenuate adipocyte lipid accretion and weight gain during periods of overconsumption of an energy-dense diet. Conversely, during caloric restriction, high calcium intake increases lipolysis and preserves thermogenesis, thereby further accelerating weight loss.[196]

Dairy Consumption. Among overweight adults, dietary patterns characterized by ample dairy consumption have a strong, inverse association with the metabolic syndrome. Dairy products, even full-fat versions, lower the odds for development of the metabolic syndrome and may ultimately reduce the risk for type 2 DM and cardiovascular disease.[195] Cheese, particularly high-quality natural cheese, can be consumed in a dietary plan akin to the heart-healthy Mediterranean diet.

The metabolic effect of dairy nutrients may be mediated by compounds intrinsic to dairy products, such as Ca^{2+}, or by the displacement of less healthful foods from the diet, such as those containing high-fructose corn syrup or *trans*–fatty acids.[25]

However, when compared with equivalent amounts of supplemental calcium, animal, epidemiologic, and clinical data demonstrate that dairy products exert a substantially greater effect on

- accelerating fat loss,
- fat distribution, and
- attenuating weight and fat gain.

Higher consumption of dairy products is also associated with

- reduced blood pressure,
- decreased platelet aggregation, and
- a lower risk for stroke.[197]

This augmented effect of dairy versus supplemental Ca^{2+} is probably attributable to additional bioactive compounds in dairy products acting synergistically with Ca^{2+} to attenuate adiposity. Among such bioactive compounds in dairy products are branched-chain amino acids and angiotensin-converting enzyme inhibitory peptides.[196] The consumption of dairy products also conveys a significant intake of minerals in addition to Ca^{2+}, such as magnesium and potassium, all of which potentially contribute to the risk reduction.[197]

In a dietary study, 32 adults aged on average 49 years with a mean BMI of 34.9 kg/m^2, placed on one of three dietary regimens incorporating 400 to 500 mg Ca^{2+}, 800 mg Ca^{2+}, or 1200 to 1300 mg Ca^{2+} with dairy, achieved body weight losses of 6.4%, 8.6%, and 10.9%, respectively, with fat losses of 4.8, 5.6, and 7.2 kg, respectively. Loss of abdominal fat was also highest in the high-Ca^{2+}/dairy group.[198]

In the Coronary Artery Risk Development in Young Adults (CARDIA) study, a population-based prospective study of 3157 adults aged 18 to 30 years monitored from 1985-1986 to 1995-1996, dairy consumption was inversely associated with the incidence of all metabolic syndrome components in individuals who were overweight (BMI ≥25 kg/m^2) at baseline, but not in leaner individuals. The adjusted odds of two or more components of the metabolic syndrome developing were 72% lower in overweight individuals in the highest than in the lowest category of dairy consumption. Each daily occasion of dairy consumption was associated with 21% lower odds of the metabolic syndrome. These associations applied to African American and white individuals and to men and women and were not explained by other dietary factors.[199]

MAGNESIUM

Magnesium deficiency has adverse cardiovascular consequences, with a negative impact on hypertension, DM, arrhythmias, atherosclerosis, and sudden death.[200]

Endothelial Function. Decreased intracellular magnesium levels impair NO release from the vascular endothelium.[201] Oral magnesium supplementation (15 mmol magnesium ion, 365 mg magnesium citrate) improves endothelial function as measured by brachial artery flow–mediated dilation. In patients with CHD, magnesium supplementation also improves exercise tolerance and quality of life after 6 months of supplementation.[202,203]

Coronary Vascular Disease. Magnesium may lessen the risk for CHD. In a study of 7172 men in the Honolulu Heart Program, the lowest daily consumption of magnesium (50 to 186 mg/day) was associated with a 1.5- to 1.8-fold increase in CHD incidence over 15 years when compared with the highest magnesium intake (340 to 1183 mg/day). The difference in incidence pertained after adjustments for age, nutrients, and other cardiovascular risk factors.[204]

Insulin Action. There appears to be an inverse association between magnesium intake and the risk for type 2 DM. Magnesium supplementation improves insulin action in elderly patients. In the Nurses' Health Study, there was a significant, inverse relationship between magnesium intake and the development of DM, particularly for women with a BMI of 25 kg/m^2 or greater. Mean insulin levels in overweight women were inversely related to magnesium intake.[205] In a 12- to 18-year follow-up study of 127,932 men and women, after adjusting for family history, age, BMI, physical activity, smoking, alcohol consumption, hypertension, and hypercholesterolemia, the relative risk for type 2 DM was 0.67 ($P < .001$) for men and 0.66 ($P < .001$) for women in the highest as compared with the lowest quintiles of magnesium intake.[206]

OTHER SPECIFIC FOOD ITEMS

Numerous epidemiologic studies have concluded that the consumption of fruits and vegetables reduces cardiovascular disease, DM, and cancer risk. The vitamin, antioxidant, mineral, fiber, and folate content of fruits and vegetables has a major impact on disease prevention and may partially explain their protective effect in lowering the incidence of cardiovascular and metabolic disease. Other compounds, such as flavonoids, phytates, lycopenes, carotenoids, and other phytochemicals in fruits and vegetables, probably also play a protective role.

The benefit of fruit or vegetable consumption rises significantly with the number of servings consumed. In a Greek study of 848 patients admitted with acute coronary syndrome and 1078 controls, individuals in the upper quintile of fruit consumption (five or more items per day) had a 72% lower risk for CHD events (odds ratio, 0.28) when compared with those in the lowest quintile (less than one item per day). Consumption of vegetables on more than 3 days per week was associated with a 70% lower risk for CHD events (odds ratio, 0.30) when compared with absent vegetable intake.[207]

Apples are rich in fiber, specifically pectin, which has a favorable impact on glucose and lipid homeostasis. Apples suppress appetite and have anti-inflammatory activity. They may lower the risk for cancer.

Asparagus is an excellent source for the antioxidant glutathione. It may lower the risk for cancer.

Avocados are rich in monounsaturated oleic acid. They are one of the richest sources of the powerful antioxidant glutathione. They have plenty of fiber, folate, vitamin B_6, and vitamin C.

Barley contains potent antioxidants, including tocotrienols.

Beans, including navy, black, kidney, pinto, soy, and lentils, are very high in fiber, with potent, beneficial effects on carbohydrate and lipid metabolism.

Beets are rich in iron and other minerals and are of benefit with obesity.

Bell peppers are rich in the antioxidant vitamin C.

Blueberries are powerful nutritional antioxidants and are rich in flavonoids, vitamin C, and dietary fiber.

Broccoli is abundant in antioxidant vitamins, carotenes, and flavonoids, including glutathione, vitamin C, β-carotene, quercetin, indoles, lutein, glucarate, and sulforaphane. It has ample fiber and chromium and may lower the risk for cancer.

Brussels sprouts possess some of the same properties as broccoli and cabbage.

Cabbage (including bok choy) contains numerous antioxidant compounds and can reduce the risk for cancer.

Carrots are a superb source of β-carotene, a powerful antioxidant. Carrots have a high soluble fiber content.

Cauliflower contains many of the same beneficial compounds as broccoli and cabbage.

Celery has a mild diuretic effect. Celery compounds reduce blood pressure in animals.

Chili peppers have antioxidant activity. They suppress appetite and increase the metabolic rate.

Cinnamon is a stimulant of insulin activity. It has mild anticoagulant activity.

Cranberries are powerful nutritional antioxidants rich in dietary fiber. Their consumption may raise levels of HDL.

Collard greens have antioxidant activity as a result of lutein, vitamin C, and β-carotene.

Eggplant has diuretic and antioxidant activity with beneficial vascular effects.

Fenugreek seed steadies carbohydrate metabolism and may have a beneficial impact on blood pressure.

Eggs are low in saturated fats and rich in nutrients, including vitamins A, D, E, and K, as well as iron. Egg whites are an excellent source of protein. Lutein in the yolk is an effective antioxidant and may be of benefit in preventing macular degeneration. Although the yolk is also rich in cholesterol, the presence of phosphatidylcholine in the yolk appears to decrease the dietary absorption of cholesterol. Eggs derived from hens fed special mash may be enriched in n-3 fatty acids. An egg a day has no significant impact on the risk for heart disease and stroke.

Elderberries are powerful nutritional antioxidants rich in flavonoids, vitamin C, and dietary fiber.[96]

Garlic has been used by the ancient Egyptians, Chinese, and Greeks for medicinal purposes to fight numerous maladies. An active flavonoid in garlic is allixin.

Garlic has many components with potential antibiotic, antiplatelet, and antithrombotic properties. It has been reported to have antihypertensive effects. Although garlic has no significant lipid-lowering efficacy, it may benefit vascular health. Meta-analysis findings also suggest that garlic may have some efficacy in the prevention of bladder, stomach, and gastrointestinal cancer.[208]

Mushrooms are valued for their promise as disease preventive agents. Diverse mushrooms have antioxidative, anti-inflammatory, vasculoprotective, anticancer, and antidiabetic properties.[209]

Mustard (including horseradish) increases the metabolic rate.

Oats are rich in fiber and exert stabilizing effects on lipid and carbohydrate metabolism.

Onions (including chives, shallots, scallions, leeks) are exceptionally strong antioxidants. Shallots, yellow and red onions, but not white onions, are the richest dietary sources of quercetin, a potent antioxidant. Onions have anti-inflammatory effects.

Oranges contain carotenoids, terpenes, and flavonoids. They are also rich in antioxidant vitamin C and β-carotene.

Parsley has high concentrations of antioxidants such as monoterpenes, phthalides, and polyacetylenes. It also has diuretic activity.

Pineapple contains an antibacterial and anti-inflammatory enzyme called bromelain.[96]

Plant sterols and stanols, such as β-sitosterol, interfere with the enteric absorption of cholesterol. They are available in margarine form and may lower LDL by up to 10% to 15%. The cholesterol-lowering effect is additive to that of statin drugs.[210]

Prickly pear is the common name of a species of cactus of the genus *Opuntia*. *Opuntia streptacantha* is best for consumption because of its taste. Both the fruit and the immature pads are consumed. The plant is high in soluble fiber such as pectin, which is implicated in slowing carbohydrate and fat absorption from the intestines. Prickly pear has anti-inflammatory activity, which may underlie its efficacy in lessening "hangover" symptoms. The plant may also improve insulin sensitivity and hepatic cholesterol metabolism.[211]

Pumpkins are extremely high in β-carotene and have antioxidant activity.

Spinach is a superb source of antioxidants and contains about four times more β-carotene and three times more lutein than broccoli does. It is rich in fiber.

Tomatoes are a major source of lycopene, an antioxidant and anticancer agent.[96]

Turmeric (Curcuma longa) root contains the active ingredient curcumin, a bright yellow flavonoid that may be responsible for its health benefits. Turmeric appears to have anti-inflammatory, antioxidant, platelet antiaggregatory, and antiproliferative effects that have an impact on inflammatory processes. It may also have anticarcinogenic effects.

Watermelons are rich in glutathione and lycopenes, which may have a vasculoprotective effect and be beneficial for prostate health.[96]

CONCLUSION

The growing understanding of the physiologic impact of nutritional factors imbues the expression "you are what you eat" with an entirely new meaning. Dietary content has implications for gene expression, membrane physicochemical characteristics, receptor signaling, oxidative stress, inflammatory pathways, immune responses, endothelial function, insulin sensitivity, mental function, and emotional state (Table 15-4). With increasing insight, one may never look at food the same way again.

It is also becoming increasingly apparent that the nutrition of our food chain has potential health implications for the consumer. Even disregarding the concerns about bovine spongiform encephalopathy, meat and dairy products derived from cattle, buffalo, and other livestock that are range-fed may be healthier than products from animal byproduct–fed animals. The nutritional environment of fish and poultry similarly appears to make a difference.

Importantly, the macrodivision of nutrients into total fat, protein, and carbohydrate components, irrespective of type, is no longer sufficient for nutritional analysis. "A rose is a rose is a rose" is an equivalence that is increasingly inapplicable to fats, proteins, or carbohydrates. Fortunately, these new insights actually enrich—and render more palatable—what is now considered a healthy diet. They also empower individuals at risk for the metabolic syndrome to tailor their nutritional intake in a physiologically appropriate manner. It goes without saying that health-conscious nutrition encompasses not only healthy food but also healthful beverage choices.

The nutritional approach to insulin resistance can be exciting and fun. Every normal individual enjoys dining and imbibing. With insulin resistance and the metabolic syndrome, nutritional choices should target reduction of oxidative stress and inflammation, as well as restoration of endothelial function and sensitivity to insulin signaling. A calorically balanced diet enriched with nutritional sources of antioxidant vitamins and flavonoids, monounsaturated fatty acids, long-chain n-3 PUFAs, minerals, folic acid, L-arginine, and fiber should improve vascular endothelial function and insulin sensitivity. Correspondingly, it is clear that consumption of saturated fatty acids should be minimized and partially hydrogenated and *trans*–fatty acids altogether avoided.

Table 15-4. Diverse Effects of Selected Diets and Nutrients

DIET/NUTRIENT	ANTIOXIDANT	ANTI-INFLAMMATORY	ANTI-COAGULANT	ENDOTHELIAL PROTECTIVE	BENEFICIAL LIPID EFFECTS	ANTIPROLIFERATIVE
DASH	N/A	N/A	N/A	N/A	+	N/A
Mediterranean	N/A	+	+	+	+	N/A
Low glycemic index	N/A	N/A	N/A	N/A	+	N/A
Vegetarian	N/A	N/A	N/A	N/A	+	N/A
High dietary fiber	N/A	+	N/A	N/A	+	N/A
High fat/protein	N/A	N/A	N/A	N/A	+	N/A
Soy protein	N/A	N/A	N/A	+	+/0	N/A
Long–chain fatty acids	–	–	–	–	–	N/A
Trans–fatty acids	–	–	–	–	–	N/A
Monounsaturated fat	+	N/A	N/A	N/A	+	N/A
n-6 Fatty acids	N/A	–	–	–	N/A	N/A
n-3 Fatty acids	+	+	+	+	+	N/A
Nuts	N/A	N/A	N/A	+	+	N/A
Tea	+	+	N/A	+	+	N/A
Wine	+	+	+	+	+	+
Cocoa	+	N/A	N/A	+	+	N/A
Flavonoids	+	+	N/A	+	N/A	N/A
Dairy	N/A	N/A	+	N/A	N/A	N/A
Magnesium	N/A	N/A	N/A	+	N/A	N/A

+, Beneficial effect; –, adverse effect; 0, neutral effect; N/A, data not available.

The greater the resistance to insulin signaling, the more insulin is secreted postprandially after a carbohydrate load to maintain glucose homeostasis. High carbohydrate intake will thus accentuate the untoward stress pathways of hyperinsulinemia. Clearly, processed, refined carbohydrates, and low-fat/high-carbohydrate diets in general, are to be avoided with insulin resistance to minimize an excessive postprandial rise in insulin. The elimination of wide postprandial glucose-insulin swings may, in addition, prevent caloric overconsumption. Overweight, insulin-resistant individuals would thus be expected to benefit from low-glycemic diets with an emphasis on healthy sources of fiber, fat, and protein.

In this respect, the glycemic index or load appears to be a better predictor of dietary metabolic effects than mere carbohydrate content. The viscous fiber content of complex carbohydrate food confers significant benefits in terms of glycemic control and lipid profile and offers the health benefits accruing to the high intake of fruits, nuts, vegetables, and legumes.

There are many unsettled questions, such as the optimal balance between n-3 and n-6 PUFAs, the implications of the amount and sources of protein, or the effects of individual phytochemicals, antioxidants, and minerals. Future studies of any specific dietary manipulations must be of adequate duration, in defined populations, to compare the effects of such manipulations on markers of oxidative stress and inflammation, on vascular function and insulin sensitivity, and on compliance, dropout rates, quality of life, and risks and benefits, with specific end points such as CHD events and the development of DM.

Successive fad diets promote rapid weight loss with an untoward, yo-yo effect of repetitive cycles of rebound weight gain. In lieu of the frustration of ill-fated weight loss efforts, maintenance of physical fitness, weight control, and smoking cessation, in conjunction with the adoption of a Mediterranean-style diet focusing on whole and unrefined foods rich in color and texture, synergistically benefit vascular function, insulin sensitivity, and lipid profile. Such dietary and fitness approaches can evolve into satisfying, pleasurable, and healthful lifestyles that can be indefinitely maintained.

ANTIHYPERTENSIVE	ANTIATHEROGENIC	CARDIOVASCULAR EVENTS	INSULIN SENSITIVITY	ADIPONECTIN	WEIGHT LOSS
+	N/A	N/A	+	N/A	N/A
N/A	N/A	+	+	N/A	N/A
N/A	N/A	N/A	+	N/A	+
N/A	N/A	N/A	+	N/A	N/A
N/A	N/A	+	+	N/A	N/A
N/A	N/A	N/A	N/A	N/A	+
N/A	N/A	N/A	N/A	N/A	N/A
N/A	N/A	–	–	N/A	–
N/A	N/A	–	–	N/A	–
N/A	N/A	+	N/A	N/A	+
N/A	N/A	N/A	N/A	N/A	N/A
+	N/A	+	+	N/A	+
N/A	N/A	+	+	N/A	N/A
+	+	+	+	N/A	+
N/A	+	+	+	+	N/A
+	N/A	N/A	N/A	N/A	N/A
N/A	N/A	+	N/A	N/A	N/A
+	N/A	+	+	N/A	+/0
N/A	N/A	+	+	N/A	N/A

GLOSSARY

ACAT2	acyl CoA:cholesterol acyltransferase 2
ADMA	asymmetric dimethylarginine
AHA	American Heart Association
ALA	alpha-linolenic acid
ATP	Adult Treatment Panel
BH_4	tetrahydrobiopterin
BMI	body mass index
CARDIA	Coronary Artery Risk Development in Young Adults
CETP	cholesteryl ester transfer protein
cGMP	cyclic guanosine 3′,5′-monophosphate
CHD	coronary heart disease
CLA	conjugated linoleic acid
CoA	coenzyme A
COMT	catechol *O*-methyltransferase
COX	cyclooxygenase
CRP	C-reactive protein
DASH	Dietary Approaches to Stop Hypertension
DDAH	dimethylarginine dimethylaminohydrolase
DHA	docosahexaenoic acid
DM	diabetes mellitus
eNOS	endothelial nitric oxide synthase
EPA	eicosapentaenoic acid
FDA	Food and Drug Administration
GLUT	glucose transporter
HDL	high-density lipoprotein
HbA_{1c}	Glycated hemoglobin A
HL	hepatic lipase
HOPE	Heart Outcomes Prevention Evaluation
ICAM	intercellular adhesion molecule
IL	interleukin
iNOS	inducible nitric oxide synthase
IRS	insulin receptor substrate
LCAT	lecithin-cholesterol acyltransferase
LDL	low-density lipoprotein
LOX	lipoxygenase
Lp	lipoprotein
LPL	lipoprotein lipase
LXR	liver X receptor
MAPK	mitogen-activated protein kinase
MCP-1	monocyte chemotactic protein-1
MI	myocardial infarction
NADH/NADPH	nicotinamide adenine dinucleotide phosphate oxidase
NCEP	National Cholesterol Education Program
NFκB	nuclear factor kappaB
NHANES	National Health and Nutrition Examination Survey
NIH	National Institutes of Health
NO	nitric oxide
PAI-1	plasminogen activator inhibitor-1
PDGF	platelet-derived growth factor
PGE_2	prostaglandin E_2
PI3K	phosphatidylinositol 3-kinase
PKB	protein kinase B
PLTP	phospholipid transfer protein
PPAR	peroxisome proliferator–activated receptor
PUFA	polyunsaturated fatty acid
RXR	retinoid X receptor
SREBP	sterol regulatory element binding protein
TNF	tumor necrosis factor
tPA	tissue plasminogen activator
VCAM	vascular cell adhesion molecule
VEGF	vascular endothelial growth factor
VLDL	very-low-density lipoprotein

REFERENCES

1. The Economist Technology Quarterly, September 6, 2003, pp 26-27
2. Storlien LH, Higgins JA, Thomas TC, et al. Diet composition and insulin action in animal models. Br J Nutr 2000; 83(suppl 1):S85-S90
3. Hu FB, Willett WC. Optimal diets for prevention of coronary heart disease. JAMA 2002;288:2569-2578
4. Clinical guidelines on the identification, evaluation, and treatment of overweight and obesity in adults—the Evidence Report. Obes Res 1998;6(suppl 2):51S-209S
5. Position of the American Dietetic Association: weight management. J Am Diet Assoc 1997;97:71-74
6. Krauss RM, Deckelbaum RJ, Ernst N, et al. Dietary guidelines for healthy American adults: a statement for health professionals from the National Committee, American Heart Association. Circulation 1996;94:1795-1800
7. Zamiska N. New diet guide: fewer grains, more veggies. Wall St J 2004;August 30:B1
8. Obarzanek E, Sacks FM, Vollmer WM, et al. DASH Research Group. Effects on blood lipids of a blood pressure-lowering diet: the Dietary Approaches to Stop Hypertension (DASH) Trial. Am J Clin Nutr 2001; 74:80-89
9. Choi HK, Atkinson K, Karlson EW, et al. Purine-rich foods, dairy and protein intake, and the risk of gout in men. N Engl J Med 2004;350:1093-1103
10. Barclay L. DASH diet improves insulin sensitivity as well as hypertension. Diabetes Care 2004;27:340-347

11. Willett WC, Sacks F, Trichopoulou A, et al. Mediterranean diet pyramid: a cultural model for healthy eating. Am J Clin Nutr 1995;61(suppl):1402S-1406S
12. Hu FB. The Mediterranean diet and mortality—olive oil and beyond. N Engl J Med 2003;348:2595-2596
13. Chrysohoou C, Panagiotakos DB, Pitsavos C, et al. Adherence to the Mediterranean diet attenuates inflammation and coagulation process in healthy adults: the Attica study. J Am Coll Cardiol 2004;44:152-158
14. Esposito K, Marfella R, Ciotola M, et al. Effect of a Mediterranean-style diet on endothelial dysfunction and markers of vascular inflammation in the metabolic syndrome. A randomized trial. JAMA 2004;292: 1440-1446
15. Trichopoulou A, Costacou T, Bamia C, Trichopoulos D. Adherence to a Mediterranean diet and survival in a Greek population. N Engl J Med 2003;348:2599-2608
16. de Lorgeril M, Renaud S, Mamelle N, et al. Mediterranean alpha-linolenic acid–rich diet in secondary prevention of coronary heart disease. Lancet 1994;343:1454-1459
17. Singh RB, Dubnov G, Niaz MA, et al. Effect of an Indo-Mediterranean diet on progression of coronary artery disease in high risk patients: a randomized single-blind trial. Lancet 2002;360:1455-1461
18. Knoops KTB, de Groot LCGPM, Kromhout D, et al. Mediterranean diet, lifestyle factors, and 10-year mortality in elderly European men and women. JAMA 2004;292:1433-1439
19. Søndergaard E, Møller JE, Egstrup K. Effect of dietary intervention and lipid-lowering treatment on brachial vasoreactivity in patients with ischemic heart disease and hypercholesterolemia. Am Heart J 2003;145:E19
20. Leeds AR. Glycemic index and heart disease. Am J Clin Nutr 2002;76(suppl):286S-289S
21. Brand-Miller JC, Thomas M, Swan V, et al. Physiological validation of the concept of glycemic load in lean young adults. J Nutr 2003;133:2728-2732
22. Frost G, Leeds AA, Dore CJ, et al. Glycaemic index as a determinant of serum HDL-cholesterol concentration. Lancet 1999;353:1269-1276
23. Simin L, Manson JE, Stampfer MJ, et al. Dietary glycemic load assessed by food-frequency questionnaire in relation to plasma high density-lipoprotein cholesterol and fasting plasma triacylglycerols in postmenopausal women. Am J Clin Nutr 2001;73:560-566
24. Minehira K, Tappy L. Dietary and lifestyle interventions in the management of the metabolic syndrome: present status and future perspective. Eur J Clin Nutr 2002;56: 1262-1269
25. Ludwig DS. Diet and development of the insulin resistance syndrome. Asia Pac J Clin Nutr 2003;12(suppl):S4
26. Bouche C, Rizkalla SW, Luo J, et al. Five-week, low–glycemic index diet decreases total fat mass and improves plasma lipid profile in moderately overweight nondiabetic men. Diabetes Care 2002;25:822-828
27. Pereira MA, Swain J, Goldfine AB, et al. Effects of a low–glycemic load diet on resting energy expenditure and heart disease risk factors during weight loss. JAMA 2004;292:2482-2490
28. Jenkins DJA, Kendall CWC, Marchie A, et al. Effects of a dietary portfolio of cholesterol-lowering foods vs lovastatin on serum lipids and C-reactive protein. JAMA 2003;290:502-510
29. Kuo CS, Lai NS, Ho LT, Lin CL. Insulin sensitivity in Chinese ovo-lactovegetarians compared with omnivores. Eur J Clin Nutr 2004;58:312-316
30. Stone NJ, Kushner R. Effects of dietary modification to reduce vascular risks and treatment of obesity. Cardiol Clin 2003;21:415-433
31. King DE, Egan BM, Geesey ME. Relation of dietary fat and fiber to elevation of C-reactive protein. Am J Cardiol 2003;92:1335-1339
32. Rimm EB, Ascherio A, Giovannucci E, et al. Vegetable, fruit, and cereal fiber intake and risk of coronary heart disease among men. JAMA 1996;275:447-451
33. Bazzano LA, He J, Ogden LG, et al. Dietary fiber intake and reduced risk of coronary heart disease in US men and women: the National Health and Nutrition Examination Survey I Epidemiologic Follow-up Study. Arch Intern Med 2003;163:1897-1904
34. Ludwig DS. The glycemic index: physiological mechanisms relating to obesity, diabetes, and cardiovascular disease. JAMA 2002;287:2414-2423
35. Eades MR, Eades MD. Protein Power. New York, Bantam Books, 1999
36. Steward HL, Bethea MC, Andrews SS, Balart LA. Sugar Busters! New York, Ballantine Publishing, 1995
37. Atkins RC. Dr. Atkins' New Diet Revolution, revised ed. New York, Avon Books, 1998
38. Foster GD, Wyatt HR, Hill JO, et al. A randomized trial of a low-carbohydrate diet for obesity. N Engl J Med 2003;348:2082-2090
39. Samaha FF, Iqbal N, Seshadri P, et al. A low-carbohydrate as compared with a low-fat diet in severe obesity. N Engl J Med 2003;348:2074-2081
40. Yancy W, Olsen MK, Guyton JR, et al. A low-carbohydrate, ketogenic diet versus a low-fat diet to treat obesity and hyperlipidemia: a randomized, controlled trial. Ann Intern Med 2004;140:769-777
41. Stern L, Iqbal N, Seshadri P, et al. The effects of low-carbohydrate versus conventional weight loss diets in severely obese adults: one-year follow-up of a randomized trial. Ann Intern Med 2004;140:778-785
42. Jiang R, Manson JE, Meigs JB, et al. Body iron stores in relation to risk of type 2 diabetes in apparently healthy women. JAMA 2004;291:711-717
43. Fung TT, Schulze M, Manson JE, et al. Dietary patterns, meat intake, and the risk of type 2 diabetes in women. Arch Intern Med 2004;164:2235-2240
44. Aude YW, Agatston AS, Lopez-Jimenez F, et al. The National Cholesterol Education Program diet vs a diet lower in carbohydrates and higher in protein and monounsaturated fat: a randomized trial. Arch Intern Med 2004;164:2141-2146
45. Appel LJ. The effects of protein intake on blood pressure and cardiovascular disease. Curr Opin Lipidol 2003;14: 55-59
46. Merz-Demlow BE, Duncan AM, Wangen KE, et al. Soy isoflavones improve plasma lipids in normocholesterolemic, premenopausal women. Am J Nutr 2000;71: 1462-1469
47. Anderson JW, Johnstone BM, Cook-Newell ME. Meta-analysis of the effects of soy protein intake on serum lipids. N Engl J Med 1995;333:276-282
48. Yildirir A, Tokgozoglu SL, Oduncu T, et al. Soy protein diet significantly improves endothelial function and lipid parameters. Clin Cardiol 2001;24:711-716
49. Steinberg FM, Guthrie NL, Villablanca AC, et al. Soy protein with isoflavones has favorable effects on endothelial function that are independent of lipid and antioxidant effects in healthy postmenopausal women. Am J Clin Nutr 2003;78:123-130
50. Cuevas AM, Irribarra VL, Castillo OA, et al. Isolated soy protein improves endothelial function in post-menopausal hypercholesterolemic women. Eur J Clin Nutr 2003;57:889-894
51. Krauss RM, Eckel RH, Howard B, et al. AHA Scientific Statement: AHA Dietary Guidelines. Revision 2000:

A statement for healthcare professionals from the nutrition committee of the American Heart Association. J Nutr 2001;131:132-146

52. Crouse JR 3rd, Morgan T, Terry JG, et al. A randomized trial comparing the effect of casein with that of soy protein containing varying amounts of isoflavones on plasma concentrations of lipids and lipoproteins. Arch Intern Med 1999;159:2070-2076
53. Bhathena SJ, Ali AA, Haudenschild C, et al. Dietary flaxseed meal is more protective than soy protein concentrate against hypertriglyceridemia and steatosis of the liver in an animal model of obesity. J Am Coll Nutr 2003;22:157-164
54. Lavigne C, Tremblay F, Asselin G, et al. Prevention of skeletal muscle insulin resistance by dietary cod protein in high fat–fed rats. Am J Physiol Endocrinol Metab 2001;281:E62-E71
55. Tremblay F, Lavigne C, Jacques H, Marette A. Dietary cod protein restores insulin-induced activation of phosphatidylinositol 3-kinase/Akt and GLUT4 translocation to the T-tubules in skeletal muscle of high-fat–fed obese rats. Diabetes 2003;52:29-37
56. Zhang X, Young HA. PPAR and the immune system—what do we know? Int Immunopharm 2002;2:1029-1044
57. Jequier E. Pathways to obesity. Int J Obes Relat Metab Disord 2002;26(suppl):S12-S17
58. Piers LS, Walker KZ, Stoney RM, et al. The influence of the type of dietary fat on postprandial fat oxidation rates: monounsaturated (olive oil) vs saturated fat (cream). Int J Obes Relat Metab Disord 2002;26:814-821
59. Yaqoob P. Lipids and the immune response: from molecular mechanisms to clinical applications. Curr Opin Clin Nutr Metab Care 2003;6:133-150
60. Coppack SW. Pro-inflammatory cytokines and inflammatory tissue. Proc Nutr Soc 2001;60:349-356
61. Carroll MF, Schade DS. Timing of antioxidant vitamin ingestion alters postprandial proatherogenic serum markers. Circulation 2003;108:24-31
62. Duplus E, Forest C. Is there a single mechanism for fatty acid regulation of gene transcription? Biochem Pharmacol 2002;64:893-901
63. Jump DB. The biochemistry of n-3 polyunsaturated fatty acids. J Biol Chem 2002;277:8755-8758
64. Thanapoulou AC, Karamanos BG, Angelico FV, et al. Dietary fat intake as risk factor for the development of diabetes. Multinational, multicenter study of the Mediterranean Group for the Study of Diabetes (MGSD). Diabetes Care 2003;26:302-307
65. Vessby B. Dietary fat, fatty acid composition in plasma and the metabolic syndrome. Curr Opin Lipidol 2003;14:15-19
66. Lehninger AL. Biochemistry, 2nd ed. New York, Worth Publishers, 1975
67. http://www.scientificpsychic.com/fitness/fattyacids.html
68. Tada N, Yoshida H. Diacylglycerol on lipid metabolism. Curr Opin Lipidol 2003;14:29-33
69. Willet WC, Stampfer MJ, Manson JE, et al. Intake of *trans* fatty acids and risk of coronary heart disease among women. Lancet 1993;341:581-585
70. Hu FB. Confronting *trans* fat. EInternal Med News 2003;36(18)
71. Tavani A, Gallus S. Alpha-linolenic acid and nonfatal acute myocardial infarction. Circulation 2003;108:e127-e128
72. Hauswirth CB, Scheeder MRL, Beer JH. High omega-3 fatty acid content in alpine cheese. The basis for an alpine paradox. Circulation 2004;109:103-107
73. Yu Y, Correll JP, Heuvel V. Conjugated linoleic acid decreases production of proinflammatory products in macrophages: evidence for a PPAR-gamma–dependent mechanism. Biochim Biophys Acta 2002:1581:89-99
74. Gaullier JM, Haise J, Hoye K, et al. Conjugated linoleic acid supplementation for 1 year reduces body fat mass in healthy overweight humans. Am J Clin Nutr 2004;79: 1118-1125
75. Dyerberg J, Bang HO, Stoffersen E, et al. Eicosapentaenoic acid and prevention of thrombosis and atherosclerosis? Lancet 1978;2:117-119
76. Botham KM, Zheng X, Napolitano M, et al. The effects of dietary n-3 polyunsaturated fatty acids delivered in chylomicron remnants on the transcription of genes regulating synthesis and secretion of very-low-density lipoprotein by the liver: modulation by cellular oxidative state. Exp Biol Med (Maywood) 2003;228: 143-151
77. Pischon T, Hankinson SE, Hotamisligil GS, et al. Habitual dietary intake of n-3 and n-6 fatty acids in relation to inflammatory markers among US men and women. Circulation 2003;108:155-160
78. Diep QN, Amiri F, Touyz RM, et al. PPARalpha activator effects on Ang II–induced vascular oxidative stress and inflammation. Hypertension 2002;40:866-871
79. Sethi S, Ziouzenkova O, Ni H, et al. Oxidized omega-3 fatty acids in fish oil inhibit leukocyte-endothelial interactions through activation of PPAR alpha. Blood 2002; 100:1340-1346
80. Stulnig TM, Huber J, Leitinger N, et al. Polyunsaturated eicosapentaenoic acid displaces proteins from membrane rafts by altering raft lipid composition. J Biol Chem 2001;276:37335-37340
81. Fan YY, McMurray DN, Ly LH, Chapkin RS. Dietary (n-3) polyunsaturated fatty acids remodel mouse T-cell lipid rafts. J Nutr 2003;133:1913-1920
82. Goodfellow J, Bellamy MF, Ramsey MW, et al. Dietary supplementation with marine omega-3 fatty acids improve systemic large artery endothelial function in subjects with hypercholesterolemia. J Am Coll Cardiol 2000;35:265-270
83. Dallongeville J, Yarnell J, Ducimetière P, et al. Fish consumption is associated with lower heart rates. Circulation. 2003;108:820-825
84. Thies F, Garry JM, Yaqoob P, et al. Association of n-3 polyunsaturated fatty acids with stability of atherosclerotic plaques: a randomised controlled trial. Lancet 2003;361:477-485
85. Hu FB, Bronner L, Willett WC, et al. Fish and omega-3 fatty acid intake and risk of coronary heart disease in women. JAMA 2002;287:1815-1821
86. Albert CM, Hennekens CH, O'Donnel CJ, et al. Fish consumption and risk of sudden cardiac death. JAMA 1998;279:23-28
87. GISSI-Prevenzione Investigators. Dietary supplementation with n-3 polyunsaturated fatty acids and vitamin E after myocardial infarction: results of the GISSI-Prevenzione trial. Gruppo Italiano per lo Studio della Sopravvivenza nell'Infarto Miocardico. Lancet 1999;354: 447-455
88. Marchioli R, Barzi F, Bomba E, et al. Early protection against sudden death by n-3 polyunsaturated fatty acids after myocardial infarction: time-course analysis of the results of the Gruppo Italiano per lo Studio della Sopravvivenza nell'Infarto Miocardico (GISSI)—Prevenzione. Circulation 2002;105:1897-1903
89. He K, Song Y, Daviglus ML, et al. Accumulated evidence on fish consumption and coronary heart disease mortality: a meta-analysis of cohort studies. Circulation 2004;109:2705-2711
90. Wang S, Sun C, Kao Q, Yu C. Effects of chromium and fish oil on insulin resistance and leptin resistance in obese developing rats. Wei Sheng Yan Jiu 2001;30:284-286

91. Santica M, Marcovina M, Kennedy H, et al. Fish intake, independent of apo(a) size, accounts for lower plasma lipoprotein(a) levels in Bantu fishermen of Tanzania: the Lugalawa study. Arterioscler Thromb Vasc Biol 1999; 19:1250-1256
92. Caron MF, Nguyen IT, Folstad JE. Treatment of very high triglycerides with fish oils: A review of 2 cases. J Pharm Technol 2002;19:14-18
93. Mozaffarian D, Psaty BM, Rimm EB, et al. Fish intake and risk of incident atrial fibrillation. Circulation 2004;110:368-373
94. Schrepf R, Limmert T, Claus Weber P, et al. Immediate effects of n-3 fatty acid infusion on the induction of sustained ventricular tachycardia. Lancet 2004;363: 1441-1442
95. Mozaffarian D, Lemaitre RN, Kuller HL, et al. Cardiac benefit of fish consumption may depend on type of fish meal consumed. The Cardiovascular Health Study. Circulation 2003;107:1372-1377
96. http://www.naturalways.com/medValFd.htm
97. Morris MC, Evans DA, Bienias JL, et al. Consumption of fish and n-3 fatty acids and risk of incident Alzheimer disease. Arch Neurol 2003;60:940-946
98. Neergaard L. Don't be scared off fish by mercury warnings. Pittsburgh Tribune 2003;Thursday, December 25:A13
99. Davis RJ. A nutty idea for your health? Wall St J 2003; December 23:D5
100. Jenkins DJA, Kendall CWC, Marchie A, et al. Dose response of almonds on coronary heart disease risk factors: blood lipids, oxidized low-density lipoproteins, lipoprotein (a), homocysteine, and pulmonary nitric oxide. A randomized, controlled, crossover trial. Circulation 2002;106:1327-1332
101. Ros E, Nunez I, Perez-Heras A, et al. A walnut diet improves endothelial function in hypercholesterolemic subjects. A randomized crossover trial. Circulation 2004;109:1609-1614
102. Jiang R, Manson JE, Stampfer MJ, et al. Nut and peanut butter consumption and risk of type 2 diabetes in women. JAMA 2002;288:2554-2560
103. Walsh N. Tea for heart disease and cancer prevention. EInternal Med News 2003;36(13)
104. Balentine DA, Wiseman SA, Bouwens LCM. The chemistry of tea flavonoids. Crit Rev Food Sci Nutr 1997;37:693-704
105. Evans JL, Goldfine ID, Maddux BA, Grodsky GM. Oxidative stress and stress-activated signaling pathways: a unifying hypothesis of type 2 diabetes. Endocr Rev 2002;23:599-622
106. Dona M, Dell'Aica I, Calabrese F, et al. Neutrophil restraint by green tea: inhibition of inflammation, associated angiogenesis, and pulmonary fibrosis. J Immunol 2003;170:4335-4341
107. Chantre P, Lairon D. Recent findings of green tea extract AR25 (Exolise) and its activity for the treatment of obesity. Phytomedicine 2002;9:3-8
108. Dulloo AG, Seydoux J, Girardier L, et al. Green tea and thermogenesis: interactions between catechin-polyphenols, caffeine and sympathetic activity. Int J Obes Relat Metab Disord 2000;24:252-258
109. Dulloo AG, Duret C, Rohrer D, et al. Efficacy of a green tea extract rich in catechin polyphenols and caffeine in increasing 24-h energy expenditure and fat oxidation in humans. Am J Clin Nutr 1999;70:1040-1045
110. McCarty MF. Hepatothermic therapy of obesity: rationale and an inventory of resources. Med Hypotheses 2001;57:324-336
111. Murase T, Nagasawa A, Suzuki J, et al. Beneficial effects of tea catechins on diet-induced obesity: stimulation of lipid catabolism in the liver. Int J Obes Relat Metab Disord 2002;26:1459-1464
112. Duffy SJ, Keaney JF Jr, Holbrook M, et al. Short- and long-term black tea consumption reverses endothelial dysfunction in patients with coronary artery disease. Circulation 2001;104:151-156
113. Yang YC, Lu FH, Wu JS, et al. The protective effect of habitual tea consumption on hypertension. Arch Intern Med 2004;164:1534-1540
114. Chyu K-Y, Babbidge SM, Zhao X, et al. Differential effects of green tea–derived catechin on developing versus established atherosclerosis in apolipoprotein E–null mice. Circulation 2004;109:2448-2453
115. Maeda K, Kuzuya M, Cheng XW, et al. Green tea catechins inhibit the cultured smooth muscle cell invasion through the basement barrier. Atherosclerosis 2003; 166:23-30
116. Sesso HD, Gaziano JM, Buring JE, Hennekens CH. Coffee and tea intake and the risk of myocardial infarction. Am J Epidemiol 1999;149:162-167
117. Hirano R, Momiyama Y, Takahashi R, et al. Comparison of green tea intake in Japanese patients with and without angiographic coronary artery disease. Am J Cardiol 2003;90:1150-1153
118. Geleijnse JM, Launer LJ, Van der Kuip DA, et al. Inverse association of tea and flavonoid intakes with incident myocardial infarction: the Rotterdam Study. Am J Clin Nutr 2002;75:880-886
119. Mukamal KJ, Maclure M, Muller JE, et al. Tea consumption and mortality after acute myocardial infarction. Circulation 2002;105:2476-2481
120. Anderson RA, Polansky MM. Tea enhances insulin activity. J Agric Food Chem 2002;50:7182-7186
121. Hosoda K, Wang MF, Liao ML, et al. Antihyperglycemic effect of oolong tea in type 2 diabetes. Diabetes Care 2003;26:1714-1718
122. Davies MJ, Judd JT, Baer DJ, et al. Black tea consumption reduces total and LDL cholesterol in mildly hypercholesterolemic adults. J Nutr 2003;133:3298S-3302S
123. Wemyss N. Wine and civilization. Bull Soc Med Friends Wine 1998;40:3-4
124. Renaud S, de Lorgeril M. Wine, alcohol, platelets, and the French paradox for coronary heart disease. Lancet 1992;339:1523-1526
125. St Leger AS, Cochrane AL, Moore F. Factors associated with cardiac mortality in developed countries with particular reference to the consumption of wine. Lancet 1979;12:1017-1020
126. Criqui M. Alcohol in the myocardial infarction patient. Lancet 1998;352:1873
127. Whitehead TP, Robinson D, Allaway S. Effect of red wine ingestion on antioxidant capacity of serum. Clin Chem 1995;41:32-35
128. Freedman JE. High-fat diets and cardiovascular disease. J Am Coll Cardiol 2003;41:1750-1751
129. Oak M-H, Chataigneau M, Keravis T, et al. Red wine polyphenolic compounds inhibit vascular endothelial growth factor expression in vascular smooth muscle cells by preventing the activation of the p38 mitogen-activated protein kinase pathway. Arterioscler Thromb Vasc Biol 2003;23:1001-1007
130. Frankel EN, Kanner J, German JB. Inhibition of oxidation of human low density lipoprotein by phenolic substances in red wine. Lancet 1993;341:454-457
131. Sierksma A, van der Gaag MS, Kluft C, Hendriks HF. Moderate alcohol consumption reduces plasma C-reactive protein and fibrinogen levels: a randomized, diet-controlled intervention study. Eur J Clin Nutr 2002;56:1130-1136

132. Greenfield JR, Samaras K, Jenkins AB, et al. Obesity is an important determinant of baseline serum C-reactive protein concentration in monozygotic twins, independent of genetic influences. Circulation 2004;109:3022-3028
133. Volpato S, Pahor M, Ferrucci L, et al. Relationship of alcohol intake with inflammatory markers and plasminogen activator inhibitor-1 in well-functioning older adults. The Health, Aging, and Body Composition Study. Circulation 2004;109:607-612
134. Imhof A, Froehlich M, Brenner H, et al. Effect of alcohol consumption on systemic markers of inflammation. Lancet 2001;357:763-767
135. Stewart SH, Mainous AG 3rd, Gilbert G. Relation between alcohol consumption and C-reactive protein levels in the adult US population. J Am Board Fam Pract 2002;15:437-442
136. Stare F. Myocardial infarction in patients with portal cirrhosis. Nutr Rev 1961;19:37
137. Leikert JF, Rathel TR, Wohlfart P, et al. Red wine polyphenols enhance endothelial nitric oxide synthase expression and subsequent nitric oxide release from endothelial cells. Circulation 2002;106:1614-1617
138. Khan NQ, Lees DM, Douthwaite JA, et al. Comparison of red wine extract and polyphenol constituents on endothelin-1 synthesis by cultured endothelial cells. Clin Sci (Lond) 1997;6:507-511
139. Hashimoto M, Kim S, Eto M, et al. Effect of acute intake of red wine on flow-mediated vasodilatation of the brachial artery. Am J Cardiol 2001;88:1457-1460
140. Goldfinger TM. Beyond the French paradox: the impact of moderate beverage alcohol and wine consumption in the prevention of cardiovascular disease. Cardiol Clin 2003;21:449-457
141. Vliegenthart R, Oei H-H, van den Elzen AP, et al. Alcohol consumption and coronary calcification in a general population. Arch Intern Med 2004;164:2355-2360
142. Mukamal KJ, Conigrave KM, Mittleman MA, et al. Roles of drinking pattern and type of alcohol consumed in coronary heart disease in men. N Engl J Med 2003; 348:109-118
143. Casani L, Segales E, Vilahur G, et al. Moderate daily intake of red wine inhibits mural thrombosis and monocyte tissue factor expression in an experimental porcine model. Circulation 2004;110:460-465
144. Stampfer MJ, Colditz GA, Willett WC, et al. A prospective study of moderate alcohol consumption and the risk of coronary disease and stroke in women. N Engl J Med 1988;319:267-273
145. Rimm EB, Giovannucci EL, Willett WC, et al. Prospective study of alcohol consumption and risk of coronary disease in men. Lancet 1991;338:464-468
146. Di Castelnuovo A, Rotondo S, Iacoviello L, et al. Meta-analysis of wine and beer consumption in relation to vascular risk. Circulation 2002;105:2836-2844
147. De Oliveira E, Silva ER, Foster D, et al. Alcohol consumption raises HDL cholesterol levels by increasing the transport rate of apolipoproteins A-I and A-II. Circulation 2000;102:2347-2352
148. Catena C, Novello M, Dotto L, et al. Serum lipoprotein(a) concentrations and alcohol consumption in hypertension: possible relevance for cardiovascular damage. J Hypertens 2003;21:281-288
149. Hannuksela ML, Liisanantti MK, Savolainen MJ. Effect of alcohol on lipids and lipoproteins in relation to atherosclerosis. Crit Rev Clin Lab Sci 2002;39:225-283
150. Zilkens RR, Puddey IA. Alcohol and type 2 diabetes—another paradox? J Cardiovasc Risk 2003;10:25-30
151. Kroenke CH, Chu NF, Rifai N. A cross-sectional study of alcohol consumption patterns and biologic markers of glycemic control among 459 women. Diabetes Care 2003;26:1971-1978
152. Sierksma A, Patel H, Ouchi N, et al. Effect of moderate alcohol consumption on adiponectin, tumor necrosis factor-alpha, and insulin sensitivity. Diabetes Care 2004;27:184-189
153. Fisher ND, Hughes M, Gerhard-Herman M. Flavanol-rich cocoa induces nitric-oxide–dependent vasodilation in healthy humans. J Hypertens 2003;21:2281-2286
154. Beecher GR. Overview of dietary flavonoids: nomenclature, occurrence and intake. J Nutr 2003;133:3248S-3254S
155. Nestel P. Isoflavones: their effects on cardiovascular risk and functions. Curr Opin Lipidol 2003;14:3-8
156. Kondo K, Matsumoto A, Kurata H, et al. Inhibition of oxidation of low-density lipoprotein with red wine. Lancet 1994;344:1152
157. http://exchange.healthwell.com/nutritionscience-news/nsn_backs/Aug_99/cancer.cfm
158. Appeldoorn CCM, Bonnefoy A, Lutters BCH, et al. Gallic acid antagonizes P-selectin–mediated platelet-leukocyte interactions. Implications for the French paradox. Circulation 2005;111:106-112
159. Widlansky ME, Gokce N, Keaney JJ, Vita JA. The clinical implications of endothelial dysfunction. J Am Coll Cardiol 2003;42:1149-1160
160. Hertog MGL, Feskens EJM, Hollman PCH, et al. Dietary antioxidant flavonoids and risk of coronary heart disease: the Zutphen Elderly Study. Lancet 1993;342:1007-1011
161. Keli SO, Hertog MG, Feskens EJ, Kromhout D. Dietary flavonoids, antioxidant vitamins, and incidence of stroke: the Zutphen study. Arch Intern Med 1996;156:637-642
162. Hertog MG, Kromhout D, Aravanis C, et al. Flavonoid intake and long-term risk of coronary heart disease and cancer in the seven countries study. Arch Intern Med 1995;155:381-386
163. Engler MM, Engler MB, Malloy MJ, et al. Antioxidant vitamins C and E improve endothelial function in children with hyperlipidemia: Endothelial Assessment of Risk from Lipids in Youth (EARLY) Trial. Circulation 2003;108:1059-1063
164. Cooke JP. Does ADMA cause endothelial dysfunction? Arterioscler Thromb Vasc Biol 2000;20:2032-2037
165. Cuevas AM, Guasch V, Castillo O, et al. A high-fat diet induces and red wine counteracts endothelial dysfunction in human volunteers. Lipids 2000;35:143-148
166. Stein JH, Keevil JG, Wiebe DA, et al. Purple grape juice improves endothelial function and reduces the susceptibility of LDL cholesterol to oxidation in patients with coronary artery disease. Circulation 1999;100:1050-1055
167. Plotnick GD, Corretti MC, Vogel RA, et al. Effect of supplemental phytonutrients on impairment of the flow-mediated brachial artery vasoreactivity after a single high-fat meal. J Am Coll Cardiol 2003;41:1744-1749
168. Gilman AG, Goodman LS, Gilman A (eds). Goodman and Gilman's The Pharmacological Basis of Therapeutics, 6th ed. New York, McMillan, 1980
169. Davis RJ. Not all forms of vitamin E should be vilified. Wall St J 2004;November 23:D9
170. Duffy SJ, Vita JA, Keany JF Jr. Antioxidants and endothelial function. Heart Failure 1999;15:135-152
171. Yusuf S, Dagenais G, Pogue J, et al. Vitamin E supplementation and cardiovascular events in high-risk patients: the Heart Outcomes Prevention Evaluation study investigators. N Engl J Med 2000;342:154-160
172. Miller ER, Pastor-Barriuso R, Dalal D, et al. Meta-analysis: high-dosage vitamin E supplementation may increase all-cause mortality. Ann Intern Med 2005;142:37-46
173. Gilligan DM, Sack MN, Guetta V, et al. Effect of antioxidant vitamins on low density lipoprotein oxidation

and impaired endothelium-dependent vasodilation in patients with hypercholesterolemia. J Am Coll Cardiol 1994;24:1611-1617
174. MRC/BHF Heart Protection Study Group. MRC/BHF Heart Protection study of antioxidant vitamin supplementation in 20,536 high-risk individuals: a randomised placebo-controlled trial. Lancet 2002;360:23-33
175. Khaw KT, Bingham S, Welch A, et al. Relation between plasma ascorbic acid and mortality in men and women in EPIC-Norfolk prospective study: a prospective population study. European Prospective Investigation into Cancer and Nutrition. Lancet 2001;357:657-663
176. Harrison DG, Cai H. Endothelial control of vasomotion and nitric oxide production. Cardiol Clin 2003;21: 289-302
177. Schindler TH, Nitzsche EU, Munzel T, et al. Coronary vasoregulation in patients with various risk factors in response to cold pressor testing. J Am Coll Cardiol 2003;42:814-822
178. Wilkinson IB, Megson IL, MacCullum H, et al. Oral vitamin C reduces arterial stiffness and platelet aggregation in humans. J Cardiovasc Pharmacol 1999;34: 690-693
179. Osganian SK, Stampfer MJ, Rimm E, et al. Vitamin C and risk of coronary heart disease in women. J Am Coll Cardiol 2003;42:246-252
180. Moini H, Packer L, Saris NE. Antioxidant and prooxidant activities of alpha-lipoic acid and dihydrolipoic acid. Toxicol Appl Pharmacol 2002;182:84-90
181. Jones W, Li X, Qu ZC, et al. Uptake, recycling, and antioxidant actions of alpha-lipoic acid in endothelial cells. Free Radic Biol Med 2002;33:83-93
182. Maddux BA, See W, Lawrence JC Jr, et al. Protection against oxidative stress–induced insulin resistance in rat L6 muscle cells by micromolar concentrations of alpha-lipoic acid. Diabetes 2001;50:404-410
183. Litherland GJ, Hajduch E, Hundai HS. Intracellular signaling mechanisms regulating glucose transport in insulin-sensitive tissues (review). Mol Membr Biol 2001;18:195-204
184. Aldini G, Carini M, Piccoli A, et al. Procyanidins from grape seeds protect endothelial cells from peroxynitrite damage and enhance endothelium-dependent relaxation in human artery: new evidences for cardio-protection. Life Sci 2003;73:2883-2898
185. Calabresi L, Gomaraschi M, Franceschini G. Endothelial protection by high-density lipoproteins: from bench to bedside. Arterioscler Thromb Vasc Biol 2003;23: 1724-1731
186. Muenzel T, Keany JF Jr. Are the ACE-inhibitors a "magic bullet" against oxidative stress? Circulation 2001; 104:1571-1574
187. Norata GD, Pirillo A, Catapano AL. Statins and oxidative stress during atherogenesis. J Cardiovasc Risk 2003;10:181-189
188. Stanger O. Physiology of folic acid in health and disease. Curr Drug Metab 2002,3:211-223
189. Hayden MR, Tyagi SC. Is type 2 diabetes mellitus a vascular disease (atheroscleropathy) with hyperglycemia a late manifestation? The role of NOS, NO, and redox stress. Cardiovasc Diabetol 2003;2:2
190. Doshi SN, McDowell IF, Moat SJ, et al. Folic acid improves endothelial function in coronary artery disease via mechanisms largely independent of homocysteine lowering. Circulation 2002;105:22-26
191. De Vriese AS, Blom HJ, Heil SG, et al. Endothelium-derived hyperpolarizing factor–mediated renal vasodilatory response is impaired during acute and chronic hyperhomocysteinemia. Circulation 2004;109:2331-2336
192. Tyagi SC: Homocyst(e)ine and heart disease: pathophysiology of extracellular matrix. Clin Exp Hypertens 1999;21:181-198
193. Napoli C, Ignarro-Williams S, de Nigris F, et al. Long-term combined beneficial effects of physical training and metabolic treatment on atherosclerosis in hypercholesterolemic mice. Proc Natl Acad Sci U S A 2004; 101:8797-8802
194. Piatti PM, Monti LD, Valsecchi G, et al. Long-term oral L-arginine administration improves peripheral and hepatic insulin sensitivity in type 2 diabetic patients. Diabetes Care 2001;24:875-880
195. Teegarden D. Calcium intake and reduction in weight or fat mass. J Nutr 2003;133:249S-251S
196. Zemel MB. Mechanisms of dairy modulation of adiposity. J Nutr 2003;133:252S-256S
197. Massey LK. Dairy food consumption, blood pressure and stroke. J Nutr 2001;131:1875-1878
198. Zemel MB, Thompson W, Milstead A, et al. Calcium and dairy acceleration of weight and fat loss during energy restriction in obese adults. Obes Res 2004;12: 582-590
199. Pereira MA, Jacobs DR Jr, Van Horn L, et al. Dairy consumption, obesity, and the insulin resistance syndrome in young adults: the CARDIA Study. JAMA 2002;287:2081-2089
200. Saris NEL, Mervaala E, Kappanen H, et al. Magnesium. An update on physiological, clinical and analytical aspects. Clin Chim Acta 2000;294:1-26
201. Pearson PJ, Evora PR, Seccombe JF, Schaff HV. Hypomagnesemia inhibits nitric oxide release from coronary endothelium: protective role of magnesium infusion after cardiac operations. Ann Thorac Surg 1998;65:967-972
202. Shechter M, Sharir M, Paul-Labrador M, et al. Oral magnesium therapy improves endothelial function in patients with coronary artery disease. Circulation 2000;102:2353-2358
203. Shechter M, Merz CNB, Stuehlinger HG, et al. Effects of oral magnesium therapy on exercise tolerance, exercise-induced chest pain, and quality of life in patients with coronary artery disease. Am J Cardiol 2003;91:517-521
204. Abbott RD, Ando F, Masaki KH, et al. Dietary magnesium intake and the future risk of coronary heart disease (the Honolulu Heart Program). Am J Cardiol 2003;92:665-669
205. Song Y, Manson JE, Buring JE, Liu S. Dietary magnesium intake in relation to plasma insulin levels and risk of type 2 diabetes in women. Diabetes Care 2004;27: 59-65
206. Lopez-Ridaura R, Willett WC, Rimm EB, et al. Magnesium intake and risk of type 2 diabetes in men and women. Diabetes Care 2004;27:134-140
207. Panagiotakos DB, Pitsavos C, Kokkinos P, et al. Consumption of fruits and vegetables in relation to the risk of developing acute coronary syndromes; the CARDIO2000 case-control study. Nutrition J 2003;2:2
208. Walsh N. Garlic disappoints for lipid-lowering. EInternal Med News 2001;34(17)
209. Stamets P. MycoMedicinals. An Informational Treatise on Mushrooms. Olympia, WA, MycoMedia Productions, a division of Fungi Perfecti, 2002
210. Miettinen TA, Gylling H. Regulation of cholesterol metabolism by dietary plant sterols. Curr Opin Lipidol 1999;10:9-14
211. Shapiro K. Natural products used for diabetes. J Am Pharm Assoc 2002;42:217-226

Pharmacology 16

With insulin resistance or the metabolic syndrome, lifestyle changes such as

- **increased regular aerobic physical activity,**
- **weight reduction,**
- **dietary changes, and**
- **smoking cessation**

should always be pursued as initial and ongoing therapeutic steps. These interventions substantially reduce the risk for subsequent cardiovascular complications and type 2 diabetes mellitus (DM). Successful implementation of lifestyle changes will synergistically complement any appropriate pharmacologic therapy that is undertaken.

After appropriate lifestyle changes have been established, what constitutes further appropriate therapy for the metabolic syndrome? The metabolic and hemodynamic derangements of the metabolic syndrome individually raise cardiovascular risk and interdependently increase premature cardiovascular disease morbidity and mortality. Primary prevention trials have demonstrated the benefit of specific therapy with aspirin, lipid-lowering agents, and antihypertensives to reduce the risk for subsequent coronary heart disease (CHD). **In view of the cumulative and additive health hazards posed by components of the metabolic syndrome, pharmacologic intervention to reduce cardiovascular risk is appropriate.**

Optimal prevention targets are still evolving. Effective pharmacologic therapy needs to target not only the manifest risk factors, such as hypertension, dyslipidemia, and the prothrombotic milieu, but also the underlying inflammation and oxidative stress, endothelial dysfunction, and insulin resistance. Successful pharmacologic intervention, directed at the metabolic syndrome, would be expected to slow, arrest, or ideally reverse vascular disease progression and may prevent up to 80.5% and 82.1% of CHD events in men and women, respectively, over a 10-year period.[1] As the progression to cardiovascular disease is slowed, so is the development of type 2 DM, as has been observed in statin and angiotensin-converting enzyme (ACE) inhibitor trials.[2,3]

An abundance of pathways lead to the metabolic syndrome, which in turn displays a multiplicity of risk factors. It is not a surprise that at present, aggressive, multitarget therapy implies a multifaceted approach. Therapy with

- **aspirin,**
- **statins or fibrates (or both),**
- **antagonists of the renin-angiotensin-aldosterone system (RAAS), and**
- **possibly insulin sensitizers,**

together with therapeutic lifestyle changes, is currently of benefit in addressing the central, pathophysiologic disturbances of the metabolic syndrome.

ASPIRIN

Salicylates were originally derived from the bark of the willow tree. Since the time of Hippocrates, they have been used as analgesics and antipyretics.[4] Aspirin has numerous antioxidant, anti-inflammatory, and antithrombotic effects that may be of benefit in vascular disease and insulin resistance.

For otherwise healthy individuals with insulin resistance, whose 10-year risk for a first coronary event is 10% or greater, the benefits of long-term aspirin therapy probably outweigh any risks according to the U.S. Preventive Services Task Force and the American Heart Association (AHA). For primary prevention in such individuals with insulin resistance, barring contraindications, an aspirin dose of 81 to 325 mg/day is currently recommended.

Antioxidant Action. Reactive oxygen species (ROS) play a role in the process of insulin resistance. Aspirin interferes with the generation of pro-oxidant species.

It blocks the generation of ROS during prostaglandin metabolism through the inhibition of cyclooxygenase (COX).[5] Aspirin also inhibits the activation of neutrophils and the associated production of superoxide. In a rat animal model of insulin resistance, chronic aspirin therapy prevented vascular superoxide production and significantly reduced insulin resistance (Fig. 16-1).[6] Aspirin may limit the oxidation of lipoproteins and fibrinogen.[4]

Anti-inflammatory Effects. Insulin resistance is engendered through an inflammatory process

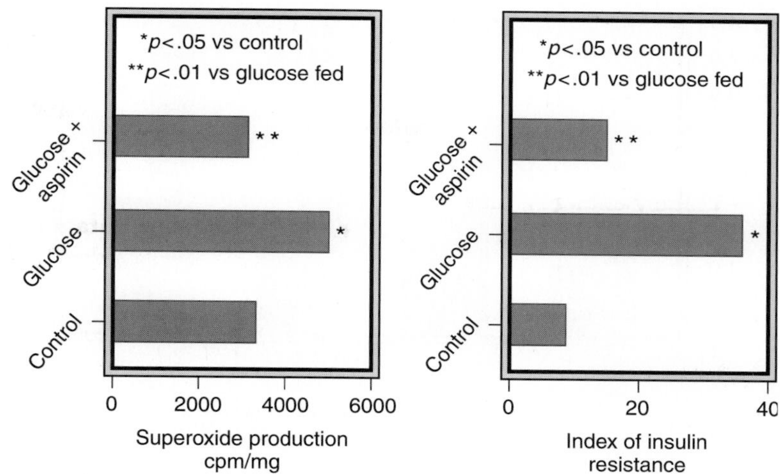

Figure 16–1. Effect of glucose feeding in the presence or absence of chronic aspirin on superoxide production and insulin resistance in a rat model of insulin resistance. *(Modified from Midaoui AE, Wu R, de Champlain J. Prevention of hypertension, hyperglycemia and vascular oxidative stress by aspirin treatment in chronically glucose-fed rats. J Hypertens 2002;20: 1407-1412.)*

and proinflammatory mediators. Aspirin functions as an anti-inflammatory agent.

Prostaglandin Synthesis. Aspirin inhibits the generation of inflammatory prostaglandins by interfering with the biosynthesis of cyclic prostanoids from arachidonic acid.

Arachidonic acid, derived from plasma membrane phospholipids, is oxidized by the enzyme COX. There are two COX isoforms:

1. COX-1 is constitutively expressed in most cells, and
2. COX-2 is induced by inflammatory stimuli and growth factors.

After the COX reaction and a number of intermediary steps, prostacyclin, thromboxane A_2, and other prostaglandins that participate in the inflammatory response are generated. Aspirin inhibits COX via irreversible acetylation of the serine moiety Ser530 of COX-1 and Ser516 of COX-2. Aspirin is 170-fold more potent at COX-1 than at COX-2 inhibition.[4]

Proinflammatory Cytokines. Nuclear factor kappaB (NFκB) is implicated in insulin resistance in animal models and in human obesity. NFκB increases the transcription of genes for proinflammatory cytokines. High doses of aspirin prevent the activation of NFκB.

In the resting cell, NFκB exists as an inactive heterodimer of two subunits, p50 and p65, complexed with the inhibitor subunit IκB. Activation of NFκB entails its disinhibition. In the process, activation of a serine kinase cascade stimulates IκB kinase, which phosphorylates IκB. IκB phosphorylation induces its proteasome-mediated degradation, which frees NFκB to translocate to the nucleus and be activated.[7]

High doses of aspirin and salicylate inhibit the β-subunit of the enzyme IκB kinase, in effect preventing activation of NFκB.[8,9]

C-Reactive Protein and Tumor Necrosis Factor-α. C-reactive protein (CRP), a marker for systemic inflammation, has significant predictive value for the development of unstable CHD and type 2 DM. In survivors of acute myocardial infarction (MI), aspirin lowered levels of CRP, as well as tumor necrosis factor-alpha (TNF-α), at a dose of 160 mg/day,[10] although the findings are controversial.[11] Aspirin use may lower the risk for acute coronary syndrome (ACS) in men with the highest quartile of CRP by 50% (Fig. 16-2).[12]

Aspirin may also inhibit the cytokine-induced expression of inducible nitric oxide synthase (iNOS).[4]

Anti–Platelet Aggregatory Activity. Aspirin may prevent acute cardiovascular events by means of its antiplatelet properties.

Insulin resistance is associated with abnormalities in platelet function. Acute thrombotic occlusion of diseased blood vessels plays a key role in triggering CHD events. Aspirin exerts its primary anti–platelet aggregatory effect via irreversible inhibition of COX, although other mechanisms may play a role.[4]

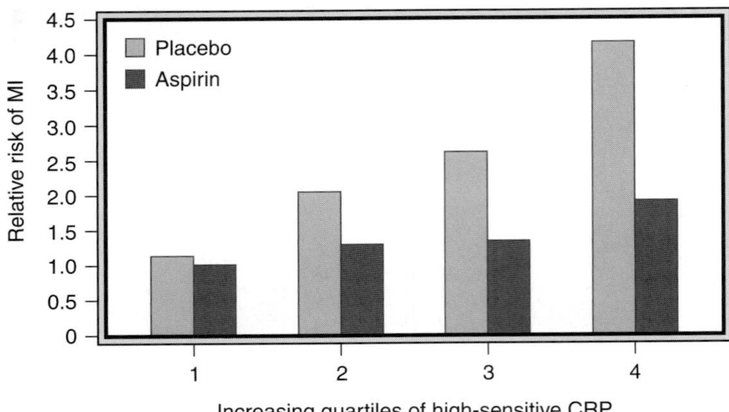

Figure 16–2. Risk of myocardial infarction in apparently healthy men on aspirin therapy: impact of elevated high-sensitivity C-reactive protein (CRP). *(Modified from Ridker PM, Cushman M, Stampfer MJ, et al. Inflammation, aspirin, and the risk of cardiovascular disease in apparently healthy men. N Engl J Med 1997;336:973-979.)*

Antiproliferative Activity. Treatment with aspirin may protect against the vascular disease of insulin resistance by inhibiting plaque growth and vascular remodeling.

Aspirin inhibits cell proliferation via transforming growth factor-β (TGF-β). TGF-β, which directly stops cell proliferation, restrains cells in the G_0 phase, inhibits the cellular uptake of growth factors such as platelet-derived growth factor (PDGF) and insulin-like growth factor, and seems to play an important role in aspirin-mediated inhibition of cell proliferation. This relationship between aspirin and TGF-β may also underlie other aspirin effects, such as cancer chemoprevention, immunomodulation, and wound healing.[13]

Prevention of Vascular Events. Aspirin is effective in the primary and secondary prevention of acute ischemic syndromes.

Five published trials, from 1988 onward, have examined the use of aspirin in primary prevention: the Physicians' Health Study (22,071 participants), the British Doctors' Trial (5139), the Thrombosis Prevention Trial (5085), the Hypertension Optimal Treatment Study (18,790), and the Primary Prevention Project (4495). These trials encompassed a total of 55,580 randomized participants with 11,466 women. They showed aspirin to be associated with a statistically significant 32% reduction in the risk for a first MI and a significant 15% reduction in the risk for all major vascular events, without significant effects on nonfatal stroke or vascular death.[14]

For secondary prevention in subjects with CHD, hypertension, and cardiovascular risk factors, aspirin reduces ischemic cardiovascular events and total mortality.[15,16]

LIPID-LOWERING THERAPY

The National Cholesterol Education Program (NCEP) Adult Treatment Panel (ATP) III recommends that all adults be screened with a fasting lipid profile that includes

- total cholesterol,
- high-density lipoprotein (HDL) cholesterol,
- low-density lipoprotein (LDL) cholesterol, and
- triglycerides.[17]

The NCEP ATP III addresses the metabolic syndrome as a secondary therapeutic target for the prevention of cardiovascular disease. ATP III uses low HDL, or

- **HDL <40 mg/dL in men and**
- **HDL <50 mg/dL in women,**

as one of its criteria for diagnosis of the metabolic syndrome.[17] A triglyceride/HDL ratio of 3.8 may serve as predictor for LDL phenotype, with 79% of phenotype B (small, dense LDL) occurring at a ratio greater than 3.8 and 81% of phenotype A (large, buoyant LDL) occurring at a ratio less than 3.8.[18] Beyond comprehensive therapeutic lifestyle changes, additional pharmacologic intervention is frequently mandated for improvement in HDL and reduction of cardiovascular risk.[17]

Targets of Lipid-Lowering Therapy. Early and aggressive lipid management is an essential risk reduction strategy for individuals with the metabolic syndrome. NCEP ATP III treatment targets include

- LDL <100 mg/dL,
- HDL >40 mg/dL, and
- triglyceride levels <150 mg/dL.

Table 16-1. LDL and Non-HDL Goals for Three ATP III Risk Categories with Triglycerides ≥200 mg/dL

	Primary Target	Secondary Targets		
RISK CATEGORY	**LDL (mg/dL)**	**NON-HDL* (mg/dL)**	**TOTAL APO B (mg/dL)**	**LDL PARTICLE CONCENTRATION (nmol/L)**
CHD or CHD risk equivalent	<100	<130	<90	<1100
≥2 Multiple risk factors	<130	<160	<110	<1400
0-1 Risk factor	<160	<190	<130	<1800

*Non-HDL = VLDL + LDL = total cholesterol – HDL; non-HDL becomes a secondary therapeutic target when serum triglycerides range from 200 to 500 mg/dL.
apo, apoprotein; ATP, Adult Treatment Panel; CHD, coronary heart disease; HDL, high-density lipoprotein; LDL, low-density lipoprotein; VLDL, very-low-density lipoprotein.
Modified from Rosenson RS. Clinical role of LDL and HDL subclasses and apolipoprotein measurement. ACC Curr J Rev 2004;13:33-37.

In fact, the American Diabetes Association recommends

- HDL >45 mg/dL for men and
- HDL >55 mg/dL for women.

When serum triglycerides range from 200 to 500 mg/dL, non-HDL cholesterol (= very-low-density lipoprotein [VLDL] + LDL = total cholesterol – HDL) becomes a secondary therapeutic target (Table 16-1).

Because of the high incidence of mixed lipid disorders, multidrug combination therapy may be needed in many individuals. Varied classes of hypolipidemic drugs are available that have a differential impact on the lipid profile (Table 16-2).

Expected CHD events in men and women over a 10-year period may be reduced by 51.2% and 50.6%, respectively, through an increase in HDL to 60 mg/dL or greater and by 46.2% and 38.1%, respectively, through a reduction in LDL to less than 100 mg/dL.[1]

Lower Low-Density Lipoprotein Target. Even lower LDL goals may be of benefit. Inflammatory conditions variably affect LDL levels, and LDL levels are frequently not elevated in a proinflammatory state. At present, the ATP III treatment algorithm has been modified for very high-risk individuals, with an LDL goal of less than 70 mg/dL suggested as a therapeutic option and a reasonable clinical strategy. This therapeutic option also applies to patients at very high risk whose baseline LDL is less than 100 mg/dL (Table 16-3).[19]

Studies of patients after ACS suggest a benefit with further LDL reduction. In the Reversing Atherosclerosis with Aggressive Lipid Lowering

Table 16-2. Lipid-Lowering Effects of Hypolipidemic Drug Classes and Mutual Interactions

DRUG CLASS	LDL REDUCTION (%)	HDL INCREASE (%)	TRIGLYCERIDE REDUCTION (%)	POTENTIAL INTERACTION WITH
Statins	–18-55	+5-16	–7-30	Fibrate: myopathy Niacin: myopathy, hepatic dysfunction Bile acid sequestrants: decreased statin absorption
Fibrates	–5-20	+11-25	–20-50	Statin: myopathy Bile acid sequestrants: decreased fibrate absorption
Niacin	–5-25	+20-35	–20-50	Statin: myopathy, hepatic dysfunction
Bile acid sequestrants	–15-30	+3-5	0/+	Statin: decreased statin absorption Fibrate: decreased fibrate absorption

HDL, high-density lipoprotein; LDL, low-density lipoprotein.

Table 16-3. Three ATP III Risk Categories to Modify LDL Goals

CHD/CHD risk equivalents* (10-year risk,† >20%)	LDL <100 mg/dL; optional, <70 mg/dL
≥2 Multiple risk factors (10-year risk, 10%-20%)	LDL <130 mg/dL; optional, <100 mg/dL
≥2 Multiple risk factors (10-year risk, <10%)	LDL <130 mg/dL
0-1 Risk factor	LDL <160 mg/dL

Very high risk favors a goal LDL less than 70 mg/dL.
HDL greater than 60 mg/dL is a negative risk factor.
*Diabetes mellitus and peripheral vascular disease are CHD risk equivalents.
†Ten-year risk calculators are available at www.nhlbi.nih.gov/guidelines/cholesterol.
ATP, Adult Treatment Panel; CHD, coronary heart disease, HDL, high-density lipoprotein; LDL, low-density lipoprotein.
Modified from Grundy SM, Cleeman JI, Merz CNB, et al. Implications of recent clinical trials for the National Cholesterol Education Program Adult Treatment Panel III Guidelines. Circulation 2004;110:227-239.

(REVERSAL) study of 502 patients with stable CHD, a baseline LDL level of 150 mg/dL, and a CRP level of 3.0 mg/L, 40 mg of pravastatin daily as standard therapy was compared with 80 mg of atorvastatin daily for 18 months. Intravascular sonography found the higher statin dose, which was associated with substantially greater LDL lowering to 79 mg/dL versus 110 mg/dL and CRP lowering to 1.8 mg/L versus 2.8 mg/L, to be superior at slowing atheroma progression. Plaque burden progressed 2.7% in the pravastatin group, but regressed 0.4% in the atorvastatin group. Further analysis showed that LDL reduction did not explain all the differences in efficacy.[20] In a study of 4162 patients in the Pravastatin or Atorvastatin Evaluation and Infection Therapy—Thrombolysis in Myocardial Infarction 22 (PROVE IT-TIMI 22) study, who had been hospitalized for ACS within the preceding 10 days, therapy with 40 mg of pravastatin daily as standard therapy was compared with 80 mg of atorvastatin daily for 2 years for their effect on reducing the risk for recurrent MI or death from coronary causes. The intensive lipid-lowering regimen with high-dose atorvastatin, in which LDL was lowered to a median level of 62 mg/dL, achieved a 16% reduction in death or major cardiovascular events when compared with the standard pravastatin regimen, which achieved a median LDL level of 95 mg/dL ($P < .001$).[21] The strategy of early and aggressive lipid lowering after ACS was also supported by findings of the A to Z trial, although the results did not achieve statistical significance.[22]

Mechanism of Low-Density Lipoprotein Reduction with Hypolipidemic Measures. Most circulating cholesterol is the result of endogenous hepatic synthesis. LDL is the major conveyor of cholesterol to the periphery. The lipoprotein's apolipoprotein (apo) B-100 binds to LDL(B,E) receptors. Upon binding of the LDL complex to the receptor, the cholesteryl esters of LDL are hydrolyzed in lysosomes to produce free cholesterol.

The intracellular accumulation of free cholesterol inhibits release of the sterol regulatory element binding protein (SREBP). SREBP increases the transcription of two genes:

1. the LDL receptor gene and
2. the gene for 3-hydroxy-3-methylglutaryl (HMG) coenzyme A (CoA) reductase, which is the rate-limiting enzyme for cholesterol synthesis.

The lowering of SREBP by free cholesterol thus engenders down-regulation of the LDL receptor and cholesterol synthesis.

On the other hand, a reduction in the hepatic cholesterol pool via dietary measures or via hypolipidemic drugs increases the release of SREBP. As a result, LDL receptors are up-regulated and LDL levels are decreased.[23,24]

HYPOLIPIDEMIC DRUGS: THE HMG-COA REDUCTASE INHIBITORS

Primary and secondary intervention trials have shown that in all populations, irrespective of cholesterol levels, reduction of LDL via HMG-CoA reductase inhibitor therapy reduces cardiovascular risk.[25-27] According to the guidelines of the NCEP, over 36 million individuals may currently be eligible for HMG-CoA reductase inhibitor therapy.[28,29]

Originally targeted to lower elevated plasma lipids, HMG-CoA reductase inhibitors may also confer clinical benefit by modulating the inflammatory processes underlying atherosclerosis and the metabolic syndrome.

Mechanism of Action. HMG-CoA reductase inhibitors, as implied by their name, inhibit HMG-CoA reductase, thereby interfering with the synthesis of cholesterol and isoprenoids.

Lipid-Lowering Effect. HMG-CoA reductase inhibitors, also termed statins, have beneficial effects on plasma lipids. They block the rate-limiting step in hepatic cholesterol synthesis, the conversion of HMG CoA to mevalonate by competitively binding to hepatic HMG-CoA reductase at nanomolar concentrations (Fig. 16-3). As a result, the intrahepatocellular free cholesterol concentration falls. There are two potential consequences of statin inhibition of cholesterol synthesis:

1. There may be less secretion of cholesterol with VLDL, and VLDL particle formation and secretion may be reduced.[30]
2. The ensuing up-regulation of hepatic LDL receptors lowers circulating levels of LDL particles.[31]

Isoprenoid Depletion. Statins have pleiotropic, beneficial effects beyond lipid lowering that may be caused by depletion of isoprenoids. By inhibiting HMG-CoA reductase, statins also interfere with the synthesis of other compounds that are derived via the mevalonate pathway, such as the isoprenoids.

Isoprenoids. Isoprenoids participate in a number of physiologic processes.[4] They mediate the isoprenylation of other signaling proteins; for example, they cause

- geranylgeranylation of the membrane-associated proteins Rho, Rab, and Rac and
- farnesylation of Ras and laminin.

Isoprenylation describes a lipid modification involving the covalent addition of geranylgeranyl or farnesyl isoprenoids to cysteine residues on

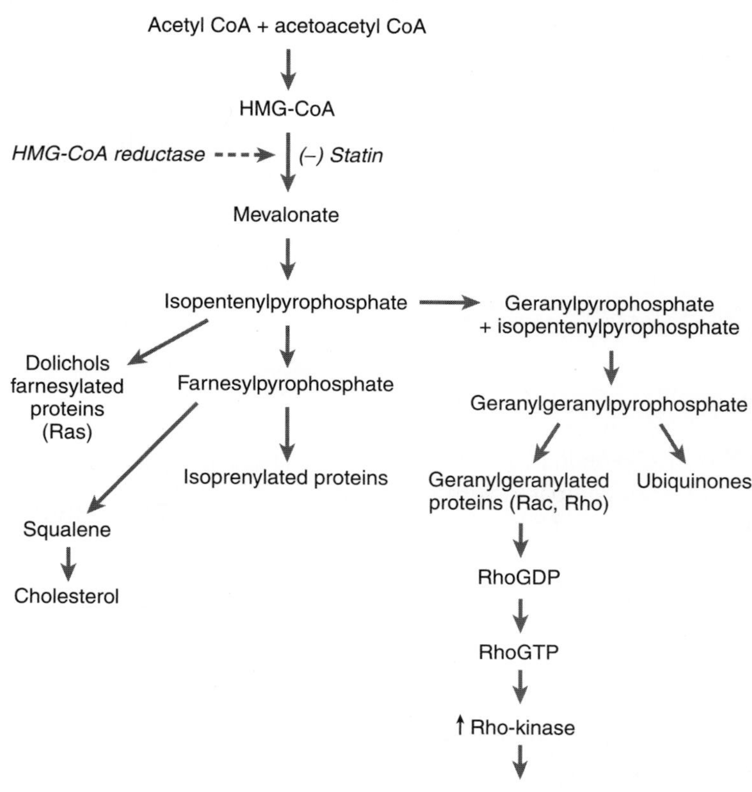

Figure 16–3. 3-Hydroxy-3-methylglutaryl coenzyme A (HMG-CoA) reductase inhibition: impact on cholesterol and isoprenoid synthesis and inflammation. GDP, guanosine 5′-diphosphate; GTP, guanosine 5′-triphosphate. *(Modified from Sowers J. Effects of statins on the vasculature: implication for aggressive lipid management in the cardiovascular metabolic syndrome. Am J Cardiol 2003;91(suppl): 14B-22B.)*

proteins in order to promote membrane-protein and protein-protein interactions.[23,32]

Rho, Rac, and Ras. Rho, Rac, and Ras are small guanosine triphosphatase (GTPase) molecules involved in cellular signaling. Isoprenylation is a necessary step in the activation of inactive, cytoplasmic guanosine diphosphate (GDP)-bound Rho/Ras to the active, plasmalemmal GTP-bound state (Fig. 16-4).[23]

Active, plasma membrane–attached Rho/Ras are implicated in

- causing changes in the actin cytoskeleton,
- allowing the assembly of focal adhesion complexes,
- increasing cell proliferation,
- increasing cell migration, and
- raising the expression of iNOS.[23]

Rac is a component of the nicotinamide adenine dinucleotide phosphate (NADH/NADPH) oxidase complex of both leukocytes and vascular cells.[33]

Statin Impact on Isoprenylation. Statins compromise the synthesis and thus deplete the cellular pools of key isoprenoids such as

- geranylgeranylpyrophosphate and
- farnesylpyrophosphate,

thereby inhibiting both geranylgeranylation and farnesylation.[23,32] As a result, statins

- inhibit lipid attachment to Rho/Ras and their subsequent membrane translocation, activation, and proinflammatory effects[34] and
- down-regulate Rac1-GTPase activity by reducing the isoprenylation and translocation of Rac1 to the cell membrane. The inhibition of Rac1 by statins decreases the NADH/NADPH oxidase–related production of ROS in vascular smooth muscle cells and cardiac myocytes.[33]

Impact of Low-Density Lipoprotein Reduction with Statins in Insulin-Resistant and Diabetic Populations. Diabetic and metabolic syndrome patients are at high risk for recurrent coronary events that can be substantially reduced by HMG-CoA reductase therapy.

Traditionally, atherosclerosis has been considered to be the result of lipid disorders. Clinical trials of statin therapy have been formulated on that construct and do not specifically address insulin resistance and the effect on diabetic individuals. Post hoc analysis of diabetic subgroups in some of these trials has demonstrated the efficacy of statins in lowering LDL and decreasing the incidence of cardiovascular disease in patients with the metabolic syndrome or DM.

The Cholesterol And Recurrent Events (CARE) study was a 5-year trial of 4139 patients who had sustained an MI an average of 10 months before study entry and who were randomized to pravastatin, 40 mg/day, or placebo. The CARE study

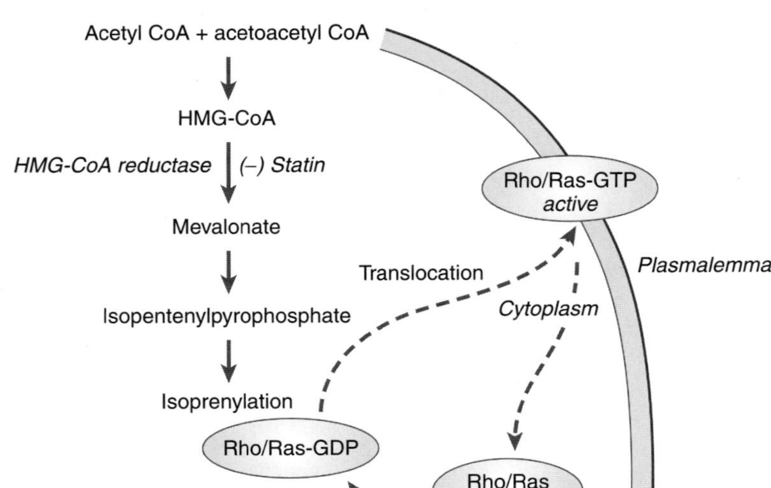

▸▸ **Figure 16–4.** The inhibitory effect of statins on Rho/Ras protein isoprenylation as a mediator of statin pleiotropic effects. GDP, guanosine 5′-diphosphate; GTP, guanosine 5′-triphosphate; HMG-CoA, 3-hydroxy-3-methylglutaryl coenzyme A. *(Modified from Sowers J. Effects of statins on the vasculature: implication for aggressive lipid management in the cardiovascular metabolic syndrome. Am J Cardiol 2003;91[suppl]: 14B-22B.)*

included 586 diabetic patients with mean baseline levels of LDL cholesterol (136 mg/dL), HDL cholesterol (38 mg/dL), and triglyceride (164 mg/dL) similar to those of the nondiabetic group. Reduction of LDL cholesterol by pravastatin was similar in diabetics and nondiabetics, as were the significant reductions in the relative risk for coronary events and revascularization procedures.[35]

In the Scandinavian Simvastatin Survival Study (4S), a secondary intervention trial involving 4444 patients with CHD and total cholesterol higher than 200 mg/dL, the prevalence of CHD was lowered and coronary events were reduced with simvastatin, 20 to 40 mg/day, versus placebo. Statin therapy also reduced coronary events in diabetic subjects and in individuals with impaired fasting glucose. Surprisingly, in 4S, statin therapy was more effective for lipid-triad subjects with high LDL cholesterol, high triglycerides, and low HDL cholesterol than for isolated high-LDL subjects.[36,37]

Similar findings were obtained with simvastatin, 40 mg, versus placebo in the Heart Protection Study (HPS), a trial involving 20,536 individuals with total cholesterol greater than 135 mg/dL and vascular disease or at high risk for such because of the presence of DM or hypertension. A substudy of 5963 type 1 and type 2 diabetics in HPS aged 40 to 80 years with an average baseline LDL level of 124 mg/dL, even in the absence of preexisting CHD or other cardiovascular disease, showed a significant reduction in the primary end point of coronary death or nonfatal MI, with comparable decreases in coronary revascularization and stroke after 5 years of therapy. An average reduction in LDL cholesterol of 39 mg/dL during the trial lessened the risk for major vascular events by 22% ($P < .0001$) in diabetics, similar to the reduction seen in nondiabetic patients, regardless of lipid concentrations or glycemic control.[38]

No benefit for diabetic or metabolic syndrome patients was seen in the Anglo-Scandinavian Cardiac Outcomes Trial (ASCOT). ASCOT tested 10,305 hypertensive patients without known CHD but with three additional cardiovascular risk factors in a lipid-lowering substudy of atorvastatin, 10 mg, versus placebo. The primary end point was fatal CHD and nonfatal MI. Secondary end points were total cardiovascular events, procedures, and coronary events. Total cholesterol decreased from 209 to 160 mg/dL and LDL from 131 to 87 mg/dL. The substudy was stopped early at 3.3 years (versus 5 years) because of a significant primary end point risk reduction of 36%, $P = .0005$. There was an approximately 35% risk reduction in all lipid cohorts, including those starting with total cholesterol less than 190 mg/dL and LDL less than 115 mg/dL. However, there was no primary end point benefit for diabetics and individuals with the metabolic syndrome.[39]

In contrast, another randomized, placebo-controlled clinical study of atorvastatin, 10 mg/day, that directly targeted diabetics, the Collaborative Atorvastatin Diabetes Study (CARDS), which included 2838 diabetic patients aged 40 to 75 years without a documented previous history of CHD but with retinopathy, albuminuria, current smoking, or hypertension, was stopped 2 years early after a median of 3.9 years' follow-up because of a significant 37% reduction in the incidence of MI, stroke, and coronary revascularization, $P = .001$.[40] At randomization, patients were selected for plasma LDL cholesterol levels of 160 mg/dL or less and triglyceride levels of 600 mg/dL or less. Assessed separately, atorvastatin, as compared with placebo, reduced ACS events by 36%, coronary revascularization by 31%, stroke by 48%, and mortality by 27%, $P = .059$.[41,42]

Statin Effect on Triglycerides. Statin therapy primarily lowers LDL levels. Statins may, however, also reduce plasma triglyceride levels by up to 35%.[43] Several mechanisms appear to be involved:

- In a rat model of hypertriglyceridemia, atorvastatin increased the expression of peroxisome proliferator–activated receptor-alpha (PPAR-α), which caused a reduction in hepatocellular triacylglycerol and plasma free fatty acid levels.[44]
- Statins stimulate lipoprotein lipase (LPL) activity.[45]
- In diabetic and nondiabetic individuals, pravastatin reduces apo C-III. Apo C-III is a small protein on the surface of apo B lipoproteins, such as VLDL, intermediate-density lipoprotein (IDL), and LDL, that inhibits LPL from hydrolyzing the triglycerides within apo B lipoproteins. As a result of statin action, LPL activity is disinhibited and atherogenic apo C-III–positive lipoproteins are reduced.[46]

Statin Effect on High-Density Lipoproteins. In addition to reducing LDL cholesterol and triglycerides, statins modestly increase the levels of

- **HDL cholesterol by up to 6% and**
- **apo A-I by at most 5% to 10%.**[43]

Statins also normalize the size distribution of HDL particles.[47]

Diverse statins have differing impact on HDL: low 10-mg doses of rosuvastatin raise HDL more effectively than do 10-mg doses of atorvastatin and pravastatin or 20 mg of simvastatin[48]; high 80-mg doses of simvastatin may be more efficacious at HDL elevation than 40- to 80-mg doses of atorvastatin.[49]

Two mechanisms contribute to a statin-mediated rise in HDL:

1. A reduction in triglyceride levels will raise HDL.
2. Statin activation of PPAR-α, via inhibition of RhoA activation, appears to play a contributory role. In human HepG2 hepatoma cells, statins, acting at the transcriptional level with a rise in human apo A-I promoter activity, increased apo A-I messenger RNA (mRNA) levels. The statin response element coincides with a PPAR-α response element that confers fibrate responsiveness. Increased statin-induced PPAR-α activity was abolished by geranylgeranylpyrophosphate but enhanced by exposure to a RhoA inhibitor. Statins and fibrates synergistically activate PPAR-α.[50]

Lipid-Independent Beneficial Effects of Statins. Beneficial effects on dyslipidemia do not account for all the observed vascular risk reduction with statins.[24] Treatment efficacy does not depend on LDL lowering alone, and benefit is derived irrespective of the baseline LDL, even when less than 100 mg/dL.[32] Time-to-event curves with statin therapy diverge earlier than predicted from cholesterol lowering alone.[25] The 70% decrease in the incidence of coronary events is out of proportion with the minimal lesion regression of 0.7% seen in the Familial Atherosclerosis Treatment Study (FATS).[51] Beneficial effects on inflammation, coagulability, and endothelial function probably contribute to the mechanism of action of these agents.

Because the cholesterol-independent, pleiotropic effects of statins are predominantly due to inhibition of isoprenoid rather than of cholesterol synthesis, the cholesterol-independent effects of statins have shifted therapeutic considerations from a focus on numerical lipid parameters to a global assessment of inflammatory activity and cardiovascular risk.

Irrespective of the underlying lipid profile, statin therapy would appear to be indicated in insulin-resistant individuals with metabolic syndrome, who are at moderate to high risk for cardiovascular events.

Structural Variation of Statins. Different statins have structural variations that determine their lipophilicity, metabolism, half-life, and lipid-lowering potency (Table 16-4). Pravastatin and rosuvastatin are hydrophilic and thus do not penetrate plasma membranes as readily as the lipophilic agents do. Hydrophilic and lipophilic agents do appear to have similar beneficial, non–lipid-lowering related effects,[23] although some differences in pleiotropic effects may pertain.[52]

Antioxidant Effect. Oxidative pathways play a role in insulin resistance. **Statins have antioxidant effects. They inhibit isoprenylation of key proteins involved in oxidant/antioxidant processes of the vessel wall.**

In endothelial and smooth muscle cell culture studies, statins suppress Rac isoprenylation, thus

Table 16-4. Doses of Available Statins Needed for a 30% to 40% Reduction in LDL as Derived from FDA Drug Package Inserts

DRUG	DOSE (mg/day)	LDL REDUCTION (%)
Atorvastatin	10	39
Lovastatin	40	31
Pravastatin	40	34
Simvastatin	20-40	35-41
Fluvastatin	40-80	25-35
Rosuvastatin	5-10	39-45

Every doubling of the dose above the standard dose achieves an approximately 6% decrease in LDL level.
FDA, Food and Drug Administration; LDL, low-density lipoprotein.
Modified from Grundy SM, Cleeman JI, Merz CNB, et al. Implications of recent clinical trials for the National Cholesterol Education Program Adult Treatment Panel III Guidelines. Circulation 2004;110:227-239.

impairing Rac translocation to the plasma membrane. Because Rac is a component of the NADH/NADPH oxidase complex, superoxide formation is suppressed. In this way, statins directly, or indirectly via modulation of angiotensin II and endothelin release, lower ROS formation.[23,33]

The antioxidant milieu established by statins has a beneficial impact. As a result, statins

- prevent the oxidative inactivation and destruction of nitric oxide (NO);
- reduce LDL oxidation, decrease activation of the lectin-like oxidized LDL receptor, and reduce the avidity of macrophages for oxidized LDL[53]; and
- increase levels of natural antioxidants such as vitamins C and E, ubiquinones, and glutathiones.[23,54]

Clinically, statins promote potent, systemic antioxidant effects through the suppression of oxidation pathways implicated in atherogenesis. In hypercholesterolemic subjects without CHD, 12 weeks of atorvastatin (10 mg/day) caused significant reductions in plasma levels of protein-bound chlorotyrosine, nitrotyrosine, and dityrosine, specific derivatives of myeloperoxidase-derived and NO-derived oxidant pathways that are up-regulated with atheroma formation. These reductions, albeit similar in magnitude to reductions in total cholesterol and apo B-100, occurred independent of decreases in lipids and lipoproteins.[33]

Anti-inflammatory Effect. Statins exert anti-inflammatory effects independent of their cholesterol-lowering properties. The anti-inflammatory actions may contribute to statin-related plaque stabilization and the reduction in CHD and DM risk for individuals with normal LDL.

Numerous potential pathways are involved.

Nuclear Factor kappaB. In vitro studies suggest direct inhibition of NFκB by statins.[4] Statins also diminish activator protein-1 (AP-1) activity. NFκB and AP-1 are transcription factors that regulate genes involved in numerous inflammatory pathways.[32]

NFκB activation, as part of the cellular oxidative and inflammatory response, entails the membrane translocation of GTP-binding proteins such as Rac to couple to the phospholipid cell membrane layer via isoprenylation. Because statins inhibit Rac membrane translocation, they undercut the resultant NFκB activation and secondary interleukin-6 (IL-6) elaboration.[4]

PPAR Activation. Activation of PPAR-γ and PPAR-α contributes to the anti-inflammatory effect of statins.

Atorvastatin activates PPAR-γ in a concentration-dependent manner. In cultured, primary human monocytes, it thus inhibited

- TNF-α production by up to 38%,
- monocyte chemoattractant protein-1 (MCP-1) by up to 85%, and
- gelatinase B by up to 73%.[55]

Similarly, in human monocytes, pravastatin increased the expression of PPAR-γ, thereby abolishing NFkB expression and significantly inhibiting matrix metalloproteinases (MMPs), MCP-1, and TNF-α.[56]

In human umbilical vein endothelial cells (HUVECs), statins induced the mRNA expression of PPAR-α and PPAR-γ associated with significant reductions in IL-1β and IL-6 mRNA. Overall, there was lower expression of adhesion molecules and reduced vascular smooth muscle cell proliferation, transmigration, and leukocyte rolling.[23]

Immunoactivation. Statins act as inhibitors of the major histocompatibility complex class II (MHC-II)-mediated immunoactivation. MHC-II expression can activate T cells. Although in contrast to MHC-I, MHC-II is constitutively expressed on only a limited number of specialized cells, such expression can be induced by interferon-γ. Statins inhibit the induction of MHC-II expression by interferon-γ.[4]

CD40 and its ligand CD154 are implicated in several immunologic pathways and mediate a wide range of proatherogenic processes. Statin treatment reduces the cell surface expression of CD40 on atheroma-associated cells in vitro and on atherosclerotic lesions in patients[57] and interferes with CD40 signaling at several levels with beneficial effect.[32]

T-Cell Activity. Atorvastatin may regulate the cytotoxic activity of T cells and the number of T cells in atherosclerotic plaque. Atorvastatin regulates one of the main mechanisms of cell death activation, expression of the Fas–Fas ligand system in T cells, via inhibition of RhoA prenylation.[58]

Infectious Agent–Related Inflammation. In a number of instances, indolent, chronic infections may be implicated in the pathophysiology of atherosclerosis and insulin resistance by inducing inflammatory modifications in vascular cells. Statins appear to limit such effects of pathogens.

Statins reduced *Chlamydia pneumoniae*–induced, macrophage-mediated signaling and transmission by interfering with Rac1 and RhoA prenylation and NFκB activation.[59]

Similarly, fluvastatin restrained cytomegalovirus (CMV) replication in HUVECs. In HUVECs infected with CMV, coincubation with fluvastatin inhibited viral antigen expression, DNA synthesis, and viral particle production, conceivably by reducing NFκB binding activity.[60]

Statins may have potential benefit in sepsis treatment. Of mice rendered septic by cecal ligation and perforation, those treated with simvastatin survived nearly four times longer than did the untreated mice. With statin therapy, the vascular inflammatory response was allayed. There was complete preservation of cardiac function, hemodynamic status, and β-adrenergic receptor sensitivity, which were severely impaired in untreated, septic mice.[61]

Clinical Studies. In patients with CHD, atorvastatin, 80 mg/day, significantly reduced cytokine and chemokine receptor mRNA levels in peripheral blood mononuclear cells with a reduction in the spontaneous release of IL-8 and macrophage inflammatory protein-1α.[62]

C-Reactive Protein. **The anti-inflammatory impact of statins decreases CRP levels independent of LDL levels.** CRP elaboration by the liver is stimulated by IL-6. IL-6 expression is enhanced by NFκB, by TNF-α, and by oxidized LDL. Statins interfere with these stimuli.[4]

In the primary prevention Pravastatin Inflammation/CRP Evaluation (PRINCE) trial of 1702 individuals, when compared with placebo, pravastatin lowered CRP by 16.9% (0.02 mg/dL) in all subgroups by 24 weeks in an LDL-independent manner.[63] In the primary prevention, 5-year Air Force/Texas Coronary Atherosclerosis Prevention Study (AFCAPS-TexCAPS) of 5742 participants, lovastatin reduced CRP by 14.8% ($P < .001$) and effectively prevented ACS events independent of baseline lipid levels when compared with placebo.[64] In the 5-year, secondary prevention CARE trial of 4139 post-MI patients, pravastatin lowered CRP by 21.6% in comparison to controls ($P = .007$), unrelated to the magnitude of lipid lowering. Risk reduction attributable to treatment was highest in patients with elevated baseline levels of CRP, suggestive of ongoing, low-grade inflammation,[65] an effect also seen with simvastatin.[66]

Statins also reduce CRP acutely in the setting of ACS. Within the first 5 days of admission for ACS, the initiation of 80 mg/day atorvastatin therapy prevented a 188% rise in CRP.[67] In the Myocardial Ischemia Reduction with Aggressive Cholesterol Lowering (MIRACL) study of subjects with unstable angina or non–Q-wave MI who were randomized to atorvastatin, 80 mg/day, or placebo within 24 to 96 hours of hospital admission and treated for 16 weeks, CRP was 34% lower with atorvastatin than with placebo. Smaller doses of statins appeared to have a lesser anti-inflammatory effect than higher doses did, and the effect was independent of plasma LDL levels.[68]

Aggressive strategies of cardiovascular risk reduction via statin therapy may need to include assessment of not only lipids but also activity of the inflammatory process. Patients who have low CRP levels with statin therapy have better clinical outcomes than do those with higher CRP levels, regardless of the associated level of LDL cholesterol. Although the PROVE IT-TIMI 22 study demonstrated the importance of achieving LDL levels less than 70 mg/dL after ACS, subsequent event-free survival was also linked to a reduction in CRP levels. In that same trial, among 3745 patients with ACS, achieving a target CRP level of less than 2 mg/L was associated with significant improvement in event-free survival, an effect present at all levels of LDL cholesterol achieved. The relationship between the reduction in LDL and CRP varied greatly from patient to patient; less than 3% of the variation in achieved CRP levels was explained by the variation in achieved LDL cholesterol levels.[69] Similarly, in the REVERSAL trial, intravascular ultrasonography showed both the magnitude of change in CRP levels and the size of change in LDL levels to be independent predictors of significantly slower rates of plaque progression after statin therapy.[70]

CD40 Ligand. Early statin therapy after ACS counters the risk for recurrent cardiovascular events associated with elevated levels of the proinflammatory, prothrombotic cytokine CD40 ligand. Of 3086 subjects enrolled in the MIRACL study of atorvastatin, 80 mg/day, versus placebo, plasma CD40 ligand was measured in 2908 patients at baseline and in 2352 at 16 weeks. Only high levels of CD40 ligand (>90th percentile) were a risk factor for a recurrent cardiovascular event. Although atorvastatin only modestly lowered the CD40 ligand level (P = .08), the CHD event risk was effectively abolished by atorvastatin, which reduced the risk by 48%.[71]

Anticoagulant Effect. The metabolic syndrome is associated with a prothrombotic and antifibrinolytic milieu. **Statins have antithrombotic effects, which contribute to the lower cardiovascular event rate with statin use.** The antithrombotic and profibrinolytic effects are independent of cholesterol levels.[4]

Statin-mediated isoprenoid depletion with inhibition of Rho protein isoprenylation

- promotes tissue plasminogen activator (tPA) synthesis,
- reduces plasminogen activator inhibitor-1 (PAI-1) production,
- reduces endothelin-1 elaboration, and
- inhibits the expression of tissue factor by macrophages.[4]

Statins also

- normalize thrombin formation;
- inhibit activation of factors V and XIII and prothrombin;
- inactivate factor Va;
- decrease levels of fibrinogen, fibrinopeptide A, fibrin degradation product D-dimer, thrombin–antithrombin III complex, and thrombomodulin[72]; and
- lower blood viscosity.[73]

Platelet Activation. Statins reduce platelet activation. Patients with hyperlipidemia and the metabolic syndrome have increased platelet reactivity. Such platelets have down-regulated NO elaboration[74] and a reduced number of prostacyclin binding sites. Statins reduce thromboxane A_2 formation. They normalize platelet responsiveness to prostacyclin and probably up-regulate platelet-derived NO production, thus interfering with platelet hyperreactivity.[4] The reduced cholesterol-to-phospholipid content of the platelet membrane with statin therapy probably contributes to impaired platelet aggregability (Table 16-5).[73]

Table 16-5. Effect of HMG-CoA Reductase Inhibition on Inflammatory Processes

PROCESS	REDUCTION
Oxidative stress	Angiotensin I expression/synthesis NADH/NADPH oxidase activity COX-2 expression Lipoxygenase products ROS
Inflammation	Angiotensin I expression/synthesis NFκB activation CRP Adhesion molecules—P-selectin
Thrombosis	Tissue factor expression and activity Fibrinogen generation Thrombin generation PAI-1 expression Blood viscosity
Platelets	Thromboxane A_2 synthesis Aggregation and endothelial adhesion

COX, cyclooxygenase; CRP, C-reactive protein; HMG-CoA, 3-hydroxy-3-methylglutaryl coenzyme A; NADH/NADPH, nicotinamide adenine dinucleotide phosphate; NFκB, nuclear factor kappaB; PAI-1, plasminogen activator inhibitor-1; ROS, reactive oxygen species.
Adapted from Sowers J. Effects of statins on the vasculature: implication for aggressive lipid management in the cardiovascular metabolic syndrome. Am J Cardiol 2003;91(suppl):14B-22B.

Vascular Function. Statins improve endothelial function and promote the production of NO. Both the lipid-lowering and the pleiotropic effects of statin therapy play a role. In hypercholesterolemia, LDL reduction in itself improves endothelial function as seen with LDL lowering via dietary intervention or the use of bile acid resins.[75,76]

Endothelial Function. Endothelial dysfunction is a hallmark of the metabolic syndrome. Abnormal functioning of the endothelium underlies insulin resistance and vascular pathology. Therapy with

HMG-CoA reductase inhibitors consistently reverses endothelial dysfunction.[77,78] **By increasing NO production, statins improve endothelial function, an effect that contributes to the lower incidence of cardiovascular events with statin therapy.** Statins may, however, vary in their efficacy to enhance the release of NO by endothelial as well as vascular smooth muscle cells.[23,79]

Statin therapy improves endothelium-dependent coronary vasomotion within 24 hours, before any significant reductions in cholesterol and CRP in patients with ACS.[80] There are various mechanisms independent of serum cholesterol levels whereby statins may enhance NO release[81]:

- Treatment of human endothelial cells with statins increases the protein and mRNA expression of endothelial NO synthase (eNOS) by increasing the half-life of eNOS mRNA without changing transcription of the eNOS gene.[81]
  The underlying cause appears to be the statin-related inhibition of isoprenoid production and Rho geranylgeranylation. Rho kinase ordinarily suppresses the expression of eNOS. Inactive Rho fails to activate Rho kinase. With failed suppression of eNOS, NO production is enhanced.[81]
- Statins may increase eNOS activity posttranslationally via activation of the phosphatidylinositol 3-kinase (PI3K)/Akt pathway[34] or through interaction with heat shock protein 90 (HSP90) (or via both means).[79]
- Statins lower plasmalemmal caveolin levels, thus decreasing the inhibition of eNOS by caveolin. For example, rosuvastatin decreased caveolin-1 expression and promoted eNOS function in mice in vivo, with concurrent improvements in blood pressure and heart rate variability.[82]

In normolipidemic rat models of hypertension, rosuvastatin reduced arterial pressure with a reduction in peripheral resistance.[83]

Vasculogenesis. In animal studies, hypercholesterolemia inhibits vasculogenesis. A reduction in cholesterol level alone may disinhibit angiogenesis and reestablish new blood vessel formation.[84]

Statin therapy may promote a proangiogenic response independent of lipid lowering. Stimulation of the Akt pathway by statins may play a role in this effect. Statins can also mobi-lize and activate endothelial progenitor cells to restore endothelial integrity and function after injury.[84,85]

Cell Proliferation. Statins have antiproliferative effects. They suppress abnormal endothelial and vascular smooth muscle cell proliferative responses to injury. They also induce apoptosis of pathologic vascular smooth muscle cells in vivo.

These effects are mediated by

- down-regulation of Bcl-2 expression,
- inhibition of the isoprenylation of Rho and Rac family GTPases that couple growth factor receptors to the intracellular mitogen-activated protein kinase (MAPK)/extracellular signal–regulated kinase (ERK) signaling pathways, and
- induction of the cell cycle inhibitor $p27^{Kip}$ (Table 16-6).[86]

Table 16-6. Effects of HMG-CoA Reductase Inhibitors on the Vasculature

SITE	INCREASE	DECREASE
Endothelial cells	eNOS expression/stability/activity eNOS-calmodulin dissociation Bone marrow–derived progenitor cells tPA	Endothelin-1 expression/synthesis Adhesion molecules—P-selectin
Vascular smooth muscle cells	Apoptosis iNOS expression and activity Na^+ pump activity	Contractility with vasoconstrictors Proliferation and migration Cytoplasmic Ca^{2+}

eNOS, endothelial nitric oxide synthase; HMG-CoA, 3-hydroxy-3-methylglutaryl coenzyme A; iNOS, inducible NOS; tPA, tissue plasminogen activator.

Adapted from Sowers J. Effects of statins on the vasculature: implication for aggressive lipid management in the cardiovascular metabolic syndrome. Am J Cardiol 2003;91(suppl):14B-22B.

Tissue Perfusion and Function. There is an increase in tissue perfusion with statin therapy. In contrast to the prompt improvement in endothelial function with statin therapy, the enhancement of tissue perfusion appears to require long-term exposure to statin effects. It reflects not only an increment in endothelially mediated, flow-dependent vasodilation, but also the cumulative impact of statin-modulated anti-inflammatory, vasculoprotective, and other effects.[87,88]

In hyperlipidemic patients with a mean age of 75 years and symptomatic peripheral vascular disease, 40 mg of simvastatin daily for 6 and 12 months significantly increased the duration of exercise until the onset of claudication by 24% and 42%, respectively.[89] Similarly, in patients with intermittent claudication, pain-free walking time improved after 12 months of treatment with 80 mg/day atorvastatin.[90] In hyperlipidemic patients undergoing statin therapy, even though an improvement in lipid profile was detectable at 6 weeks, improvements in myocardial perfusion were delayed and detectable only at 6 months. Furthermore, the enhancement of tissue perfusion was not closely correlated to improvements in lipid profile.[91] In moderately hypercholesterolemic subjects without heart disease, 6-month therapy with atorvastatin improved myocardial contractile reserve as assessed by pulsed-wave tissue Doppler imaging during low-dose dobutamine infusion.[87] Short-term, 14-week therapy with 10 mg/day simvastatin was of symptomatic benefit even for patients with symptomatic, nonischemic, dilated cardiomyopathy. Patients treated with simvastatin had a lower New York Heart Association (NYHA) functional class than did those receiving placebo, with significant improvement in left ventricular ejection fraction and lower plasma concentrations of TNF-α, IL-6, and brain natriuretic peptide.[88]

Atherogenesis. **Statins reduce atherogenesis beyond the impact attributable to cholesterol lowering alone, largely as a result of their anti-inflammatory effects.**

One such anti-inflammatory effect entails the down-regulation of angiotensin II type 1 (AT_1) receptors in vascular smooth muscle by HMG-CoA reductase inhibitors. As a result, statins ameliorate angiotensin II–induced vascular injury.[92] In angiotensin II–dependent animal models, statins have antihypertrophic and antifibrotic effects.[93]

In a rabbit model of atherosclerosis, simvastatin elicited regression of atherosclerotic lesions.[94] In an apo E*3-Leiden mouse model of diet-induced hypercholesterolemia and atherosclerosis, rosuvastatin significantly reduced aortic atheroma cross-sectional lesion area in excess of the reduction effected via cholesterol lowering alone. Concurrently, rosuvastatin suppressed the expression of MCP-1 and TNF-α in the vessel wall while lowering plasma concentrations of serum amyloid A and fibrinogen, independent of its cholesterol-lowering effect.[95]

Inhibition of NFκB activity and Rho prenylation may underlie the statin-related reduction in plaque destabilization via matrix-degrading MMP enzymes. MMPs are regulated by proinflammatory cytokines such as TNF-α, IL-1, and CD40L. HMG-CoA reductase inhibitors lower the expression and function of the

- interstitial collagenases MMP-1 and MMP-13,
- gelatinases MMP-2 and MMP-9, and
- stromelysin MMP-3

in macrophages, the major source of MMPs in lesions, as well as in most other cell types involved in atherogenesis. Additionally, statins augment the expression of endogenous tissue inhibitors of MMP (TIMPs) in vascular cells and macrophages and thereby enhance vascular lesion stability.[32]

Clinically, lipid-lowering therapy with simvastatin for 12 months is associated with some regression of coronary atherosclerosis. In 40 male patients with hypercholesterolemia, CHD, and a nonsignificant coronary artery lesion in a not previously revascularized coronary artery, 12 months of 40 mg/day simvastatin induced a significant reduction of 6.3% (P = .002) in plaque and media volume on serial intravascular ultrasound studies, along with significant reductions in total and LDL cholesterol.[96]

Metabolic Syndrome. Treatment with statins may increase insulin sensitivity. The anti-inflammatory, antioxidant, and vasculoprotective effects of statins would be expected to have a favorable impact on insulin sensitivity and the onset of type 2 DM.

Insulin Resistance. **Statins enhance sensitivity to insulin signaling.**

In 20 nonobese, normoglycemic, normotensive patients with hyperlipidemia, fasting serum insulin levels were significantly higher than those in reference subjects. Treatment with fluvastatin, 40 mg once daily for 3 months, improved insulin sensitivity as assessed by the homeostasis assessment model (HOMA).[97] In 35 dyslipidemic, normoglycemic patients, fluvastatin, 40 mg/day for 8 weeks, improved insulin resistance. The change in HOMA-evaluated insulin resistance was not correlated with alterations in triglyceride, LDL, HDL, or total cholesterol levels.[98] In 33 subjects with impaired glucose tolerance, 40 mg atorvastatin per day versus placebo over a 16-week period decreased CRP significantly in the atorvastatin-treated group and produced a trend toward significant improvement in insulin sensitivity.[99] In 195 elderly type 2 diabetic patients with mean age of 67 years, treatment for 8 weeks with simvastatin or atorvastatin versus placebo significantly lowered plasma total LDL, HDL, and triglyceride concentrations while improving insulin resistance.[100]

New-Onset Type 2 Diabetes Mellitus. Statin therapy may delay the onset of type 2 DM.

In the primary prevention West of Scotland Coronary Prevention Study trial of 6595 high-risk patients, assignment to pravastatin therapy slowed progression of CHD, with concomitant prevention of the onset of type 2 DM by 30% in high-risk individuals ($P = .042$).[3]

Other Statin Effects. Statins have numerous beneficial effects in other conditions linked to inflammation.

Autonomic Function. Autonomic dysfunction, characterized by sympathetic predominance and vagal withdrawal, is associated with the metabolic syndrome. Statins may improve autonomic dysfunction.

Atorvastatin, 10 mg/day, ameliorated autonomic dysfunction in patients with the metabolic syndrome, with a small reduction in systolic blood pressure.[101] Analogously, simvastatin, in a rabbit model of heart failure, resulted in normalization of sympathetic outflow and reflex regulation, as assessed by plasma norepinephrine levels, direct recordings of renal sympathetic nerve activity, and baroreflex function.[102]

Cardiac Arrhythmias. Statin therapy may reduce the incidence of cardiac arrhythmias.

The use of statins appears to be protective against atrial fibrillation. In a canine sterile pericarditis model of atrial fibrillation, atorvastatin prevented the maintenance of atrial fibrillation by inhibiting inflammation.[103] In a sample of 449 patients with chronic, stable CHD without atrial fibrillation monitored prospectively for an average of 5 years, statin therapy was associated with a significantly reduced risk for development of atrial fibrillation independent of the reduction in serum cholesterol levels.[104] In 62 patients with lone, persistent atrial fibrillation lasting 3 months or longer who underwent successful external cardioversion, the use of statins was associated with a significant decrease in the risk for arrhythmia recurrence after successful cardioversion.[105]

Data from the Antiarrhythmics Versus Implantable Defibrillators (AVID) trial revealed a reduction in ventricular tachycardia or fibrillation in ischemic cardiomyopathy with lipid-lowering therapy, suggestive of an antiarrhythmic effect. Seventy-nine percent of these patients were receiving statin therapy; 19%, fibrates; and 3%, bile acid resins.[106]

Psychological Well-Being. Statin use may benefit psychological well-being and lower the risk for depression.

In a retrospective study of the United Kingdom General Practice Research Database, the adjusted odds ratio of depression was 0.4 for current statin use when compared with nonuse.[107] In contrast to other vigorous lipid-lowering modalities, long-term statin therapy, particularly via lipophilic agents, caused a progressive, cumulative reduction in levels of depression, anxiety, and hostility. The effect was independent of the degree of cholesterol lowering.[108]

Other Effects. The pleiotropic properties of statins favorably affect a variety of other conditions.

Statins appear to be of benefit for renal and bone health.[24] Their use is associated with a reduction in the risk for dementia and Alzheimer's disease, osteoporosis, macular degeneration, and breast and other cancers, with salutary effects on multiple sclerosis and nonischemic cardiomyopathy.[109-113]

HYPOLIPIDEMIC DRUGS: THE FIBRIC ACID DERIVATIVES

Fibric acid derivatives, or fibrates, such as clofibrate, ciprofibrate, bezafibrate, fenofibrate, and gemfibrozil, are considered to be PPAR-α activators. They were synthesized originally as metabolically stable analogues of branched-chain fatty acids. When compared with the efficacy of eicosapentaenoic acid, fibrates are strong activators of PPAR.[114]

Therapy to reduce LDL does not address the most common lipid disorder in the metabolic syndrome: low plasma levels of HDL and hypertriglyceridemia. Fibrates are used for the treatment of hypertriglyceridemia with or without hypoalphalipoproteinemia.

Clinical Trials. Trials have shown clinical benefit with fibrate therapy for cardiovascular disease.

The Veterans Affairs High Density Lipoprotein Cholesterol Intervention Trial (VA-HIT) confirmed that the use of 1200 mg/day of gemfibrozil in 2531 patients with CHD, LDL 140 mg/dL or greater, triglyceride 300 mg/dL or less, and HDL 40 mg/dL or less, over a median duration of 5.1 years, was associated with a 22% reduction in death from CHD and nonfatal MI. Subgroup analysis of 627 diabetics showed a 24% reduction in CHD-related death. The absolute CHD risk reduction was 4% to 5% for the entire cohort and 8% for patients with DM. Although triglycerides decreased by 24.5% and HDL rose by 7.5%, this occurred without a lowering of LDL. There was, however, no reduction in rates of coronary revascularization, unstable angina-related hospitalizations, or total mortality.[115]

Beneficial effects of fibrates have been documented in other angiographic and clinical end point trials, such as the Bezafibrate Coronary Atherosclerosis Intervention Trial (BECAIT); the St. Mary's, Ealing, Northwick Park Diabetes (SENDCAP) study; the Lopid Coronary Angiographic Trial (LOCAT); the Bezafibrate Infarction Prevention (BIP) study; and the Diabetes Atherosclerosis Intervention Study (DAIS).[116,117] It is, however, not yet clear whether targeted therapy to raise HDL or to lower triglycerides is of greater importance.

Mechanism of Action. Fibrate therapy lowers triglyceride and LDL levels while increasing HDL.

Peroxisome Proliferator–Activated Receptors. Fibrates are PPAR-α activators and thus have a direct effect on at least five genes that determine lipoprotein synthesis, structure, and function. Clofibrate and fenofibrate activate both PPAR-α and PPAR-γ, albeit with a 10-fold selectivity preference for PPAR-α. Bezafibrate has no particular selectivity for any PPAR subtype and induces transcriptional activation of PPAR-α/retinoid X receptor-alpha (RXR-α), PPAR-δ/RXR-α, and PPAR-γ/RXR-α. Currently used fibrates have relatively low affinity for PPAR-α and thus require high oral doses for clinical efficacy.[116]

Acetyl CoA Carboxylase. Inhibition of acetyl CoA carboxylase (ACC), the rate-limiting enzyme for malonyl CoA formation, is another important target for the fibric acid derivatives.

ACC exists as two major isoforms, ACC1 or ACC-α, implicated in fatty acid synthesis, and ACC2 or ACC-β, implicated in the control of mitochondrial beta oxidation.

The ACC isoforms can be regulated by fibrates via

- repressed ACC gene expression through the activation of PPAR-α,
- allosteric inhibition by fibroyl CoA esters, and
- activation of adenosine 5′-monophosphate (AMP)-activated protein kinase (AMPK), which phosphorylates and inactivates ACC in cardiac and skeletal myocytes.[118]

Fibrate interaction with ACC-α and ACC-β is an important aspect of the lipid-lowering effects of fibrates:

- inhibition of hepatic fatty acid synthesis: fibrate inhibition of ACC-α decreases the synthesis of a lipid component of VLDL;
- activation of fatty acid beta oxidation: fibrate inhibition of ACC-β lowers malonyl CoA levels and disinhibits fatty acid oxidation, thus partitioning fatty acids away from esterification and toward oxidation, as evidenced by the increased production of ketone bodies.[118]

Triglycerides. Fibrates decrease plasma triglyceride levels as a result of their aforementioned interactions with ACC and PPAR-α. By inhibiting ACC, fibrates lower hepatic VLDL triglyceride synthesis (28% for gemfibrozil).[116,119]

Fibrate-mediated PPAR-α activation enhances LPL activity, thus increasing fatty acid uptake and the clearance of VLDL and chylomicron remnants and in the process reducing plasma triglyceride levels. Fibrates

- induce the gene transcription of LPL and
- decrease the synthesis of apo C-III, an inhibitor of LPL, thereby effectively increasing LPL lipolytic activity, particularly in the liver. The reduced apo C-III content of triglyceride-rich lipoproteins facilitates their clearance.

As a result, gemfibrozil increases the fractional catabolic rate of VLDL triglyceride by 92%.[116,119]

Low-Density Lipoprotein. Fibrates may have an impact on LDL levels and phenotype. The lower plasma levels of triglyceride-rich lipoproteins lessen the transfer of cholesteryl esters from HDL to VLDL, which may instead transfer to LDL. This renders LDL more enriched in cholesteryl esters and less dense, thereby enhancing its binding affinity to the LDL receptor. Consequently, there is increased clearance of LDL with lowering of LDL plasma levels.[119]

High-Density Lipoprotein. On average, fibrates increase HDL levels by 10% to 15%. Fibrates increase both the number of HDL carriers for reverse cholesterol transport and the cellular expression of receptors for HDL.

The fibrate-mediated increase in HDL derives

- indirectly from a reduction in plasma levels of triglyceride-rich lipoproteins, which decreases HDL catabolism, and
- directly from the induction of hepatic apo A-I and apo A-II expression, which increases HDL synthesis.[120]

Fibrates, via PPAR-α activation, up-regulate the expression of HDL receptors, specifically, the

- adenosine triphosphate–binding cassette A1 (ABCA-1) transporter and
- scavenger receptor B1 (SR-B1)/CLA-1 in human macrophages,

thus promoting cholesterol efflux from foam cells and cholesterol uptake by hepatocytes.[116,121]

Insulin Resistance and New-Onset Diabetes Mellitus. PPAR-α agonists improve insulin sensitivity. Bezafibrate may reduce the incidence and delay the onset of type 2 DM in patients with impaired fasting glucose.

Three hundred three nondiabetic patients with CHD, 42 to 74 years of age with a fasting blood glucose level of 110 to 125 mg/dL, were treated with either 400 mg/day bezafibrate retard (156 patients) or placebo (147 patients) and evaluated over a 6.2-year follow-up period. New-onset DM occurred in 80 (54.4%) patients from the placebo group versus 66 (42.3%) from the bezafibrate group ($P = .04$), at 3.8 ± 2.6 years for placebo versus 4.6 ± 2.3 years for bezafibrate ($P = .004$). Bezafibrate therapy was associated with a hazard ratio of 0.70 for the new onset of DM.[122]

Statin-Fibrate Combination. Combination therapy with statins and fibrates may be considered in individuals with combined low HDL, high triglyceride, and high LDL levels. Combination therapy (fenofibrate 200 mg/day, simvastatin, 10 mg/day) decreases apo C-II and apo C-III in parallel with impressive reductions in triglyceride-rich, apo B–containing lipoproteins.[123] Such therapy requires very careful monitoring because of an increased risk for drug-induced myopathy, a risk that may be lessened by lower-dose statin therapy. Avoidance of gemfibrozil, which raises plasma levels of statins, may also lessen the incidence of myopathy. This adverse pharmacokinetic interaction with statins has not been observed with fenofibrate or bezafibrate.[123]

Other. Fibrates (fenofibrate, 200 mg/day), like statins, may also improve autonomic dysfunction in the metabolic syndrome, with a small reduction in systolic blood pressure.[101]

Potential Adverse Effects. An extreme net flux of cholesterol from extrahepatic tissues to the liver induced by excessive PPAR-α ligand activation may conceivably represent a disruptive change in global lipid homeostasis. It could result in loss of cholesterol and other lipids from peripheral tissues, especially from plasma membrane caveolae. Excessive tissue loss of cholesterol might perturb normal cellular signaling and result in tissue atrophy. On the other hand, the increased cholesterol content in the hepatocyte plasma membrane might actually enhance hepatocyte signaling and play a role in the hepatic hypertrophy and hepatocarcinogenesis associated with long-term PPAR ligand treatment in animal models.[124] Fibrates induce hepatic peroxisome proliferation and hepatomegaly and are nongenotoxic hepatocarcinogens in rodents.[116]

HYPOLIPIDEMIC DRUGS: NICOTINIC ACID

An important alternative for fibrate therapy in individuals with low HDL and high triglyceride levels is nicotinic acid, or niacin, which in combination with statin therapy has a lower potential risk for myopathy than the fibrate-statin combination does.

Nicotinic acid lowers the plasma concentration of triglyceride and is the most effective agent for increasing HDL levels. It can raise HDL by up to 30% and augments peripheral glucose uptake and oxidation.[120,121,125]

Clinical Studies. Nicotinic acid has beneficial effects on CHD.

The Familial Atherosclerosis Treatment Study (FATS) demonstrated regression of CHD associated with a shift in LDL density.[126] Positive results were also reported in the Stockholm Ischemic Heart Disease Secondary Prevention Study[127] and in the Coronary Drug Project. With intermediate-release niacin, there was a nonsignificant reduction in nonfatal MI and a significant reduction in total mortality after 15 years of follow-up.[128] In a 1-year study, extended-release niacin (1000 mg/day) added to background statin therapy in 167 patients with known CHD and HDL less than 45 mg/dL increased HDL by 21%. Common carotid intima-media thickness remained unchanged in the niacin group but increased significantly in the placebo group. The difference in the progression of intima-media thickness was significant only in subjects without insulin resistance.[129] The HDL-Atherosclerosis Treatment Study (HATS), which used a combination of niacin with simvastatin, achieved a 26% increase in total HDL and a 65% increase in the HDL2 subfraction. When compared with placebo, the treatment arm had a 90% lower incidence of major clinical cardiovascular events, $P = .03$.[130]

Mechanism of Action. Nicotinic acid lowers triglyceride levels and raises HDL, with beneficial effects on LDL density.

Triglycerides and Low-Density Lipoprotein. Nicotinic acid decreases circulating triglyceride by inhibiting adipose lipolysis and increasing triglyceride clearance. It favorably affects LDL levels and phenotype.

Nicotinic acid is an inhibitor of adipocyte lipolysis. It thus reduces the release of free fatty acids into plasma and their return to the liver. Acute elevations in plasma free fatty acids up-regulate hepatic de novo lipogenesis. The niacin-related reduced free fatty acid flux to the liver thus partially explains its triglyceride-lowering effect inasmuch as it diminishes the production of hepatic VLDL and apo B–containing lipoproteins such as IDL and LDL, in general. There is also increased clearance of triglycerides from plasma.

The curtailed generation of large, triglyceride-rich VLDL, in turn, lowers the formation of small, dense LDL. In fact, niacin induces increased LDL buoyancy.[120,121,125]

High-Density Lipoprotein. Nicotinic acid raises HDL by lowering triglyceride levels and diminishing apo A-I catabolism.

Because of the reduction in triglycerides, nicotinic acid secondarily increases HDL levels. The large, cardioprotective HDL2ab lipoprotein is further augmented by nicotinic acid as it reduces apo A-I catabolism, thereby limiting apo A-I uptake by the liver without impairing the transfer of cholesteryl ester into the liver. As a result, the capacity of apo A-I to carry on reverse cholesterol transport is enhanced.[120,121,125]

Other. The long-term benefit of nicotinic acid is mitigated by an increase in insulin resistance over time with a secondary rebound in plasma free fatty acids and worsening hyperglycemia. In fact, the effect of nicotinic acid on cardiovascular outcomes in patients with the metabolic syndrome and DM is not known. At present, nicotinic acid is a second-line agent to be used with caution in that setting. Other adverse effects include flushing, hyperuricemia, and hepatic dysfunction. Acipimox, an analogue of nicotinic acid with a longer duration of action, may share the beneficial metabolic effects of nicotinic acid without the adverse rebound effects.[131]

Patients taking a combination of statins with niacin need to be monitored for signs or symptoms of myopathy.

HYPOLIPIDEMIC DRUGS: EZETIMIBE

Modulation of cholesterol absorption in the intestine can profoundly alter cholesterol levels. Ezetimibe interferes with the enteric absorption of cholesterol. Ezetimibe is absorbed and recycled in the enterohepatic circulation as its glucuronide derivative, which itself inhibits cholesterol absorption as well. It lowers serum cholesterol levels by 18% to 25%, presumably by reducing chylomicron delivery of cholesterol to the liver, diminishing hepatocyte cholesterol content, and up-regulating LDL receptor activity.[132]

Ezetimibe's action may entail the disruption of an intestinal sterol transport complex. In larval and adult zebra fish intestinal epithelium, ezetimibe disrupts the formation of a protein heterodimer formed as annexin complexes with caveolin-1.[133]

HYPOLIPIDEMIC DRUGS: BILE ACID SEQUESTRANTS

Bile acid sequestrants act on the exogenous pathway of cholesterol metabolism. In the intestinal lumen, these agents bind bile acids, thereby increasing their fecal excretion and reducing their enterohepatic recirculation. As a result, there is increased de novo hepatic cholesterol synthesis, enhanced conversion of cholesterol into bile acids, and up-regulation of hepatic LDL receptors with lowering of circulating LDL. The efficacy of LDL lowering with bile acid sequestrants is 7% to 32%.[134]

Up-regulated hepatic cholesterol synthesis also entails greater VLDL secretion from the liver. This may engender resultant hypertriglyceridemia and thus limit the applicability of these agents in individuals with dyslipidemia secondary to insulin resistance.[134]

Up to 30% of individuals taking these drugs have unpleasant gastrointestinal side effects. These agents require multiple daily dosing. Administration needs to be separated by 3 hours from other drugs, such as statins, fibrates, warfarin, cyclosporine, hypoglycemic agents, β-blockers, thyroid hormone, and certain diuretics, to avoid a significant decrement in drug absorption.[134]

HYPOLIPIDEMIC DRUGS: INVESTIGATIONAL AGENTS

The cholesteryl ester transfer protein (CETP) inhibitor torcetrapib has boosted HDL by 45% to 55% in phase II trials.

In 19 subjects with low HDL levels, partial CETP inhibition by 28% to 65% with torcetrapib markedly raised HDL levels and also lowered LDL levels, both when administered as monotherapy and when administered in combination with a statin. Treatment with 120 mg of torcetrapib once daily increased plasma concentrations of HDL by 61% ($P < .001$), and 120 mg twice-daily dosing increased it by 106% ($P < .001$). Torcetrapib, 120 mg/day, in conjunction with atorvastatin raised HDL by 46% ($P = .001$) while reducing LDL levels by 17% ($P = .02$). Additionally, torcetrapib significantly altered the distribution of cholesterol among HDL and LDL subclasses, with an increase in the mean particle size of HDL and LDL in each cohort.[135]

Phase II trials with a torcetrapib-atorvastatin combination to look at changes in carotid intimal-medial thickness as a primary end point are under way.[136]

ANTAGONISM OF THE RENIN-ANGIOTENSIN-ALDOSTERONE SYSTEM

The RAAS plays a major role in inflammation and endothelial dysfunction, in hypertension and atherogenesis, and in disturbances in glucose metabolism and the progression to type 2 DM. There is crosstalk between angiotensin II and insulin signaling at multiple levels. This renders antagonism of the RAAS an appropriate target for intervention.

Hypertension. Hypertension is common with insulin resistance and is one of the diagnostic criteria for the metabolic syndrome. Improvement in hypertension contributes to the reduction in cardiovascular risk. Blood pressure targets are generally set at 130/80 mm Hg in higher-risk individuals. A 10–mm Hg reduction in systolic blood pressure in the United Kingdom Prospective Diabetes Study (UKPDS) reduced cardiovascular risk by 12%.[137] A 67% risk reduction was achieved in the Hypertension Optimal Treatment (HOT) study only for diabetic individuals whose diastolic blood pressure was lowered to less than 80 mm Hg.[138] Control of blood pressure to levels less than 120 mm Hg for systolic and less than 80 mm Hg for diastolic pressure may prevent 28.2% and 45.2% of expected CHD events in men and women, respectively, over a period of 10 years.[1] Therapeutic lifestyle changes via weight loss, exercise activities, healthy dietary choices, and sodium restriction should always be considered as first-line therapy before pharmacologic intervention.

Angiotensin Antagonism. Angiotensin was originally thought to be solely a potent hormonal vasoconstrictor. Therapy to antagonize angiotensin II effects has thus had as its initial focus vasodilation with ensuing blood pressure and afterload reduction. With increasing insight into the manifold impact of angiotensin II on oxidative and inflammatory processes and tissue remodeling in the vasculature, myocardium, brain, kidneys, skeletal muscle, and adipose tissue, the beneficial pleiotropic effects of such therapy have been increasingly appreciated.[139]

RENIN-ANGIOTENSIN-ALDOSTERONE SYSTEM ANTAGONISTS: THE ANGIOTENSIN-CONVERTING ENZYME INHIBITORS

Traditionally, ACE inhibitors elicit their effects by inhibiting the conversion of angiotensin I to angiotensin II, thus diminishing the local and systemic adverse effects of the latter. However, nearly 40% of angiotensin I may be converted to angiotensin II via non-ACE pathways, a bypass mechanism that may increase with hyperinsulinemia (Fig. 16-5).[140]

Additionally, ACE inhibitors block the role of ACE in the kallikrein-kinin system. The ACE enzyme has significant affinity for bradykinin and catalyzes its degradation. ACE inhibitors inhibit the breakdown of bradykinin, thereby increasing the local, vascular effects of this partial antagonist to angiotensin II action via an increase in the production of NO and prostaglandin E_2 (Fig. 16-6).[4,141]

ACE inhibitors are the first-line therapeutic agents for treating hypertension in patients with insulin resistance and the metabolic syndrome.[142]

Antioxidant Effects. ACE inhibitors have antioxidant effects.

Angiotensin II is one of the most potent endogenous stimuli for the generation of superoxide via stimulation of the vascular and leukocyte membrane NADH/NADPH oxidase system. Interruption of this mechanism by ACE inhibitors reduces the generation of ROS and decreases plasma markers of oxidative stress.[142,143] ACE inhibitors reduce oxidation of LDL and decrease activation of the lectin-like oxidized LDL receptor.[53]

Figure 16–5. The renin-angiotensin-aldosterone system and sites of action for β-adrenergic blockers, angiotensin-converting enzyme (ACE) inhibitors, angiotensin II type 1 (AT_1) receptor blockers, and aldosterone antagonists.

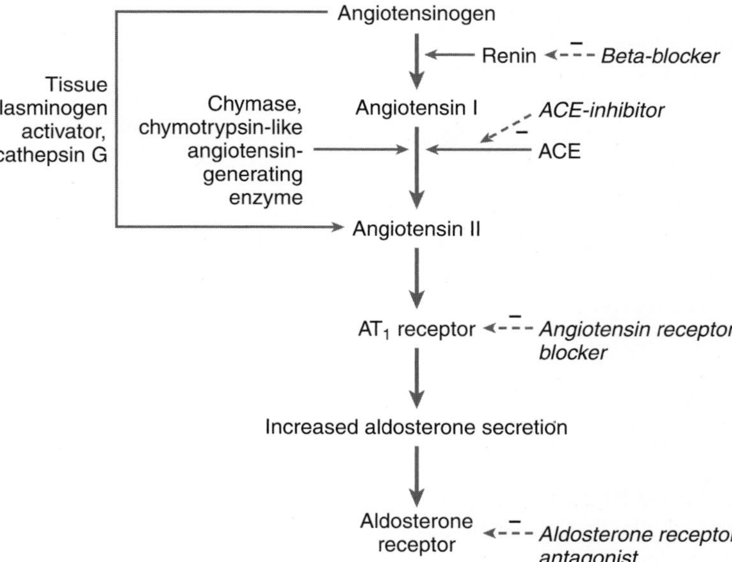

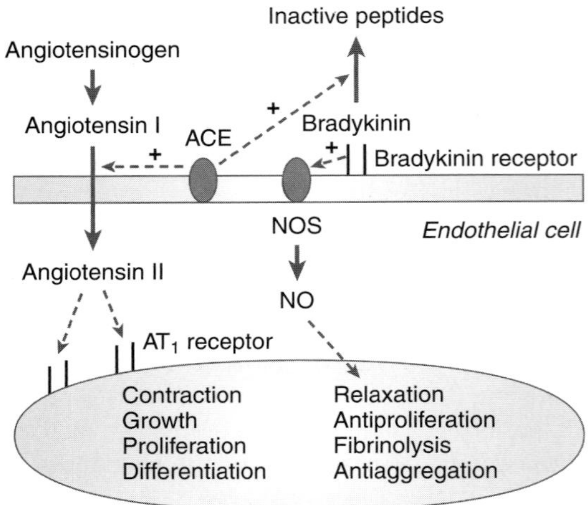

Figure 16–6.
Endothelial cell angiotensin-converting enzyme (ACE): angiotensin II production and bradykinin degradation. AT-1, angiotensin II type 1; NO, nitric oxide; NOS, NO synthase. *(Modified from Calles-Escandon J, Cipolla M: Diabetes and endothelial dysfunction: a clinical perspective. Endocr Rev 2001;22:36-52.)*

Anti-inflammatory Effects. ACE inhibitors have anti-inflammatory effects directly by diminishing angiotensin II–related proinflammatory pathways and indirectly through bradykinin effects.[144]

In vitro, ACE inhibitors lead to reduced activation of the NFκB and AP-1 signaling pathways and reduce vascular inflammation. They blunt the release of inflammatory cytokines such as IL-6 and reduce the concentration of CRP.[4,53,145]

ACE inhibitors also enhance the concentration of anti-inflammatory cytokines such as IL-10.[4] Their anti-inflammatory effects are additive to the effects of statins.[146]

Antithrombotic Effects. ACE inhibitors lower the tendency toward thrombosis and enhance fibrinolysis.

In vitro, ACE inhibitors blunt the release of plasma markers of thrombosis.[4,53] The ACE inhibitor–mediated increase in bradykinin facilitates endogenous fibrinolysis.[4,147]

Vascular Health. ACE inhibitor therapy enhances endothelial function. Such therapy has beneficial hemodynamic effects and is protective of vascular health.[142]

ACE inhibitors improve endothelial-derived NO production, smooth muscle relaxation, and vascular compliance. Several mechanisms are involved. ACE inhibitors

- decrease circulating and vascular angiotensin II levels, as well as secondary sympathetic activation and endothelin-1 elaboration, thereby blunting the adverse vascular effects of these vasoconstrictors;
- lessen the oxidant inactivation of NO; and
- increase bradykinin levels. Bradykinin activates eNOS in a calcium-independent fashion, stimulating the production of NO. Bradykinin is also implicated in boosting prostacyclin and endothelium-derived hyperpolarizing factor levels.[4,147]

ACE inhibitors decrease the activation of MMP-2 and MMP-9 and improve plaque stability.[4,53]

Clinical Studies. Although ACE inhibitors may not reverse atherogenesis, clinically they stabilize and slow the progression of atherosclerotic lesions and thus reduce clinical cardiovascular events and stroke.[142] Interestingly, in the setting of optimized and intensive medical and interventional therapy, with sufficient lowering of LDL levels, ACE inhibitors may fail to further reduce the rate of cardiovascular events.[144]

The randomized, controlled Heart Outcomes Prevention Evaluation (HOPE) trial was conducted from 1994 to 1999 in 9297 individuals 55 years or older without left ventricular dysfunction or heart failure, but with vascular disease (known CHD, stroke, peripheral vascular disease) or with DM and one other risk factor. The use of ramipril, 10 mg/day, was associated with a significant, absolute reduction of 3.8% for death, unstable angina, MI, and stroke.[2]

In the European Trial On Reduction of Cardiac Events with Perindopril in Stable Coronary Artery Disease (EUROPA), 12,218 patients with a mean age of 60 years and previous MI, angiographic CHD, coronary revascularization, or a positive stress test received either perindopril, 8 mg once daily, or placebo. During the mean follow-up of 4.2 years, there was a 20% relative risk reduction in the primary end point of cardiovascular death, MI, or cardiac arrest with perindopril.[148]

In the Trial on Reversing Endothelial Dysfunction (TREND) involving patients with CHD but without left ventricular systolic dysfunction, quinapril improved endothelial function only in patients whose LDL concentration exceeded 125 mg/dL.[144,149]

For patients with CHD and intact left ventricular systolic function in the Quinapril Ischemic Event Trial (QUIET), quinapril reduced the progression of CHD and the cardiovascular event rate only in subjects with elevated levels of LDL, but it had no impact on the overall rate of cardiovascular events.[144,150]

The Prevention of Events with Angiotensin Converting Enzyme Inhibition (PEACE) trial tested 8290 patients, 64 years old on average, with stable CHD, with intact left ventricular systolic function, and without DM. Treatment and placebo patients were all receiving aggressive medical and interventional therapy. Patients randomly assigned to trandolapril, 4 mg/day, had no reduction in cardiovascular morbidity or mortality relative to placebo patients.[151]

Insulin Resistance. ACE inhibitors improve insulin sensitivity and glucose metabolism.[139]

There are numerous mechanisms whereby ACE inhibitors may improve glucose metabolism.

Anti-inflammatory and Antioxidant Effects. The anti-inflammatory and antioxidant effects of ACE inhibitors may enhance metabolic and vascular insulin sensitivity and contribute to the reduction in risk for development of type 2 DM.

Vascular Effects. The vasculoprotective effects of ACE inhibitors, via enhancement of the bradykinin-NO pathway, may improve nutritive microvascular tissue perfusion and insulin delivery to metabolically active tissues, thereby enhancing glucose metabolism, especially in skeletal muscle.

In type 2 diabetic mice, the administration of an ACE inhibitor, temocapril, significantly decreased plasma glucose and insulin concentrations. Translocation of glucose transporter 4 (GLUT4) to the plasma membrane was significantly enhanced without influencing insulin receptor substrate-1 (IRS-1) phosphorylation. The beneficial effects were antagonized by administration of a bradykinin B_2 receptor antagonist, Hoe140, or a NOS inhibitor, L-NAME.[152]

Intracellular Signaling. Angiotensin II inhibits intracellular insulin signaling at multiple levels. ACE inhibitors may limit the negative crosstalk between angiotensin II and insulin pathways.

ACE inhibitors improved insulin sensitivity in a tissue culture system. GLUT4 protein and hexokinase activity were correspondingly increased.[153]

Adiponectin. Hypoadiponectinemia is related to insulin resistance. ACE inhibition increases adiponectin concentrations with improvement in insulin sensitivity.[154]

Two-week therapy with temocapril, 4 mg/day, in individuals with essential hypertension significantly decreased blood pressure and increased adiponectin levels.[154]

Clinical Impact on New-Onset Type 2 Diabetes Mellitus. Clinically, ACE inhibitors reduce insulin resistance and lower the development of type 2 DM. ACE inhibition should be considered the preferred therapy for insulin-resistant individuals with hypertension and established CHD.[139,155]

Clinical Studies. A number of ACE inhibitors appear to lower rates of new-onset type 2 DM in high-risk individuals.

The Captopril Prevention Project (CAPP) in hypertensive patients demonstrated a 14% lower incidence of newly diagnosed type 2 DM in the patient group receiving captopril rather than placebo.[156]

In a retrospective analysis of 291 nondiabetic heart failure patients at one center of the Studies of Left Ventricular Dysfunction (SOLVD) trial, DM developed in 40 patients during 2.9 ± 1.0 years of follow-up. Although baseline characteristics were similar in the enalapril and placebo groups, DM developed in 9 (5.9%) in the enalapril group and 31 (22.4%) in the placebo group ($P < .0001$). Enalapril use was associated with a hazard ratio of 0.22 for new-onset DM.[157]

In the Antihypertensive and Lipid-Lowering Treatment to Prevent Heart Attack (ALLHAT) trial, the ACE inhibitor lisinopril, as well as the calcium channel blocker amlodipine, was associated with a significantly lower risk for new-onset type 2 DM when compared with the thiazide-type diuretic chlorthalidone, which caused hypokalemia, glucose intolerance, and DM.[158]

In a subset of 5720 HOPE trial patients older than 55 years without known DM but with vascular disease, monitored for a mean of 4.5 years, a significant reduction in the incidence of type 2 DM occurred with therapy. DM developed in

102 individuals (3.6%) in the ramipril group versus 155 (5.4%) in the placebo group. Effectively, ramipril treatment was associated with a 34% reduction in new-onset DM, and the relative risk for development of DM was 0.66% for the ramipril group ($P < .001$).[155]

Other Angiotensin-Converting Enzyme Inhibitor Effects. ACE inhibitors are protective of renal dysfunction and have antiarrhythmic effects.

Clinical Impact on Renal Disease. ACE inhibition should be considered the preferred therapy for insulin-resistant individuals with hypertension, renal disease, or microalbuminuria.

ACE inhibitor therapy favorably modulates microalbuminuria, a symptom of endothelial dysfunction.[155] Ramipril and other ACE inhibitors have a nephroprotective effect and slow the progression of both diabetic and nondiabetic renal disease unrelated to the antihypertensive effects of the drugs.[159,160]

In 3577 people older than 55 years with DM and vascular disease but not proteinuria included in the HOPE study, ramipril therapy lowered overt nephropathy by 24%, $P = .027$. The benefit exceeded that attributable to the reduction in blood pressure alone.[161]

Arrhythmia. ACE inhibitors reduce the incidence of atrial fibrillation in patients with left ventricular dysfunction. The underlying mechanism may reflect a direct antiarrhythmic effect. Alternatively, an indirect effect, mediated through the reduction in left atrial filling pressure or neurohormonal mechanisms, may be at play.[162]

RENIN-ANGIOTENSIN-ALDOSTERONE SYSTEM ANTAGONISTS: THE ANGIOTENSIN II RECEPTOR BLOCKERS

For individuals intolerant of ACE inhibition, angiotensin II receptor blockers (ARBs) are an appropriate therapeutic alternative for antihypertensive therapy and for cardiovascular and diabetic risk reduction. Although the mechanisms of action of ACE inhibitors and ARBs differ (see Fig. 16-5), their clinical effects are similar.[163] ARBs have been shown to improve outcomes for patients with heart failure who are already receiving ACE inhibition.[164]

At least two types of angiotensin receptors have been identified in humans, AT_1 and AT_2 receptors. The AT_1 receptor is present in many tissues and organs, including the heart, blood vessels, kidneys, and adipocytes. The AT_2 receptor is expressed mainly in the fetus and has low levels of expression after birth. Most known physiologic and pathophysiologic effects of angiotensin II appear to be mediated through the AT_1 receptor, which is selectively and competitively blocked by ARBs with high affinity and slow dissociation.[165]

With ARB blockade of the AT_1 receptors, the potential physiologic effects of AT_2 receptor stimulation may come into play.[165] AT_2 receptor stimulation mediates vasodilation and antiproliferative activity, possibly via NO and bradykinin generation, and antagonizes the AT_1 receptor actions of angiotensin II. AT_2 receptor activation also enhances renal sodium excretion, renin release, and dilation of renal afferent arterioles (Fig. 16-7).[165]

ARBs exhibit a number of pleiotropic effects.

Antioxidant Effect. By antagonizing the prooxidant effects of angiotensin II, the ARBs, like ACE inhibitors, exert an antioxidant effect.

ARBs reduce circulating markers of oxidative stress.[166,167] They decreased a marker of oxidative stress, thiobarbituric acid reactive substance, in an animal model and reduced 8-isoprostane levels in patients with hypercholesterolemia.[84]

Anti-inflammatory Effect. Akin to the action of ACE inhibitors, ARBs block inflammatory pathways instigated by activation of AT_1 receptors. ARBs reduce circulating markers of inflammation.[166,167] Their anti-inflammatory actions complement statin effects.[146]

ARBs may exert a greater systemic anti-inflammatory effect than ACE inhibitors do. In a clinical study of 48 patients with CHD conducted 6 to 8 weeks after coronary angioplasty, 3 months of therapy with either enalapril, 20 mg/day, or irbesartan, 300 mg/day, increased levels of the anti-inflammatory IL-10 and reduced serum MMP-9 protein and activity. However, only AT_1 blockade also lowered levels of CRP and IL-6 and diminished platelet aggregation.[168]

Vasculoprotective Effect. ARBs are vasculoprotective by antagonizing the vascular RAAS,

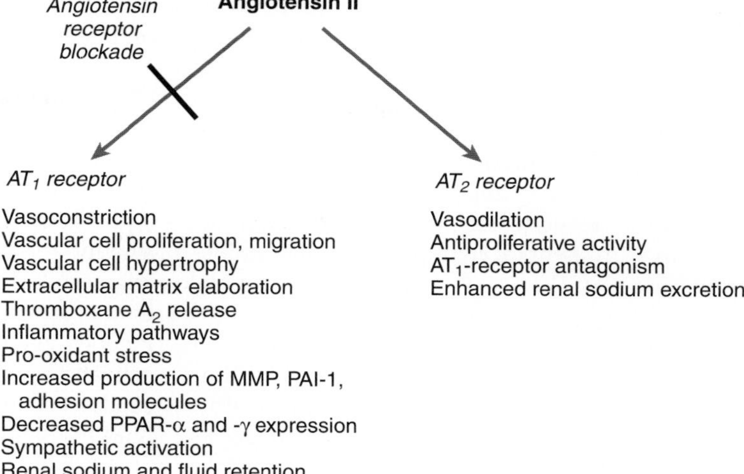

Figure 16–7. Angiotensin II receptor blockade of the AT_1 receptor enhancing AT_2 receptor effects. MMP, matrix metalloproteinase; PAI-1, plasminogen activator inhibitor-1; PPAR, peroxisome proliferator–activated receptor.

which plays a pivotal role in the development of endothelial dysfunction and the acceleration of atherosclerosis.

Endothelial Function. ARBs improve endothelial function, probably via antioxidant and anti-inflammatory effects. The concomitant elevation in plasma and tissue angiotensin II levels with ARB therapy may provide vascular protection not only by reducing AT_1 receptor–mediated effects but also via unopposed stimulation of the AT_2 receptor.[169]

AT_1 receptor blockade via candesartan in hypertensive patients reversed endothelial dysfunction together with a reduction in measures of oxidative stress, inflammation, and thrombosis. These effects were independent of a blood pressure–lowering effect (Fig. 16-8).[170] In patients with mild to moderate hypertension, the administration of losartan, 100 mg/day, irbesartan, 300 mg/day, and candesartan, 16 mg/day, significantly improved the brachial flow–mediated dilator response to reactive hyperemia and reduced levels of malondialdehyde, an index of oxidative stress, when compared with placebo. Irbesartan and candesartan lowered plasma levels of PAI-1, and only candesartan lowered plasma levels of MCP-1.[171] AT_1 receptor antagonism via losartan and irbesartan improved endothelial function in patients with CHD.[172]

Antiatherosclerotic Effects. Specific blockade of the RAAS may confer antiatherosclerotic effects.

In a comparison of equihypotensive doses of irbesartan with the calcium antagonist amlodipine on diabetes-induced plaque formation in apo E–null mice for 20 weeks, irbesartan, but not amlodipine attenuated the development of atherosclerosis, with a reduction in plaque

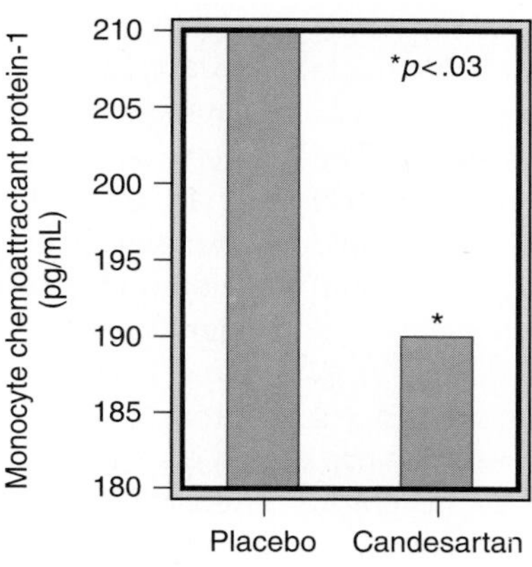

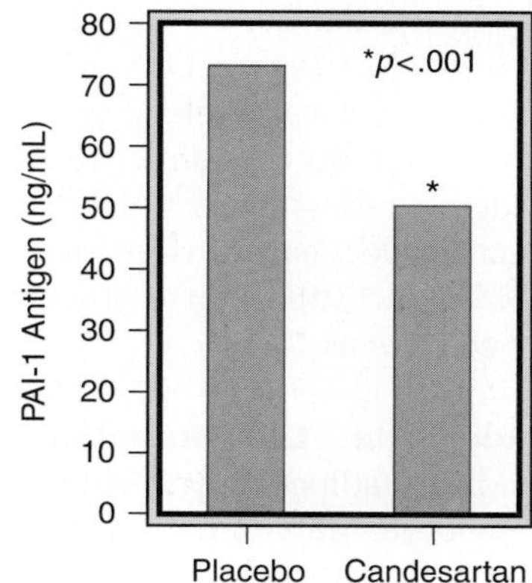

Figure 16–8. Pleiotropic effects of candesartan in hypertensive patients: reduction in plasma levels of monocyte chemoattractant protein-1 and plasminogen activator inhibitor-1 (PAI-1). *(Modified from Koh KK, Ahn JY, Han SH, et al. Pleiotropic effects of angiotensin II receptor blocker in hypertensive patients. J Am Coll Cardiol 2003;42: 905-910.)*

collagen content, cellular proliferation, and macrophage infiltration. Irbesartan more effectively mitigated the DM-induced overexpression of the AT_1 receptor, PDGF-B, MCP-1, and vascular cell adhesion molecule-1 (VCAM-1) in the aorta despite equipotent blood pressure reduction.[173]

In the Losartan Intervention For Endpoint Reduction in Hypertension (LIFE) trial comparing losartan with atenolol therapy, with hydrochlorothiazide (HCTZ) used as a second agent in both groups, despite equipotent blood pressure lowering, losartan prevented or retarded the progression of CHD events. Losartan reduced the combined end point of cardiovascular death, stroke, or MI by 24% and total mortality by 39% when compared with atenolol.[174]

Insulin Sensitivity. Angiotensin II inhibits intracellular insulin signaling. Additionally, with activation of the RAAS, multiple mechanisms for the initiation and progression of inflammation and oxidative stress contributing to insulin resistance come into play. **AT_1 receptor antagonism improves insulin sensitivity.**[175]

In a fructose-fed rat model of insulin resistance, short- and long-term AT_1 receptor blockade with losartan preserved glucose tolerance and insulin sensitivity.[176] In a mouse genetic model of the metabolic syndrome, treatment with an ARB inhibited the development of hyperinsulinemia, hypertension, obesity, cardiac hypertrophy, and atherosclerosis.[177]

In addition to pathways shared with ACE inhibitors, several mechanisms contribute to the enhancement of insulin sensitivity by ARBs.

MAPK Activation. ARBs may activate MAPK in skeletal muscle and thereby enhance glucose uptake.

In Otsuka Long-Evans Tokushima Fatty rats, a model of type 2 DM, AT_1 receptor blockade improved local skeletal muscle insulin resistance, but not systemic insulin resistance. The augmented glucose uptake in skeletal muscle may have been attributable to ARB-mediated MAPK activation or to other, non–PI3K-related mechanisms.[178]

Adipocyte Differentiation. Angiotensin II reduces adipose conversion and inhibits preadipocyte differentiation via the AT_1 receptor. AT_1 receptor blockade markedly enhances adipogenesis, which may have a favorable impact on insulin sensitivity.[179]

PPAR-γ Activation. Lipophilic ARBs, akin to partial PPAR-γ agonists, may activate PPAR-γ and regulate PPAR-γ target genes in vivo.[180]

In 3T3-L1 adipocytes, the ARBs irbesartan and telmisartan induced and activated PPAR-γ activity, thereby promoting PPAR-γ–dependent adipocyte differentiation. This effect also occurred in the absence of AT_1 receptors and was thus independent of receptor blocking actions. PPAR-γ activation pertained primarily to lipophilic ARBs capable of intracellular penetration in order to bind to the nuclear receptors.[180]

Adiponectin. ARBs, like ACE inhibitors, may reverse hypoadiponectinemia and thus enhance sensitivity to insulin signaling.

In patients with essential hypertension, therapy with candesartan, 8 mg/day for 2 weeks, lowered blood pressure significantly while increasing the adiponectin concentration.[154]

Clinical Studies. ARBs clinically improve insulin sensitivity and lessen the new onset of type 2 DM.

Candesartan cilexetil improves insulin sensitivity and exerts a sympathoinhibitory effect. The Candesartan Role on Obesity and on Sympathetic System (CROSS) study examined the antihypertensive, neuroadrenergic, and metabolic effects of AT_1 receptor blockade via candesartan cilexetil (8 to 16 mg once daily) in comparison to a diuretic HCTZ (25 to 50 mg once daily) in 127 obese, hypertensive individuals aged 50.7 ± 5.1 years. Candesartan cilexetil caused significant reductions in both mean blood pressure and muscle sympathetic nerve activity. Candesartan also caused a significant increase in insulin sensitivity, in contrast to HCTZ, which while achieving similar blood pressure reductions, did not affect sympathetic nerve activity and worsened insulin sensitivity.[181]

In the LIFE trial comparing losartan with atenolol therapy, losartan prevented or retarded the progression of CHD events together with a significant 25% reduction in the development of type 2 DM when compared with the atenolol group.[174]

In the 15,245-patient Valsartan Antihypertensive Long-Term Use Evaluation (VALUE) antihypertensive trial in high-risk adults with a mean age of 67 years, valsartan therapy (80 to 160 mg/day), after a mean of 4 years, was associated with a 20% lower incidence of new-onset DM than calcium channel blocker therapy with amlodipine (5 to 10 mg/day) was (13.1% versus 16.4%), whereas both therapies had an equivalent incidence of cardiac morbidity and mortality.[182]

The Candesartan in Heart Failure Assessment of Reduction in Mortality and Morbidity (CHARM) Overall Programme trial demonstrated a 22% reduction in the development of type 2 DM. A total of 7601 patients with chronic heart failure were monitored for 37.7 months while taking an average of 24 mg/day of candesartan versus placebo. The hazard ratio for the development of diabetes was 0.78, $P = .020$.[164]

Nephroprotection. ARBs may slow the progression of nephropathy. ARB therapy may be nephroprotective not only through reduction of AT_1 receptor–mediated oxidative stress but also through stimulation of the AT_2 receptor.[169]

The Irbesartan Diabetic Nephropathy Trial (IDNT), the Reduction of Endpoints in NIDDM with the Angiotensin II Antagonist Losartan (RENAAL) trial, and the LIFE trial support the use of ARBs in patients with nephropathy secondary to type 2 DM. ARB therapy significantly lowered the progression to end-stage renal disease (losartan) and proteinuria (losartan, irbesartan), effects that were independent of the hypotensive effects of these agents.[183]

RENIN-ANGIOTENSIN-ALDOSTERONE SYSTEM ANTAGONISTS: THE ALDOSTERONE ANTAGONISTS

Aldosterone is implicated in the pathogenesis of vascular inflammation, endothelial dysfunction, and insulin resistance. Traditional therapies, such as ACE inhibitors and ARBs, may not be effective in maintaining long-term suppression of aldosterone. Spironolactone, a nonselective aldosterone receptor blocker, effectively lowers elevated blood pressure, improves endothelial dysfunction, reduces left ventricular hypertrophy, and lowers the incidence of fatal arrhythmias.[184] However, spironolactone, because of its interaction with other steroid receptors, has unacceptable side effects for patients. As a result, eplerenone, a selective aldosterone blocker, is of interest to examine for its efficacy not only in cardiovascular but also in metabolic risk reduction in a patient population with elevated inflammatory markers, endothelial dysfunction, and insulin resistance.

β-ADRENERGIC BLOCKADE

Blockade of β-adrenergic receptors has successfully reduced the risk for sudden death in post-MI patients and in those with hypertension and heart failure. These effects have been assumed to derive from the antiarrhythmic and antihypertensive effects of β-adrenergic blockade, together with the beneficial impact on myocardial oxygen consumption and remodeling.[185]

With ischemic heart disease, congestive heart failure, and post-MI status, the cardiovascular benefits attending β-blockade are well established, and such use is well tolerated. β-blockade has been associated with a deterioration in insulin sensitivity. However, the cardiovascular benefits attending β-blockade far outweigh the risks of increased insulin resistance. In insulin-resistant states, should an indication for β-blocker therapy exist, it may be more favorable to use β_1-selective agents or, preferably, vasodilating β-blockers.[186]

Antiatherogenic Effect. Both animal and epidemiologic studies have implicated stress as an etiologic factor in atherosclerosis.[187] **Preliminary animal and human data suggest that β-adrenergic blockade of the sympathetic nervous system may have a favorable impact on vascular remodeling and exert a direct, antiatherosclerotic effect.**[185]

In addition to reduced sympathetic activity and improved hemodynamic parameters, direct effects on the vascular endothelium and interference with stress-induced mitogenic and inflammatory pathways via β-blockade all play a role.[185]

- β-Blocker therapy inhibited the development of stress-induced atherosclerosis in cynomolgus monkeys.[188]
- β-Blockers have additive effects to those of statins in reducing the rate of progression of carotid intima-media thickness of carotid plaque. In the Beta-Blocker Cholesterol-Lowering Asymptomatic Plaque Study (BCAPS), 793 subjects 49 to 70 years old

with asymptomatic carotid plaque were treated with either 25 mg metoprolol CR/XL or placebo in the setting of lipid-lowering therapy. That dose caused only a mean 2.5 beat per minute reduction in heart rate with no effect on lipids or blood pressure. At 18- and 36-month follow-up, the progression of maximal intima-media thickness in the carotid artery was significantly lower in the treatment versus the control group, together with a significant reduction in the combined end point of all-cause mortality, nonfatal MI, or stroke.[189]

- In a similar patient cohort, albeit with hyperlipidemia, in the Effects of Long-Term Treatment of Metoprolol CR/XL on Surrogate Variables for Atherosclerotic Disease (ELVA) trial, metoprolol CR/XL, 100 mg/day, was compared with placebo against background therapy with fluvastatin, 40 mg/day. At 1 and 3 years' follow-up, there was a highly significant difference in the rate of progression of carotid artery intima-media thickness favoring the addition of β-blockade to background lipid-lowering therapy.[190]

Insulin Sensitivity. Despite the beneficial effect of β-blockade on cardiovascular disease, **β-adrenergic blockade has traditionally been reported to worsen insulin resistance and to constitute a risk factor for the development of DM.[191] However, vasodilating β-blockers may actually improve insulin sensitivity and delay the onset of type 2 DM.**

Metabolic Effects of β-Adrenergic Blockade. Counteracting some of the metabolic and vascular effects of β_2-adrenergic stimulation, β-blockade reduces

- peripheral microvascular, nutritive blood flow, thereby compromising glucose and insulin delivery to insulin-sensitive tissues;
- lipolysis and energy expenditure, thus favoring weight gain; and
- insulin secretion.

In fact, blockade of β-adrenergic receptors reduces glucose uptake in skeletal muscles by up to 32% with a mild increase in plasma glucose and hyperinsulinemia.[186]

Impact of β_1-Selective β-Blockers on Insulin Resistance. Both nonselective and selective β_1-blockers increase insulin resistance and impair glucose-stimulated insulin release. Although β-blockers can be ranked according to their negative impact on insulin sensitivity, with propranolol being the worst, followed by metoprolol, atenolol, and pindolol, overall the use of β-blockers by hypertensive patients is associated with a 28% higher incidence of DM when compared with no therapy at all.[192,193]

Impact of Vasodilating β-Blockers on Insulin Sensitivity. In contrast to conventional β-blockers, vasodilating β-blockers may have no adverse effect on insulin action or may actually improve it. The vasodilator-mediated enhancement in skeletal muscle blood flow and other ancillary properties of these agents may be playing a role.

- Celiprolol has β_2-stimulating properties. It induces vasodilation and may improve insulin action.[194]
- In contrast to conventional β-blockers, α_1-adrenergic receptor blockers increase insulin sensitivity, particularly in insulin-resistant patients. Carvedilol is considered to be an α_1-, β_1-, and β_2-adrenergic receptor blocker with ancillary vasodilatory, anti-ischemic, and antioxidant effects. The net impact of carvedilol is, effectively, an improvement in insulin sensitivity.[193]

Additional Benefits of Vasodilating β-Blockers in Insulin Resistance. Vasodilating and antioxidant β-blockers may have other beneficial and vasculoprotective effects in insulin-resistant individuals. Their use may be associated with

- improvements in the lipid profile,
- less oxidation of LDL,
- less vascular smooth muscle proliferation,
- reduced platelet aggregation,
- lower blood viscosity, and
- a reduction in microalbuminuria.[186]

Clinical Studies. Clinically, carvedilol appears to improve insulin sensitivity and endothelial function. It may also decrease the incidence of type 2 DM.

In a randomized, double-blind, parallel-group trial (The Glycemic Effects in Diabetes Mellitus: Carvedilol-Metoprolol Comparison in Hypertensives—GEMINI) conducted for 35 weeks to compare the effects of carvedilol and metoprolol tartrate on glycemic control in 1235 participants aged 36 to 85 years with hypertension and type 2 DM who were receiving RAAS blockers, carvedilol did not affect glycemic control and improved some components of the metabolic syndrome relative to metoprolol. Although blood pressure was similar between groups, mean glycated hemoglobin A (HbA_{1c}) increased with metoprolol ($P < .001$) but remained unchanged with carvedilol. Insulin sensitivity improved with carvedilol ($P = .004$) but not with metoprolol, with a significant between-group difference. Progression to microalbuminuria was less frequent with carvedilol (6.4%) than with metoprolol (10.3%) ($P = .04$).[195]

In the Carvedilol Or Metoprolol European Trial (COMET), 3029 patients with NYHA class II to IV heart failure were randomized to receive carvedilol, 25 mg, or metoprolol tartrate, 50 mg, twice a day. Doses actually achieved were 42 mg of carvedilol and 85 mg of metoprolol per day. Primary end points showed a 17% significant reduction in mortality with carvedilol versus metoprolol. Among the secondary end points from COMET, treatment with carvedilol versus metoprolol tartrate produced significant reductions in cardiovascular mortality, fatal stroke, and new-onset DM.[196]

INSULIN-SENSITIZING THERAPY: THIAZOLIDINEDIONES OR GLITAZONES

Thiazolidinediones (TZDs) were initially developed for their antioxidant properties because of a structural similarity to α-tocopherol. They are synthetic ligands that bind to and activate PPAR-γ, a transcription factor that regulates the expression of specific genes, predominantly in fat cells. PPAR-γ ligands increase the transcription of genes coding for

- LPL,
- fatty acid transporter protein,
- fatty acyl CoA synthase,
- adipocyte lipid binding protein 2,
- malic enzyme,
- glucokinase, and
- GLUT4.

The TZDs enhance insulin sensitivity primarily at the level of adipose tissue with some effect on the liver and secondary effects on skeletal muscle.[197,198]

Thiazolidinediones in Clinical Use. Type 2 DM is currently the only approved indication for therapy with TZDs.

Reductions in cardiovascular events have not yet been demonstrated with TZD insulin-sensitizing therapy. Cardiovascular outcome trials are needed to confirm that the TZD-induced improvements in CHD risk factors do, in fact, translate into lower cardiovascular morbidity and mortality with a reduction in the onset of type 2 DM. However, insulin-sensitizing therapy might be considered in insulin-resistant individuals with severe atherogenic dyslipidemia, evidence of significant vascular inflammation, or established CHD.[199]

TZDs have been tested as experimental therapies with variable success in other insulin-resistant conditions, such as nonalcoholic fatty liver disease, polycystic ovary syndrome, and lipodystrophies.[200]

After the withdrawal of troglitazone because of hepatic toxicity, which does not seem to be a clinical class effect, there are currently two TZDs in clinical use, although other agents are in development:

1. rosiglitazone is PPAR-γ specific, and
2. pioglitazone appears to bind to both PPAR-γ and PPAR-α. Pioglitazone is metabolized via the hepatic P-450 CYP3A4 enzymes.

Partial PPAR-γ Activation. TZDs are considered PPAR-γ activators. They may actually decrease the expression of PPAR-γ mRNA, akin to the actions of ligands for other nuclear receptors such as the glucocorticoid and thyroid receptor. However, there is no associated change in the expression of genes that are positively regulated by PPAR-γ, thus suggesting that mechanisms such as PPAR-γ phosphorylation, by increasing activation, may compensate for the drop in expression.[201]

Mechanism of Insulin Sensitization. Because PPAR-γ exists primarily in fat cells, TZD action is largely centered on adipose tissue. TZD use is also associated with other beneficial anti-inflammatory and vasculoprotective effects that may be conducive to restoring insulin sensitivity.

It remains unclear whether all the improvements in insulin sensitivity are a direct TZD effect or derive secondarily from alterations in lipid storage, inflammation, plasma free fatty acids, and adipokines.

Adipogenesis and Fatty Acid Steal. TZDs exert their insulin-sensitizing actions in part via "fatty acid steal," which involves stimulation of free fatty acid storage in adipose tissue and sparing of other tissues such as the liver, skeletal muscle, and pancreatic beta cells from lipotoxicity. In effect, they lower ectopic fat deposition in nonadipose tissue, thereby decreasing one of the mechanisms leading to insulin resistance.[200]

TZDs, via PPAR-γ activation, have a potent adipogenic effect. In the process, TZDs promote the differentiation and proliferation of fat cells by increasing the number of small adipocytes and the mass of subcutaneous adipose tissue. By augmenting the amount of subcutaneous, peripheral fat, the lipid storage capacity of adipose tissue is enlarged, which allows the appropriate uptake and storage of fatty acids in adipose tissue. With greater adipose storage capacity, ectopically stored triacylglycerol is redistributed out of skeletal muscle and the liver into the peripheral adipocyte pool. In this manner, nonadipose insulin-sensitive tissues, such as skeletal muscle and the liver, as well as pancreatic beta cells, are released from the deleterious, metabolic effects of ectopic lipid storage. There is also an increase in overall fatty acid oxidation with an improvement in insulin signaling in skeletal muscle and the liver.[200,202]

Free Fatty Acids. The TZDs interfere with the release of free fatty acids, major mediators of systemic insulin resistance.

Acting via PPAR-γ2, TZDs induce LPL in adipose tissue, thus increasing the appropriate uptake of free fatty acids into adipocytes for storage as triacylglycerol. There is a corresponding reduction in circulating free fatty acid levels.[203] The anti-inflammatory impact of PPAR-γ activation with adipogenic and antilipolytic effect contributes to the lowering of free fatty acid levels.

Inflammation. As PPAR-γ agonists, TZDs are anti-inflammatory, which may favor insulin sensitivity.

TZDs modulate insulin sensitivity by altering adipokine release: release of proinflammatory adipokines is diminished, whereas adiponectin levels are enhanced. TZDs cause a reduction in proinflammatory cytokines such as TNF-α, CRP, IL-6, and MMP-9. They have a favorable impact on monocyte and macrophage function (Table 16-7).[200,204,205]

Oligonucleotide microarrays in differentiated 3T3-L1 adipocytes have indicated that rosiglitazone and pioglitazone each regulate the expression of more than 100 genes that cluster together. Various adipokines, such as adiponectin, TNF-α, resistin, and 11β-hydroxysteroid dehydrogenase, are among the genes that are regulated by PPAR-γ agonists in rodents[200]:

- Some of the insulin-sensitizing effect of TZDs may be mediated by a reduction in the expression of resistin analogues and in circulating levels of TNF-α and leptin.[200]
- TZDs may increase the production of adiponectin in white adipocytes by lowering TNF-α expression.[206]
  Adiponectin, an adipokine produced exclusively by adipose tissue, is insulin sensitizing and antiatherogenic. Adiponectin levels are low in patients with obesity and type 2 DM. TZDs increase adiponectin expression in adipocytes in vitro. In vivo treatment with TZDs markedly increases circulating adiponectin levels.[200]

Table 16-7. Thiazolidinedione Impact on Pro-oxidant, Inflammatory, and Prothrombotic Processes

Suppression of reactive oxygen species generation
Reduction of intranuclear nuclear factor kappaB
Enhanced expression of inhibitor kappaB alpha
Reduction in levels of
  Tumor necrosis factor-alpha
  C-reactive protein
  Monocyte chemoattractant protein-1
  Intercellular adhesion molecule-1
  Plasminogen activator inhibitor-1
Increase in interleukin-10

Modified from Dandone P, Aljada A. A rational approach to pathogenesis and treatment of type 2 diabetes mellitus, insulin resistance, inflammation, and atherosclerosis. Am J Cardiol 2002;90(suppl):27G-33G.

- In adipose tissue, TZDs repress expression of 11β-hydroxysteroid dehydrogenase type 1, the enzyme that produces cortisol in adipose tissue. TZDs thus diminish local glucocorticoid receptor effects and visceral adiposity.

In the liver and in adipose tissue, 11β-hydroxysteroid dehydrogenase type 1 catalyzes the interconversion of inactive cortisone to active cortisol. The full-blown metabolic syndrome develops in mice that overexpress 11β-hydroxysteroid dehydrogenase 1 in adipose tissue. In such mice, TZDs decrease visceral-omental fat accumulation, thereby alleviating features of the metabolic syndrome. However, no data on the effects of TZDs on 11β-hydroxysteroid dehydrogenase 1 activity or expression in humans are available.[200,207]

Vascular Effects. TZDs have a number of beneficial vascular effects (Table 16-8).

Endothelial Function. TZDs may improve endothelial function.

Table 16-8. Thiazolidinedione Impact on Cardiovascular Risk Factors

Adiposity	Reduced visceral-omental adiposity
	Enhanced subcutaneous adipogenesis
Hypertension	Improved insulin-mediated vasodilation
	Decreased endothelin-1 expression
	Attenuated vascular smooth muscle contractility
Dyslipidemia	Lowered triglyceride levels
	Raised high-density lipoprotein levels
	Increased low-density lipoprotein particle size
Hypercoagulability	Reduced plasminogen activator inhibitor-1 levels
	Lower fibrinogen levels
Atherogenesis	Decreased carotid intimal inflammation
	Attenuated intima-media thickness
	Lessened renal artery/mesangial cell proliferation

Modified from Fonseca VA. Management of diabetes mellitus and insulin resistance in patients with cardiovascular disease. Am J Cardiol 2003;92(suppl):50J-60J.

TZD use is associated with a reduction in microalbuminuria.[204,205] In patients with type 2 DM, rosiglitazone monotherapy was associated with a decrease in the ratio of urinary albumin to creatinine. In a double-blind, placebo-controlled study, troglitazone therapy produced improvements in flow-mediated vasodilation in a subgroup of patients with newly diagnosed type 2 DM.[200]

Hypertension. PPAR ligands may reduce systemic blood pressure.[204,205]

They may produce their antihypertensive effect in vivo partly by blocking the translocation of Rho to the cell membrane and inhibiting the Rho/Rho kinase pathway. Specifically, pioglitazone and troglitazone up-regulate the cytosolic expression of Src homology region 2–containing protein tyrosine phosphatase-2 (SHP-2), a protein tyrosine phosphatase that dephosphorylates Vav. Vav is a GTP/GDP exchange factor that up-regulates Rho kinase activity. Dephosphorylation of Vav inhibits Rho kinase activation.[208]

Vascular Remodeling. TZD therapy limits the extent of vascular remodeling and smooth muscle cell migration.[204,205]

A placebo-controlled study with rosiglitazone showed reduced progression of intima-media thickness of the common carotid artery in patients with type 2 DM.[200]

Therapy with rosiglitazone may reduce in-stent restenosis in diabetic patients with CHD who are undergoing coronary stent implantation. In a prospective, randomized, case-controlled trial involving 95 diabetic patients with CHD who were randomly assigned to either control or rosiglitazone, rosiglitazone therapy for 6 months lowered the fasting insulin concentration and significantly reduced CRP when compared with control. The rate of in-stent restenosis, as determined by quantitative coronary angiography performed at study entry and again at 6-month follow-up, was significantly reduced in the rosiglitazone group when compared with control at 17.6% versus 38.2%, $P = .030$, with a significantly lower degree of diameter stenosis than in the control group.[209]

Fibrinolysis and Atherogenesis. TZDs may diminish atherogenic and thrombogenic processes.

TZDs enhance fibrinolysis with a reduction in PAI-1 levels.

In a rabbit model of atherosclerosis, the combination of a PPAR agonist, L-805645, with simvastatin had additive effects on the regression of atherosclerotic lesions: decreased macrophage content, lower MMP activity, and increased smooth muscle cell/collagen content of lesions.[94]

Manifestations of Insulin Sensitization. TZD-mediated insulin sensitization has a number of beneficial subcellular and global metabolic manifestations. Overall, TZDs may reduce the rate of conversion from insulin resistance to type 2 DM and may exert protective effects against DM-related glomerular dysfunction and diabetic nephropathy.[204,205]

Subcellular Effects. PPAR-γ activation by TZDs improves intracellular insulin signaling.

- There is increased insulin-induced phosphorylation of IRS-1 and activation of Akt kinase to enhance insulin action.[203]
- By increasing the level of Cbl-associated protein (CAP), PPAR-γ activation via TZDs facilitates tyrosine phosphorylation of Cbl by the insulin receptor, thereby engendering increased Cbl activation of PI3K and atypical protein kinase C (PKC) for facilitated glucose uptake via GLUT4 translocation.[210]
- TZDs increase glucose transport activity in skeletal muscle and raise insulin-stimulated glycogen synthesis in muscle.[203]

Metabolic Manifestations. TZDs have a beneficial impact on numerous carbohydrate and lipid derangements deriving from insulin resistance. They may be of potential benefit for the full spectrum of the metabolic syndrome.

Carbohydrate Metabolism. TZDs consistently lower fasting and postprandial glucose and insulin concentrations in clinical studies. The reduction in insulin concentration is consistent with an insulin-sensitizing effect of the TZDs.

In human, insulin-resistant states, TZDs decrease postprandial and postabsorptive glycemia and insulinemia. They decrease HbA_{1c} by 1.0% to 1.5% and glucose by 45 to 60 mg/dL. A reduction in insulin concentration has been confirmed by direct measurements in human in vivo studies. TZDs increase insulin-stimulated glucose uptake in peripheral tissues, with a 20% to 40% rise in insulin-induced glucose utilization in skeletal muscle. They augment adipose and hepatic insulin sensitivity. Pancreatic insulin secretory responses increase.[200,211]

Lipid Metabolism. TZD therapy may lower circulating levels of triglycerides, raise levels of HDL, and improve the LDL phenotype.

TZD therapy with troglitazone or pioglitazone decreases circulating triglyceride levels, especially if markedly elevated, by increasing the lipolysis and clearance of triglyceride-rich lipoproteins into adipose tissue. TZD therapy increases HDL levels by as much as 10% to 20%.[200,212]

TZD effects on LDL levels are variable. LDL levels tend to remain unchanged with pioglitazone monotherapy and to increase by 8% to 16% in studies with rosiglitazone.[200] TZDs transition small, oxidized LDL complexes to larger, buoyant, less atherogenic particles.[212]

Thiazolidinedione Side Effects. Until further exploration of the effects of TZDs on myocardial metabolism and function in cardiomyopathy, TZDs are currently contraindicated for use in persons with NYHA class III to IV congestive heart failure. They should not be prescribed in the setting of familial adenomatous polyposis coli because of the risk for colonic carcinoma.[213] As with PPAR-α agonists, it is important to consider the systemic signaling effects of PPAR-γ agonists rather than focus on the limited metabolic effects alone.[124]

Increased Adipose Weight Gain. A major effect, and thus side effect, of TZD action is adipogenic differentiation leading to weight gain and expansion of the subcutaneous fat depot. Augmented food consumption may also play a role.[214] Fat mass accretion may amount to 1 to 4 kg/yr, 2 to 3 kg for every 1% decrease in HbA_{1c} values.[200,202] Chronic TZD therapy may, however, decrease the mass of visceral/omental fat, thus mitigating the potentially negative, systemic metabolic effects of fat expansion.[212]

Fluid Retention. Another side effect of TZDs is fluid retention. It is manifested primarily as peripheral edema secondary to plasma volume expansion with dilutional cytopenia, specifically, slight decreases in the hemoglobin level and hematocrit. Edema has been reported in 4% to 6% of patients undergoing treatment with TZDs and in up to 17% of users with systolic or diastolic ventricular dysfunction. In the latter group, fluid retention as a result of combined TZD-insulin therapy has required overnight hospitalization for heart failure in 9.9% of NYHA class II and III patients with left ventricular ejection fractions less than 40%, an occurrence particularly common in individuals older than 64 years. This increase in the incidence of heart failure has caused a warning to that effect to be included with the prescription information for rosiglitazone (Avandia) and pioglitazone (Actos).[200,215]

The reasons for fluid retention and peripheral edema with TZD use are probably multifactorial. There appears to be a reduction in renal excretion of sodium with an increase in sodium and free water retention:

- TZDs have both L-type voltage- and receptor-dependent calcium channel blocking ability and suppress PKC in vascular smooth muscle cells, thereby causing arterial vasodilation. Troglitazone dilates afferent and efferent glomerular arterioles and thus decreases glomerular capillary pressure and glomerular filtration.[216]
- TZDs may interact synergistically with insulin to facilitate sodium reabsorption, with a subsequent increase in extracellular volume.
- Increased sympathetic nervous system activity, altered interstitial ion transport, alterations in endothelial permeability, and PPAR-mediated expression of vascular permeability growth factor represent other possible mechanisms for edema with these agents.[217]

Cardiac Hypertrophy. Cardiac hypertrophy with increases in cardiac size and weight may occur with TZD therapy. Similar consequences are seen with insulin therapy, and these side effects may reflect improved insulin action.[202,218]

Proinflammatory, Atherogenic Effects. Under certain conditions, TZDs can promote the induction of proinflammatory cytokines. This effect may occur when ligand-activated PPAR-γ interacts with the cognate *cis*-element PPAR response element (PPRE) in the promoter region of a target gene.

PPAR activators may at times enhance the development of vascular lesions and can thus exhibit a potential proatherogenic effect.[219]

Tumerogenic Effects. Preclinical studies in a murine animal model have suggested that TZDs are tumor producing.[213]

Investigational Venues. Dual PPAR-α and PPAR-γ agonists may be better insulin sensitizers than isolated PPAR-γ agonists are. Combined PPAR-α/γ activation appears to be a promising approach to partially reverse insulin resistance and prevent the onset of type 2 DM. This approach combines

1. the PPAR-α–mediated catabolism of fatty acids via enhanced myocyte and hepatic fatty acid oxidation, with lipid-lowering and cardioprotective effects, and
2. the PPAR-γ–mediated adipogenesis, with glucose-lowering and insulin-sensitizing effects.

This dual approach corrects the abnormalities in both lipid and glucose metabolism and avoids the problem of body fat weight accretion seen with monotherapy via PPAR-γ ligands. As many as eight combination PPAR-α and PPAR-γ agonists are currently under clinical development, including two in phase III trials.[200] In prevention and treatment studies using Zucker diabetic fatty rats, PPAR-α/γ activation via ragaglitazar more effectively improved insulin sensitivity than did PPAR-γ activation alone via rosiglitazone.[214] Muraglitazar (BMS 298585), developed by Bristol-Myers, has had positive results in final-stage human trials involving 4500 diabetics; it has shown beneficial effects on blood glucose, as well as on levels of triglycerides and HDL.[220]

INSULIN-SENSITIZING THERAPY: BIGUANIDES AND AMPK ACTIVATORS

Activation of AMPK may improve insulin sensitivity and enhance glucose uptake. AMPK is a target of the biguanide insulin sensitizer metformin, which increases the activity of both catalytic subunits of AMPK.[221] In addition to its small peripheral insulin-sensitizing effect, metformin mainly inhibits hepatic gluconeogenesis.[222]

Combinations of TZDs and biguanides, such as rosiglitazone maleate and metformin hydrochloride, are available. Currently, it is as yet premature to resort to medical therapy with insulin sensitizers for the prevention of DM in the setting of insulin resistance and glucose intolerance.

Clinical Impact. Metformin decreases cardiovascular risk and delays the onset of type 2 DM[223]:

- Metformin improves endothelial function.[223]
- Metformin decreases cardiovascular events in patients with type 2 DM independent of glycemic control.[224]
- The Diabetes Prevention Program (DPP) reported on a trial of more than 3000 individuals with glucose intolerance in the absence of DM. The three treatment arms were metformin alone, exercise plus weight loss (7% weight loss and 150 minutes of exercise per week), and placebo. Over 2.8 years of follow-up, there was a 31% reduction in the onset of DM with metformin and 58% with lifestyle change, relative to placebo.[225]

As is seen with chronic AMPK activation, lactic acidosis may be a rare complication of metformin therapy.[222]

Investigational Venue. Alternative pharmacologic stimulation of AMPK may well be explored for the treatment of insulin resistance and DM. 5′-Aminoimidazole-4-carboxamide ribonucleoside (AICAR) is an analogue of adenosine. It is taken up in skeletal muscle, adipocytes, and hepatocytes and is phosphorylated to form the corresponding monophosphorylated nucleotide, which mimics the allosteric activating effects of 5′-AMP on AMPK. The metabolic effects of AICAR are thus consonant with AMPK activation and entail an increase in GLUT4 translocation and fatty acid oxidation.[221]

Currently, excessive amounts of AICAR are required to achieve a pharmacologic effect. Hepatic hypertrophy develops in rats chronically exposed to AICAR. AICAR causes excessive muscle glycogen accumulation, which may itself impair insulin sensitivity. Excessive uptake of glucose, which in the absence of exercise remains unoxidized, induces plasma lactate accumulation and lactic acidosis.[226]

INCRETIN MIMETICS

Incretins are potent insulin secretagogues that increase insulin secretion in excess of that elicited by the absorbed nutrients and thus regulate postprandial glucose metabolism and glucose assimilation.

Two incretins or gut hormones,

1. glucose-dependent insulinotropic peptide (GIP, also known as gastric inhibitory polypeptide) and
2. glucagon-like peptide-1 (GLP-1),

are secreted from the upper and lower small intestinal mucosa, respectively, in response to the ingestion of a meal.

Interference with incretin function induces glucose intolerance. Incretin function is, in fact, greatly impaired in type 2 DM because of impaired secretion of GLP-1 and a severely compromised insulinotropic effect of GIP in these patients.[227]

Both GLP-1 and GIP are rapidly inactivated in the circulation by the enzyme dipeptidyl peptidase IV (DPP-IV).[228]

Glucagon-like Peptide-1. GLP-1 is the most potent, naturally occurring incretin. It is one of the five separately processed domains of preproglucagon. The cellular and hemodynamic actions of GLP-1 are similar to those of glucagon. It has inotropic effects. Akin to glucagon, it causes G protein–coupled receptor activation and adenylate cyclase stimulation.[229] GLP-1 inhibits the secretion of glucagon. It slows gastric emptying and thereby reduces appetite and food intake.[227]

GLP-1 augments insulin secretion. It stimulates the formation of new pancreatic beta cells in rodents via enhanced beta cell proliferation and greater differentiation of duct progenitor cells into mature beta cells.[227]

GLP-1 incretin appears to have insulinomimetic effects. These effects may be attributable to the metabolite GLP-1(9-36) amide, which is biologically active and may increase glucose uptake through non–insulin-dependent mechanisms, independent of increased insulin levels. The metabolite is also a potent suppressor of glucagon activity.[230]

A continuous infusion of GLP-1 in type 2 diabetic patients has impressive insulin-sensitizing effects. GLP-1 is associated with reduced insulin resistance in skeletal muscle and adipose tissue and improvement in insulin-mediated glucose uptake.[230]

Incretin-Mimetic Therapy. Two approaches have been taken to use the insulinotropic and glucose-lowering actions of GLP-1 as a therapeutic agent:

1. development of DPP-IV–resistant analogues and
2. inhibition of DPP-IV.[228]

Exenatide. Exenatide is a synthetic copy of exendin-4, the toxin in Gila monster saliva, and has properties similar to those of human GLP-1. Exenatide improves the function of pancreatic beta cells and thereby stimulates insulin secretion. It improves blood sugar control, slows the movement of food through the gastrointestinal tract, decreases food intake, reduces weight gain, or causes weight loss. Because exenatide is enzymatically digested in the intestines, it requires twice-daily injections, before breakfast and before dinner.

Exenatide has been studied in type 2 diabetic volunteers. Twenty-seven percent of the volunteers experienced nausea while taking the drug, and no beneficial effect was seen on lipid profiles.[231] In a phase III clinical study, two daily injections of exenatide (5 or 10 μg) or placebo was administered to 336 patients with type 2 DM. At 30 weeks, HbA_{1c} levels were reduced by 0.9% in exenatide versus placebo patients, $P < .01$. The treatment group also experienced a 5.5-lb weight loss, $P < .05$. Forty-five percent of patients experienced nausea versus 23% of the placebo group.[232]

DPP-IV Inhibitor. LAF237, an oral inhibitor of DPP-IV, prevents the inactivation of endogenous GLP-1 and thus increases circulating levels of active GLP-1. In 3-month studies, both when used alone and when added to metformin in type 2 DM patients, twice-daily 25-mg doses of LAF237 caused a sustained reduction in glucose and HbA_{1c} levels. Side effects have been hypoglycemia, mild atrioventricular block, and lower extremity edema.[233,234]

ANTIOBESITY PHARMACOTHERAPY

Efforts at weight loss via dietary and exercise measures frequently fail because of high recidivism rates. Thus, pharmacotherapy for obesity may be considered an option. Pharmacotherapy can be contemplated for individuals with a body mass index (BMI)

- ≥30 kg/m^2 or
- ≥27 kg/m^2 with comorbid conditions.

Expectations for Antiobesity Pharmacotherapy. The following points should be considered with antiobesity pharmacotherapy:

1. Antiobesity pharmacotherapy is expected to be a life-long treatment.
2. Individuals undergoing treatment who experience no weight loss within a month of initiation of therapy may be refractory to a specific pharmacologic approach.
3. The loss of 10% of body weight is considered a successful intervention.
4. Weight loss tends to plateau after 6 months.
5. Some individuals regain weight after a year on therapy.
6. The biochemistry governing food-seeking behavior and fuel storage is essential for survival, and the neurotransmitters modulating appetite and weight control participate in other physiologic functions. Pharmacologic interference with such processes can be expected to have significant side effects.

Approved Anorexics. Currently approved agents for obesity pharmacotherapy include principally sibutramine and orlistat. Clinical experience with these agents indicates only a modest antiobesity impact with some attendant clinical benefit.[235]

Sibutramine. Sibutramine is a schedule IV anorexic that functions as a combined serotonin and norepinephrine reuptake inhibitor.

By affecting the monoamine system in the hypothalamus, sibutramine suppresses appetite and increases satiety. It also enhances thermogenesis.

It may be associated with a dose-related increase in hypertension, heart rate, and cardiovascular morbidity. Headaches, xerostomia, anorexia, and constipation may also occur.[236]

Orlistat. Orlistat is a pancreatic lipase inhibitor that causes weight loss through malabsorption.

At therapeutic dosages, orlistat blocks the absorption of 30% of dietary fat. Less than 1% of the drug is absorbed.

The drug is active in the gastrointestinal lumen as a potent, slowly reversible inhibitor of pancreatic, gastric, and carboxylester lipases, as well as phospholipase A_2. These lipases are required for the hydrolysis of dietary triglycerides and prevent the intestines from digesting and absorbing fatty acids.[236]

Although orlistat use may improve the lipid metabolic profile,[237] side effects can be troublesome and include severe abdominal cramping, diarrhea, flatus with discharge, fecal urgency, oily spotting, and evacuation. These side effects may abate after the first 4 weeks of therapy and may be limited by the concomitant use of a gel-forming fiber such as psyllium mucilloid.[235]

A vitamin supplement may prevent deficiencies in fat-soluble vitamins such as D and E and β-carotene.

Investigational Anorexics

Axokine. Axokine is a genetically modified and less potent version of ciliary neurotrophic factor that was developed as a treatment of amyotrophic lateral sclerosis but was found ineffective. A side effect of the medication is weight loss.

Axokine appears to have a mechanism of action analogous to that of leptin. The receptors for axokine and leptin share significant homology, and both receptors act on the same central pathways for appetite control in the arcuate nucleus. In contrast to leptin, resistance to axokine does not appear to occur even in obese individuals. Axokine seems to have long-term effects on the brain by apparently blocking the usual recidivism to weight loss. It is administered subcutaneously. Some side effects are injection site erythema, nausea, and a dry cough.[235]

Leptin. Although leptin has been ineffectual in inducing weight loss because of the occurrence of leptin resistance in obesity, leptin administered after weight loss may aid in preventing rebound weight gain.[238]

Melanocortin Receptor-4–Targeted Compounds. Leptin's appetite-suppressing actions are mediated in part via the melanocortin receptors. Melanocortin receptor-4–targeted compounds are being developed and appear to cause weight loss in rodents, with clinical studies planned for the future.[235]

Neuropeptide Y Antagonists. Neuropeptide Y (NPY) is a 36–amino acid neurotransmitter with complex effects on feeding, anxiety, circadian rhythms, reproduction, pituitary-adrenocortical function, and thermoregulation. It acts via at least six receptors, Y1 to Y6. Acting via the Y5 receptor, NPY is the most powerful appetite stimulant known. NPY5 antagonists might be effective antiobesity agents.[239]

Peptide YY3-36. Peptide YY3-36, or PYY, is synthesized by intestinal cells in response to food intake. Its central effects are a reduction in appetite. Preliminary studies with the agent are under way. Injection of the hormone 2 hours preprandially limits spontaneous food intake by 26%, with continued efficacy for 12 hours (Fig. 16-9).[240]

Selective β3-Adrenergic Receptor Agonists. Whereas α2-adrenergic receptors are antilipolytic, β3-adrenergic receptors enhance the resting metabolic rate and lipolysis. Over the last few decades, numerous agents manipulating the sympathetic nervous system have been tried. A selective β3-receptor agonist, BRL 35135, may show some promise. It induces weight loss and increases nonoxidative glucose disposal while improving glucose tolerance and decreasing hyperinsulinemia.[241,242]

Rimonabant. The endocannabinoid system seems to play a critical role in the regulation of appetite. Blockade of cannabinoid receptors has anorexigenic effects.

The Endocannabinoid System. During fasting, the oxyntic mucosa of the gastrointestinal tract expresses and releases a cannabinoid CB1 agonist as an appetite-stimulating, orexigenic factor in the short-term regulation of food intake.[243] The use of cannabis, or marijuana, is in general associated with food craving. There are cannabinoid receptors in adipose tissue, as well as in the enteric and central nervous system. Endocannabinoid systems control brain reward processes and, in particular, the capacity for explicit stimuli to precipitate food-seeking behavior. There is a possible link between

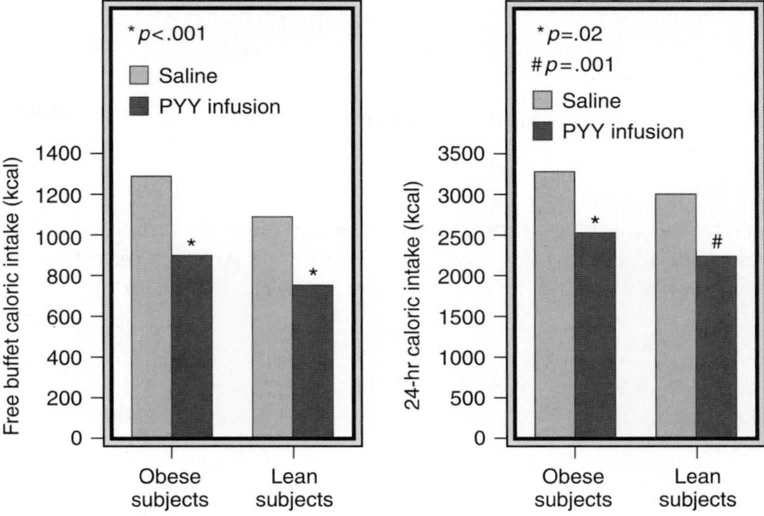

▶▶ **Figure 16–9.** Impact of peptide YY3-36 (PYY) versus saline infusion on free buffet and 24-hour caloric intake in obese and lean subjects. *(Modified from Batterham RL, Cohen MA, Ellis SM, et al. Inhibition of food intake in obese subjects by peptide YY3-36. N Engl J Med 2003;349:941-948.)*

cannabinoid processes and dopaminergic D_3 and/or D_2 receptor–mediated transmission in the corticolimbic structures.[244]

Cannabinoid Receptor Antagonism. Rimonabant (SR141716, Acomplia), has been developed as a selective antagonist to the cannabinoid CB1A receptor. It suppresses appetite.[235] Rimonabant's anorexigenic effects may involve dopaminergic D_3 receptor–mediated processes.

In rodent animal models, rimonabant reduced the intake of palatable food, as well as the self-administration of several addictive drugs.[244] Clinical rimonabant studies have shown increased smoking abstinence and a significant reduction in body weight with rimonabant when compared with placebo.

Weight Loss. In the weight loss trial Rimonabant in Obesity (RIO) Lipids, presented at the American College of Cardiology meeting in 2004, of 1000 patients with an average BMI of 34 kg/m² monitored for 1 year on a 600 calorie reduction diet who were treated with 20 mg or 5 mg of rimonabant versus placebo, 62% of patients completed the study. Weight loss at 1 year was 8 kg, 4 kg, and 2 kg, respectively, for the 20-mg, 5-mg, and placebo groups, with a 9-cm decrease in abdominal girth (Fig. 16-10). On active therapy, patients more readily tolerated the caloric restriction.

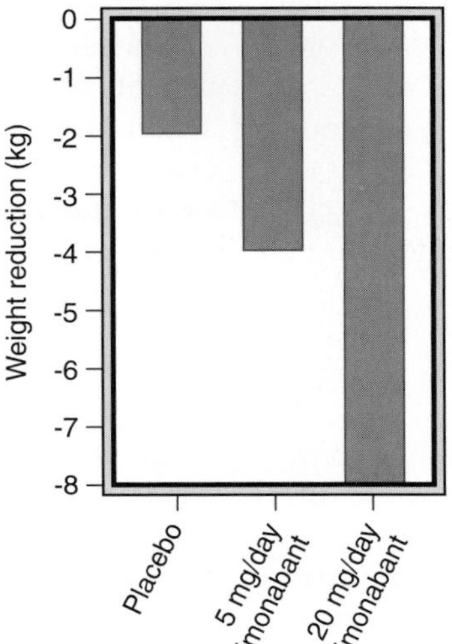

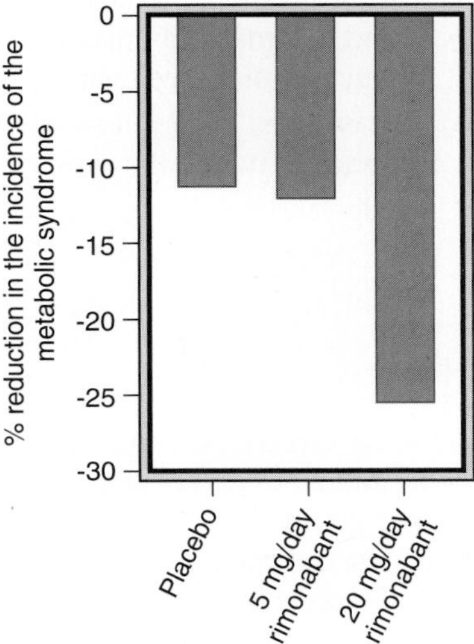

▶▶ **Figure 16–10.** Effect of 1-year therapy with 5-mg and 20-mg daily doses of the selective endocannabinoid receptor antagonist rimonabant on weight reduction and incidence of the metabolic syndrome in overweight individuals (BMI ≥34 kg/m²). *(Adapted from Anthenelli RM, Despres J-P. Effects of rimonabant in the reduction of major cardiovascular risk factors. Results from the RIO-LIPIDS Trial (Weight reducing and metabolic effects in overweight/obese patients with dyslipidemia). American College of Cardiology Scientific Sessions, 2004.)*

Table 16-9. Pleiotropic Effects of Selected Antiplatelet, Lipid-Modulating, Antihypertensive, Insulin-Sensitizing, and Anorexigenic Medications

	ANTIOXIDANT	ANTI-INFLAMMATORY	ANTICOAGULANT	ENDOTHELIAL PROTECTIVE	ANTIPROLIFERATIVE
Aspirin	+	+	+	N/A	+
Statins	+	+	+	+	+
Fibrates	N/A	N/A	N/A	N/A	N/A
Niacin	N/A	N/A	N/A	N/A	N/A
Ezetimibe	N/A	N/A	N/A	N/A	N/A
ACE inhibitors	+	+	+	+	N/A
ARBs	+	+	N/A	+	N/A
Vasodilating β-blockers	+	N/A	N/A	N/A	N/A
Thiazolidinediones	N/A	+	+	+	+
Biguanides	N/A	N/A	N/A	+	N/A
Rimonabant	N/A	N/A	N/A	N/A	N/A

+, Beneficial effect; –, adverse effect; 0, neutral effect; N/A, data not available.
ACE, angiotensin-converting enzyme; ARBs, angiotensin II receptor blockers.

In the follow-up RIO–North America study of 3045 subjects on reduced-calorie diets presented at the AHA Scientific Sessions in 2004, rimonabant, 20 mg/day, was used for 2 years and compared with 1 year of therapy followed by 1 year of placebo. The resulting average 17-lb weight loss and 3.2-inch decrease in waistline was maintained principally in the treatment group.[245]

Metabolic Effects. Rimonabant in the RIO trials had beneficial effects on glucose and lipid metabolism, principally at the 20-mg/day dose, when compared with placebo.

- Rimonabant increased adiponectin levels by an average of 41%.
- Rimonabant significantly reduced glucose and normalized insulin levels in an oral glucose tolerance test.
- There was a significant decline in the incidence of metabolic syndrome.
- Triglycerides decreased by 15% on average.
- HDL levels increased significantly.
- LDL particle size increased from the small to the less atherogenic, large form.

Adverse Effects. Adverse events leading to drug discontinuation occurred in 13% of patients in the 20-mg group versus 7.2% in the placebo group. The most common adverse effects, occurring principally within the first year of use, were depression, anxiety, irritability, nausea, and diarrhea. Serious adverse events were relatively rare in all groups.[245,246]

CONCLUSION

Aspirin, statins, ACE inhibitors, ARBs, fibrates, TZDs, and biguanides combat elements of the metabolic syndrome that lead to vascular disease and type 2 DM. A recent study of patients with ACS demonstrated not just an additive effect, but synergism as well when combination therapy with antiplatelet agents, statins, ACE inhibitors, and β-blockers was used. The combination of therapies was independently associated with lower 6-month mortality. Depending on the number of appropriate agents used, there was a 72% to 87% reduction in mortality.[247]

Conceivably, such incremental, synergistic benefit may apply to treatment of the metabolic syndrome and render the concept of a "polypill" containing a combination of appropriate agents rather attractive for insulin-resistant patients. A "polypill" would aid in improving patient compliance while simultaneously reducing multiple risk factors.[247]

Few data exist on the effects of specific drug interventions in nondiabetic individuals with the metabolic syndrome, and there are no data regarding any potential pharmacologic synergism with polypharmacy. Because most clinical trials that have shown clinical benefit have included subjects with characteristics of the metabolic syndrome, the study results may pertain

ANTIHYPERTENSIVE	ANTIATHEROGENIC	CARDIOVASCULAR EVENTS	INSULIN SENSITIVITY	ADIPONECTIN
N/A	N/A	+	N/A	N/A
?/+	+	+	+	N/A
N/A	N/A	+	+	N/A
N/A	N/A	+	–	N/A
N/A	N/A	N/A	N/A	N/A
+	N/A	+	+	+
+	+	+	+	+
+	+	+	+	N/A
+	+	N/A	+	+
N/A	N/A	+	+	N/A
N/A	N/A	N/A	+	+

to insulin-resistant individuals. However, there is a clear-cut need for prospective, controlled studies to address the efficacy of specific pharmacologic interventions, and possible synergisms, in insulin-resistant individuals with respect to the traditional study end points of mortality, cardiovascular events, and new-onset type 2 DM.

This raises the question of how such insulin-resistant individuals should be defined and how treatment efficacy should be monitored beyond the traditional study end points. Inflammation and oxidative stress underlie endothelial dysfunction, insulin resistance, atherosclerosis, and DM. Baseline testing and periodic reassessment of appropriate measures for inflammation and oxidant stress, endothelial function, and insulin resistance would offer more sensitive physiologic determinants of efficacy to complement the established end points.[246]

It is of interest that the beneficial, pleiotropic effects of numerous pharmaceutical agents act "behind the scenes" and are independent of the original pharmacologic targets at which they were directed (Table 16-9). Yes, ACE inhibitors reduce angiotensin-mediated vasoconstriction and statins lower LDL levels, but they, importantly, also reduce inflammatory activation. Pharmacologic efficacy may therefore not necessarily equate with traditional targets, and individually tested drug actions may not represent a class effect. In the future, clinical dose titration of drugs may need to resort to additional, nontraditional measures, such as markers of inflammation and oxidative stress, to gauge efficacy.

Therapies focusing on restoring endothelial function and insulin sensitivity will require elucidation of the regulatory, molecular mechanisms underlying normal and dysfunctional physiology. The rational development of new therapies will depend on these insights. For example, preserving the integrity of caveolae as functioning signaling modules may be critical for normal functioning of insulin and NO pathways, with endothelial dysfunction intimately linked to insulin resistance.

The metabolic syndrome comprises the cardiovascular and metabolic manifestations of a chronic proinflammatory process with oxidant stress. It is an inflammatory vascular disease in its inception and in its complications. Therefore, antioxidant and anti-inflammatory therapies should be helpful in reversing the underlying pathophysiology and protecting the integrity of the endothelium and insulin signaling pathways. Currently, therapeutic modalities include

- RAAS antagonism, which reduces oxidant stress and is anti-inflammatory, and
- statin therapy, which has anti-inflammatory and antioxidant effects.

In fact, a number of trials of patients with CHD have shown that antioxidant and anti-inflammatory RAAS antagonists and statins not only prevent cardiovascular events but also reduce the new onset of type 2 DM.

According to NCEP guidelines, any three of the following criteria define the presence of the metabolic syndrome:

- enlarged waistline,
- hypertension,
- elevated triglyceride level,
- decreased HDL level, and
- impaired fasting glucose level.

The gravity of the metabolic syndrome as a predictor of adverse outcomes increases with the number and the severity of its constituent elements. Each component is a risk factor in its own right. Beyond the additive effect of these components on cardiovascular risk, there is a synergism compounding the threat to cardiovascular health.

Currently, therapy needs to first address the individual's major metabolic disturbance. Taking each aspect of the metabolic syndrome individually:

- Enlarged waistline—reflective of excessive visceral/omental adipose tissue, with adipose insulin resistance triggered by inflammation, elaborating proinflammatory adipokines while reducing adiponectin levels and creating a prothrombotic milieu.

  Potential therapeutic considerations:

  1. inflammation—statins/RAAS antagonism,
  2. prothrombotic state—aspirin,
  3. visceral fat—PPAR-γ ligand, and
  4. obesity—antiobesity pharmacotherapy.

- Hypertension—reflective of endothelial dysfunction and vascular insulin resistance triggered by inflammation, sympathetic and RAAS hyperactivity, and oxidative stress. Risk factor for further cardiovascular disease.

  Potential therapeutic considerations:

  1. endothelial dysfunction—RAAS antagonism,
  2. RAAS—RAAS antagonism,
  3. sympathetic hyperactivity—vasodilating β-adrenergic blockade, and
  4. oxidative stress—statins.

- Dyslipidemia—reflective of hepatic insulin resistance triggered by inflammation. Risk factor for further vascular disease.

  Potential therapeutic considerations:

  1. inflammation—statin therapy;
  2. triglycerides—fibrates, PPAR-γ ligand, niacin;
  3. HDL—fibrates, PPAR-γ ligand, niacin;
  4. small, dense LDL—statins, fibrates, PPAR-γ ligand, niacin; and
  5. insulin resistance—PPAR-γ ligand.

- Impaired glucose metabolism—reflective of skeletal muscle insulin resistance triggered by inflammation. Risk factor for hyperglycemia, further inflammatory activation, further oxidant stress, type 2 DM, and macrovascular and microvascular disease.

  Potential therapeutic considerations:

  1. inflammation—statin therapy;
  2. oxidant stress—RAAS antagonism;

Table 16-10. Interventions to Reduce Cardiovascular Events and Incident Diabetes Mellitus in the Metabolic Syndrome

Mental stress	Stress relaxation techniques Moderate exercise Adequate sleep
Visceral/omental adiposity	Exercise Adequate sleep Weight loss Thiazolidinediones Antiobesity pharmacotherapy Bariatric surgery
Oxidant stress	Moderate exercise Diet rich in antioxidants RAAS antagonism Statins
Proinflammatory state	Eradicate chronic infection, e.g., periodontitis Smoking cessation Moderate exercise Weight loss Mediterranean-type diet Statins Aspirin RAAS antagonism Thiazolidinediones Fibrates
Endothelial dysfunction	Moderate exercise Stress relaxation techniques Sauna Mediterranean diet rich in antioxidants, n-3 fatty acids Statins RAAS antagonism Thiazolidinediones Biguanides

(Continued)

Table 16-10. Interventions to Reduce Cardiovascular Events and Incident Diabetes Mellitus in the Metabolic Syndrome—Cont'd

Insulin resistance	Moderate exercise Adequate sleep Weight loss Mediterranean diet rich in antioxidants, n-3 fatty acids RAAS antagonism Thiazolidinediones Biguanides
Hypertension	Moderate exercise Weight loss DASH diet RAAS antagonism Vasodilating β-blockers Calcium channel blockers Thiazolidinediones
Dyslipidemia	Exercise Weight loss Mediterranean high-fiber diet rich in n-3 fatty acids Statins Fibrates Thiazolidinediones
Hypercoagulability	Mediterranean diet Aspirin Thiazolidinediones

DASH, Dietary Approaches to Stop Hypertension; RAAS, renin-angiotensin-aldosterone system.

3. insulin resistance—PPAR-γ ligand, biguanide therapy; and
4. hyperglycemia—further diabetic therapy.

While targeting first the predominant disturbance, such as hypertension or dyslipidemia, therapy needs to expand until all pertinent factors are comprehensively covered. Endothelial dysfunction, dyslipidemia, vascular instability, ongoing inflammation, hypertension, left ventricular dysfunction, and the prothrombotic milieu must all eventually be addressed. Controlling all risk factors may prevent more than 80% of cardiovascular events in at-risk populations.[1]

In the future, if borne out by clinical trials and well tolerated for chronic therapy, a number of additional pharmacologic approaches hold promise:

- suitable AMPK activators and combination PPAR-α/γ agonists may be of interest for enhancing sensitivity to insulin and improving both carbohydrate and lipid metabolism;
- therapies that increase adiponectin should have a similar metabolic impact and have a vasculoprotective effect;
- therapy targeting HDL, e.g., via CETP inhibition, may have potent vasculoprotective effects; and
- selective endocannabinoid receptor antagonism may be a powerful tool for the prevention and reversal of caloric overconsumption.

Pharmacologic therapy, underpinned by determined therapeutic lifestyle changes (Tables 16-10 and 16-11), may reverse insulin resistance and delay or prevent the devastating consequences of the metabolic syndrome. Ultimately, an aggressive, comprehensive, multifaceted therapeutic approach will not only benefit cardiovascular and metabolic health but also aid in the prevention of other related medical problems such as cancer, frailty in aging, and dementia.

Table 16-11. Summary of Lifestyle and Medical-Surgical Approaches to the Metabolic Syndrome

Patient Self-Directed Efforts

Moderate daily exercise
Stress relaxation techniques
Adequate sleep
Hygiene for avoidance of chronic infections, e.g., dental prophylaxis
Mediterranean low-glycemic, high-fiber, antioxidant, high–n-3 fatty acid diet
Avoidance of weight gain
Weight loss
Smoking avoidance or cessation

Medical Intervention

Identification and eradication of chronic source of infection/inflammation
Aspirin
Statins
RAAS antagonist
PPAR-α ligands
PPAR-γ ligands
Biguanides
Antiobesity pharmacotherapy

Surgical Intervention

Eradication of chronic source of infection/inflammation
Bariatric surgery

PPAR, peroxisome proliferator–activated receptor; RAAS, renin-angiotensin-aldosterone system.

GLOSSARY

ABCA-1	Adenosine triphosphate–binding cassette A1
ACC	acetyl CoA carboxylase
ACE	angiotensin-converting enzyme
ACS	acute coronary syndrome
AFCAPS-TexCAPS	Air Force/Texas Coronary Atherosclerosis Prevention Study
AHA	American Heart Association
AICAR	5′-aminoimidazole-4-carboxamide ribonucleoside
ALLHAT	Antihypertensive and Lipid-Lowering Treatment to Prevent Heart Attack
AMP	adenosine 5′-monophosphate
AMPK	5′-AMP–activated protein kinase
AP-1	activator protein-1
apo	apolipoprotein
ARB	angiotensin II receptor blocker
ARBITER	Arterial Biology for Investigation of the Treatment Effects of Reducing Cholesterol
ASCOT	Anglo-Scandinavian Cardiac Outcomes Trial
AT_1	angiotensin II type 1
AT_2	angiotensin II type 2
ATP	Adult Treatment Panel
AVID	Antiarrhythmics Versus Implantable Defibrillators
BCAPS	Beta-Blocker Cholesterol-Lowering Asymptomatic Plaque Study
BECAIT	Bezafibrate Coronary Atherosclerosis Intervention Trial
BIP	Bezafibrate Infarction Prevention
BMI	body mass index
CAP	Cbl-associated protein
CAPP	Captopril Prevention Project
CARDS	Collaborative Atorvastatin Diabetes Study
CARE	Cholesterol And Recurrent Events
CETP	cholesteryl ester transfer protein
CHARM	Candesartan in Heart Failure Assessment of Reduction in Mortality and Morbidity
CHD	coronary heart disease
CMV	cytomegalovirus
CoA	coenzyme A
COMET	Carvedilol Or Metoprolol European Trial
COX	cyclooxygenase
CROSS	Candesartan Role on Obesity and on Sympathetic System
CRP	C-reactive protein
DAIS	Diabetes Atherosclerosis Intervention Study
DM	diabetes mellitus
DPP	Diabetes Prevention Program
DPP-IV	dipeptidyl peptidase IV
ELVA	Effects of Long-Term Treatment of Metoprolol CR/XL on Surrogate Variables for Atherosclerotic Disease
eNOS	endothelial NOS
ERK	extracellular signal–regulated kinase
EUROPA	European Trial on Reduction of Cardiac Events with Perindopril in Stable Coronary Artery Disease
FATS	Familial Atherosclerosis Treatment Study
GDP	guanosine 5′-diphosphate
GEMINI	The Glycemic Effects in Diabetes Mellitus: Carvedilol-Metoprolol Comparison in Hypertensives
GIP	glucose-dependent insulinotropic peptide
GLP	glucagon-like peptide
GLUT	glucose transporter
GTP	guanosine 5′-triphosphate
HATS	HDL-Atherosclerosis Treatment Study
HCTZ	hydrochlorothiazide
HDL	high-density lipoprotein
HbA_{1c}	glycated hemoglobin A
HMG	3-hydroxy-3-methylglutaryl
HOMA	homeostasis assessment model
HOPE	Heart Outcomes Prevention Evaluation
HOT	Hypertension Optimal Treatment
HPS	Heart Protection Study
HSP90	heat shock protein 90
HUVEC	human umbilical vein endothelial cell
IDL	intermediate-density lipoprotein
IDNT	Irbesartan Diabetic Nephropathy Trial
IL	interleukin
iNOS	inducible NOS
IRS	insulin receptor substrate
LDL	low-density lipoprotein

LIFE	Losartan Intervention For Endpoint Reduction in Hypertension
LOCAT	Lopid Coronary Angiographic Trial
LPL	lipoprotein lipase
MAPK	mitogen-activated protein kinase
MCP	monocyte chemoattractant protein
MHC	major histocompatibility complex
MI	myocardial infarction
MIRACL	Myocardial Ischemia Reduction with Aggressive Cholesterol Lowering
MMP	matrix metalloproteinase
NADH/NADPH	nicotinamide adenine dinucleotide phosphate oxidase
NCEP	National Cholesterol Education Program
NFκB	nuclear factor kappaB
NO	nitric oxide
NOS	nitric oxide synthase
NPY	neuropeptide Y
NYHA	New York Heart Association
PAI-1	plasminogen activator inhibitor-1
PDGF	platelet-derived growth factor
PEACE	Prevention of Events with Angiotensin Converting Enzyme Inhibition
PI3K	phosphatidylinositol 3-kinase
PKC	protein kinase C
PPAR	peroxisome proliferator–activated receptor
PPRE	PPAR response element
PRINCE	Pravastatin Inflammation/CRP Evaluation
PROVE IT-TIMI 22	Pravastatin or Atorvastatin Evaluation and Infection Therapy—Thrombolysis in Myocardial Infarction 22
PYY	peptide YY3-36
QUIET	Quinapril Ischemic Event Trial
RAAS	renin-angiotensin-aldosterone system
RENAAL	Reduction of Endpoints in NIDDM with the Angiotensin II Antagonist Losartan
REVERSAL	Reversing Atherosclerosis with Aggressive Lipid Lowering
RIO	Rimonabant in Obesity
ROS	reactive oxygen species
RXR	retinoid X receptor
4S	Scandinavian Simvastatin Survival Study
SENDCAP	St. Mary's, Ealing, Northwick Park Diabetes
SHP-2	Src homology region 2–containing protein tyrosine phosphatase-2
SOLVD	Studies Of Left Ventricular Dysfunction
SR	scavenger receptor
SREBP	sterol regulatory element binding protein
TGF	transforming growth factor
TIMP	tissue inhibitor of MMP
TNF	tumor necrosis factor
tPA	tissue plasminogen activator
TREND	Trial on Reversing Endothelial Dysfunction
TZD	thiazolidinedione
UKPDS	United Kingdom Prospective Diabetes Study
VA-HIT	Veterans Affairs High Density Lipoprotein Cholesterol Intervention Trial
VALUE	Valsartan Antihypertensive Long-Term Use Evaluation
VCAM	vascular cell adhesion molecule
VLDL	very-low-density lipoprotein

REFERENCES

1. Wong ND, Pio JR, Franklin SS, et al. Preventing coronary events by optimal control of blood pressure and lipids in patients with the metabolic syndrome. Am J Cardiol 2003;91:1421-1426
2. The Heart Outcomes Prevention Evaluation Study Investigators. Effects of an angiotensin-converting enzyme inhibitor, ramipril, on cardiovascular events in high-risk patients. N Engl J Med 2000;342:145-153
3. Freeman DJ, Norrie J, Sattar N, et al. Pravastatin and the development of diabetes mellitus: evidence for a protective treatment effect in the West of Scotland Coronary Prevention Study. Circulation 2001;103:357-362
4. Schieffer B, Drexler H. Role of 3-hydroxy-3-methylglutaryl coenzyme A reductase inhibitors, angiotensin-converting enzyme inhibitors, cyclooxygenase-2 inhibitors, and aspirin in antiinflammatory and immunomodulatory treatment

of cardiovascular disease. Am J Cardiol 2003;91(suppl): 12H-18H

5. Metz SA. Anti-inflammatory agents as inhibitors of prostaglandin synthesis in man. Med Clin North Am 1981;65:713-757
6. Midaoui AE, Wu R, de Champlain J. Prevention of hypertension, hyperglycemia and vascular oxidative stress by aspirin treatment in chronically glucose-fed rats. J Hypertens 2002;20:1407-1412
7. Evans JL, Goldfine ID, Maddux BA, Grodsky GM. Oxidative stress and stress-activated signaling pathways: a unifying hypothesis of type 2 diabetes. Endocr Rev 2002;23:599-622
8. Yuan M, Konstantopoulos N, Lee J, et al. Reversal of obesity- and diet-induced insulin resistance with salicylates or targeted disruption of IkB. Science 2001;293:1673-1677
9. Kim JK, Kim YJ, Fillmore JJ, et al. Prevention of fat-induced insulin resistance by salicylate. J Clin Invest 2001;108: 437-446
10. Solheim S, Arnesen H, Eikvar L, et al. Influence of aspirin on inflammatory markers in patients after acute myocardial infarction. Am J Cardiol 2003;92:843-845
11. Azar RR, Klayme S, Germanos M, et al. Effects of aspirin (325mg/day) on serum high-sensitivity C-reactive protein, cytokines, and adhesion molecules in healthy volunteers. Am J Cardiol 2003;92:236-238
12. Ridker PM, Cushman M, Stampfer MJ, et al. Inflammation, aspirin, and the risk of cardiovascular disease in apparently healthy men. N Engl J Med 1997;336:973-979
13. Redondo S, Santos-Gallego CG, Ganado P, et al. Acetylsalicylic acid inhibits cell proliferation by involving transforming growth factor-β. Circulation 2003;107: 626-629
14. Eidelman RS, Hebert PR, Steven M, et al. An update on aspirin in the primary prevention of cardiovascular disease. Arch Intern Med 2003;163:2006-2010
15. Hennekens CH. Update on aspirin in the treatment and prevention of cardiovascular disease. Am Heart J 1999; 137:S9-S13
16. de Gaetano G. Low dose aspirin and vitamin E in people at cardiovascular risk: a randomized trial in general practice. Collaborative Group of the Primary Prevention Project. Lancet 2001;357:89-95
17. Expert Panel on Detection, Evaluation, and Treatment of High Blood Cholesterol in Adults. Executive Summary of The Third Report of The National Cholesterol Education Program (NCEP) Expert Panel on Detection, Evaluation, and Treatment of High Blood Cholesterol in Adults (Adult Treatment Panel III). JAMA 2001;285: 2486-2497
18. Hanak V, Munoz J, Teague J, et al. Accuracy of the triglyceride to high-density lipoprotein cholesterol ratio for prediction of the low-density lipoprotein phenotype B. Am J Cardiol 2004;94:219-222
19. Grundy SM, Cleeman JI, Merz CNB, et al. Implications of recent clinical trials for the National Cholesterol Education Program Adult Treatment Panel III Guidelines. Circulation 2004;110:227-239
20. Nissen SE, Tuzcu EM, Schoenhagen P, et al. Effect of intensive compared with moderate lipid-lowering therapy on progression of coronary atherosclerosis: a randomized controlled trial. JAMA 2004;291:1071-1080
21. Cannon CP, Braunwald E, McCabe CH, et al. Intensive versus moderate lipid lowering with statins after acute coronary syndromes. N Engl J Med 2004;350:1495-1504
22. de Lemos JA, Blazing MA, Wiviott SD, et al. For the A to Z Investigators. Early intensive vs a delayed conservative simvastatin strategy in patients with acute coronary syndromes. JAMA 2004;292:1307-1316
23. Sowers J. Effects of statins on the vasculature: implication for aggressive lipid management in the cardiovascular metabolic syndrome. Am J Cardiol 2003;91(suppl): 14B-22B
24. McFarlane SI, Muniyappa R, Francisco R, Sowers JR. Pleiotropic effects of statins: lipid reduction and beyond. J Clin Endocrinol Metab 2002;87:1451-1458
25. Shepherd J, Cobbe SM, Ford I, et al. West of Scotland Coronary Prevention Study Group. Prevention of coronary heart disease with pravastatin in men with hypercholesterolemia. N Engl J Med 1995;333:1301-1307
26. Randomized trial of cholesterol lowering in 4444 patients with coronary heart disease: the Scandinavian Simvastatin Survival Study (4S). Lancet 1994;344:1383-1389
27. Sacks FM, Moye LA, Davis BR, et al. Relationship between plasma LDL concentrations during treatment with pravastatin and recurrent coronary events in the cholesterol and recurrent events trial. Circulation 1998; 97:1446-1452
28. http://www.clinicacayanga.f2s.com/Chol_guide_2001.htm
29. Lauer MS, Fontanarosa PB. Updated guidelines for cholesterol management. JAMA 2001;285:2508-2509
30. Arad Y, Ramakrishnan R, Ginsberg HN. Lovastatin therapy reduces low density lipoprotein apo B levels in subjects with combined hyperlipidemia by reducing the production of apo B containing lipoproteins: implications for the pathophysiology of apo B production. J Lipid Res 1990;31:567-582
31. Uauy R, Vega GL, Grundy SM, Bilheimer DM. Lovastatin therapy in receptor negative homozygous familial hypercholesterolemia: lack of effect on lipoprotein concentrations or turnover. J Pediatr 1988;113:387-392
32. Schoenbeck U, Libby P. Inflammation, immunity, and HMG-CoA reductase inhibitors. Statins as antiinflammatory agents? Circulation 2004;109(suppl II):II18-II26
33. Shishehbor MH, Brennan M-L, Aviles RJ, et al. Statins promote potent systemic antioxidant effects through specific inflammatory pathways. Circulation 2003;108: 426-431
34. Barandier C, Ming XF, Rusconi S, Yang Z. PKC is required for activation of ROCK by RhoA in human endothelial cells. Biochem Biophys Res Commun 2003;304: 714-719
35. Goldberg RB, Mellies MJ, Sacks FM, et al. Cardiovascular events and their reduction with pravastatin in diabetic and glucose-intolerant myocardial infarction survivors with average cholesterol levels: subgroup analyses in the cholesterol and recurrent events (CARE) trial. The Care Investigators. Circulation 1998;98:2513-2519
36. Haffner SM, Alexander CM, Cook TJ, et al. Reduced coronary events in simvastatin-treated patients with coronary heart disease and diabetes or impaired fasting glucose levels: subgroup analyses in the Scandinavian Simvastatin Survival Study. Arch Intern Med 1999;159: 2661-2667
37. Ballantyne CM, Olsson AG, Cook TJ, et al. Influence of low high-density lipoprotein cholesterol and elevated triglyceride on coronary heart disease events and response to simvastatin therapy in 4S. Circulation 2001;104: 3046-3051
38. Collins R, Armitage J, Parish S, et al. MRC/BHF Heart Protection Study of cholesterol-lowering with simvastatin in 5963 people with diabetes: a randomized placebo-controlled trial. Lancet 2003;361:2005-2016
39. Sever PS, Dahlof B, Poulter NR, et al. Prevention of coronary and stroke events with atorvastatin in hypertensive patients who have average or lower-than-average cholesterol concentrations, in the Anglo-Scandinavian Cardiac Outcomes Trial—Lipid Lowering Arm (ASCOT-LLA): a

multicentre randomised controlled trial. Lancet 2003; 361:1149-1158
40. Winslow R. Pfizer's hopes: antismoking pill, Lipitor, for diabetes. Wall St J 2003;June 17:B1
41. Colhoun HM, Thomason MJ, Mackness MI, et al. Design of the Collaborative AtoRvastatin Diabetes Study (CARDS) in patients with type 2 diabetes. Diabet Med 2002;19:201-211
42. Colhoun HM, Betteridge DJ, Durrington PN, et al. CARDS investigators. Primary prevention of cardiovascular disease with atorvastatin in type 2 diabetes in the Collaborative Atorvastatin Diabetes Study (CARDS): multicentre randomised placebo-controlled trial. Lancet 2004;364:685-696
43. The Diabetes Atorvastatin Lipid Intervention (DALI) Study Group. The effect of aggressive versus standard lipid lowering by atorvastatin on diabetic dyslipidemia: the DALI study: a double-blind, randomized, placebo-controlled trial in patients with type 2 diabetes and diabetic dyslipidemia. Diabetes Care 2001;24:1335-1341
44. Roglans N, Sanguino E, Peris C, et al. Atorvastatin treatment induced peroxisome proliferator–activated receptor alpha expression and decreased plasma nonesterified fatty acids and liver triglyceride in fructose-fed rats. J Pharmacol Exp Ther 2002;302:232-239
45. Mead JR, Irvine SA, Ramji DP. Lipoprotein lipase: structure, function, regulation, and role in disease. J Mol Med 2002;80:753-769
46. Lee S-J, Sacks FM. Effect of pravastatin on intermediate-density and low-density lipoproteins containing apolipoprotein CIII in patients with diabetes mellitus. Am J Cardiol 2003;92:121-124
47. Asztalos BF, Schaefer EJ. High-density lipoprotein subpopulations in pathologic conditions. Am J Cardiol 2003;91(suppl 7A):12E-17E
48. Blasetto J, Stein E, Brown WV, et al. Efficacy of rosuvastatin compared with other statins in hypercholesterolemic patients and in special population groups. Am J Cardiol 2003;91(suppl 5A):3C-10C
49. Illingworth DR, Crouse JR Jr, Hunninghake DB, et al. A comparison of simvastatin and atorvastatin up to maximal recommended doses in a large multicenter randomized clinical trial. Curr Med Res Opin 2001;17:43-50
50. Martin G, Duez H, Blanquart C, et al. Statin-induced inhibition of the Rho-signaling pathway activates PPARalpha and induces HDL apoA-I. J Clin Invest 2001; 107:1423-1432
51. Brown BG, Hillger L, Zhao XQ, et al. Types of change in coronary stenosis severity and their relative importance in overall progression and regression of coronary disease. Observation from the FATS Trial. Familial Atherosclerosis Treatment Study. Ann N Y Acad Sci 1995;748:407-418
52. Chong PH, Seeger JD, Franklin C. Clinically relevant differences between statins: implication for therapeutic selection. Am J Med 2001;111:390-400
53. Szmitko P, Wang CH, Weisel RD, et al. Biomarkers of vascular disease linking inflammation to endothelial activation. Circulation 2003;108:2041-2048
54. Vaughan CJ, Gotto AM, Basson CT. The evolving role of statins in the management of atherosclerosis. J Am Coll Cardiol 2000;35:1-10
55. Grip O, Janciauskiene S, Lindgren S. Atorvastatin activates PPAR-gamma and attenuates the inflammatory response in human monocytes. Inflamm Res 2002;51:58-62
56. Zelvyte I, Dominaitiene R, Crisby M, Janciauskiene S. Modulation of inflammatory mediators and PPARgamma and NFkappaB expression by pravastatin in response to lipoproteins in human monocytes in vitro. Pharmacol Res 2002;45:147-154
57. Mulhaupt F, Matter CM, Kwak BR, et al. Statins (HMG-CoA reductase inhibitors) reduce CD40 expression in human vascular cells. Cardiovasc Res 2003;59: 755-756
58. Blanco-Colio LM, Muñoz-García B, Martín-Ventura JL, et al. 3-Hydroxy-3-methylglutaryl coenzyme A reductase inhibitors decrease Fas ligand expression and cytotoxicity in activated human T lymphocytes. Circulation 2003;108:1506-1513
59. Dechend R, Gieffers J, Dietz R, et al. Hydroxymethylglutaryl coenzyme A reductase inhibition reduces *Chlamydia pneumoniae*–induced cell interaction and activation. Circulation 2003;108:261-265
60. Potena L, Frascaroli G, Grigioni F, et al. Hydroxymethylglutaryl coenzyme A reductase inhibition limits cytomegalovirus infection in human endothelial cells. Circulation 2004;109:532-536
61. Merx MW, Liehn EA, Janssens U, et al. HMG-CoA reductase inhibitor simvastatin profoundly improves survival in a murine model of sepsis. Circulation 2004;109: 2560-2565
62. Waehre T, Damas JK, Gullestad L, et al. Hydroxymethylglutaryl coenzyme A reductase inhibitors downregulate chemokines and chemokine receptors in patients with coronary artery disease. J Am Coll Cardiol 2003; 41:1460-1467
63. Albert MA, Danielson E, Rifai N, Ridker PM, for the PRINCE Investigators. Effect of statin therapy on C-reactive protein levels. The Pravastatin Inflammation/CRP Evaluation (PRINCE): a randomized trial and cohort study. JAMA 2001;286:64-70
64. Ridker PM, Rifai N, Clearfield M, et al, for the Air Force/Texas Coronary Atherosclerosis Prevention Study Investigators. Measurement of C-reactive protein for the targeting of statin therapy in the primary prevention of acute coronary events. N Engl J Med 2001;344:1959-1965
65. Ridker PM, Rifai N, Pfeffer MA, et al, for the Cholesterol and Recurrent Events (CARE) investigators. Long-term effects of pravastatin on plasma concentration of C-reactive protein. Circulation 1999;100:230-235
66. Plenge JK, Hernandez TL, Weil KM, et al. Simvastatin lowers C-reactive protein within 14 days. An effect independent of low-density lipoprotein cholesterol reduction. Circulation 2002;106:1447-1452
67. Correia LCL, Sposito AC, Lima JC, et al. Anti-inflammatory effect of atorvastatin (80mg) in unstable angina pectoris and non–Q-wave acute myocardial infarction. Am J Cardiol 2003;92:298-301
68. Kinlay S, Schwartz GG, Olsson AG, et al. High-dose atorvastatin enhances the decline in inflammatory markers in patients with acute coronary syndromes in the MIRACL study. Circulation 2003;108:1560-1566
69. Ridker PM, Cannon CP, Morrow D, et al, for the Pravastatin or Atorvastatin Evaluation and Infection Therapy—Thrombolysis in Myocardial Infarction 22 (PROVE IT-TIMI 22) Investigators. C-reactive protein levels and outcomes after statin therapy. N Engl J Med 2005;352:20-28
70. Nissen SE, Tuzcu EM, Schoenhagen P, et al, for the Reversal of Atherosclerosis with Aggressive Lipid Lowering (REVERSAL) Investigators. Statin therapy, LDL cholesterol, C-reactive protein, and coronary artery disease. N Engl J Med 2005;352:29-38
71. Kinlay S, Schwartz GG, Olsson AG, et al, for the Myocardial Ischemia Reduction with Aggressive Cholesterol Lowering (MIRACL) Study Investigators. Effect of atorvastatin on risk of recurrent cardiovascular events after an acute coronary syndrome associated with high soluble CD40 ligand in the Myocardial Ischemia

Reduction with Aggressive Cholesterol Lowering (MIRACL) study. Circulation 2004;110:386-391
72. George SJ, Dhond AJ, Alderson SM, Ezekowitz MD. Neuroprotective effects of statins may not be related to total and low-density lipoprotein cholesterol lowering. Am J Cardiol 2002;90:1237-1239
73. Standley PR, Ali S, Bapna C, et al. Increased platelet cytosolic calcium responses to low density lipoprotein in type II diabetes with and without hypertension. Am J Hypertens 1993;6:938-943
74. Selwyn AP. Prothrombotic and antithrombotic pathways in acute coronary syndromes. Am J Cardiol 2003;91 (suppl):3H-11H
75. Harrison DG, Armstrong ML, Frieman PC, Heistad DD. Restoration of endothelium-dependent relaxation by dietary treatment of atherosclerosis. J Clin Invest 1987; 80:1808-1811
76. Leung WH, Lau CP, Wong CK. Beneficial effect of cholesterol-lowering therapy on coronary endothelium-dependent relaxation in hypercholesterolemic patients. Lancet 1993;341:1496-1500
77. Egashira K, Hirooka Y, Kai H, et al. Reduction in serum cholesterol with pravastatin improves endothelium-dependent coronary vasomotion in patients with hypercholesterolemia. Circulation 1994;89:2519-2524
78. Treasure CB, Klein JL, Weintraub WS, et al. Beneficial effects of cholesterol-lowering therapy on the coronary endothelium in patients with coronary artery disease. N Engl J Med 1995;332:481-487
79. Laufs U. Beyond lipid-lowering: effects of statins on endothelial nitric oxide. Eur J Clin Pharmacol 2003; 58:719-731
80. Wassman S, Faul A, Hennen B, et al. Rapid effect of 3-hydroxy-3-methylglutaryl coenzyme A reductase inhibition on coronary endothelial function. Circ Res 2003;93:e98-e103
81. Laufs U, Endres M, Liao JK. Regulation of endothelial NO production by Rho GTPase. Med Klin (Munich) 1999;94:211-218
82. Pelat M, Dessy C, Massion P, et al. Rosuvastatin decreases caveolin-1 and improves nitric oxide–dependent heart rate and blood pressure variability in apolipoprotein E-/- mice in vivo. Circulation 2003;107:2480-2486
83. Susic D, Varagic J, Ahn J, et al. Beneficial pleiotropic vascular effects of rosuvastatin in two hypertensive models. J Am Coll Cardiol 2003;42:1091-1097
84. Hirai N, Kawano H, Yasue H, et al. Attenuation of nitrate tolerance and oxidative stress by an angiotensin II receptor blocker in patients with coronary spastic angina. Circulation 2003;108:1446-1450
85. Llevadot J, Murasawa S, Kureishi Y, et al. HMG-CoA reductase inhibitor mobilizes bone marrow–derived endothelial progenitor cells. J Clin Invest 2001;108:399-405
86. Nishimura T, Vaszar LT, Faul JL, et al. Simvastatin rescues rats from fatal pulmonary hypertension by inducing apoptosis of neointimal smooth muscle cells. Circulation 2003;108:1640-1645
87. Bountioukos M, Rizzello V, Krenning BJ, et al. Effect of atorvastatin on myocardial contractile reserve assessed by tissue Doppler imaging in moderately hypercholesterolemic patients without heart disease. Am J Cardiol 2003;92:613-616
88. Node K, Fujita M, Kitakaze M, et al. Short-term statin therapy improves cardiac function and symptoms in patients with idiopathic dilated cardiomyopathy. Circulation 2003;108:839-843
89. Aronow WS, Nayak D, Woodworth S, Ahn C. Effect of simvastatin versus placebo on treadmill exercise time until the onset of intermittent claudication in older patients with peripheral arterial disease at six months and at one year after treatment. Am J Cardiol 2003; 92:711-712
90. Mohler ER, Hiatt WR, Mark A, Creager MA. Cholesterol reduction with atorvastatin improves walking distance in patients with peripheral arterial disease. Circulation 2003;108:1481-1486
91. Schwartz RG, Pearson TA, Kalaria VG, et al. Prospective serial evaluation of myocardial perfusion and lipids during the first six months of pravastatin therapy. J Am Coll Cardiol 2003;42:600-610
92. Ichiki T, Takeda K, Tokunou T, et al. Downregulation of angiotensin II type 1 receptor by hydrophobic 3-hydroxy-3-methylglutaryl coenzyme A reductase inhibitors in vascular smooth muscle cells. Arterioscler Thromb Vasc Biol 2001;21:1896-1901
93. Takemoto M, Node K, Nakagami H, et al. Statins as antioxidant therapy for preventing cardiac myocyte hypertrophy. J Clin Invest 2001;108:1429-1437
94. Corti R, Osende JI, Fallon JT, et al. The selective peroxisomal proliferator–activated receptor-gamma agonist has an additive effect on plaque regression in combination with simvastatin in experimental atherosclerosis. J Am Coll Cardiol 2004;43:464-473
95. Kleemann R, Princen HMG, Emeis JJ, et al. Rosuvastatin reduces atherosclerosis development beyond and independent of its plasma cholesterol-lowering effect in APOE*3-Leiden transgenic mice: evidence for antiinflammatory effects of rosuvastatin. Circulation 2003; 108:1368-1374
96. Jensen LO, Thayssen P, Pedersen KE, et al. Regression of coronary atherosclerosis by simvastatin: a serial intravascular ultrasound study. Circulation 2004;110: 265-270
97. Cingozbay BY, Top C, Terekeci H, et al. Effects of fluvastatin treatment on insulin sensitivity in patients with hyperlipidaemia. J Int Med Res 2002;30:21-25
98. Sonmez A, Baykal Y, Kilic M, et al. Fluvastatin improves insulin resistance in nondiabetic dyslipidemic patients. Endocrine 2003;22:151-154
99. Costa A, Casamitjana R, Casals E, et al. Effects of atorvastatin on glucose homeostasis, postprandial triglyceride response and C-reactive protein in subjects with impaired fasting glucose. Diabet Med 2003;20: 743-745
100. Paolisso G, Barbagallo M, Petrella G, et al. Effects of simvastatin and atorvastatin administration on insulin resistance and respiratory quotient in aged dyslipidemic non–insulin-dependent diabetic patients. Atherosclerosis 2000;150:121-127
101. Melenovsky V, Wichterle D, Simek J, et al. Effect of atorvastatin and fenofibrate on autonomic tone in subjects with combined hyperlipidemia. Am J Cardiol 2003;92: 337-341
102. Pliquett RU, Cornish KG, Peuler JD, et al. Simvastatin normalizes autonomic neural control in experimental heart failure. Circulation 2003;107:2493-2498
103. Kumagai K, Nakashima H, Saku K. The HMG-CoA reductase inhibitor atorvastatin prevents atrial fibrillation by inhibiting inflammation in a canine sterile pericarditis model. Cardiovasc Res 2004;62:105-111
104. Young-Xu Y, Jabbour S, Goldberg R, et al. Usefulness of statin drugs in protecting against atrial fibrillation in patients with coronary artery disease. Am J Cardiol 2003;92:1379-1383
105. Siu CW, Lau CP, Tse HF. Prevention of atrial fibrillation recurrence by statin therapy in patients with lone atrial fibrillation after successful cardioversion. Am J Cardiol 2003;92:1343-1345

106. Mitchell LB, Powell JL, Gillis AM, et al; AVID Investigators. Are lipid-lowering drugs also antiarrhythmic drugs? An analysis of the Antiarrhythmics Versus Implantable Defibrillators (AVID) Trial. J Am Coll Cardiol 2003;42:81-87
107. Yang CC, Jick S, Jick H. Lipid-lowering drugs and the risk of depression and suicidal behavior. Arch Intern Med 2003;163:1926-1932
108. Young-Xu Y, Chan KA, Liao JK, et al. Long-term statin use and psychological well-being. J Am Coll Cardiol 2003;42:690-697
109. Marx J. Bad for the heart, bad for the mind? Science 2001;294:508-509
110. Hall NF, Gale CR, Syddal H, et al. Risk of macular degeneration in users of statins: cross sectional study. BMJ 2001;323:375-376
111. Wang PS, Solomon DH, Mogun H, Avorn J. HMG-CoA reductase inhibitors and the risk of hip fractures in elderly patients. JAMA 2000;283:3205-3210
112. Cauley JA, Zmuda JM, Lui LY, et al. Lipid-lowering drug use and breast cancer in older women: a prospective study. J Womens Health 2003;12:749-756
113. Topol E. Intensive statin therapy—a sea change in cardiovascular prevention. N Engl J Med 2004;350: 1562-1564
114. Jump DB. The biochemistry of n-3 polyunsaturated fatty acids. J Biol Chem 2002;277:8755-8758
115. Rubins HB, Robins SJ, Collins D, et al. Gemfibrozil for the secondary prevention of coronary heart disease in men with low levels of high-density lipoprotein cholesterol. Veterans Affairs High-Density Lipoprotein Cholesterol Intervention Trial Study Group. N Engl J Med 1999;341:410-418
116. Fruchart J-C, Staels B, Duriez P. PPARs, metabolic disease and atherosclerosis. Pharmacol Res 2001;44:345-352
117. Pineda-Torra I, Chinetti G, Duval C, et al. Peroxisome proliferator–activated receptors: from transcriptional control to clinical practice. Curr Opin Lipidol 2001; 12:245-254
118. Munday MR, Hemingway CJ. The regulation of acetyl-CoA carboxylase—a potential target for the action of hypolipidemic agents. Adv Enzyme Regul 1999;39: 205-234
119. Ruotolo G, Howard BV. Dyslipidemia of the metabolic syndrome. Curr Cardiol Rep 2002;4:494-500
120. Sprecher DL, Watkins TR, Behar S, et al. Importance of high-density lipoprotein cholesterol and triglyceride levels in coronary heart disease. Am J Cardiol 2003;91: 575-580
121. Rader DJ. Effects of nonstatin lipid drug therapy on high-density lipoprotein metabolism. Am J Cardiol 2003;91(suppl):18E-23E
122. Tenenbaum A, Motro M, Fisman EZ, et al. Peroxisome proliferator–activated receptor ligand bezafibrate for prevention of type 2 diabetes mellitus in patients with coronary artery disease. Circulation 2004;109: 2197-2202
123. Vega GL, Ma PTS, Cater NB, et al. Effects of adding fenofibrate (200mg/day) to simvastatin (10mg/day) in patients with combined hyperlipidemia and metabolic syndrome. Am J Cardiol 2003;91:956-960
124. Xie Y, Yang Q, DePierre JW. The effects of peroxisome proliferators on global lipid homeostasis and the possible significance of these effects to other responses to these xenobiotics: an hypothesis. Ann N Y Acad Sci 2002; 973:17-25
125. Morgan JM, Capuzzi DM, Baksh RI, et al. Effects of extended-release niacin on lipoprotein subclass distribution. Am J Cardiol 2003;91:1432-1436
126. Zambon A, Hokanson JE, Brown BG, Brunzell JD. Evidence for a new pathophysiological mechanism for coronary artery disease regression: hepatic-lipase mediated changes in LDL density. Circulation 1999;99: 1959-1964
127. Carlson LA, Rosenhammer G. Reduction of mortality in the Stockholm Ischaemic Heart Disease Secondary Prevention Study by combined treatment with clofibrate and nicotinic acid. Acta Med Scand 1988;223: 405-418
128. Canner PL, Berge KG, Wenger NK, et al. Fifteen year mortality in Coronary Drug Project patients: long-term benefit with niacin. J Am Coll Cardiol 1986;8: 1245-1255
129. Taylor AJ, Sullenberger LE, Lee HJ, et al. Arterial Biology for the Investigation of the Treatment Effects of Reducing Cholesterol (ARBITER) 2. A double-blind, placebo-controlled study of extended-release niacin on atherosclerosis progression in secondary prevention patients treated with statins. Circulation 2004;110: 3512-3517
130. Brown BG, Zhao XQ, Chait A, et al. Simvastatin and niacin, antioxidant vitamins, or the combination for the prevention of coronary disease. N Engl J Med 2001; 345:1583-1592
131. Fulcher GR, Walker M, Catalano C, et al. Metabolic effects of suppression of nonesterified fatty acid levels with acipimox in obese NIDDM subjects. Diabetes 1992;41:1400-1408
132. Catapano AL. Ezetimibe: a selective inhibitor of cholesterol absorption. Eur Heart J 2001;3:E6-E10
133. Smart EJ, De Rose RA, Farber SA. Annexin 2–caveolin 1 complex is a target of ezetimibe and regulates intestinal cholesterol transport. Proc Natl Acad Sci U S A 2004; 101:3450-3455
134. Illingworth DR. Achievement of low-density lipoprotein cholesterol goals: new strategies to address new guidelines. Cardiol Clin 2003;21:363-375
135. Brousseau ME, Schaefer EJ, Wolfe ML, et al. Effects of an inhibitor of cholesteryl ester transfer protein on HDL cholesterol. N Engl J Med 2004;350:1505-1515
136. Jancin B. New nonstatin drugs to redefine lipid lowering. Int Med News 2004;37:101
137. Adler AI, Stratton IM, Neil HA, et al. Association of systolic blood pressure with macrovascular and microvascular complications of type 2 diabetes (UKPDS 36): prospective observational study. BMJ 2000;321:412-419
138. Hansson L, Zanchetti A, Carruthers SG, et al. Effects of intensive blood pressure lowering and low-dose aspirin in patients with hypertension: principal results of the Hypertension Optimal Treatment (HOT) randomized trial: HOT Study Group. Lancet 1998;351: 1755-1762
139. McFarlane SI, Kumar A, Sowers JR. Mechanisms by which angiotensin-converting enzyme inhibitors prevent diabetes and cardiovascular disease. Am J Cardiol 2003;91(suppl):30-37
140. Rincon-Choles H, Kasinath BS, Gorin Y, et al. Angiotensin II and growth factors in the pathogenesis of diabetic nephropathy. Kidney Int Suppl 2002;82:8-11
141. Brown NJ, Vaughan DE. Angiotensin-converting enzyme inhibitors. Circulation 1998;97:1411-1420
142. Higgins JP. Can angiotensin-converting enzyme inhibitors reverse atherosclerosis? South Med J 2003;96: 569-579
143. Griendling KK, Minieri CA, Ollerenshaw JD, Alexander RW. Angiotensin II stimulates NADH and NADPH oxidase activity in cultured vascular smooth muscle cells. Circ Res 1994;74:1141-1148

144. Pitt B. ACE inhibitors for patients with vascular disease without left ventricular dysfunction—May they rest in PEACE? N Engl J Med 2004;351:2115-2117
145. Ridker PM. Clinical application of C-reactive protein for cardiovascular disease detection and prevention. Circulation 2003;107:363-369
146. Lauten WB, Khan QA, Rajagopalan S, et al. Usefulness of quinapril and irbesartan to improve the antiinflammatory response of atorvastatin and aspirin in patients with coronary heart disease. Am J Cardiol 2003;91: 1116-1119
147. Prasad A, Husain S, Quyyumi AA. Abnormal flow-mediated epicardial vasomotion in human coronary arteries is improved by angiotensin-converting enzyme inhibition: a potential role of bradykinin. J Am Coll Cardiol 1999;33:796-804
148. Fox KM; EURopean trial On reduction of cardiac events with Perindopril in stable coronary Artery disease Investigators. Efficacy of perindopril in reduction of cardiovascular events among patients with stable coronary artery disease: randomised, double-blind, placebo-controlled, multicentre trial (the EUROPA study). Lancet 2003;362:782-788
149. Mancini GB, Henry GC, Macaya C, et al. Angiotensin-converting enzyme inhibition with quinapril improves endothelial vasomotor dysfunction in patients with coronary artery disease. Circulation 1996;94:258-265
150. Pitt B, O'Neill B, Feldman R, et al. The QUinapril Ischemic Event Trial (QUIET): evaluation of chronic ACE inhibitor therapy in patients with ischemic heart disease and preserved left ventricular function. Am J Cardiol 2001;87:1058-1063
151. The PEACE Trial Investigators. Angiotensin-converting-enzyme inhibition in stable coronary artery disease. N Engl J Med 2004;351:2058-2068
152. Shiuchi T, Cui TX, Wu L, et al. ACE inhibitor improves insulin resistance in diabetic mouse via bradykinin and NO. Hypertension 2002;40:329-334
153. Jacob S, Henriksen EJ, Fogt DL, Dietze GJ. Effects of trandolapril and verapamil on glucose transport in insulin-resistant rat skeletal muscle. Metabolism 1996;45:535-541
154. Furuhashi M, Ura N, Higashiura K, et al. Blockade of the renin-angiotensin system increases adiponectin concentrations in patients with essential hypertension. Hypertension 2003;42:76-81
155. Yusuf S, Gerstein H, Hoogwerf B, et al, for the HOPE Study Investigators. Ramipril and the development of diabetes. JAMA 2001;286:1882-1885
156. Hansson L, Lindholm LH, Niskanen L, et al. Effect of angiotensin-converting enzyme inhibition compared with conventional therapy on cardiovascular morbidity and mortality in hypertension: the Captopril Prevention Project (CAPPP) randomised trial. Lancet 1999;353: 611-616
157. Vermes E, Ducharme A, Bourassa MG, et al. Enalapril reduces the incidence of diabetes in patients with chronic heart failure: insight from the Studies Of Left Ventricular Dysfunction (SOLVD). Circulation 2003;107:1291-1296
158. Punzi HA, Punzi CF. Metabolic issues in the Antihypertensive and Lipid-Lowering Heart Attack Trial Study. Curr Hypertens Rep 2004;6:106-110
159. Lewis EJ, Hunsicker LG, Bain RP, Rohde RD. The effect of angiotensin-converting-enzyme inhibition on diabetic nephropathy. N Engl J Med 1993;329:1456-1462
160. Jafar TH, Schmid CH, Landa M, et al. Angiotensin-converting-enzyme inhibitors and progression of nondiabetic renal disease. Ann Intern Med 2001;135:73-87
161. Heart Outcomes Prevention Evaluation Study Investigators. Effects of ramipril on cardiovascular and microvascular outcomes in people with diabetes mellitus: results of the HOPE study and MICRO-HOPE substudy. Lancet 2000;355:253-259
162. Vermes E, Tardif J-C, Bourassa MG, et al. Enalapril decreases the incidence of atrial fibrillation in patients with left ventricular dysfunction: insights from the Studies Of Left Ventricular Dysfunction (SOLVD) trials. Circulation 2003;107:L2926-L2931
163. Laverman G, Ruggenenti P, Remuzzi G. Angiotensin-converting enzyme inhibition or angiotensin receptor blockade in hypertensive diabetics? Curr Hypertens Rep 2003;5:364-367
164. Pfeffer MA, Swedberg K, Granger CB, et al. Effects of candesartan on mortality and morbidity in patients with chronic heart failure: the CHARM-Overall programme. Lancet 2003;362:759-766
165. Prasad A, Quyyumi AA. Renin-angiotensin system and angiotensin receptor blockers in the metabolic syndrome. Circulation 2004;110:1507-1512
166. Wassman S, Hilgers S, Laufs U, et al. Angiotensin II type 1 receptor antagonism improves hypercholesterolemia-associated endothelial dysfunction. Arterioscler Thromb Vasc Biol 2002;22:1208-1212
167. Hornig B, Landmesser U, Kohler C, et al. Comparative effect of ACE inhibition and angiotensin II type 1 receptor antagonism on bioavailability of nitric oxide in patients with coronary artery disease: role of superoxide dismutase. Circulation 2001;103:799-805
168. Schieffer B, Bunte C, Witte J, et al. Comparative effects of AT_1-antagonism and angiotensin-converting enzyme inhibition on markers of inflammation and platelet aggregation in patients with coronary artery disease. J Am Coll Cardiol 2004;44:362-368
169. Strawn WB. Pathophysiological and clinical implications of AT(1) and AT(2) angiotensin II receptors in metabolic disorders: hypercholesterolaemia and diabetes. Drugs 2002;62(Spec No 1):31-41
170. Koh KK, Ahn JY, Han SH, et al. Pleiotropic effects of angiotensin II receptor blocker in hypertensive patients. J Am Coll Cardiol 2003;42:905-910
171. Koh KK, Han SH, Chung W-J, et al. Comparison of the effects of losartan, irbesartan, and candesartan on flow-mediated brachial artery dilation and on inflammatory and thrombolytic markers in patients with systemic hypertension. Am J Cardiol 2004;93:1432-1435
172. Prasad A, Halcox JP, Waclawiw MA, Quyyumi AA. Angiotensin type 1 receptor antagonism reverses abnormal coronary vasomotion in atherosclerosis. J Am Coll Cardiol 2001;38:1089-1095
173. Candido R, Allen TJ, Lassila M, et al. Irbesartan but not amlodipine suppresses diabetes-associated atherosclerosis. Circulation 2004;109:1536-1542
174. Lindholm LH, Ibsen H, Dahlof B, et al. Cardiovascular morbidity and mortality in patients with diabetes in the Losartan Intervention For Endpoint reduction in hypertension study (LIFE): a randomised trial against atenolol. Lancet 2002;359:1004-1010
175. Motley ED, Eguchi K, Gardner C, et al. Insulin-induced Akt activation is inhibited by angiotensin II in the vasculature through protein kinase C-alpha. Hypertension 2003;41:775-780
176. Iyer SN, Katovich MJ. Effect of acute and chronic losartan treatment on glucose tolerance and insulin sensitivity in fructose-fed rats. Am J Hypertens 1996;9:662-668
177. Ortlepp JR, Breuer J, Eitner F, et al. Inhibition of the renin-angiotensin system ameliorates genetically

determined hyperinsulinemia. Eur J Pharmacol 2002; 436:145-150

178. Ishizawa K, Yoshizumi M, Tsuchiya K, et al. Effects of losartan in combination with or without exercise on insulin resistance in Otsuka Long-Evans Tokushima Fatty rats. Eur J Pharmacol 2001;430:359-367
179. Janke J, Engeli S, Gorzelniak K, et al. Mature adipocytes inhibit in vitro differentiation of human preadipocytes via angiotensin type 1 receptors. Diabetes 2002;51: 1699-1707
180. Schupp M, Janke J, Clasen R, et al. Angiotensin type 1 receptor blockers induce peroxisome proliferator–activated receptor-gamma activity. Circulation 2004;109: 2054-2057
181. Grassi G, Seravalle G, Dell'Oro R, et al. Comparative effects of candesartan and hydrochlorothiazide on blood pressure, insulin sensitivity, and sympathetic drive in obese hypertensive individuals: results of the CROSS study. J Hypertens 2003;21:1761-1769
182. Julius S, Kjeldsen SE, Webel M, et al. Outcomes in hypertensive patients at high risk of cardiovascular risk treated with regimens based on valsartan or amlodipine: the VALUE randomized trial. Lancet 2004;363:2022-2031
183. Keane WF, Kurokawa K, Lyle PA, et al. Treatment of type 2 diabetic patients with kidney disease with AT1-receptor antagonists: lessons from recent trials. Clin Exp Nephrol 2002;6:175-181
184. Stier CT Jr, Koenig S, Lee DY, et al. Aldosterone and aldosterone antagonism in cardiovascular disease: focus on eplerenone (Inspra). Heart Dis 2003;5:102-118
185. Wikstrand J, Berglund G, Hedblad B, Hulthe J. Antiatherosclerotic effects of beta-blockers. Am J Cardiol 2003;91(suppl):25H-29H
186. Kirpichnikov D, McFarlane SI, Sowers JR. Heart failure in diabetic patients: utility of beta-blockade. J Card Fail 2003;9:333-344
187. Kaplan JR, Manuck SB. Status, stress and atherosclerosis: the role of the environment and individual behavior. Ann NY Acad Sci 1999;896:145-161
188. Kaplan JR, Manuck SB, Adams MR, et al. Inhibition of coronary atherosclerosis by propranolol in behaviorally predisposed monkeys fed an atherogenic diet. Circulation 1987;76:1364-1372
189. Hedblad B, Wikstrand J, Janzon L, et al. Low dose metoprolol CR/XL and fluvastatin slow progression of carotid intima-media thickness: main results from the Beta-Blocker Cholesterol-Lowering Asymptomatic Plaque Study (BCAPS). Circulation 2001;103:1721-1726
190. Wiklund O, Hulthe J, Wikstrand J, et al. Effect of controlled release/extended release metoprolol on carotid intima-media thickness in patients with hypercholesterolemia: a 3-year randomized study. Stroke 2002;33: 572-577
191. Sowers JR, Bakris GL. Antihypertensive therapy and the risk of type 2 diabetes mellitus. N Engl J Med 2000; 342:969-970
192. Gress TW, Nieto FH, Shahar E, et al. Hypertension and antihypertensive therapy as risk factors for type 2 diabetes mellitus. Atherosclerosis Risk in Communities Study. N Engl J Med 2000;342:905-912
193. Bobbio M, Ferrua S, Opasich C, et al. Survival and hospitalization in heart failure patients with or without diabetes treated with beta-blockers. J Card Fail 2003; 9:192-202
194. Malminiemi K, Laine H, Knuuti MJ, et al. Acute effects of celiprolol on muscle blood flow and insulin sensitivity: studies using (^{15}O)-water, (^{18}F)-fluorodeoxyglucose and positron emission tomography. Eur J Clin Pharmacol 1997; 52:19-26
195. Bakris GL, Fonseca V, Katholi RE, et al. Metabolic effects of carvedilol vs metoprolol in patients with type 2 diabetes mellitus and hypertension. A randomized controlled trial. JAMA 2004;292:2227-2236
196. Poole-Wilson PA, Swedberg K, Cleland JG, et al. Comparison of carvedilol and metoprolol on clinical outcomes in patients with chronic heart failure in the Carvedilol Or Metoprolol European Trial (COMET): randomised controlled trial. Lancet 2003; 362:7-13
197. Goldstein BJ. Current views on the mechanism of action of thiazolidinedione insulin sensitizers. Diabetes Technol Ther 1999;1:267-275
198. Kahn CR, Chen L, Cohen SE. Unraveling the mechanism of action of thiazolidinediones. J Clin Invest 2000; 106:1305-1307
199. Viberti G, Kahn SE, Greene DA, et al. A Diabetes Outcome Progression Trial (ADOPT): an international multicenter study of the comparative efficacy of rosiglitazone, glyburide, and metformin in recently diagnosed type 2 diabetes. Diabetes Care 2002;25: 1737-1743
200. Yki-Järvinen H. Thiazolidinediones. N Engl J Med 2004;351:1106-1118
201. Perrey S, Ishibashi S, Yahagi N, et al. Thiazolidinedione- and tumor necrosis factor alpha–induced downregulation of peroxisome proliferator–activated receptor gamma mRNA in differentiated 3T3-L1 adipocytes. Metabolism 2001;50:36-40
202. Gorson DM. Significant weight gain with rezulin therapy. Arch Intern Med 1999;159:99
203. Girard J. PPAR-gamma et insulino-resistance. Ann Endocrinol 2002;63:1S19-1S22
204. Fonseca VA. Management of diabetes mellitus and insulin resistance in patients with cardiovascular disease. Am J Cardiol 2003;92(suppl):50J-60J
205. Wang T-D, Chen W-J, Lin J-W, et al. Effects of rosiglitazone on endothelial function, C-reactive protein, and components of the metabolic syndrome in non-diabetic patients with the metabolic syndrome. Am J Cardiol 2004;93:362-365
206. Mayerson AB, Hundal RS, Dufour S, et al. The effects of rosiglitazone on insulin sensitivity, lipolysis, and hepatic and skeletal muscle triglyceride content in patients with type 2 diabetes. Diabetes 2002;51:797-802
207. Akazawa S, Sun F, Ito M, et al. Efficacy of troglitazone on body fat distribution in type 2 diabetes. Diabetes Care 2000;23:1067-1071
208. Wakino S, Hayashi K, Kanda T, et al. Peroxisome proliferator–activated receptor gamma ligands inhibit Rho/Rho kinase pathway by inducing protein tyrosine phosphatase SHP-2.Circ Res 2004;95:e45-e55
209. Choi D, Kim SK, Choi SH, et al. Preventative effects of rosiglitazone on restenosis after coronary stent implantation in patients with type 2 diabetes. Diabetes Care 2004;27:2654-2660
210. Farese RV. Function and dysfunction of aPKC isoforms for glucose transport in insulin-sensitive and insulin-resistant states. Am J Physiol Endocrinol Metab 2002; 283:E1-E11
211. Matthaei S, Stumvoll M, Kellerer M, Haring HU. Pathophysiology and pharmacological treatment of insulin resistance. Endocr Rev 2000;21:585-618
212. Thomas JC, Taylor KB. Effects of troglitazone on lipoprotein subclasses in patients who are insulin resistant. Diabetes 2001;50(Suppl 2):A455

213. Saez E, Tontonoz P, Nelson MC, et al. Activators of the nuclear receptor PPARgamma enhance colon polyp formation. Nat Med 1998;4:1058-1061
214. Brand CL, Sturis J, Gotfredsen CF, et al. Dual PPARalpha/gamma activation provides enhanced improvement of insulin sensitivity and glycemic control in ZDF rats. Am J Physiol Endocrinol Metab 2002; 284:E841-E854
215. Tang WHW, Francis GS, Hoogwerf BJ, Young JB. Fluid retention after initiation of thiazolidinedione therapy in diabetic patients with established chronic heart failure. J Am Coll Cardiol 2003;41:1394-1398
216. Nikolaidis LA, Levine TB. Peroxisome proliferator activator receptors (PPAR), insulin resistance, and cardiomyopathy. Friends or foe for the diabetic patient with heart failure. Cardiol Rev 2004;12:158-170
217. Nesto RW, Bell D, Bonow RO, et al. Thiazolidinedione use, fluid retention, and congestive heart failure: a consensus statement from the American Heart Association and American Diabetes Association. October 7, 2003. Circulation 2003;108:2941-2948
218. Evans DJ, Pritchard-Jones K, Trotman-Dickinson B. Insulin oedema. Postgrad Med J 1986;62:665-668
219. Zhang X, Young HA. PPAR and the immune system—what do we know? Int Immunopharm 2002;2:1029-1044
220. Martinez B. Bristol-Myers diabetes drug produces positive test results. Wall St J 2004;Nov 18:A6
221. Zierath JR. Invited review: Exercise training–induced changes in insulin signaling in skeletal muscle. J Appl Physiol 2002;93:773-781
222. Innerfield RJ. Metformin-associated mortality in U.S. studies. N Engl J Med 1996;334:1611-1613
223. Mather KJ, Verma S, Anderson TJ. Improved endothelial function with metformin in type 2 diabetes mellitus. J Am Coll Cardiol 2001;37:1344-1350
224. UK Prospective Diabetes Study (UKPDS) Group. Effect of intensive blood-glucose control with metformin on complications in overweight patients with type 2 diabetes (UKPDS 34). Lancet 1998;352:854-865
225. Knowler WC, Barrett-Connor E, Fowler SE, et al, for the Diabetes Prevention Program Research Group. Reduction in the incidence of type 2 diabetes with lifestyle intervention or metformin. N Engl J Med 2002;346:393-403
226. Winder WW. AMP-activated protein kinase: possible target for treatment of type 2 diabetes. Diabetes Technol Ther 2000;2:441-448
227. Holst JJ, Orskov C. Incretin hormones—an update. Scand J Clin Lab Invest Suppl 2001;234:75-85
228. Vahl TP, D'Alessio DA. Gut peptides in the treatment of diabetes mellitus. Expert Opin Investig Drugs 2004; 13:177-188
229. Taegtmeyer H. Cardiac metabolism as a target for the treatment of heart failure. Circulation 2004;110:894-896
230. Nikolaidis LA, Elahi D, Hentosz T, et al. Recombinant glucagon-like peptide-1 increases myocardial glucose uptake and improves left ventricular performance in conscious dogs with pacing-induced dilated cardiomyopathy. Circulation 2004;110:955-961
231. Chase M. This gut reaction aids weight loss. Wall St J 2003;June 17:D4
232. DeFronzo RA, Ratner RE, Han J, et al. Effects of exenatide (exenolin-4) on glycemic control and weight over 30 weeks in metformin-treated patients with type 2 diabetes. Diabetes Care 2005;28:1092-1100
233. Ahren B. New strategy in type 2 diabetes tested in clinical trials. Glucagon-like peptide 1 (GLP-1) affects basic causes of the disease. Lakartidningen 2005; 102:545-549
234. Ahren B, Landin-Olsson M, Jansson PA, et al. Inhibition of dipeptidyl peptidase-4 reduces glycemia, sustains insulin levels, and reduces glucagon levels in type 2 diabetes. J Clin Endocrinol Metab 2004;89:2078-2084
235. Gura T. Obesity drug pipeline not so fat. Science 2003;299:849-852
236. Stone NJ, Kushner R. Effects of dietary modification to reduce vascular risks and treatment of obesity. Cardiol Clin 2003;21:415-433
237. Lucas CP, Boldrin MN, Reaven GM. Effect of orlistat added to diet (30% of calories from fat) on plasma lipids, glucose, and insulin in obese patients with hypercholesterolemia. Am J Cardiol 2003;91:961-964
238. Grady D. Why we eat (and eat and eat). New York Times 2002;November 26;D1-D2
239. Inui A. Neuropeptide Y feeding receptors: are multiple subtypes involved? Trends Pharmacol Sci 1999;20: 43-46
240. Batterham RL, Cohen MA, Ellis SM, et al. Inhibition of food intake in obese subjects by peptide YY3-36. N Engl J Med 2003;349:941-948
241. Cawthorne MA, Sennitt MV, Arch JS, Smith SA. BRL 35135, a potent and selective atypical beta-adrenoceptor agonist. Am J Clin Nutr 1992;55(suppl 1):252S-257S
242. Jequier E. Pathways to obesity. Int J Obes Relat Metab Disord 2002;26(suppl 2):S12-S17
243. Konturek SJ, Konturek JW, Pawlik T, Brzozowski T. Brain-gut axis and its role in the control of food intake. J Physiol Pharmacol 2004;55(1 Pt 2):137-154
244. Duarte C, Alonso R, Bichet N, et al. Blockade by the cannabinoid CB1 receptor antagonist, rimonabant (SR141716), of the potentiation by quinelorane of food-primed reinstatement of food-seeking behavior. Neuropsychopharmacology 2004;29:911-920
245. Winslow R. Drug helps patients shed pounds, keep them off. Wall St J 2004;November 10:D13
246. Van Gaal LF, Rissanen AM, Scheen AJ, et al; RIO-Europe Study Group. Effects of the cannabinoid-1 receptor blocker rimonabant on weight reduction and cardiovascular risk factors in overweight patients: 1-year experience from the RIO-Europe Study. Lancet 2005;365:1389-1397
247. Mukherjee D, Fang J, Chetcuti S, et al. Impact of combination evidence-based medical therapy on mortality in patients with acute coronary syndromes. Circulation 2004;109:745-749

Index

Note: Page numbers followed by the letter f refer to figures and those followed by t refer to tables.

A

B

C

D

E

F

H

I

N

O

Q

R

S

T

U

V

W